Boh's Pharmacy Practice Manual: A Guide to the Clinical Experience

FOURTH EDITION

Boh's Pharmacy Practice Manual: A Guide to the Clinical Experience

FOURTH EDITION

EDITOR

Susan M. Stein, DHEd, MS, BS Pharm, RPh
Associate Dean, College of Health Professions
Professor, School of Pharmacy
Pacific University
Hillsboro, Oregon

Wolters Kluwer
Health
Philadelphia • Baltimore • New York • London
Buenos Aires • Hong Kong • Sydney • Tokyo

Acquisitions Editor: Sirkka Howes
Product Development Editor: Stephanie Roulias
Production Project Manager: David Orzechowski
Senior Designer: Stephen Druding
Manufacturing Coordinator: Margie Orzech
Production Services/Compositor: SPi Global

Fourth Edition

351 West Camden Street
Baltimore, MD 21201

Two Commerce Square
2001 Market Street
Philadelphia, PA 19103

9 8 7 6 5 4 3 2 1

Printed in China

Library of Congress Cataloging-in-Publication Data

Boh's pharmacy practice manual : a guide to the clinical experience / editor, Susan M. Stein.—Fourth edition.

p. ; cm.

Pharmacy practice manual

Includes bibliographical references and index.

ISBN 978-1-4511-8967-4

I. Stein, Susan M. (Susan Marie), 1966- editor of compilation. II. Title: Pharmacy practice manual.

[DNLM: 1. Pharmacy Service, Hospital—methods—Handbooks. 2. Clinical Clerkship—methods—Handbooks. 3. Pharmacy—methods—Handbooks. QV 735]

RS122.5

615.1068—dc23

2013035992

DISCLAIMER

Care has been taken to confirm the accuracy of the information present and to describe generally accepted practices. However, the authors, editors, and publisher are not responsible for errors or omissions or for any consequences from application of the information in this book and make no warranty, expressed or implied, with respect to the currency, completeness, or accuracy of the contents of the publication. Application of this information in a particular situation remains the professional responsibility of the practitioner; the clinical treatments described and recommended may not be considered absolute and universal recommendations.

The authors, editors, and publisher have exerted every effort to ensure that drug selection and dosage set forth in this text are in accordance with the current recommendations and practice at the time of publication. However, in view of ongoing research, changes in government regulations, and the constant flow of information relating to drug therapy and drug reactions, the reader is urged to check the package insert for each drug for any change in indications and dosage and for added warnings and precautions. This is particularly important when the recommended agent is a new or infrequently employed drug.

Some drugs and medical devices presented in this publication have Food and Drug Administration (FDA) clearance for limited use in restricted research settings. It is the responsibility of the health care provider to ascertain the FDA status of each drug or device planned for use in his or her clinical practice.

To purchase additional copies of this book, call our customer service department at **(800) 638-3030** or fax orders to **(301) 223-2320.** International customers should call **(301) 223-2300.**

Larry E. Boh

1953–2001

Larry E. Boh passed away days before the publication of the second edition. Larry was respected and much admired by his students and fellow professors for his immeasurable contributions to the pharmacy profession.

PREFACE

Pharmacy practice and our health care system are evolving before our eyes: our education and practice standards must keep pace. Pharmacists are inspired by an inherent desire to care for patients, a fascination with pharmacokinetics and pharmacotherapy, and a passion to help. We have a wonderful profession, and each of us carries a responsibility to nurture and support the next generation of pharmacists and the practice it becomes.

We proudly bring you the fourth edition of *Boh's Pharmacy Practice Manual: A Guide to the Clinical Experience*. The title maintains a link to honor an inspiring, brilliant mentor: Larry Boh. Larry had a powerful, lasting impact on many successful clinical pharmacists practicing today. As editor of the first edition (*Clinical Clerkship Manual*) and the second edition (*Pharmacy Practice Manual: A Guide to the Clinical Experience*), he motivated knowledgeable, talented contributing editors to create an anthology that provided practitioners a valuable reference throughout their career. The fourth edition further expanded and restructured chapters to support current as well as emerging practitioners. A purposeful emphasis was placed on providing resources to practitioners of all degrees. Many chapters were expanded to include updated standards of care while others were condensed and focused to maximize value. The pharmacy profession provides us a unique opportunity to improve the quality and value of our patients' lives. We hope you find this book an indispensable tool in that endeavor and encourage you to never stop learning, questioning, or striving to expand your knowledge and impact on patient care.

Susan M. Stein

ACKNOWLEDGMENTS

I wish to acknowledge and thank the contributing authors and colleagues from the previous editions of "the Boh book." The memory of Larry Boh and his passion to pay it forward to the next generation, to support and challenge future practitioners to provide their patients with the best care available is evident throughout this text.

To the talented contributing authors of the fourth edition, thank you so very much for your dedication and for sharing your expertise and valuable resources in creating this indispensable resource. Through this compilation, your knowledge, insight, and experience will support clinicians far beyond your spheres of influence. We all will gain from your excellence as clinical practitioners.

To the publishing staff at Lippincott Williams & Wilkins, thank you for your endless persistence, guidance, and insight in bringing this book to press in our vision. Your investment in our profession is greatly appreciated.

Finally, I wish to thank Danny, my husband, honey bunny, and pathfinder. Without his support and wisdom, this book would not be in your hands.

This book is in memory of Larry E. Boh and Martin F. Stein, my mentors in pharmacy and life.

CONTRIBUTORS

Roberta A. Aulie, PharmD
Residency Program Director
Department of Pharmacy
St. Mary's Hospital
Madison, Wisconsin

David T. Bearden, PharmD
Clinical Associate Professor
Chair, Department of Pharmacy Practice
College of Pharmacy
Oregon State University
Portland, Oregon

Robert M. Breslow, BS Pharm, BCPS
Clinical Associate Professor
School of Pharmacy
University of Wisconsin
Madison, Wisconsin

Molly E. Bruvold, PharmD
Pharmacist Specialist
VA Medical Center
Indianapolis, Indiana

Kristina L. Butler, PharmD, BCPS
Manager, Clinical Pharmacists
Clinical Pharmacy Department
Providence Medical Group
Portland, Oregon

Kam L. Capoccia, PharmD, BCPS
Clinical Assistant Professor
Department of Pharmacy Practice
College of Pharmacy
Western New England University
Springfield, Massachusetts

Shelley L. Chambers-Fox, BS Pharm, PhD
Clinical Pharmacist
Community Health Association of Spokane
Pullman, Washington

Breanne Chipman, PharmD
Clinical Pharmacist
Operating Room Services
Department of Pharmacy Services
Legacy Health Systems
Portland, Oregon

Sandra B. Earle, PharmD
Associate Professor
Assessment Coordinator
College of Pharmacy
University of Findlay
Findlay, Ohio

Kate Farthing, PharmD, BCPS, FASHP
Pharmacy Clinical Coordinator
Quality & Patient Safety
Legacy Good Samaritan Medical Center
Portland, Oregon

William E. Fassett, PhD, RPh
Professor
Department of Pharmacotherapy
College of Pharmacy
Washington State University
Spokane, Washington

Devon Flynn, PharmD, BCPS, AAHIVP
HIV Clinical Pharmacist
Oregon Health & Science University
Portland, Oregon

Melanie Petilla Foeppel, PharmD, BCACP
Assistant Professor
Director of Post-Graduate Training
School of Pharmacy
Pacific University
Hillsboro, Oregon

Jeffery Fortner, PharmD
Assistant Professor
School of Pharmacy
Pacific University
Hillsboro, Oregon

Brad S. Fujisaki, PharmD, BCPS
Associate Professor
School of Pharmacy
Pacific University
Hillsboro, Oregon

Kenneth C. Jackson II, PharmD
Professor
School of Pharmacy
Wingate University
Wingate, North Carolina

Jennifer M. Jordan, PharmD, BCPS
Associate Professor
School of Pharmacy
Pacific University
Hillsboro, Oregon

Marianne Krupicka, PharmD
Pharmacy Clinical Coordinator
Randall Children's Hospital
Legacy Health Systems
Portland, Oregon

Pauline A. Low, PharmD
Adjunct Professor
School of Pharmacy
Pacific University
Hillsboro, Oregon

Linda Garrelts MacLean, BS Pharm, CDE
Associate Dean for Advancement
Clinical Associate Professor of Pharmacotherapy
College of Pharmacy
Washington State University
Spokane, Washington

Kristine B. Marcus, BS Pharm, BCPS
Associate Professor
School of Pharmacy
Pacific University
Hillsboro, Oregon

Patricia M. Mossbrucker, BS Pharm
Medication Management Program
Kaiser Permanente
Portland, Oregon

Daniel R. Neal, PharmD
Director of Pharmacy
VA Roseburg Healthcare System
Roseburg, Oregon

Teresa A. O'Sullivan, PharmD, BCPS
Director of Experiential Education
Acting Assistant Professor, Department of Pharmacy
School of Pharmacy
University of Washington
Seattle, Washington

Katherine E. Rotzenberg, PharmD
Drug Information Pharmacist
Department of Pharmacy
St. Mary's Hospital
Madison, Wisconsin

Gordon Sacks, PharmD, FCCP, BCNSP
Department Head and Professor
Department of Pharmacy Practice
Harrison School of Pharmacy
Auburn University
Auburn, Alabama

Kathleen A. Skibinski, MS, BS Pharm
Project Director (HCIA)
Pharmacy Society of Wisconsin
Madison, Wisconsin

Susan M. Stein, DHEd, MS, BS Pharm, RPh
Associate Dean, College of Health Professions
Professor, School of Pharmacy
Pacific University
Hillsboro, Oregon

Ty Vo, PharmD, BCPS
Drug Information and Formulary
Kaiser Permanente
Portland, Oregon

Diana Wells, PharmD, BCPS
Assistant Clinical Professor
Department of Pharmacy Practice
Harrison School of Pharmacy
Auburn University
Auburn, Alabama

Jonathan R. White, PharmD, BCPS
Clinical Pharmacy Specialist
Primary Care
Providence Medical Group
Portland, Oregon

Megan Willson, PharmD, CDE
Clinical Assistant Professor
Department of Pharmacotherapy
Washington State University
Spokane, Washington

Ann K. Wittkowsky, PharmD, CACP, FASHP, FCCP
Clinical Professor
School of Pharmacy
University of Washington
Director
Anticoagulation Services
University of Washington Medical Center
Seattle, Washington

CONTENTS

1

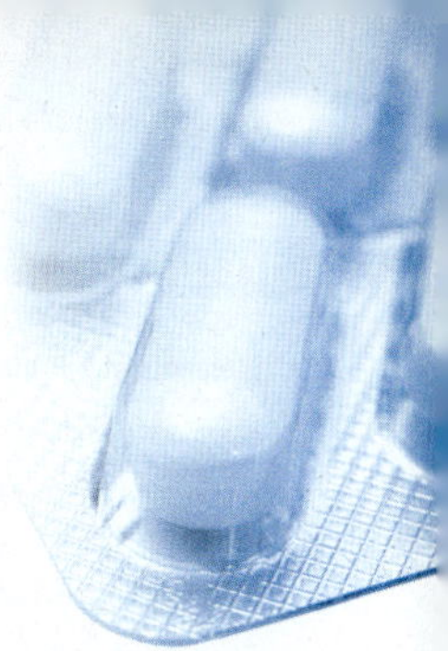

Professionalism in Pharmacy

Susan M. Stein, William E. Fassett, and Jeffery Fortner

Professionalism is an all-encompassing concept that conjures images of how to make a positive impression on patients, other health care professionals, and the public. According to the American Association of Colleges of Pharmacy (AACP) Professionalism Task Force, traits of a professional include[1]

- Knowledge and skills
- A commitment to self-improvement and lifelong learning
- A service-minded orientation
- Pride in the profession and a dedication to advance its value to society
- Creating a covenantal relationship with those served
- Alertness, creativity, initiative, and innovation
- Conscientiousness, integrity, and trustworthiness
- Flexibility and punctuality
- Accountability for his/her performance
- Ethically sound decision making and moral behavior
- Leadership

Developing professionalism, or professional socialization, begins with taking pride in the profession and growing this pride throughout the didactic and clinical components of education and beyond.[2] The authors encourage use of the Professional Self-Assessment (Table 1.1) both now and as you develop in your career. Maintaining professionalism provides the gateway to successful delivery and acceptance of clinical pharmacy practice.

Professionalism and Trust

Imagine yourself boarding an airplane for a flight in the middle of a stormy day. When the pilots and flight attendants look sharp and

TABLE 1.1 Professional Self-Assessment

Elements of a Professional	Self-assessment of Element
Knowledge and skills	
A commitment to self-improvement and lifelong learning	
A service-minded orientation	
Pride in the profession and dedication to advance its value to society	
Create a covenantal relationship with those served	
Alertness, creativity, initiative, and innovation	
Conscientiousness, integrity, and trustworthiness	
Flexibility and punctuality	
Accountability for his/her performance	
Ethically sound decision making and moral behavior	
Leadership	

act sharp, is the quality of your trip improved? Are you more likely to trust them and follow their directions when your life may depend on it?

Now, consider what it is like to be sick. Your illness impairs your ability to function, to work, to enjoy life, and perhaps to keep on living. Patients with grave or potentially disabling illnesses must rely on strangers—physicians, nurses, laboratory technicians, pharmacists, and others—to do for them things they cannot do for themselves. As retold by Zaner, "A man with lung cancer emphasized: 'When the doctor told me I had this tumor, frankly, it alarmed me, but he did it in such a way that it left me with a feeling of confidence.' A diabetic underscored the point: 'if you can't communicate and you can't understand your disease, then you don't have confidence in the medical help you are getting [citations omitted].'"[3]

So much of success in health care depends on patient trust in his or her health care provider that establishing a trusting relationship is the very first principle in the Code of Ethics for Pharmacists (see Box 1.1). The critical first step to earn patient trust is to act professionally.

BOX 1.1 Code of Ethics for Pharmacists

Preamble

Pharmacists are health professionals who assist individuals in making the best use of medications. This Code, prepared and supported by pharmacists, is intended to state publicly the principles that form the fundamental basis of the roles and responsibilities of pharmacists. These principles, based on moral obligations and virtues, are established to guide pharmacists in relationships with patients, health professionals, and society.

I. A pharmacist respects the covenantal relationship between the patient and pharmacist.
Considering the patient–pharmacist relationship as a covenant means that a pharmacist has moral obligations in response to the gift of trust received from society. In return for this gift, a pharmacist promises to help individuals achieve optimum benefit from their medications, to be committed to their welfare, and to maintain their trust.

II. A pharmacist promotes the good of every patient in a caring, compassionate, and confidential manner.
A pharmacist places concern for the well-being of the patient at the center of professional practice. In doing so, a pharmacist considers needs stated by the patient as well as those defined by health science. A pharmacist is dedicated to protecting the dignity of the patient. With a caring attitude and a compassionate spirit, a pharmacist focuses on serving the patient in a private and confidential manner.

III. A pharmacist respects the autonomy and dignity of each patient.
A pharmacist promotes the right of self-determination and recognizes individual self-worth by encouraging patients to participate in decisions about their health. A pharmacist communicates with patients in terms that are understandable. In all cases, a pharmacist respects personal and cultural differences among patients.

IV. A pharmacist acts with honesty and integrity in professional relationships.
A pharmacist has a duty to tell the truth and to act with conviction of conscience. A pharmacist avoids discriminatory practices, behavior or work conditions that impair professional judgment, and actions that compromise dedication to the best interests of patients.

CONTINUED

BOX 1.1 Code of Ethics for Pharmacists *(continued)*

V. A pharmacist maintains professional competence.
A pharmacist has a duty to maintain knowledge and abilities as new medications, devices, and technologies become available and as health information advances.

VI. A pharmacist respects the values and abilities of colleagues and other health professionals.
When appropriate, a pharmacist asks for the consultation of colleagues or other health professionals or refers the patient. A pharmacist acknowledges that colleagues and other health professionals may differ in the beliefs and values they apply to the care of the patient.

VII. A pharmacist serves individual, community, and societal needs.
The primary obligation of a pharmacist is to individual patients. However, the obligations of a pharmacist may at times extend beyond the individual to the community and society. In these situations, the pharmacist recognizes the responsibilities that accompany these obligations and acts accordingly.

VIII. A pharmacist seeks justice in the distribution of health resources.
When health resources are allocated, a pharmacist is fair and equitable, balancing the needs of patients and society.

Adopted by the membership of the
American Pharmaceutical Association
October 27, 1994

Reprinted from the American Pharmacists Association from http://www.pharmacist.com/code-ethics. Copyright 1994 APhA, Accessed April 11, 2013, with permission.

Professionalism and Performance

Many philosophers, Aristotle prime among them, have noted that to become a person whose actions are worthy of respect, including self-respect, it is important at the outset to behave in a respectable manner. But this is much more than merely acting the part. Behaving consistently in the way you wish to become forms good habits and reinforces the desired behavior. Professionalism describes in part the way you act to create in others an image of you as a "pro." But being professional is in and of itself a desirable way to act. People who behave professionally are significantly more likely to deliver high quality care. Perhaps as important, you will find that when patients and other professionals trust you, their confidence in you helps build your own self-assurance.

A recent popular phrase describes well how a person behaves professionally to become professional: he or she "talks the talk and walks the walk."

Embracing Change

Whether personal or professional, change is often uncomfortable, but is also inevitable. Like most professions, pharmacy today looks quite different from pharmacy 40 years ago. The unremitting efforts of three generations of pharmacists and student pharmacists to move the profession forward have now positioned pharmacy to be the profession responsible for providing patient care that insures optimal medication therapy outcomes.[4,5] As you progress through the next 30 years of your career, you will be involved in many changes too. The most successful professionals are those who embrace change by adapting to new expectations, accepting new responsibilities, and capitalizing on new opportunities. Most professionals tend to perform better, and gain more satisfaction, in their work when it is at least somewhat challenging. At the same time, it is also easy to fall into a routine and establish a "comfort zone" with your work. An insightful preceptor once said, "If you ever feel very comfortable in your work, it's time to consider a change, because being too comfortable makes you prone to mistakes." Since mistakes in pharmacy can be devastating, embrace change knowing the discomfort makes you a better professional.

Positive First Impressions

One's outward physical appearance greatly influences his or her effectiveness. Presenting yourself as awake, alert, and well-groomed (clean shaven or groomed facial hair, no body odor, clean hair, etc.) to your patients creates a positive impression. Companies and institutions have dress codes, and professional associations use statements such as "business casual," "business dress," and "casual" to describe appropriate and acceptable dress at their meetings. These recommendations prepare the individual to meet expectations and be accepted professionally. What you wear creates an immediate impression, and the goal is to be professional. Remember to know the dress code of each facility or event to confirm expectations. Also, it is advised to overdress if unsure. By the way, no one expects young health care professionals to spend a lot of money on business attire; you can "dress for success" and stay within your budget. An online Google search for the phrase "dress for success for less" will provide you with several sources of useful information. See Table 1.2 for some specific suggestions.

TABLE 1.2 Dress Code Suggestions

Dress Code	Men	Women	Avoid
Clinical experiences	White lab coat and name tag (unless otherwise directed by preceptor), professional dress	White lab coat and name tag (unless otherwise directed by preceptor), professional dress	Anything worn or torn Anything unclean or wrinkled Anything interpreted as revealing or suggestive Blue jeans, sweatshirts Athletic shoes, sandals
Professional dress	Dress pants, buttoned shirt, tie, suits	Dress pants or skirts, blouse, suits	Anything worn or torn Anything unclean or wrinkled Anything interpreted as revealing or suggestive Blue jeans, sweatshirts Athletic shoes, sandals
Business casual	Dress pants, buttoned shirt, collared shirt	Dress pants, blouse	Anything worn or torn Anything unclean or wrinkled Anything interpreted as revealing or suggestive Blue jeans, sweatshirts Athletic shoes, sandals
Business dress	Suit or sport coat with pressed slacks	Suit or skirt with dressy top, dress	Too casual Anything worn or torn Anything unclean or wrinkled Anything interpreted as revealing or suggestive Blue jeans, sweatshirts Athletic shoes, sandals
Casual	Casual pants, collared shirt	Casual pants, collared shirt, or casual top	Anything worn or torn Anything unclean or wrinkled Anything interpreted as revealing or suggestive

Professional Behavior

Impressions are also created based on an individual's behavior and attitude. When you arrive at work, how you interact with others and how you shake hands are behaviors that can influence how others perceive you. See Table 1.3 for examples of appropriate and inappropriate behavior. Seek clarification if there is a misunderstanding. If you find that some of your habits fall in the "inappropriate" category—figure out how to change, and do it as soon as you can.

Communication

Effective communication is the ability to share ideas and receive information using verbal, written, and visual skills. The importance of effective communication in health care also influences first impressions and cannot be overemphasized. It involves patients, caregivers, and other health care providers. Miscommunication can be fatal. Frequent use of good communication skills improves effectiveness. Tables 1.4 and 1.5 provide examples of effective communication styles and techniques to improve effectiveness.

Particular types of patients may require different communication techniques. See Table 1.5 for techniques to improve communication effectiveness with these patient groups.

Confidentiality

Respecting patient confidentiality and that of others is an integral part of professionalism. Confidential information may be shared or discussed only in appropriate environments and only with appropriate individuals. The federal Health Insurance Portability and Accountability Act (HIPAA) specifies appropriate confidentiality guidelines. Use the following online link for more information: http://www.cms.hhs.gov/HIPAAGenInfo/. Understand this also: Those confidential conversations you have with colleagues concerning their personal issues or workplace concerns must be treated with great care. You should reveal to others the private matters you discuss with friends or colleagues only when patient care or safety, or equally important legal or ethical

(*Text continued on page 12*)

TABLE 1.3 Appropriate and Inappropriate Behavior Examples

Appropriate	Inappropriate
Prompt: on time or even early; call if delayed and provide estimated time of arrival	Late/inconsistent about being on time; not calling if late; not showing up
Identify and introduce yourself when interacting with others: "Hello, my name is Daphne and I am the pharmacist"	Crashing into a conversation: "Why didn't anyone prescribe vancomycin?!"
Strong, firm handshake	Not offering your hand for handshake greeting, "wet and wimpy" handshake
Consistent in actions and communication: clear pronunciation; articulate	Inconsistent actions and poor communication; mumbling; not answering questions
Positive attitude: willing to try new things, willing to participate: "Can I help?"	Negative attitude: unwilling to try new things, actively participate: "That's not my job."
Confidence and willingness to learn more: "I would like to learn more about that"	Overconfidence, arrogance: "I already know that"
Respectful: nonjudgmental and respectfully agree or disagree: "I can see your point; thanks for the clarification"	Disrespectful and judgmental; "You are wrong"; "That's not what the book says"; "You are not as smart as the other pharmacist"
Empathetic: "This must be hard for you"	Not concerned: "It's not my problem"
Involved, self-directed, and proactive: "What can I do to help?"	Stand around, wait for someone to tell you what to do next, reactive
Good time management: on time, plan out day and responsibilities, efficient, well rested	Poor time management: late, rush through responsibilities and decisions, little or no sleep
Prioritize conflicts, projects, requests, presentations; maintain focus	Double-booked meetings at same time, late projects, lack of prioritization, lack of focus
Character:	
• Honesty and integrity—your own words, your own work, confidentiality • Accountability—to yourself, patients, other health care professionals • Responsibility—for you, your actions, your time, your knowledge	• Plagiarize, gossip, use someone else's work and claim as your own • Blame others for your lack of completing a task, knowledge, promptness, etc. • Not able to accept and own responsibility

TABLE 1.4 Effective and Ineffective Communication Examples

Effective	Ineffective
Verbal:	
• Enunciate	• Mumble
• Project your voice	• Talk softly or away from the individual
• Avoid colloquialisms, idioms, clichés	• Examples: "burning fever," "cold fish"
• Speak slowly, regular cadence	• Speak too quickly or irregular cadence
• Ask open-ended questions (answer other than yes/no): "Which…, How…"	• Ask only yes or no type questions: "Do you…"
• Ask direct questions/requests to gather detailed information: "Describe how your pain feels today."	• Ask generalizations: "How is it going?"
Nonverbal:	
• Eye contact when being spoken to or when asking a question	• Looking away or not paying attention when addressed
• Proxemics (spatial relationships): lean toward but not too close	• Crowding or too far away, barrier between the individual and you
• Ask permission to touch a patient	• Touching without receiving permission
• Body language: open posture, warm smile, alert eyes	• Crossed arms, furrowed brow, repeatedly clearing throat
Active listening:	
• Use all senses to absorb information	• Not paying attention to information shared
• Focus, document information acquired	• Not documenting information obtained
• Listen, not just hearing	• Forget details or improvise information
• Retain and remember	• Respond with what you want to hear
• Respond with reflection and clarifications, use pictures	• Introduce multiple topics and confuse issues
• Stay with one topic	• Interrupt and rush information retrieval
• Do not interrupt	• Finish others' sentences and assume
• Do not complete sentences	• Interrupt, project lack of interest
• "Gate": listen more effectively with sympathy (pity/compassion) versus empathy (identify with what patient feels)	• Disregard feelings of the other; not care, not interested, not involved
• Respect others' thoughts and ideas	• Disrespectful: "It isn't possible to have that side effect with that drug…you are wrong"
Oral communication or presentation:	
• Relax, prepare, practice	• Rush preparation, do not practice
• Organize your thoughts	• Disorganized information
• Concise and clear	• Ramble, disjoint flow
Written communication:	
• Organized	• Disorganized, inconsistent
• Appropriate spelling, grammar	• Do not proofread, poor grammar, typos
• Referenced correctly	• Poor or missing references, plagiarized
• Efficiently written	• Difficult to read, disjoint, too long

(continued)

TABLE 1.4 Effective and Ineffective Communication Examples *(continued)*

Effective	Ineffective
Interaction with patient or health care professional:	
• Environment—appropriate location and time to discuss confidential information • Preparation—what to say, how to say it, goal of the interaction, summarize • Greeting—introduce self and describe intent • Present your statement and discuss—state purpose, provide information, encourage discussion, provide recommendation, obtain answer • Closure and documentation—summarize and potential follow-up/monitoring	• Too loud, not private, in the middle of the hallway, too busy • Disorganized, not planned, no goal • Forget to introduce self, forget to describe intent • Blurt recommendation with no information, demand answer with no discussion, forget to obtain answer • No closure or fail to document

Source: Hosley JH, Molle E. *A Practical Guide to Therapeutic Communication for Health Professionals*. St. Louis, MO: Saunders Elsevier; 2006. Ref.[6]; and Herrier RN, Boyce RW. Communicating more effectively with physicians, Part 2. *J Am Pharm Assoc*. 1996;NS36(9):547–548.[7]

TABLE 1.5 Patient-Dependent Communication Techniques

Patient Population	Technique
Geriatric	• Respectful, not condescending • Address with surname and title (Mr., Ms., etc.) • Maintain eye contact throughout, sit down if individual is seated • Increase font size of instructions and labels (>14 font) • Speak clearly and directly, slowly paced, avoid mumbling • Medication adherence tools when appropriate (medication box, reminder timer, pictures, calendar/time chart for marking doses taken) • Provide seating if waiting for interaction to occur
Pediatric	• Interact with parent/guardian if child too young, uninterested • Address both parent/guardian and child • Interact with child calmly, respectfully, maintain eye contact at child's level, keep it simple, use examples or pictures
Deaf	• Eye contact prior to conversation; touch hand to gain attention • Directly in front of individual with eye contact throughout interaction • Avoid turning away from patient until interaction completed • Speak clearly, calmly, without exaggerated facial expressions, short words and phrases, keep it simple • Visual aids to emphasize important points or instructions (inhaler, diagram, pictures, instruction sheet, label instructions, etc.) • Learn sign language to improve trust and rapport

TABLE 1.5 Patient-Dependent Communication Techniques *(continued)*

Patient Population	Technique
Language barrier	• Learn greetings and other phrases in other languages to improve trust and rapport ("Please," "Thank you," "Good day") • Interpreter if necessary (online, telephone, or in person) • Normal tone of voice and slower speed, not louder and faster • Short, simple words ("pain" rather than "discomfort") and phrases, repeat as needed, stay with one topic until receptive • Yes/no questions for ease of translation • Avoid slang and idioms • Written information, labeled instructions, posted signs in appropriate language
Cultural barrier	• Verbal signs of misunderstanding (confusion, anxiety): explain in a different format • Confidentiality expectations may vary • Matriarchal or patriarchal society may determine decision maker • Time sensitivity may vary: late for appointments • Eye contact may vary: decrease eye contact to decrease anxiety • Diet may vary; confirm before making recommendations
Cognitive issue	• Interact with caregiver if possible • Keep phrases short, increase yes/no questions • Avoid correcting the individual or creating conflict • Avoid distractions and keep length of interaction short • Obtain information through observation and listening
Hostility	• Remain calm, focus on intent of interaction • Avoid arguing or further escalating the interaction • Obtain information through observation and listening • Redirect to complete interaction effectively • Set limits to what is appropriate and what will not be tolerated • Know policies and procedures of the facility, access to security • Document when interaction completed
Other (financial, etc.)	• Avoid judging patient based on financial status, ability to afford • Avoid berating obvious value of prevention: provide care and education respectfully • Provide support and access if possible (medication assistance programs, medication adherence tools, etc.) • Recognize potential conflict in perceived weakness of illness, avoid emphasizing, focus on providing information

Source: Hosley JH, Molle E. *A Practical Guide to Therapeutic Communication for Health Professionals*. St. Louis, MO: Saunders Elsevier; 2006. Ref.[6]; and Herrier RN, Boyce RW. Communicating more effectively with physicians, Part 2. *J Am Pharm Assoc*. 1996;NS36(9):547–548.[7]

issues, require. In most cases, more damage is done to otherwise effective teams by gossip than by any other interpersonal factors.

Cultural Diversity

The concept of cultural diversity is discussed frequently, generally focusing on recognizing and accepting differences between individuals deriving from cultural influences. Differences can include knowledge, values, beliefs, and behaviors. Recommendations for appropriately and effectively working with culturally diverse patients and health care professionals are listed in Table 1.6.

Professional or Academic Misconduct

Inappropriate or illegal behavior is the opposite of professionalism. Depending on the degree of the infringement or action, a student or resident may be penalized with failure of a course or clinical experience or even expulsion from an academic program. A licensed professional may receive a fine, license suspension, license revocation, or be banned from the profession. To avoid the possibility of losing the privilege to practice pharmacy, educate yourself. Be aware of and follow policies and procedures and laws. See Table 1.7 for additional information regarding misconduct.

TABLE 1.6 Cultural Diversity Recommendations

Cultural Diversity Recommendations
• Learning about cultural diversity is a lifelong process • Be genuinely respectful in your interactions with others • Look inside, look outside, and recognize the differences • Unfamiliar behavior is an opportunity for learning • Assumptions provide recognition but should not be acted on • Accept that values may be entrenched; therefore, modify tools to be effective • Promote culturally diverse educational techniques • Learn a language's common phrases to build trust and rapport • Refer patients to community cultural resources • If needed, use an interpreter or bilingual family member • Visual aids will likely improve communication

Source: Zweber A. Cultural competence in pharmacy practice. *Am J Pharm Educ.* 2002;66:172–176.[8]

TABLE 1.7 Misconduct Examples

Misrepresenting, falsifying, or altering data	Falsifying records (i.e., to steal controlled substances)
Plagiarizing a report or article	Abusing controlled substances
Cheating on an examination	Using illicit drugs
Stealing supplies, medication, journals, etc.	Breaking the law (civil, criminal, or administrative) in any way
Selling products in violation of policy	Compromising ethics or integrity
Sharing confidential information (patient, financial, contractual, etc.)	

Plagiarizing, most commonly defined as using another author's original material and claiming it as your own, should be avoided. Be diligent and reference sources appropriately. See Table 1.8 for types of plagiarism and Chapter 5 for additional information.

Sexual Harassment and Discrimination

Sexual harassment has broad interpretations and can occur in many different environments. Academia, organizations, and corporations have extensive policies and procedures describing sexual harassment and guidance regarding an incident. Federal and state laws also address this issue. A description of sexual harassment by the U.S. Equal Employment Opportunity Commission is provided in Table 1.9.

TABLE 1.8 Tips to Avoid Plagiarism

Four common types of plagiarism:

- Direct: lifting passages in their entirety without quotations
- Mosaic: intertwining ideas of original author with own without giving credit
- Paraphrase: using different words to provide the same idea without giving credit to the original author
- Insufficient: providing credit to the original author for only a portion of the material used

Source: Iverson C, Flanagin A, Fontanarosa PB, et al. *American Medical Association Manual of Style. A Guide for Authors and Editors*. 9th ed. Philadelphia, PA: Williams & Wilkins; 1998.[9]

TABLE 1.9 Definition of Sexual Harassment

Harassment can include "sexual harassment" or unwelcome sexual advances, requests for sexual favors, and other verbal or physical harassment of a sexual nature
Harassment does not have to be of a sexual nature, however, and can include offensive remarks about a person's sex. For example, it is illegal to harass a woman by making offensive comments about women in general
Both victim and the harasser can be either a woman or a man, and the victim and the harasser can be the same sex.
Although the law does not prohibit simple teasing, offhand comments, or isolated incidents that are not very serious, harassment is illegal when it is so frequent or severe that it creates a hostile or offensive work environment or when it results in an adverse employment decision (such as the victim being fired or demoted).
The harasser can be the victim's supervisor, a supervisor in another area, a coworker, or someone who is not an employee of the employer, such as a client or customer.

Reprinted from the U.S. Equal Employment Opportunity Commission[10]

This behavior is unacceptable and illegal. The key to the definition is the victim's interpretation of an individual's actions. Examples may include the following:

- Offensive sexual comments directed at particular individuals.
- Offensive comments about another person's body.
- Any offensive sexual advances.
- Engaging in offensive touching of another person.
- Engaging in or attempting to develop a romantic or sexual relationship with an individual who is a supervisor or who is in a less powerful position.

If an incident of sexual harassment is suspected or does occur, it should be reported promptly to the proper administrator with documentation and details. Ideally, report the information to the preceptor, Assistant/Associate Dean, manager, or supervisor outlined in the policy. If this individual is involved in the harassment, report to the next individual in rank. The allegation will be investigated thoroughly and possibly break a cycle of unacceptable and illegal behavior.

It is also unprofessional and illegal in virtually all health care settings to discriminate against others based on factors such as race, color, creed, religion, nationality, disability, ancestry, age, socioeconomic status, gender, or sexual orientation. In the opinion of the authors, if this concept is not inherently sensible to you, you probably should not be seeking to become a pharmacist.

Sexual Relationships or Misconduct with Patients or Key Parties

Legal concerns over discrimination and sexual harassment have arisen in employment and educational settings, but even otherwise consenting relationships among adults may be problematic in patient care because of the imbalance of power inherent in these relationships.[11,12] Of course, it is unprofessional to take advantage of one's position as a health care provider to sexually harass a patient, or to inappropriately touch or otherwise take sexual advantage of a patient or caregiver. However, state regulatory boards generally consider it unprofessional conduct to engage in consensual sexual relationships with patients or key parties (i.e., spouse, parent, etc., of patient)[13] and may specify a minimum time period that must elapse since the termination of a provider–patient relationship before the provider may seek to enter into a consensual relationship with the former patient. For example, one state's rules prohibit pharmacists, technicians, or intern pharmacists from even suggesting a dating relationship with a current patient and for 2 years after the professional relationship ends.[14] Our advice is to seek the counsel of an experienced mentor before entering into a possible personal relationship with a person you have met first as a patient.

Code of Ethics for Pharmacists and Oath of a Pharmacist

Two documents exist that reinforce the commitment pharmacists have to their patients and the health care community. The American Pharmacists Association created the Code of Ethics for Pharmacists (Box 1.1). It is updated regularly to reflect current practice. The American Pharmaceutical Association Academy of Students of Pharmacy/American Association of Colleges of Pharmacy Council of Deans (APhA-ASP/AACP-COD) Task Force on Professionalism created the Pledge of Professionalism (Box 1.2) and Oath of a Pharmacist (Box 1.3) through a joint effort. Although students often recite this statement on graduation, it should be followed and practiced throughout their training to further emphasize their commitment to the profession of pharmacy.

BOX 1.2 Pledge of Professionalism

As a student of pharmacy, I believe there is a need to build and reinforce a professional identity founded on integrity, ethical behavior, and honor. This development, a vital process in my education, will help ensure that I am true to the professional relationship I establish between myself and society as I become a member of the pharmacy community. Integrity must be an essential part of my everyday life, and I must practice pharmacy with honesty and commitment to service.

To accomplish this goal of professional development, I as a student of pharmacy should:

DEVELOP a sense of loyalty and duty to the profession of pharmacy by being a builder of community, one able and willing to contribute to the well-being of others and one who enthusiastically accepts the responsibility and accountability for membership in the profession.

FOSTER professional competency through lifelong learning. I must strive for high ideals, teamwork, and unity within the profession in order to provide optimal patient care.

SUPPORT my colleagues by actively encouraging personal commitment to the Oath of Maimonides and a Code of Ethics as set forth by the profession.

INCORPORATE into my life and practice, dedication to excellence. This will require an ongoing reassessment of personal and professional values.

MAINTAIN the highest ideals and professional attributes to ensure and facilitate the covenantal relationship required of the pharmaceutical caregiver.

The profession of pharmacy is one that demands adherence to a set of rigid ethical standards. These high ideals are necessary to ensure the quality of care extended to the patients I serve. As a student of pharmacy, I believe this does not start with graduation; rather, it begins with my membership in this professional college community. Therefore, I must strive to uphold these standards as I advance toward full membership in the profession of pharmacy. Developed by the American

BOX 1.2 Pledge of Professionalism *(continued)*

Pharmaceutical Association Academy of Students of Pharmacy/ American Association of Colleges of Pharmacy Council of Deans (APhA-ASP/AACP-COD) Task Force on Professionalism; June 26, 1994.

Reprinted with permission from the American Pharmacists Association and the American Association of Colleges of Pharmacy from http://www.aacp.org/resources/studentaffairspersonnel/studentaffairspolicies/Documents/pledgeprofessionalism.pdf. Copyright 1994 APhA/ACCP. Accessed April 11, 2013.

BOX 1.3 Oath of a Pharmacist

"I promise to devote myself to a lifetime of service to others through the profession of pharmacy. In fulfilling this vow:

I will consider the welfare of humanity and relief of suffering my primary concerns.

I will apply my knowledge, experience, and skills to the best of my ability to assure optimal outcomes for my patients.

I will respect and protect all personal and health information entrusted to me.

I will accept the lifelong obligation to improve my professional knowledge and competence.

I will hold myself and my colleagues to the highest principles of our profession's moral, ethical, and legal conduct.

I will embrace and advocate changes that improve patient care.

I will utilize my knowledge, skills, experiences, and values to prepare the next generation of pharmacists.

I take these vows voluntarily with the full realization of the responsibility with which I am entrusted by the public."

The revised Oath was adopted by the AACP House of Delegates in July 2007 and has been approved by the American Pharmacists Association. AACP member institutions should plan to use the revised Oath of a Pharmacist during the 2008–2009 academic year and with spring 2009 graduates.

Reprinted with permission from the American Association of Colleges of Pharmacy http://www.aacp.org/resources/studentaffairspersonnel/studentaffairspolicies/Documents/OATHOFAPHARMACIST2008-09.pdf. Accessed April 9, 2013.

Giving Back to Your Profession

An important part of being a professional is helping in the development and growth of your field by either giving back, or paying it forward, to your profession. Many professionals such as classmates, faculty, and preceptors at your college or school likely helped you to get to where you are now. There are many ways to give back, like donating money to your alma mater or your preferred pharmacy organization, but arguably, the most valuable donation is your time. You can help in the development of new professionals and the growth of your profession by engaging in a variety of activities such as

- Becoming a licensed preceptor and mentoring pharmacy students at your practice site
- Offering to assist with clinical skills activities at your local pharmacy school or college
- Sponsoring student attendance at state or national pharmacy association meetings
- Offering to assist with admissions interviews at your local pharmacy school or college
- Volunteering as a guest lecturer at your local pharmacy school or college

If you remember a certain preceptor, faculty, or practitioner who was particularly helpful to you, pay it forward by being that person to a future pharmacist.

Summary

Being a professional and acting professionally are characteristics that develop over time. The examples and recommendations in this chapter are just the beginning of resources available to help improve and polish a pharmacist. If you observe and emulate those around you whom you admire, commit yourself to continuous personal improvement, and treat others with respect, you will succeed as a pharmacy professional.

References

1. Popovich NG, Hammer DP, Hansen DJ, et al. Report of the AACP professionalism task force. *Am J Pharm Educ.* 2011;75(10):Article S4.
2. American Pharmacists Association. White paper on pharmacy student professionalism. APhA—Academy of Students of Pharmacy—American

Association of Colleges of Pharmacy Council of Deans Task Force on Professionalism. *J Am Pharm Assoc*. 2000;40(1):96–102.
3. Zaner RM. Trust and the patient-physician relationship. In: Pellegrino ED, Veatch RM, Langan JP, eds. *Ethics, Trust, and the Professions*. Washington, DC: Georgetown University Press; 1991:49.
4. Fassett WE. Ethics, law, and the emergence of pharmacists' responsibility for patient care. *Ann Pharmacother*. 2007;41:1264–1267. doi 10.1345/aph.1K267.
5. Joint Commission of Pharmacy Practitioners. Vision of Pharmacy Practice 2015. http://www.pharmacist.com/vision-and-mission-pharmacy-profession. Accessed April 9, 2013.
6. Hosley JH, Molle E. *A Practical Guide to Therapeutic Communication for Health Professionals*. St. Louis, MO: Saunders Elsevier; 2006.
7. Herrier RN, Boyce RW. Communicating more effectively with physicians, Part 2. *J Am Pharm Assoc*. 1996;NS36(9):547–548.
8. Zweber A. Cultural competence in pharmacy practice. *Am J Pharm Educ*. 2002;66:172–176.
9. Iverson C, Flanagin A, Fontanarosa PB, et al. *American Medical Association Manual of Style. A Guide for Authors and Editors*. 9th ed. Philadelphia, PA: Williams & Wilkins; 1998.
10. U.S. Equal Employment Opportunity Commission. Sexual Harassment. Available at http://www.eeoc.gov/laws/types/sexual_harassment.cfm. Accessed April 9, 2013.
11. Anonymous. Sexual misconduct in the practice of medicine. *JAMA*. 1991; 266:2741–2745.
12. Anonymous. Sexual or romantic relationships between physicians and key third parties. Report 11—A-98, Council on Ethical and Judicial Affairs, American Medical Association. Available at http://www.ama-assn.org/resources/doc/ethics/ceja_11a98.pdf. Accessed April 9, 2013.
13. Federation of State Medical Boards of the U.S., Inc. Addressing Sexual Boundaries: Guidelines for State Medical Boards. Available at http://www.fsmb.org/pdf/GRPOL_Sexual%20Boundaries.pdf. Accessed April 9, 2013.
14. Washington Administrative Code § 246-16-100. Available at http://apps.leg.wa.gov/wac/default.aspx?cite=246-16-100. Accessed April 9, 2013.

Other Suggested Readings and Resources

American Association of Colleges of Pharmacy (AACP). Professionalism: pharmacy student professionalism resources: pharmacy professionalism toolkit for students and faculty. www.aacp.org/resources/studentaffairspersonnel/studentaffairspolicies/Documents/Version_2%200_Pharmacy_Professionalism_Toolkit_for_Students_and_Faculty.pdf. Available at Accessed April 11, 2013.

American Society of Health-System Pharmacists. ASHP statement on professionalism. *Am J Health Syst Pharm*. 2008;65:172–174. Available at http://www.ashp.org/DocLibrary/BestPractices/EthicsStProf.aspx. Accessed April 29, 2013.

Hammer DP, Berger BA, Beardsley RS, et al. Student professionalism. *Am J Pharm Educ.* 2003;67:Article 96.

Hosley J, Molle JH. *A Practical Guide to Therapeutic Communication for Health Professionals.* St. Louis, MO: Saunders Elsevier; 2006.

Kerr RA, Beck DE, et al. Building a sustainable system of leadership development for pharmacy: Report of the 2008–2009 Argus Commission. *Am J Pharm Educ.* 2009;73(8):Article S5.

http://www.ncbi.nlm.nih.gov/pmc/articles/PMC2830040/pdf/ajpeS5.pdf. Accessed April 29, 2013.

Rantucci MJ. *Pharmacists Talking with Patients: A Guide to Patient Counseling.* 2nd ed. Philadelphia, PA: Lippincott Williams & Wilkins; 2007.

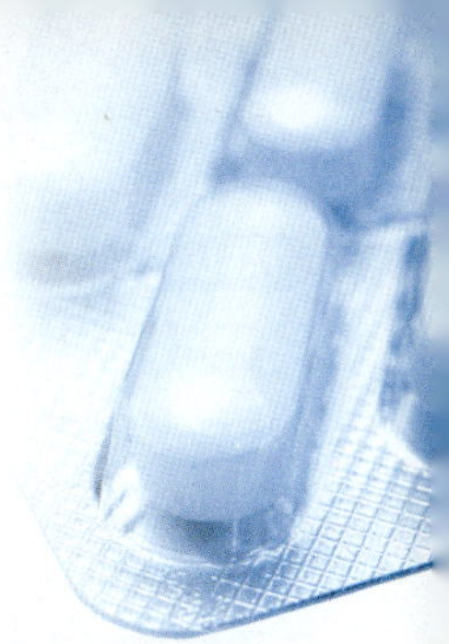

2

Patient Safety

Susan M. Stein and Kate Farthing

Ensuring patient safety is the goal of all health care professionals. It is the responsibility of each health care professional to educate, review, and promote patient safety in all venues at all times. A report by the Institute of Medicine (IOM) in 2000 released the following figures: An estimated 44,000 to 98,000 deaths occur per year due to medical errors, equated to a jumbo jet crashing each day. The report brought patient safety to the forefront of the public domain, and it has remained there since.[1,2] This chapter is designed to provide tools to promote patient safety.

Patient Safety

Patient safety is ensured in the absence of medical error or accidental injury. Medical errors can be described as errors, misadventures, or variances or system failures. An error can be defined as an unintended act or an act that does not achieve its intended outcome. Harm may or may not be the result. Additionally, a close call or near miss is encouraged to be included in error analysis.[1–3]

Medication Errors

Defining types of errors can be useful in analysis and system redesign. See Table 2.1 for a list of types of medication errors compiled by the American Society of Health Systems Pharmacists (ASHP).[4]

Report Error, Analyze Error, and Improve the System

Report Error

Improving patient safety is dependent on sharing close calls or errors that have occurred. By sharing details with others, future

TABLE 2.1 Examples of Types of Medication Errors

Error	Example
Prescribing error	Incorrect drug, dose, route, or formulation, including contraindication due to allergy
Omission error	Missed dose
Wrong time error	Not administered within dosing time
Unauthorized drug error	Drug administered not prescribed
Improper dose error	Dose administered not prescribed
Wrong dosage form error	Dosage form administered not prescribed
Wrong drug preparation error	Drug preparation or compounding error
Wrong administration technique	Route or rate different from prescribed or recommended
Deteriorated drug error	Expired or deteriorated drug administered
Monitoring error	Appropriate drug monitoring not completed
Compliance error	Patient adherence incorrect

Source: American Society of Hospital Pharmacists. ASHP guidelines on preventing medication errors in hospitals. *Am J Hosp Pharm.* 1993;50:305–314.

errors can be prevented or a deficient device can be identified and patient safety improved. This can be done using various resources listed below:

- US Pharmacopeia (USP)—Institute for Safe Medication Practices (ISMP) Medication Errors Reporting Program (MERP)
  - www.ismp.org/orderforms/reporterrortoISMP.asp
  - Operated by the USP and ISMP, MERP is a repository of medication errors. If appropriate, the information is shared with U.S. Food and Drug Administration (FDA) and drug manufacturers. The reporter's name and affiliation are kept confidential unless permission is granted.
- FDA MedWatch
  - www.fda.gov/medwatch/
  - Maintained by the FDA, MedWatch provides another opportunity to report problems with medications or devices. Also links to manufacturers, provides alerts, recalls, and reports when appropriate to health care professionals and the public.

Analyze Error

The most common cause of error is in the medication process itself, and careful analysis of the process can increase safety and reliability of the system. Some tools used to analyze errors are the following:

Root Cause Analysis (RCA)

This tool is used to analyze an error after it has occurred and learn from it. See Table 2.2 for basic steps used in this process.

Failure Mode Effects and Analysis

Another technique helpful in improving systems is a proactive tool called failure mode effects and analysis (FMEA). See Table 2.3 for details. What-if scenarios are analyzed to identify weak links in the system. Analysis of likely errors and steps to prevent them or limit their effects are introduced into the system.

Improve the System

Creating systems and following step-by-step processes decrease the potential for error. This can be viewed as mistake-proofing the system.[2] Continual evaluation to improve systems to maximize efficiency and quality of care is an overarching goal. Involving all interested stakeholders in the development process results in broad support and ultimate success.

TABLE 2.2 Basic Steps of Root Cause Analysis

Error	Comments
Describe the event	Details (when, where, how, who, etc.) Facilitated meeting with all involved Tools: white board and sticky notes to track the error of a wrong drug administered
Identify the proximate cause	All actions that led to the error and explain why it happened Tools: examine order sets, dispensing processes
Identify the contributing factors	Factors that increase the potential for the actions to occur Tools: examine staffing, environments
Create an action plan	Created to decrease potential for proximate causes in the future Tools: redesign systems

TABLE 2.3 Failure Mode and Effects Analysis Process

Step	Comments
Identify each step in the process or system	"What is each individual step in the process?"
Identify failure modes	"What could go wrong?"
Identify failure causes	"What could cause the failure to occur?"
Identify failure effects	"What could be the consequence of this failure?"
Identify the likelihood of failure effects	"What is the most likely error?"
Identify the likelihood of detection of failure	
Modify the system to prevent the most serious and common errors	

Source: Cohen MR, ed. *Medication Errors*. Washington, DC: American Pharmacists Association (APhA); 2007.
Patient Safety. Institute for Healthcare Improvement. http://www.ihi.org/knowledge/Pages/Tools/FailureModesandEffectsAnalysisTool.aspx. Accessed May 16, 2013.

Examples of systems to increase patient safety include the following[2,5,6]:

- Patient confirmation
  - Verbalize the patient's name, procedure to be completed, or medication to be administered.
- Order sets or preprinted orders
  - Order sets or preprinted orders provide standardized drugs and dosages, administration routes, and rates and communication orders with periodic review for clinical accuracy and evidence-based best practice.
  - Example: postsurgery orders for orthopedic patients
- Standardization
  - Standardized drug concentrations, which limit variation in drug concentrations available. Dosage adjustment is obtained via altering the rate of administration.
    - Examples: heparin, 25,000 units in 500 mL 0.9% sodium chloride; dopamine, 250 mg in 250 mL 0.9% sodium chloride
  - Standardized procedures or drugs available for use in a patient care setting
  - Standardized available generic companies to ensure quality drug formulation

- Read back order confirmation
  - Verbally read back an oral order that has been transcribed to writing prior to completing verbal conversation.
- Two- or three-person drug order or calculation confirmation
  - Double signature for all chemotherapy orders
  - Require triple sign-off system for all surgery patients to confirm procedure type, correct patient, correct limb, and so on.
- Read three times
  - Read the drug name three times prior to dispensing the drug to the patient.
- Use bar-coding bracelets
  - Bar code swipe prior to medication administration to confirm correct drug for correct patient
- Use color-coding systems
  - Use color-coded bracelet to identify patients with specific drug, food, or latex allergies in a health care facility.
  - Use color-coded patient slippers to identify fall-risk patients.
  - Use color-coded drug labels to delineate different drug names or concentrations.
- The five rights
  - Right drug, right dose, right route, right time, right patient
- Medication reconciliation
  - Five-step process: List current medications, list medications to prescribe, compare the two lists, select the most clinically appropriate medications, and communicate the new list to patient and caregivers. See Figure 2.1 for an example of a typical patient medication list.[7]

Each system improvement creates a barrier or safeguard to prevent an error. This system of preventative tools has been referred to as the Swiss Cheese model by James Reason.[8] With proactive methods in

Drug name (brand & generic)	Dose (strength & form)	How often taking this dose	Start/Stop	Reason for taking	Prescribing doctor
Furosemide (Lasix)	*40 mg tablet*	*Twice daily*	*01/01/2013 start*	*High blood pressure*	*Smith*

FIGURE 2.1 An example of a typical patient medication list.

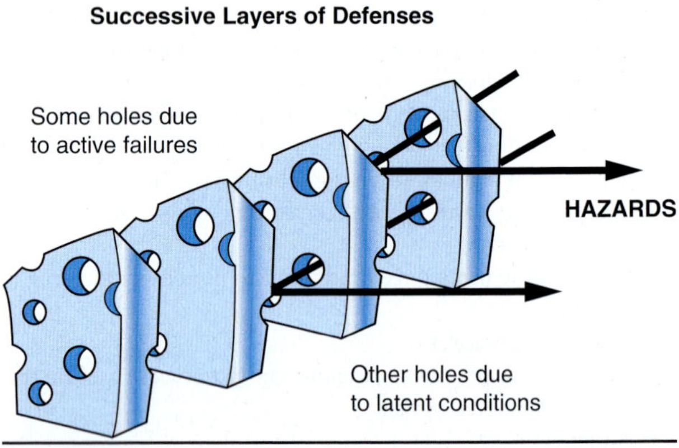

FIGURE 2.2 Swiss cheese model. (Reprinted with permission from Reason, J. *Human Error*. Cambridge, UK: Cambridge University Press, 1990.)

place, such as the use of order sets, bar code scanning, and readback techniques, we create barriers to avoid medication errors and patient harm (Fig. 2.2). There are times when our systems fail, human mistakes occur, and the processes in place to prevent error break down, resulting in an error reaching the patient (Fig. 2.2).

Culture of Safety

Establishing a culture of safety to support patient safety is critical. The culture of safety acknowledges that everyone on the health care team shares responsibility to maintain and support patient safety. It acknowledges an open environment to discuss patient safety and de-emphasizes enforcing safety through punitive tactics. The culture of safety supports open discussion and incentives for system analysis and improvement. A decrease in reporting and improvement in the system is seen in a punitive environment.[9]

Our limitations as human beings are important to recognize and acknowledge. Despite the best of intentions, we do make mistakes. Additionally, patients expect us to perform without error. These conditions work in unison to increase the pressure on health care providers to perform. The best tool to aid in preventing this vicious cycle is to embrace a culture of safety.[10–12]

The following are examples of expectations and limitations:

- Recognize the patient and his or her rights and expectations
  - Be cognizant of working with patients as human beings.
  - Patients expect safety at all times.
- Recognize the limitations of our abilities as human beings to work error free
  - Human beings make mistakes.

Useful Web Sites and Highlights

- Institute of Safe Medical Practices
  - www.ismp.org/
  - Independent nonprofit agency serving as a repository of medication alerts
  - Resources
    - High Alert Medications List
    - Error-Prone Abbreviations
    - Do Not Crush List
- National Patient Safety Organization
  - www.npsf.org/
  - Independent nonprofit with goal of improving patient safety
  - Resources
    - Online patient safety resources: www.npsf.org/rc/mp/opsr/
- Institute for Healthcare Improvement
  - www.ihi.org/IHI/Topics/PatientSafety/
  - Independent nonprofit agency focused on improving health care worldwide
  - Resources
    - Patient safety
    - Reducing mortality
- The Joint Commission (TJC)
  - http://www.jointcommission.org/topics/patient_safety.aspx/
  - Independent for-profit agency providing accreditation to health care organizations
  - Resources
    - National patient safety goals
    - Infection control
    - Speak up initiatives

    - Universal protocol for preventing wrong site, wrong procedure, wrong person surgery
- Agency for Healthcare Research and Quality (AHRQ)
  - www.ahrq.gov/
  - Federal agency within the Department of Health and Human Services responsible for improving the safety and efficacy of health care
  - Resources
    - Patient fact sheet: five steps to safer health care www.ahrq.gov/consumer/5steps.htm
- National Center for Patient Safety (NCPS)
  - www.patientsafety.gov/index.html
  - Federal organization serving the Veterans Health Administration in promoting patient safety
  - Resources
    - Provides links to other national and international Web resources
- Institute of Medicine (IOM)
  - http://www.iom.edu/
  - Independent nonprofit that provides advice regarding evidence-based informed health decisions
  - Resources
    - http://www.iom.edu/Reports/2006/Preventing-Medication-Errors-Quality-Chasm-Series.aspx

Summary

Frequent monitoring of primary literature and patient safety Web sites is advised to produce a valuable collection of resources. Use them wisely and often. Remain vigilant. Do not become apathetic, overconfident, or distracted. Remember, compromises to patient safety are often the result of poorly designed systems or failure to follow procedures.

References

1. Kohn L, Corrigan J, Donaldson M, eds. *To Err Is Human: Building a Safer Health System*. Washington, DC: Committee on Quality of Health Care in America, Institute of Medicine. National Academy Press; 2000.
2. Cohen MR, ed. *Medication Errors*. Washington, DC: American Pharmacists Association (APhA); 2007.

3. Botwinick L, Bisognano M, Haraden C. *Leadership Guide to Patient Safety. IHI Innovation Series White Paper.* Cambridge, MA: Institute for Healthcare Improvement; 2006. Available at www.IHI.org.
4. American Society of Hospital Pharmacists. ASHP guidelines on preventing medication errors in hospitals. *Am J Hosp Pharm.* 1993;50:305–314.
5. Institute for Safe Medication Practices. The “five rights.” 1999 August 17. Available at http://www.ismp.org/Newsletters/acutecare/articles/19990407.asp.
6. Cohen MR, Smetzer JL. Lack of standard dosing methods contribute to IV errors. *Hosp Pharm.* 2007;42(12):1100–1101.
7. American Society of Health-System Pharmacists. ASHP Medication Reconciliation Toolkit. 2013. Available at http://www.ashp.org/menu/PracticePolicy/ResourceCenters/PatientSafety/ASHPMedicationReconciliationToolkit_1.aspx. Accessed May 10, 2013.
8. Reason J. Human error: models and management. *BMJ.* 2000;320:768–770.
9. McIntyre N, Popper K. The critical attitude in medicine: the need for a new ethics. *Br Med J (Clin Res Ed).* 1989;287:1919–1923.
10. Patient Safety. Institute for Healthcare Improvement. Available at: www.ihi.org/IHI/Topics/PatientSafety/. Accessed December 26, 2007.
11. Patient Safety. Institute for Healthcare Improvement. Available at: http://www.ihi.org/knowledge/Pages/Tools/FailureModesandEffectsAnalysisTool.aspx. Accessed May 16, 2013.
12. Grout J. Mistake-Proofing the Design of Health Care Processes. (Prepared under an IPA with Berry College). AHRQ Publication No. 07-0020. Rockville, MD: Agency for Healthcare Research and Quality; May 2007.

3

The Law and the Clinical Practice of Pharmacy

William E. Fassett

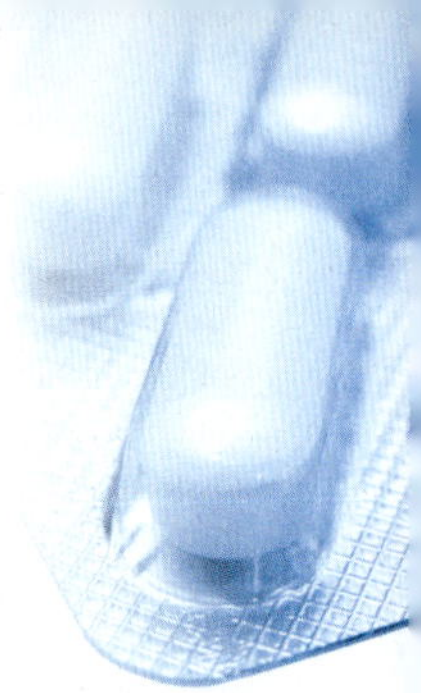

The Law's Proper Place in Clinical Decision Making

If pharmacists think about the law at all during their daily work, many do so by asking the question, "What does the law allow me to do for this patient?" This is a good question, but it must not be the first question asked in any clinical situation. This chapter begins with the assertion that the first question to be considered in any patient clinical encounter is "What does this patient need from me at this time to ensure optimal outcomes from his or her drug therapy?"

Many pharmacists who engage in a formal evaluation of a patient's care needs do so using a structured documentation process and format developed for use in the Problem-Oriented Medical Record.[1] Known by the acronym SOAP, standing for Subjective, Objective, Assessment, and Plan, each of its elements is intended to help organize the medical record. However, SOAP also serves as a process for clinical decision making. Although it has been criticized as the ideal approach to clinical diagnosis,[2,3] it remains widely taught in U.S. doctor of pharmacy programs. So, we start by using the SOAP outline to summarize the points at which legal considerations may arise during clinical decision making in Table 3.1.

Note how late in the process it is before most legal limitations appear as possible considerations. To reiterate, pharmacists are not lawyers but primary care providers; their first responsibility is to consider how best to meet patient needs and then to make sure they are doing so in a legally appropriate manner.

Quite a few legal considerations arise as pharmacists are engaged in activities necessary to maintain their license to practice or for the

TABLE 3.1 Summary of Legal Issues Arising During Clinical Decision Making

SOAP Element	Typical Elements	Potential Legal Considerations
Subjective data	Chief complaint Patient's symptoms and feelings Patient's self-reported history	Does the pharmacist have permission to take or review history?
Objective data	Physical exam Laboratory data Diagnostic procedures Medication use record	Does the pharmacist have permission to examine the patient and/or permission to obtain records?
Assessment	Identify drug therapy–related problems For each problem, identify a desired outcome, expressed in measurable terms For each problem/outcome, list available therapeutic alternatives Rank available therapeutic alternatives	Has the pharmacist considered clinical, economic, and humanistic outcomes (particularly professional standards, quality of life, and moral and ethical issues) when ranking alternatives?
Plan	With patient, select preferred alternative Prepare patient to be able to adhere to plan Follow up	Has the pharmacist considered whether the plan can be legally implemented? What documentation or record-keeping requirements are essential to implementing the plan? If the pharmacist is acting as the prescribing practitioner, has he or she obtained informed consent from the patient?

operation of a practice site. However, this chapter focuses primarily on laws relating to the routine clinical functions needed to implement pharmaceutical care for specific patients.

How to Use This Chapter

The rest of this chapter consists primarily of summary tables. Every state must consider a set of important issues when it decides how pharmacy should be practiced within its borders. These decisions by the states interact with federal law governing drugs, devices, and controlled substances. The two most important federal laws are the Food,

Drug, and Cosmetic Act (FDCA) and the Controlled Substances Act (CSA). In the following tables, federal law—where appropriate—is set out, and then typical options among the states are listed. The reader should identify those options chosen by his or her state, using the check boxes or the additional space provided.

Practice of Pharmacy

Pharmacists' Scope of Practice

State laws define the scope of practice of pharmacists. Table 3.2 summarizes the major functions of pharmacists allowed in the states. As of early 2013, 43 states allow some form of prescribing by pharmacists under protocol, and all states permit pharmacists to administer drugs or at least some vaccines.[4]

Use of Pharmacy Technicians

Most states permit, either explicitly or implicitly, the use of ancillary personnel, such as pharmacy technicians, when under the direction of a pharmacist. Table 3.3 indicates typical activities that are allowed

TABLE 3.2 Actions the Pharmacist May Perform

	Your State?	
	Yes	No
Interpreting prescription or orders for legend drugs and devices	*	
Compounding, packaging, labeling, and dispensing drugs	*	
Providing information on the hazards and uses of drugs	*	
Maintaining proper records of drugs purchased and dispensed	*	
Monitoring of drug therapy: May include ordering of laboratory tests, drug blood levels, and/or assessing vital signs. Note any special requirements:		
Administering drugs generally: "Administration" generally includes application of a drug to the body of a patient by injection, inhalation, ingestion, or other means	*	
Administering immunizations: Note any special requirements:	*	
Prescribing under protocol: Note any special requirements:	*	

*Allowed in most states

TABLE 3.3 Typical Functions of Pharmacy Technicians

	Your State? Yes	Your State? No
Packaging, pouring, or placing drugs in containers for dispensing	*	
Reconstituting prescription medications subject to verification of accuracy	*	
Affixing required labels	*	
Entering information into the pharmacy computer subject to verification	*	
Prepackaging and labeling multidose and unit-dose packages, subject to verification	*	
Picking doses for unit-dose cart fill for hospital and nursing homes, subject to verification	*	
Recording patient or medication information in the computer subject to verification	*	
Bulk compounding subject to verification	*	
Reconstitution of single or multiple units that will be given to a patient as a single dose, subject to verification	*	
Addition of a single ingredient to a prepared unit of another drug, subject to verification	*	
Initiating or accepting oral or electronic refill information from prescribers that does not change the prescription in any way	*	
Mixing more than one ingredient into a parenteral medication, subject to verification		
Checking nursing units for nonjudgmental tasks such as sanitation and outdated medications, subject to pharmacist review of problems found		
Checking unit-dose medications in a tech-check-tech program		
Stocking of dispensing machines		
Are technicians required to have special training for any of the above functions?		
Are technicians required to pass national certifying exam?		*
Are technicians required to complete continuing education?		*
Is there a limit on the ratio of technicians to pharmacists in your state? If so, is it different for community pharmacy settings than for inpatient or other settings?	*	
Notes:		

*Most states

by pharmacy technicians. Note that states may permit some activities in an institutional setting that are not permitted in community pharmacy practice.

Functions That Technicians May *Not* Perform

Many states are explicit concerning activities or decisions that must be performed by pharmacists (or interns) and may *not* be delegated to technicians. In most states, allowing a nonpharmacist to perform these functions is considered permitting the unlicensed practice of pharmacy and a cause for discipline. Table 3.4 lists functions that technicians are usually prohibited from undertaking.

TABLE 3.4 Typical Functions Prohibited to Be Performed by Pharmacy Technicians

	Prohibited in Your State?	
	Yes	**No**
Receipt of a verbal prescription other than a refill authorization	*	
Receive or transfer a prescription to another pharmacy	*	
Provide a prescription or medication to a patient without a pharmacist's verification of accuracy of the prescription	*	
Deliver a prescription to the patient when the pharmacist is absent from the pharmacy	*	
Consultation with the patient regarding the prescription and/or regarding any information in the patient medication record	*	
Consultation with the prescriber regarding the patient and the patient's prescription	*	
Interpretation of the data in the patient medication record system	*	
Ultimate responsibility for the correctness of a dispensed prescription	*	
Signing of documents or registry books that require a pharmacist's signature	*	
Professional communications with physicians, dentists, nurses, and other health care practitioners	*	
Making the offer to counsel as required by OBRA-90		

*Most states

Privileges of Pharmacy Interns

Intern pharmacists may generally perform any function that can be performed by pharmacists, while under a pharmacist's supervision. Some states are more restrictive than others regarding how closely interns must be supervised, and states interpret certain federal laws differently. For example, Drug Enforcement Administration (DEA) regulations governing transfer of refill information between pharmacies for Schedule III, IV, and V controlled substances specify that the transfer must be "communicated directly between two licensed pharmacists."[5] Boards of Pharmacy differ whether that phrase excludes interns from transferring controlled substances prescriptions. Table 3.5 lists some of the functions that may not be allowed in all states.

Dispensing or Delivering Prescription Drugs to Patients

Although distributive functions related to drug dispensing are increasingly being performed by technicians and with the aid of pharmacy automation, it remains a critical clinical responsibility of pharmacists to supervise the distribution system and to evaluate the appropriateness and correctness of every order or prescription that is processed for a patient.

Requirements of a Valid Prescription

Dispensing or delivering prescription drugs in the absence of a legally valid order or prescription is prohibited by the federal FDCA, by the CSA, and by the laws of every state; it is called diversion. Table 3.6

TABLE 3.5 Possible State Restriction of Intern's Activities

	Your State	
	Yes	No
May interns transfer or receive transfers of prescriptions for controlled substances in Schedule III, IV, or V?		
May interns sign the log book for sale of OTC Schedule V drugs?		
Does the supervising pharmacist need to recheck every prescription filled by an intern?		
Are there other restrictions on what interns may do?		

TABLE 3.6 Four Questions to Ask Before Filling a Prescription

	Rx Checklist	
	Yes	No
Is it issued for a specific patient? Note: A prescription issued with "for office use" in the patient name field is not valid		
Is it issued by an authorized prescriber?		
Was it issued in the due course of the prescriber's professional practice? • Did a bona fide physician–patient relationship exist? • Is the prescription within the prescriber's scope of practice?		
Is it for a legitimate medical purpose?		

Note: If "No" for any question, then the prescription is not valid.

summarizes the four conditions that are necessary to make a prescription valid.

Tamper-Proof Prescription Pads

Under a recent amendment to the U.S. Patriot Act, prescriptions written for Medicaid patients must be written on tamper-proof prescription pads, effective April 1, 2008. This rule does not apply to Medicaid prescriptions that are faxed, telephoned, or electronically prescribed.

Illegible Prescriptions

Prescriptions that cannot be easily read and interpreted by pharmacists are legally invalid in several states, and in some states, this rule applies to any prescription that is written in cursive handwriting. Pharmacists should always confirm with the prescriber the exact details of any prescription that is hard to read.

Legitimate Medical Purpose

In one sense, all that is needed to meet a legitimate medical purpose is that the prescriber intends the drug to treat a bona fide patient care need. If the pharmacist knows or should know that the intended use is for recreational drug use, or solely to maintain an addiction (exceptions are drugs dispensed as part of an opioid addiction treatment program), then the pharmacist cannot legally fill the prescription.

Unapproved Indications

Manufacturers may not promote drugs for any use not included in the approved package insert; however, practitioners may prescribe drugs for off-label uses for individual patients, and pharmacists may lawfully fill those prescriptions. Pharmacists may also dispense generic equivalents for uses that are indicated only in the labeling of the brand name drug (e.g., a prescription written generically for bupropion may be filled with a generic bupropion tablet for smoking cessation, even though only Zyban includes that indication in its approved labeling). Table 3.7 summarizes special situations regarding off-label use.

Required Information on Prescriptions

Certain elements must be present on a prescription at the time it is presented to a pharmacist. These generally require the date written; the name of the patient; the prescription itself, the name, address, and signature of the physician (if written); and, for controlled substances, the prescriber's DEA number. Other elements must be added and recorded when the prescription is filed in the pharmacy after dispensing. Table 3.8 summarizes these elements.

Who May Prescribe Legend Drugs?

Under both the FDCA and the CSA, persons authorized to prescribe drugs are those individuals who are licensed by the jurisdiction in which they practice. All states license physicians, dentists,

TABLE 3.7 Special Situations Regarding Off-Label Use

	Rx Checklist	
	Yes	No
Is the prescription with an off-label use intended for a Medicare or Medicaid patient? • If so, is the proposed use listed as a generally recognized use supported by evidence in USP-DI or AHFS? If No, do not fill. Note: if Yes, may require prior authorization		
Is the off-label use specifically prohibited by state law? If Yes, do not fill. • C-II stimulants used for weight loss? Anabolic steroids used for muscle building?		
Is the prescription for a patient with third-party insurance and the intended use considered experimental? If Yes, may require prior authorization		

TABLE 3.8 Elements Required on a Filled Prescription

	Your State?	
	Yes	**No**
Prescriber's name, address	* †††	
Patient's name	* †††	
Patient's address (on Rx or in the patient information system)	* ††	
Date written	* †††	
Name of drug, dosage form, strength, and quantity/duration of therapy	* †††	
Prescriber's directions to the patient	* †	
Signature of prescriber if it is a written Rx	* †††	
Prescriber's DEA number if it is for a controlled substance	* ††	
Specification regarding generic substitution		
Any refill information	*	
Any additional instructions	*	
A serial number placed by the pharmacist	* †	
The date filled	*	
The initials of the responsible pharmacist who filled the Rx	*	
The identity of the actual drug dispensed (e.g., NDC number)		
Other requirements in your state:		

*Required in most states
†Required by the FDCA
††Required by the CSA
DEA, Drug Enforcement Administration; NDC, National Drug Code

podiatrists, and veterinarians, and most states accept prescriptions written by these prescribers who practice outside the state. Midlevel practitioners, as they are called by the DEA, practice in most states, but their scope of practice varies. Therefore, out-of-state prescriptions from nurse practitioners, physician's assistants, optometrists, naturopaths, and pharmacists are not usually accepted. Table 3.9 summarizes the various health professionals who may prescribe drugs and devices in most states. The DEA maintains a summary of controlled substances prescribing privileges for midlevel practitioners on its Web site.[6]

TABLE 3.9 Prescriptive Authority of Various Health Professionals

		Your State?	
		Yes	No
Physicians (MD or DO)	All drugs, all classes for human patients, regardless of where the prescriber is licensed	✔	
Dentists (DDS or DMD)	All drugs, all classes, for human patients for head and neck conditions, regardless of where the prescriber is licensed	✔	
Podiatrists (DPM or PodD)	All drugs, all classes, for human patients, for conditions of the ankles and feet, regardless of where the prescriber is licensed	✔	
Veterinarians (DVM)	All drugs, all classes, for non–human animals, regardless of where the prescriber is licensed	✔	
Midlevel Practitioners			
Nurse Practitioners (ARNP), Clinical Nurse Specialists (CNS)	Legend drugs if appropriate to the scope of specialty and practice	*	
	• Out-of-state ARNP prescriptions allowed for legend drugs		
	• Out-of-state ARNP prescriptions allowed for controlled substances		
	• C-II	*	
	• C-III, IV, V	*	
	• Independent practice	*	
Nurse Midwife (CNM) (An ARNP specialty in most states)	Legend if appropriate to the care of the preterm and postpartum patient, and the newborn, only in state where licensed	*	
	• C-II	*	
	• C-III, IV, V	*	
	• Independent practice	*	
Nurse Anesthetists (CRNA)	Most drugs if used for preanesthesia or during anesthesia, only in state where licensed	*	
	• C-II	*	
	• C-III, IV, V	*	
	• Independent practice		*
Physicians' Assistants (PA, PA-C)	All drugs, all classes approved by supervising physician	*	
	• Out-of-state PA prescriptions allowed for legend drugs		
	• Out-of-state PA prescriptions allowed for controlled substances		
	• C-II	*	
	• C-III, IV, V	*	
	• Independent practice		*

(continued)

TABLE 3.9 Prescriptive Authority of Various Health Professionals *(continued)*

		Your State?	
		Yes	**No**
Optometrists (OD)	Legend drugs needed to screen for glaucoma, diagnosis, and treatment of minor ophthalmic conditions, only in state where licensed	*	
	• Topical ophthalmic drugs for diagnosis	*	
	• Oral and topical legend drugs used to treat ophthalmic conditions	*	
	• C-II within scope of practice		*
	• C-III within scope of practice	*	
	• C-IV within scope of practice	*	
	• C-V within scope of practice	*	
Naturopaths (ND)	Drug used in traditional naturopathic practice, which are usually limited to drugs derived from natural sources, only in state where licensed	*	
	• Homeopathic remedies, herbals	*	
	• Legend drugs		*
	• C-II within scope (e.g., codeine)		*
	• C-III or IV within scope (e.g., codeine, testosterone)		*
	• C-V within scope (e.g., codeine)		*
Licensed Midwife (not an ARNP)	May order and administer certain drugs used for delivery or neonatal care, may administer drugs ordered or prescribed for use in delivery, only in state where licensed	*	
	• May prescribe or dispense diaphragms	*	
	• May prescribe prenatal vitamins		*
	• May prescribe oral contraceptives		*
	• Independent practice	*	
Pharmacists	Prescribe legend under protocol, consistent with the scope of the authorizing prescriber, only in state where licensed	*	
	• Controlled substances within scope of authorizing prescriber		*

✔All states
*Most states

New and Refill Prescriptions

New Prescriptions

Many states make a distinction in their laws between "new" prescriptions and "refills." This is often especially important when interpreting the rules for patient counseling. Many pharmacists consider a new prescription to be one for a drug the patient has not received before. However, this is more properly seen as a new drug for the patient. Legally, a "new" prescription is one that requires the pharmacy to assign it a new prescription number. When prescriptions expire in accordance with the law, such as after 6 months for Schedule III or Schedule IV drugs, they become "new" prescriptions when reauthorized by the prescriber.

Refill Prescriptions

Refills are repeated dispensing of a drug that uses the same prescription number as a previously filled prescription. A prescription may be refilled if authorized by the prescriber, either at the time the prescription was first written or later, as long as the prescription has not expired.

Prescription Invalidation

Prescriptions become invalid after some time period in most states. Most states set a limit on how long a prescription is valid after the date written (e.g., 1 year). Federal law limits refills on Schedule III and IV drugs to five refills within 6 months after the date written, but federal law does not place a limit on how long a Schedule II prescription is valid (see "Controlled Substances"). States may also limit the total number of allowed refills.

It is often stated that when a prescriber dies or loses his or her license, the prescriptions written by that prescriber are no longer valid. Federal law does not create such a rule—as long as the prescriber was authorized at the time the prescription was written, it is a valid prescription. Some states have dealt with this specifically, either by regulation or by a formal Board policy. Table 3.10 provides an opportunity to record your state's rules on how long prescriptions are valid.

Prescription Transfers Between Pharmacies

When a prescription has refills remaining, and has not expired, you may transfer the prescription and its refill information to another pharmacy, which may dispense the remaining refills. Once transferred

TABLE 3.10 Time Limit After Which Prescriptions Are No Longer Valid

	Your State's Rule?				
	1 Month	**6 Months**	**1 Year**	**Never Expire**	**Other Time Period**
Noncontrolled prescription drugs				**	
Schedule II				**	
Schedules III and IV		* **			
Schedule V				**	
If a prescriber dies or loses his or her license, how long are his or her prescriptions valid?				**	

*Most states
**Federal law

to another pharmacy, the prescription may not be filled in your pharmacy, unless it is transferred back, whereupon it is treated as a new prescription. Tables 3.11 and 3.12 summarize steps pharmacists must take when transferring or receiving transferred prescriptions.

TABLE 3.11 Steps to Take When Transferring a Prescription to Another Pharmacy

		Rx Checklist
Record that the prescription has been transferred in the medication record system.		
Record the name and address of the pharmacy to which it was transferred.		
Record the full name of the pharmacist or intern to whom it was transferred.		
Other requirements in your state:		
If the prescription is for a C-3, C-4, or C-5 drug, you must also:	Locate the original hard copy of the Rx and write "Void" on its face. Record the DEA number of the pharmacy to which it was transferred.	

DEA, Drug Enforcement Administration

TABLE 3.12 Steps to Take When Receiving a Prescription from Another Pharmacy

		Rx Checklist
Write the word "Transfer" on your copy of the prescription		
Record the name and address of the other pharmacy		
Record the full name of the pharmacist or intern who provided you with the information (obtain both first and last name)		
Record the other pharmacy's prescription number		
Record all the other information needed for the prescription (prescriber, patient, drug, strength, quantity, directions)		
Record the following dates:	Date of the transfer	
	Date Rx was first written	
	Date Rx was last refilled	
Record the number of refills originally allowed		
Record the number of refills remaining		
Other requirements in your state:		
If the prescription is for a C-3, C-4, or C-5 drug, you must also		
	Record the DEA number of the pharmacy from whom it was received	
	Record the DEA number of the prescriber	
	Record dates and locations of all previous fillings of the Rx	
	Record the name, address, DEA number, and serial number of the original prescription and pharmacy, if it is different from the transferring pharmacy	

DEA, Drug Enforcement Administration

Pharmacists working in chains that share a common database among all their pharmacies are able in most states and under federal law to simply refill the prescription at their location and record the refill in the medication record system.

Drug Classifications

Legally, drugs marketed in the United States are classified as prescription-only (legend drugs), nonprescription, or "behind-the-counter"—a relatively new classification. (The FDA is currently reviewing testimony and comments concerning "conditions for safe use," under which otherwise prescription-only drugs could be made accessible without prescription.) Drugs may also be controlled substances, whether prescription (Rx)-only or over-the-counter (OTC). Finally, certain drugs that are precursors for methamphetamine are now subject to special requirements to reduce their availability for the production of methamphetamine.

Prescription Legend Drugs

Prescription-only drugs are also known as legend drugs, because their labels were formerly required to bear the legend, "Caution: Federal law prohibits dispensing without prescription." These drugs may now be labeled "Rx only." Prescriptions may be telephoned, faxed, written, or e-prescribed and are generally refillable without limit as long as the prescription is valid.

OTC Drugs

OTC or nonprescription drugs are those that may be sold to the public without a prescription and must bear a complete label as required by the FDA. They may be prescribed and dispensed with a prescription label only if this is pursuant to a valid prescription.

Methamphetamine Precursors

OTC sales of drugs containing pseudoephedrine (or ephedrine or phenylpropanolamine—which are not generally available) must be recorded in a log by the pharmacy or retailer unless they are combination products in liquid formulations. Products subject to the record requirement may not be accessible to the public. Any person selling these products must have completed an online training program. Under federal law, the log book must contain a statement to the purchaser of the penalties for violating the purchase limits set forth by federal law.

An electronic log book or record system may also be used, and many states (23 as of June 2013) now require the use of a national service known as the National Precursor Log Exchange, or NPLEx. The system requires the seller to enter the purchaser's identifying information and returns a message indicating if the purchaser has exceeded the purchase limits. The system will allow the seller to override the sales block if he or she feels in danger and sends an alert to law enforcement for follow-up investigation.[7]

Tables 3.13 and 3.14 summarize the federal requirements for the log book and maximum purchase limits and provide an opportunity to record your state's limits.

Controlled Substances

Controlled substances are drugs or their precursors that have a significant potential for abuse. They are divided into five schedules, depending on their medical use and potential for abuse.

Persons or firms who prescribe or dispense controlled substances must be registered with the DEA, and prescribers must place their DEA number on all prescriptions. Schedule II drugs must be ordered on special order forms.

Table 3.15 summarizes the five schedules under the CSA. You should also access and review the Pharmacist's Manual on the DEA Web site for more information on the federal laws and regulations governing controlled substances.[8]

TABLE 3.13 Limits on OTC Sales of Methamphetamine Precursors to a Single Purchaser

	Federal Law	Your State
Sales/day	3.6 g	
Sales/month	9 g	
Possession	No limit	
Package size	3.6 g	
Package type	Blister, 2 units/blister	
Sales limited to 18 years or over?	No	
Other requirements in your state?		

TABLE 3.14 Methamphetamine Precursor Sales Log Requirements

	Federal Law	Your State
Purchaser's name	Yes	
Purchaser's address	Yes	
Date of birth	No	
Type of ID	No	
Name of drug	Yes	
Quantity sold	Yes	
Date of purchase	Yes	
Time of purchase	Yes	
Is use of NPLEx electronic database required?	No	*
Other requirements in your state?		

*Most states

Is It Legitimate?

Controlled substances prescriptions are valid only if they are issued for a "legitimate medical purpose," and the pharmacist bears a "corresponding responsibility" with the prescriber to ensure that this condition is met. Thus, with each controlled substances prescription, the pharmacist must independently determine whether the prescription is legitimate. It is important, however, to remember that the pharmacist is foremost a primary care provider, not a law enforcement officer: Deciding whether to dispense or not dispense a controlled substance must be examined in light of the needs of the patient.

Red Flags Indicating a Possible Problem with a Prescription

The DEA and other authorities[8,9] recognize several characteristics that should alert a pharmacist to a possible forged or illegitimate prescription. Table 3.16 summarizes common red flags that may appear on individual prescriptions, and Table 3.17 summarizes some common behaviors of chronic pain patients that may indicate a need for increased vigilance. These red flags are not definitive, but if present require the pharmacist to validate the order or prescription and/or promote referral of the patient to treatment for possible addiction.

TABLE 3.15 Controlled Substances Requirements

CSA Schedule	Basis for Inclusion	Examples	How Prescribed	Prescriptions Expire		Refill Limits	
				Federal Law	Your State	Federal Law	Your State
I	No medical use, high potential for abuse	Heroin, LSD, psilocybin, marijuana	May not be prescribed	N/A	N/A	N/A	N/A
II	High potential for abuse	Meperidine, oxycodone, methylphenidate, amphetamines	Requires written prescription	Never		No refills	
III	Moderate potential for abuse; mostly narcotic combinations	APAP with codeine; hydrocodone with APAP	Written or oral	6 months from date written		Five refills	
IV	Moderate potential for abuse; nonnarcotics mostly	Benzodiazepines Testosterone	Written or oral	6 months from date written		Five refills	
V	Codeine ≤ 10 mg/dose plus other ingredients; antidiarrheals; low potential for abuse	Lomotil; Tylenol with codeine Elixir; codeine cough syrups; Lyrica (pregabalin)	Written or oral	Never		No limit	

CSA, Controlled Substances Act; LSD, lysergic acid diethylamide; N/A, not applicable

TABLE 3.16 Red Flags That Suggest a Forged, Altered, or Otherwise Invalid Prescription

	Rx Checklist	
	Yes	No
Does the prescription look "too good?"		
Does the quantity, directions, or dosage differ from usual medical usage?		
Do the abbreviations differ from standard medical abbreviations?		
Are the directions written in full with no abbreviations? (Actually a desirable practice for prescribers, but still an unusual event.)		
Is the prescription written in different color inks or different handwriting?		

Note: The greater the number of "Yes" checks, the greater the need for pharmacist vigilance and verification of the prescription.

TABLE 3.17 Chronic Pain Patients Red Flags

	Rx Checklist	
	Yes	No
Does the patient appear to be "doctor shopping" (obtaining multiple prescriptions for the same or similar drugs from multiple prescribers)?		
Does it appear that the patient is altering or forging prescriptions?		
Are you aware of the patient selling his or her prescription drugs?		
Does the patient insist on specific brand name narcotics and refuse generics in situations where the use of generics is indicated?		
Are there multiple episodes of lost, stolen, or accidently destroyed prescriptions and/or drugs?		
Are you aware of the patient taking or using another person's drugs?		

Note: The greater the number of "Yes" checks, the greater the need for the pharmacist to work with prescribers to ensure that the patient is not becoming addicted.

White Flags Indicating a Need by the Pharmacist to Ensure Patient Care

If the pharmacist, reacting to a red flag, delays or refuses dispensing of a prescription, the patient may suffer inappropriately if the pharmacist's decision is incorrect. Therefore, pharmacists who mistakenly refuse to dispense a legitimate prescription for controlled substances may find themselves being named in a lawsuit. As a general rule, before deciding not to dispense a prescription, the pharmacist should engage in a direct conversation with the prescriber concerning his or her decision not to dispense. Table 3.18 summarizes questions a pharmacist should ask before deciding not to dispense or to contact authorities.[10]

TABLE 3.18 White Flags That Suggest This Person Should be Treated as a Patient, Not a Felon

	Rx Checklist	
	Yes	**No**
Did the information regarding the validity of the prescription come directly from the prescriber?		
• If No, did the party inform you that the prescription is unequivocally fraudulent *and* that their response is *not* just based on a lack of information in the patient record? (If No, don't call the police.)		
Did you discuss with the prescriber that you were intending to call the police?		
• If Yes, did the prescriber agree that was appropriate? (If No, be careful about calling the police.)		
Has the patient previously established a relationship with you or the pharmacy?		
• If Yes, did your profile review suggest that the prescription is consistent with a pattern of reasonable treatment? (If Yes, do not call the police.) • If Yes, did you ask the patient about any discrepancies with the prescription? (If No, be careful about calling the police.) • If Yes, did the patient's explanation resolve issues? (If Yes, do not call the police.)		
Are you expecting the police to investigate further? (If Yes, confirm this with the police, if contacted.)		
• If No, do you believe they can rely on *your* information to conclude the prescription is fraudulent? (If No, be careful about calling the police.)		
Are you prepared to defend your decision in court? (If No, do not call the police.)		

Prescription Drug Monitoring Programs

As of mid-2013, all states but Missouri operate or plan to implement prescription drug monitoring programs (PDMPs), which are statewide electronic databases that collect designated data on substances dispensed in the state. All dispensers are required to provide information to the PDMP (including most physicians who dispense drugs), and for most pharmacies, the process is handled automatically by the prescription dispensing system. Prescribers and pharmacists, as well as authorized law enforcement personnel, may access the PDMP to help evaluate a patient's utilization of the designated substances. Some states require only controlled substance data, but others collect information on at least some noncontrolled substances. Summaries of state PDMP requirements are maintained by the National Alliance for Model State Drug Laws.[11]

Behind-the-Counter Drugs

Behind-the-counter (BTC) drugs may be sold without a prescription but must either be sold by a pharmacist or at least not displayed to the public. Currently, BTC drugs comprise only methamphetamine precursors (see "Methamphetamine Precursors") and the original Plan B (levonorgestrel 0.75 mg tablet) emergency contraception product. In June 2013, the FDA approved the marketing of Plan B One-Step (levonorgestrel 1.5 mg tablet) without prescription to persons of any age. However, the original Plan B may be sold without prescription only to persons aged 15 or over but may be dispensed to women under 15 only on prescription. Because the pharmacist will be held responsible for the sale of the original Plan B to a minor, he or she should require proof of age before selling the product without a prescription. Most states prohibit technicians from making this kind of decision.

Drug Product Selection

Drug product selection activities by pharmacists may take two forms: generic substitution or therapeutic substitution. Virtually all states permit pharmacists to substitute generic equivalent drugs for brand name drugs under specified conditions. Therapeutic substitution is commonplace in most states in hospitals and health maintenance organizations (HMOs) by use of formularies. Many states also allow for therapeutic substitution in community settings, but the mechanisms vary widely.

Generic Substitution

Pharmacists who make the effort to provide a generically equivalent drug to patients instead of a more expensive brand name drug are performing an important patient care function and fulfilling an ethical obligation to the patient, since doing so contributes to the patient's economic welfare without compromising the patient's clinical outcomes. In many states, performing a generic substitution when permitted is also mandated by state law.

In virtually all states, a generic equivalent is a drug that meets the following criteria: (i) it is the same chemical entity as the prescribed drug; (ii) it is in the same dosage form; and (iii) it is bioequivalent, which means it has statistically the same pharmacokinetic parameters of area under the curve (AUC) and time to peak concentration (T_{max}) when compared in vivo with the prescribed drug.

States generally allow the pharmacist to substitute the generic drug for the brand name drug *if* such a substitution results in a lower price to the patient and *if* the prescriber has not determined that the brand name drug is medically necessary.

How Do States Require the Prescriber to Prevent or Allow Substitution?

The states have essentially three options for specifying how prescribers should allow or prevent generic substitution:

1. Prohibit substitution unless the prescriber specifically allows it. In these states, prescriptions often have a check box (e.g., "☑ Substitution Permitted") to allow substitution. If the box is not checked, the pharmacist must dispense the prescribed brand name or call the physician for permission to substitute. In these states, when a prescription is verbally ordered by brand name, the pharmacist must then ask about generic substitution.
2. Allow substitution unless the prescriber specifically prohibits it. In these states, the prescriber must write "Dispense as Written" or "DAW" to prohibit substitution. A check box (e.g., "☑, DAW") is often allowed. In these states, when a prescription is verbally ordered by brand name, the prescriber must also specify to dispense as ordered if he or she wants to prohibit generic substitution.

3. Require the prescriber to specifically allow or specifically prohibit substitution on each prescription. Some states use a two-line prescription blank, and the prescriber must sign on the "Dispense as Written" line or the "Substitution Permitted" line. In these states, it is incumbent on the pharmacist to determine the prescriber's wishes about generic substitution when prescriptions are ordered by telephone.

Table 3.19 summarizes these options.

How May Pharmacists in a Given State Determine if a Drug Product May Be Substituted?

States also generally have three approaches to specifying how pharmacists know whether a given drug may be considered a substitutable generic equivalent to the brand name product:

1. The state may specify a list of drugs that may *never* be substituted. This list usually is composed of drugs with a "narrow therapeutic index." Such a list is termed a "negative formulary," and if the prescribed brand name drug is on the list, pharmacists may substitute a generic equivalent only by calling the prescriber to obtain prior approval.
2. The state may specify a list of drugs that are eligible for substitution, and any drug products not on that list are excluded unless the prescriber specifically approves the substitution. Such a list is called

TABLE 3.19 Options for Specifying Whether Generic Substitution Is Allowed

	Rx Checklist	
	Yes	**No**
Must you dispense the brand name prescribed unless the prescriber indicates "substitution permitted?" • If Yes, did you ask about substitution on a phoned Rx?		
May you substitute a lower-cost generic equivalent unless the prescriber has specified "DAW" in some way?		
Must the prescriber sign one line on a two-line blank on every written prescription? • If Yes, did you ask the prescriber about his or her substitution preferences on a phoned Rx?		

"DAW, "Dispense as Written"

a "positive formulary." Some states develop their own restrictive list, but for most states, the FDA Orange Book is accepted.

3. The state may set the requirements for a generic equivalent and allow the pharmacist to use such information as appropriate to determine whether the proposed substitution is appropriate. In these states, the Orange Book is one recognized source that a pharmacist may rely on.

Table 3.20 provides a checklist for determining if your state allows a particular generic to be substituted.

Labeling of Drugs and Medicines

Distributing or dispensing a drug without approved labeling makes the drug misbranded—this is prohibited by both federal and state laws. The federal FDCA and FDA regulations establish required labeling for drugs. OTC drugs must contain a drug facts label. Prescription drugs must contain approved professional labeling and, where required, informational labeling for patients (patient package inserts). FDA regulations require Medication Guides that must be included when

TABLE 3.20 Determining Whether a Product Is Generically Equivalent and Eligible for Substitution

	Your State?	
	Yes	No
Does your state have a list of "narrow therapeutic index" drugs that cannot be the subject of generic substitution? • If Yes, is the prescribed drug on the list? • If Yes, did you obtain prior authorization from the prescriber to substitute a generic drug? (If No, dispense as written.)		
Does your state require the generic drug to be on a list of approved drugs? • If Yes, is the proposed substitution on the list? • If No, did you obtain prior authorization for the substitution from the prescriber? (If No, dispense as written.)		
Does your state allow the pharmacist to use judgment based on any reliable evidence for determining that the generic drug is bioequivalent to the prescribed drug? • If Yes, do you have such evidence (e.g., AB rated in the Orange Book)? (If No, dispense as written or obtain prior authorization to dispense the generic drug.)		

dispensing a growing number of prescription drugs. A pharmacist may deliver a drug to another practitioner or pharmacy only with its FDA-approved labeling intact or to a patient with intact OTC labeling or with a prescription label when dispensed pursuant to a prescription. Federal laws specify a minimum set of elements on the labels for outpatient prescriptions and have only a few requirements for hospital drugs. Surprisingly to most pharmacists, federal law requires only the patient name and directions for use if the prescriber includes them on the prescription. States, however, have very specific requirements for drug labels, depending on the setting.

Labeling includes not only the actual label on the bottle but also the written information supplied to the patient with the container. The tables that follow indicate only what is required on the actual container or package label.

Ambulatory Prescriptions

The clinical goal of labeling for outpatient prescriptions is to give the patient information needed to use the drug appropriately. A pharmacist must always ask which information is needed by the patient and which is best supplied in writing. It is important to *always* provide patients with patient package inserts or other labeling beyond the prescription label that will help them use the drug effectively. Also, many pharmacies provide information on their labels regarding how many refills are left, when the prescription needs to be renewed, and how to contact a pharmacist for additional information, even if this is not required by their state law. See Table 3.21 for details.

Federal Side Effects Statement

A recent revision to the FDCA requires pharmacists to provide the following side effects statement to all patients receiving outpatient prescriptions: "Call your doctor for medical advice about side effects. You may report side effects to FDA at 1-800-FDA-1088." This may be placed on the label, the cap of the prescription container, a separate printed sheet, or in a Medication Guide or patient information leaflet (PIL).[12]

Beyond-Use Date

A little fewer than half of U.S. jurisdictions require a beyond-use date be placed on the label of a prescription drug dispensed to an outpatient. As a general rule, the USP indicates that a pharmacist must

TABLE 3.21 Elements Required on Label of Ambulatory Patient Prescriptions

	Federal Law	Your State
Pharmacy name	✔	✔
Pharmacy address	✔	✔
Prescription number (serial number)	✔	✔
Prescriber name	✔	✔
Date filled (federal law requires date prescribed or date filled)	✔	✔
Patient name	✔†	*
Prescriber's directions for use	✔†	*
"Side effects statement" (if not provided otherwise; see discussion)	✔	✔
"Caution: Federal law prohibits dispensing of this drug to any person other than the person for whom it was prescribed."	✔††	*††
Drug name and strength		*
Pharmacist's initials		*
Necessary auxiliary and/or precautionary labels (e.g., Shake well, Take with food, Take on an empty stomach, May cause drowsiness, etc.)		*
Pharmacy telephone number		
Quantity dispensed		
Beyond-use date (see discussion) • If required, is the maximum ❑ 1 year ❑ Manufacturer's date ❑ Other: _______		
Other requirements in your state:		

✔Required
†Only if included in prescription
††Controlled substances only
*Most states

put a beyond-use date on the prescription label, based on information from the manufacturer or from the relevant USP monograph. If stability data are lacking for a particular packaging option, the USP indicates that the beyond-use date should be no longer than 1 year from dispensing or the manufacturer's expiration date, whichever is earlier.[13]

Compliance Packaging

An important clinical service for many patients is to provide medication in custom packaging to help ensure compliance. Examples of this type of packaging include medi-sets, blister packs (like bingo cards), or strip packaging. When dispensed directly to patients, these must generally be labeled with the same information as required on a standard prescription vial. Because this packaging is not usually child resistant, permission to use non–child-resistant containers must be obtained from the patient or patient's agent.

Long-Term Care

Pharmacies serving nursing home patients typically choose from one of three types of distribution systems: unit dose, modified unit dose, and traditional prescription containers. Child-resistant containers (CRCs) are not required for nursing homes, except when medications are sent home with a patient for short excursions or on discharge.

Unit Dose

Unit dose systems involve individual patient cassettes (small drawers) labeled for each patient, with individual unit-dose packages placed into them. Cassettes are usually transported in carts, and one set of carts is at the nursing home, while a second set is at the pharmacy being prepared for the next set of doses. Carts then are exchanged at a set interval (often 48 hours to 7 days). Most states allow unused unit doses to be redispensed.

Traditional Prescriptions and Modified Unit Dose

Traditional prescription containers are usually dispensed with a 30-day supply of medication. Modified unit dose (MUD) packaging, often in the form of bingo card-type blister packs, may be dispensed in 1-week to 30-day supplies. Drugs dispensed in traditional containers cannot be reused if discontinued and must be destroyed. Many states allow the return and reuse of drugs in MUD packaging when the pharmacist can determine that the package has not been damaged or tampered with. However, once a drug has been placed in MUD packaging, it may be inconsistent with USP requirements to repackage it into another MUD container. Table 3.22 summarizes typical requirements for nursing home labeling.

TABLE 3.22 Labeling and Return Requirements for Nursing Home Distribution Systems

	Your State?		
	Traditional Prescription	MUD	UD
Name and strength of medication	*	*	*
Quantity	*	*	*
Lot number			*
Expiration date	*	*	*
Patient name	*	*	†
Patient location			
Directions for use			
Controlled substances schedule number			
May unused drugs be returned for credit and reused?		*	*
Other requirements in your state:			

*Most states
†On individual patient cassette
MUD, modified unit dose; UD, unit dose

Inpatient Medications

Table 3.23 summarizes typical requirements for labeling of inpatient drugs in hospitals.

Child-Resistant Containers

The federal Poison Prevention Packaging Act requires that certain household substances be packaged in CRCs. A copy of the publication *Poison Prevention Packaging: A Guide for Healthcare Professionals* can be found at www.cpsc.gov//PageFiles/114277/384.pdf.

It is important to understand that CRCs are designed so that 90% of elderly adults can open them if shown how. When you realize that one in six children younger than 4 years who are poisoned by prescription drugs have obtained them from a container belonging to a grandparent or great-grandparent,[14] it will become clear that pharmacists owe

TABLE 3.23 Labeling Requirements for Hospital Inpatient Drugs

	Your State?
Inpatient Oral Drugs	
Drug name	*
Strength	*
Expiration date, if applicable	*
Auxiliary labeling as applicable	*
Other requirements in your state:	
Hospital Parenteral Drugs	
Name and concentration of base solution	*
Name and amount of added drugs	*
Name and location of patient	*
Appropriate expiration dating	*
Initials of personnel who prepared the solution	
Other requirements in your state:	

*Most states

their elderly patients a chance to learn how to open CRCs before agreeing to dispense with easy-open caps.

OTC Drugs

Most OTC drugs do not require CRCs. Those that do include oral drugs containing aspirin, ibuprofen, naproxen, iron salts, diphenhydramine, fluoride, lidocaine, loperamide, and newer drugs that have been switched to OTC status since 2001 (e.g., omeprazole, ranitidine, cetirizine). Caustic substances (strong acids or bases) and hydrocarbons also require CRCs.

Manufacturers may exempt one package in each product line, providing it is labeled "Not for Use in Households with Small Children."

Legend Drugs

All oral prescription drugs require CRCs when dispensed by prescription, with a small list of exceptions. The most important exceptions include nitroglycerine sublingual tablets and chewable and sublingual isosorbide tablets containing ≤10 mg per tablet.

Pharmacists may dispense prescriptions without CRCs only when authorized by (a) the patient; (b) the patient's agent—which cannot be pharmacy personnel; or (c) the prescriber, if indicated individually on each prescription. Some states require the authorization by the patient or agent to be in writing, although this is not required by federal law.

Patient Medication Records

All but five jurisdictions (Alaska, Colorado, Guam, Maryland, and Puerto Rico)[4] mandate that pharmacies maintain patient medication records that record medications used by and dispensed to patients, along with patient information needed to properly screen prescriptions for problems and to monitor drug use. Federal law governing Medicaid (OBRA-90)[15] requires states to ensure that pharmacies maintain these records for all Medicaid patients and use the information contained in them to perform prospective drug use review (P-DUR).

Required Elements

Table 3.24 summarizes typical required elements for patient medication record systems.

Drug Use Review

OBRA-90 requires pharmacists to screen new orders against the patient drug history prior to dispensing, an activity known as P-DUR. This is required for all Medicaid patients, and states that require counseling for non-Medicaid patients (all but eight) generally require P-DUR for all patients as well. It is expected that a pharmacist who detects a problem through P-DUR will take an appropriate action to resolve the problem before delivering the drug to the patient. In some cases, patient interviews can resolve apparent issues, but often a call to the prescriber is necessary. Failure to carry out required P-DUR and properly resolve discovered problems is a growing cause of lawsuits against pharmacists.[16] Tables 3.25 and 3.26 summarize requirements for P-DUR and provide a checklist for P-DUR for individual prescriptions.

Privacy

Patients have an expectation of privacy in their relationships with pharmacists. Principle II of the Code of Ethics for Pharmacists states that "A pharmacist promotes the good of every patient in a caring,

TABLE 3.24 Elements Required in Patient Medication Records

	Medicaid Patients	Your State?
Is a patient medication record or patient profile required?	✔	*
Patient full name	✔	*
Patient address (required on all CSA prescriptions)	†	*
Patient age or date of birth	†	*
Patient telephone number	†	
Patient gender	†	*
Clinically important medical conditions	†	*
Drug allergies or drug reactions	†	*
• If none, must this be indicated (e.g., "NKA")?	*	
A list of drugs and devices previously used by the patient	†	
• OTCs used by patient		
• Prescription drugs obtained from other pharmacies	†	
• Devices obtained from other sources	†	
• Medications or devices dispensed by this pharmacy	✔	*
• Prescription number		*
• Date dispensed		*
Name, strength, dosage form		*
Quantity dispensed		*
Prescriber name or ID		*
Dispenser's initials		
Pharmacists' comments on the patient's drug therapy	✔	
Authorization for use of non-CRCs		
Other elements in your state:		

✔Must make reasonable attempt to obtain
*Most states
CSA, Controlled Substances Act; NKA, no known allergies; OTC, over-the-counter

compassionate, and confidential manner."[17] As a general rule, health providers caring for patients are entitled to know details of the patient's conditions and therapy necessary for that provider to provide patient care, including receiving payment for services and ensuring quality of care, but for no other purposes, unless the patient has

TABLE 3.25 Prospective Drug Use Review

	Medicaid Patients	Your State?
Is P-DUR required for all patients?	✔	*
• New prescriptions?	✔	*
• Refill prescriptions?		

P-DUR, prospective drug use review
✔Required
*Most states

TABLE 3.26 Elements Specified by OBRA-90 When P-DUR Is Required

	Rx Checklist	
	Yes	No
Is the drug in this order contraindicated in this patient? • If Yes, the product should *not* be dispensed.		
Is this prescription or order for a drug that duplicates therapy the patient is already receiving? • If Yes, did you determine that the other therapy has been discontinued? • Or, did you determine that the other therapy is appropriate and desired?		
Does the drug in this order potentially react adversely with any of the patient's medical conditions? • If Yes, did you determine that the physician is aware and believes the benefits outweigh the risk?		
Does the drug in this order pose possible adverse drug interactions? • If Yes, have you ruled out the possibility based on dose, separation of doses, order of dosing, or other basis? • Or, did you determine that the prescriber is aware of the interaction and believes the benefits outweigh the risk?		
Does the dose or duration of treatment prescribed in this order appear to be too high or too low? • If Yes, have you contacted the prescriber to correct the dose or duration? • Or, have you determined that the prescriber is aware of the normal dose and has confirmed this particular dose or duration?		
Is there information suggesting the patient may be allergic or cross-allergic to the drug in this order? • If Yes, have you ruled out the possibility based on patient history, interview, or confirmation with the prescriber? • Or, did you determine that the prescriber is aware of the possibility and believes the benefits outweigh the risks?		

(continued)

TABLE 3.26 Elements Specified by OBRA-90 When P-DUR Is Required *(continued)*

	Rx Checklist	
	Yes	No
Does the patient's drug use history suggest that he or she is underusing or overusing the drug in this order, or otherwise misusing the drug? • If Yes, have you identified a documented reason that explains the apparent abuse/misuse and determined that it is not an actual problem? • Or, have you educated the patient on the proper use and believe that he or she is equipped to take the drug properly in the future? • Or, have you confirmed with the prescriber the apparent misuse or abuse and the prescriber has confirmed that the prescription should be filled at this time?		

OBRA-90, Omnibus Budget Reconciliation Act of 1990; P-DUR, prospective drug use review

consented. This has been formalized under federal law by the Privacy Rule enacted under provisions of the Health Insurance Portability and Accountability Act of 1996 (HIPAA).[18] Under these rules, pharmacists may use protected health information (PHI)—information about the patient's health care that identifies the patient—for providing treatment, for obtaining payment, or for health care operations (TPHCO). Any other release of PHI requires written authorization of the patient, the patient's guardian, or the patient's agent.

Prior to use of PHI, a pharmacist must provide the patient with a Notice of Privacy Practices (NOPP), which explains how the pharmacy will use PHI and gives patients information about their rights under HIPAA or applicable state law. The patient must acknowledge receipt of the NOPP in writing. Provision of the NOPP must be done on the first visit.

Each provider must appoint a Privacy Officer who deals with requests from patients for access to their records and requests for modification of their records. Pharmacists must know the identity of their pharmacy's Privacy Officer and be able to refer patients to that person.

Special considerations exist for patient records for minors. Normally, parents or legal guardians may have access to a minor's records and may consent to care for the minor. However, when state law provides the minor with the right to consent to a given type of care, the minor then gains control over his or her PHI, and parents may not see such information without the minor's consent. In many states, minors may consent to emergency treatment or treatment for sexually transmitted diseases, reproductive health (including contraception), substance abuse, or mental health, often at age 13 or older. Also, minors who are considered emancipated as the result of court action, or are minors married to an adult, usually control their own PHI. Table 3.27 provides a checklist for the most common factors affecting a release of information about a given patient.

Providing Information and Counseling to Patients

OBRA-90 requires states to ensure that pharmacists make an "offer to counsel" all Medicaid patients with each new prescription. Most states extend the requirement to counsel patients to all patients. Most states also require pharmacists to provide additional written material that may be necessary to ensure proper medication use, and federal law requires certain written information to be provided with specific drug products.

Required Patient Counseling

Most states allow the pharmacist to use judgment in determining which information to provide to a patient concerning his or her drug therapy.

Offer to Counsel

All states permit patients or their agents to decline counseling, and most require that the pharmacist at least make an offer on new prescriptions. Some states allow the offer to be made by a technician, and a few allow the offer to be made by a sign in the pharmacy. A few states mandate counseling and do not allow counseling to be satisfied by an "offer." Table 3.28 summarizes these options for advising patients that there is information available from the pharmacist.

Elements of Counseling

The goal of patient counseling is to ensure that the patient has the information and understanding necessary to properly use his or her medication. OBRA-90 provides guidelines for the content of

TABLE 3.27 Privacy Checklist, Prior to Release of Patient PHI to Another Person or Entity

	Yes	No
Has the patient received and acknowledged the NOPP?		
Treatment (if Yes to any of the following, release is allowed) Is the release to another provider known to be caring for the patient? Is this a prescription transfer to another pharmacy at the patient's request? Is the release to a caregiver or patient's agent? Is the release to a person specifically listed by the patient as eligible to receive information? Is the release to a former provider, *and* the patient has not specifically requested that information not be provided to that provider? Has the patient specifically requested the release in writing?		
Payment (if Yes to any of the following, release is allowed) Is the release to a third-party payer to determine eligibility for payment? Is the release a finished claim to a third-party payer? Is the release to a credit card company used by the patient to pay for a professional service, in response to a justification of the charge, and contains the minimum information necessary? Is the release to a collection agency of the minimum information necessary to collect patient debts to the provider? Has the patient specifically allowed the release in writing (e.g., on a claim form or release to a third party)?		
Release of information concerning minors		
Does the minor control the information? If Yes Is it for treatment that the minor was allowed to consent to? • Or, is the minor emancipated or married to an adult and thus allowed to consent to health care in your state? If No Does it meet the criteria for release for TPHCO? • Or, did the minor specifically allow the release in writing? If No Does it meet the criteria for release for TPHCO? • Or, has a parent or legal guardian specifically allowed the release in writing?		

PHI, protected health information; NOPP, Notice of Privacy Practices; TPHCO, treatment, payment, health care operations

TABLE 3.28 Patient Counseling Requirements

	Medicaid Patients	Your State?
Is patient counseling required for		
Medicaid patients?	✔	✔
All other patients?		*
New prescriptions?	✔	*
Refill prescriptions?		*
May the pharmacist use judgment in deciding to counsel?		*
The offer to counsel		
Is not allowed, but counseling must be done		
May only be made by the pharmacist face to face	*	*
May be made by a technician		
May be made by a sign in the pharmacy		
Documentation of counseling		
Is required when counseling is given and/or when it is refused		
Is required only if patient or agent refuses counseling		
Is not required	*	*

✔Required
*Most states

counseling. Dr. Bruce Berger has provided a detailed checklist for the patient counseling session, with suggestions for pharmacist actions at each step of the process[19]; Table 3.29 is an example Rx checklist that could be used to record completion of such counseling for a given prescription on a given visit. The pharmacist can record that a given element was completed at that visit, that the patient was already aware of the information, that the element is deferred for a future visit, or that the element is not applicable for this medication.

Written Drug Information

Most pharmacies' computer systems produce PILs with new prescriptions for outpatients. This is a required element of many state laws. Certain drug products have product information for patients that is mandated by federal law in one of three ways: (i) particular regulations governing a class of drugs (e.g., oral contraceptives and estrogens); (ii) patient information specified in the official product labeling that was agreed to by the manufacturer when the drug was approved; or (iii) Medication Guides for specific products required by FDA regulations.

TABLE 3.29 RX Counseling Checklist

Patient: **Rx No:** **Pharmacist:**	**Date of Visit:**			
	Completed	**Patient Aware**	**Defer**	**N/A**
Name and description of medication				
Route of administration				
Dose and regimen				
Maximum daily dose				
Dosage form				
Duration of therapy				
Special directions and precautions for preparing or taking				
Commonly experienced: • Side effects • Adverse effects • Drug interactions • Contraindications • How to avoid the above • What to do if the above are encountered				
Techniques for self-monitoring				
Proper storage				
Refill information and how to obtain refills				
What to do if a dose is missed				
❑ Counseling declined: "The pharmacist advised me of an opportunity to learn more about my medication, but I have chosen to decline this offer"	Patient or agent signature:			

Whenever federal law specifies specific patient information, the pharmacist is required to provide this information to the patient with every prescription (new or refill) and on request.

Always remember, too, that most states require the labels of prescription containers to contain appropriate caution labels (e.g., "Take with Food" or "May Cause Drowsiness") to alert patients to critical information on proper use or storage of the drug. Table 3.30 is a checklist for determining when written information should be provided.

TABLE 3.30 RX Checklist for Written Information

	Yes	No
Do any of the following conditions apply to this drug? Is the product an oral contraceptive or estrogen? Is there a required MedGuide for this product? (www.fda.gov/cder/offices/ods/medication_guides.htm) Is there a patient package insert included with the product labeling (e.g., inhalers, injectables)? If yes • Provide to patient with each dispensing of the drug		
Does your pharmacy produce a PIL for this product? If yes • Provide to patient as required by state law or as indicated by patient need		

Concluding Comment

State and federal laws and regulations have evolved over the last 105 years in response to real problems in the manufacture, promotion, dispensing, prescribing, and use of medications. They set a minimum standard of behavior for producers, prescribers, and dispensers and provide patients with important rights regarding their medical records and the information they should be provided by providers. However, strict adherence to the letter of the law, and doing nothing more, will neither ensure optimum patient care nor continue to earn for pharmacists their respect as a trusted profession. Only competent and consistent provision of pharmaceutical care to every patient can continue to assure our profession's high esteem.

References

1. Wood LL. *Medical Records, Medical Education, and Patient Care*. Chicago, IL: Year Book Medical; 1971.
2. Delitto A, Snyder-Mackler L. The diagnostic process: examples in orthopedic physical therapy. *Phys Ther*. 1995;73(3):203–211.
3. Bossen C. Evaluation of a computerized problem-oriented medical record in a hospital department: does it support daily clinical practice? *Int J Med Inform*. 2007;76(8):592–600.
4. *Survey of State Pharmacy Laws, 2012*. Chicago, IL: National Association of Boards of Pharmacy; 2012.
5. Title 21 Code of Federal Regulations (CFR) Section 1306.25(a)(1).

6. U.S. Department of Justice Drug Enforcement Agency Office of Diversion Control: Mid-Level Practitioners Authorization by State. Available at www.deadiversion.usdoj.gov/drugreg/practioners/index.html. Accessed January 13, 2008.
7. National Precursor Log Exchange. Available at www.nplexservice.com/faq.html. Accessed June 28, 2013.
8. U.S. Department of Justice Drug Enforcement Agency Office of Diversion Control:Pharmacist's Manual. Available at www.deadiversion.usdoj.gov/pubs/manuals/pharm2/index.html. Accessed February 27, 2008.
9. Seeger VB. Is it legitimate? Strategies for assessing questionable prescriptions and DEA considerations. APHA Annual Meeting, Orlando, FL; April 4, 2005.
10. Fassett WE. Is it legitimate? Accessing controlled substances prescriptions. APHA Annual Meeting, Orlando, FL; April 4, 2005.
11. National Alliance for Model State Drug Laws. Available at www.namsdl.org. Accessed June 28, 2013.
12. Title 21 CFR Section 209.1–209.11; 73 FR 404, January 3, 2008.
13. USP Pharmacist's Pharmacopeia. 1st ed. Rockville, MD: The United States Pharmacopeial Convention; 2005:12.
14. Safe Kids, USA. Available at www.usa.safekids.org/tier3_cd.cfm?folder_id=540&content_item_id=1152. Accessed March 15, 2013.
15. Omnibus Budget Reconciliation Act of 1990, Pub. L. 101–508.
16. Pharmacists Mutual Claims Study 2007. Available at www.phmic.com/web.nsf/pages/DrugReview.html. Accessed March 22, 2008.
17. APhA. Code of Ethics for Pharmacists. Washington, DC: American Pharmacists Association. Available at www.pharmacist.com/AM/Template.cfm?Section=Search1&template=/CM/HTMLDisplay.cfm&ContentID=2903.
18. Health Insurance Portability and Accountability Act of 1996. Pub. L. 104–191.
19. Berger B. Effective patient counseling. *US Pharm.* 1999;24(2). Available at www.uspharmacist.com/oldformat.asp?url=newlook/files/Phar/ACF59D.cfm&pub_id=8&article_id=157.

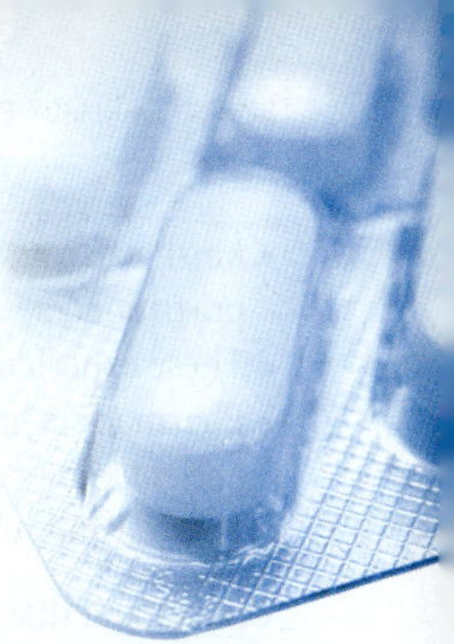

4

Patient Consultation in the Cycle of Patient Care

Megan Willson and Linda Garrelts MacLean

Clear communication is the foundation for effective patient consultation. This chapter describes, highlights, and illustrates important elements of successful patient encounters, including communication techniques. To be effective during patient consultations, the pharmacist must

- View the patient as a whole person, not just a set of symptoms or medications
- Be knowledgeable about diseases and medications
- Use certain verbal and nonverbal skills relating to consultative techniques

Pharmacist–patient consultation sessions encompass a broad range of activities including the following:

- Medication counseling
- Medication therapy management (MTM)
- Clinical interviewing to
  - Gather and evaluate information, obtain a medical history, and assess symptoms
  - Develop a care plan including patient goals
  - Implement the care plan with the patient
  - Determine what follow-up and monitoring will be necessary. An overview of the principles associated with medication counseling, MTM, and specific communication skills follows.

Getting Started

Know your patient. Maintain a broad perspective regarding the patient's involvement with the health care system.

- Patients transition between various care settings frequently, from hospital to home to nursing home to clinic and back to the hospital.

- Most patients have already been counseled by other health care practitioners.
- These experiences factor into every subsequent encounter.
- Pharmacists must work from where the patient is and from what the patient knows and thinks about his or her medications including the cultural and religious medication beliefs.

Understand that patients may:

- Not be totally honest with health care providers
- Minimize or exaggerate their needs for medication, especially analgesics
- Have an agenda to obtain a medication they have seen on television or heard about through a friend
- Not really want to get well
- Not be in agreement about care or the diagnosis
- Have limited health literacy
- Have social and economic factors affecting health care decisions
- Have cultural and religious beliefs that impact health care decisions and practices

Establish rapport between pharmacist and patient:

- Introduce yourself to the patient.
- State the purpose of the consultation.
- If you are not familiar with the patient, identification should be verified by either asking for identification or simply asking, "And you are…?"
- Counsel the caregiver if the patient's hearing is impaired or cognitively impaired.
- Work with the interpreter if a language barrier exists.
- Use a private space for cases in which sensitive information is to be discussed.
- Face the patient and maintain the appropriate interpersonal distance (1.5 to 2 ft).[1]
- Verify what the patient knows using teachback.
- Do not overload or overwhelm the patient with too much information.
- Keep information brief and to the point.
- Allow the patient to openly discuss issues of concern.
- Offer your availability for further assistance.
- Avoid medical terminology that the patient may not understand.
- Simplify medication regimen if possible.

Unique Environment Pearls: The Institutional Setting

Plan: think beyond the *acute* problem to the *chronic* care issues.

- Begin planning discharge counseling on medications at the time of the patient's admission.
- A complete and an accurate home medication list is an essential component for care of the patient in the hospital; it serves to prevent errors after discharge as well. Community pharmacies are a great resource to obtain a medication list and information about adherence.
- Consider adherence issues and drug use patterns that might have led to the admission.
- With the patient, determine strategies to overcome the difficulties identified.
- Pharmacists' intervention through medication review, discharge counseling, and follow-up by phone has been shown to favorably affect the rate of preventable adverse drug events 30 days after discharge.[2]

The REAP mnemonic can be used to plan discharge medication consultation in the hospital setting:

- *R*eason for admission:
  - Is it due to a drug-related problem or nonadherence?
  - How many and what kinds of diseases does the patient have?
  - What medications are currently prescribed?
  - Assess the patient's physical, emotional, and mental states in light of the patient history.
- *E*valuate current medication regimen for drug-related problems, including nonadherence:
  - Prioritize questioning, beginning with the most important medications that relate to the primary problem (e.g., insulin or hypoglycemic use in a patient who has diabetes) or high-risk medications.
  - Prioritize questioning, also focusing on those drugs with a multiple daily dosing regimen and those with special administration techniques, such as inhalers.
- *A*ssess the patient's knowledge base and skills to self-medicate; assess compliance-promoting strategies.
- *P*lan to avoid drug-related problems after discharge and achieve outcome goals.

The discharge counseling session includes review of the following for each prescribed medication:

- Indication
- Dosage
- Administration
- Self-monitoring
- Goals of therapy
- Follow-up laboratory tests if necessary
- Follow-up appointments if necessary

Consumer and patient satisfaction is becoming increasingly more important as health care reforms continue. Beginning in 2002, Centers for Medicaid and Medicare Services and the Agency for Healthcare Research and Quality developed the Hospital Consumer Assessment of Healthcare Providers and Systems (HCAHPS) Survey to collect patient perception of the hospital stay. Several medication-related items are asked during the survey identifying a need for pharmacist to counsel on new medications while in the hospital. Key information that needs to be delivered to the patient includes medication indication as well as side effects of the new medication.[3]

Match Your Message to Your Patient

It is important to be aware of the Transtheoretical Model of Health Behavior Change and the stages of readiness to change[4] and how these can relate to the patients' willingness to accept information and make changes to improve their health. Once you discern where your patient is in this continuum, as a pharmacist you can be certain to frame information appropriately.

STAGES

- Precontemplation: No intention of making a change in the future.
  - Discussion of proper medication use is often fruitless.
  - Example: The patient has not begun thinking of initiating insulin therapy or how it might affect his life.
- Contemplation: Thought of making a change. Likely in the next 6 months.
  - This is a great time to begin exploring reasons for not making the change and to give information about the benefits of the action.

- Example: The patient has thought about how the insulin might fit into his daily schedule or how he might be able to afford the prescription.

- Preparation: An action is planned to begin shortly, likely in the next month.
  - Help the patient develop an action plan. Set a start date and remember to provide lots of encouragement.
  - Example: the patient picks up the prescription for insulin and testing supplies.
- Action: The change or plan has been implemented.
  - Example: The patient is checking his blood sugar and injecting insulin.
- Maintenance: The action is occurring, but the patient is at risk of relapse.
  - Identify the patient's potential barriers.
  - Work with the patient to develop plans to overcome identified barriers or solutions if relapse occurs. Termination: the action has become a habit.[4]
  - Work with the patient to identify the next goal.

Recognize Connections

Significant information can be gleaned from a patient interview when the pharmacist understands the relationship between disease state and any associated mental and physical deficits, medication, and adherence.

- Cognitive limitations as a result of medical conditions may affect the patient's ability to self-administer and take medications correctly. Example:
  - Stroke and dementia can cause changes in mentation that preclude the patient from accurately filling a 7-day medication box.
  - Involving patients' caregivers and family members is a useful strategy to assist patients in their medication-taking behaviors.
- Physical limitations as a result of medical conditions may affect the patient's ability to apply a patch, topical medications, or eye drops. Examples:
  - Weakness associated with stroke may make it difficult to open packaging or apply topical medications.

    - Rheumatoid arthritis may prevent a patient from inserting eye drops.
- Medication actions, such as frequent urination caused by a diuretic, can deter a patient from taking medication.
- Blindness and cataracts can prevent patients from reading labels and instructions on medication bottles.
- Uncover deficits in the patient's ability to self-medicate through open-ended questions and demonstration of skills such as the following:
    - What is the name of your new medicine?
    - Could you show how you will apply the patch medication that has been prescribed for you? I have a patch that does not contain any active ingredient—we can work with it right here. Let us start by having you open up the package....

Realize that patients often worry more about the bad effects from medications than dosage or even indication. Recognize this association and consider using the following guidelines on side effect consultation:

- Counsel on the most common side effects.
- Counsel on the adverse reactions that are most serious and could be life threatening.
- Advise what to do if an adverse reaction is suspected.
- Provide additional information about Internet resources for the patient to access.

Medication Counseling Techniques

The pharmacist–patient consultation program (PPCP) techniques developed by the Indian Health Service three decades ago, and further refined through pharmacists' collaboration, remain a solid practice model for medication consultation. This interactive method of consultation seeks to *verify* what the patient knows about the medication and *fill in the gaps* with only the most basic information when needed.[5] Research shows that people forget 90% of what is heard within 60 minutes of hearing it.[6] By making the patient an *active* participant in the process, learning is enhanced. Two sets of questions, one for new prescriptions (Prime Questions) and the other for refill medications (Show and Tell Questions), are used in this model to engage the patient in a dynamic, structured care session.

The Prime Questions for New Prescriptions

(1) What did the doctor tell you (were you told) the medication is for?
What problem or symptom is it supposed to help?
What is it supposed to do?
(2) How did your doctor tell you (were you told) to take the medication?
How often? How much? How long?
What does X times a day mean to you?
What did your doctor say to do if you miss a dose?
(3) What did the doctor tell you (were you told) to expect?
What good effects? Bad effects? Precautions to take?
What should you do if a bad reaction occurs?

Show-and-Tell Questions for Refill Prescriptions

(1) What do you take this medication for?
(2) How have you been taking it?
(3) What kinds of problems are you having with it?

Verify that the Patient Has Understood

(1) Determine that the patient has sufficient knowledge to self-medicate.
(2) "Just to make sure I didn't leave anything out, please go over with me how you are going to use the medication."

Handling Difficulties During Counseling

Some common barriers and the skills to manage them are listed in Table 4.1. These relate to functional and/or emotional issues. Functional barriers have specific strategies for management, whereas emotional barriers require the use of active listening skills and reflecting listening responses with empathy. Reflective listening helps to affirm what the patient is saying but truly gets at the real meaning.

TABLE 4.1 Common Barriers Affecting Consultation

Barrier	Helpful Techniques
Language barrier	Identify the barrier with open-ended questions. Use pictures; contact translator
Counseling a third party	Be careful regarding confidentiality; ask for identification; provide written supplements; ask the patient to call
Hearing impaired	Use print material; move to a quiet space; speak more loudly Use final verification technique
Vision impaired	Use interactive dialogue, final verification Provide large-print material
Mental disorder	Identify problem early with open-ended questions Counsel the caregiver; repeat information and use final verification Provide written supplements

Examples of reflecting listening responses include the following:

- "Sounds like you're (frustrated, mad, happy) about your visit with the doctor."
- "I can see that this is (frustrating, worrisome) for you."
- "You seem very (concerned, worried) about how the disease or the medication might affect you."

Table 4.2 illustrates some examples of how pharmacists can balance meeting patients' needs with their own.

Table 4.3 addresses different strategies and examples on how you can deal with resistance in patients.

What Not to Do

When dealing with patients, the pharmacist must remember to do many things. The following list contains some things that the pharmacist must remember *not* to do:

- Do not expect the perfect patient.
  - Patients may take medications in ways different than the textbook indicates. They may take medications that are ineffective. It is the pharmacist's duty to discover if current therapies are helping, and then as a pharmacist, use your judgments about the drug regimen. The patient should be counseled accordingly.

TABLE 4.2 Setting Limits in the Encounter

Example	Useful Skills for the Pharmacist
The patient is overly talkative.	Take control by piggybacking onto one of the patient's comments (e.g., "I know you don't like hospitals, so let's talk about how your medicines can keep you out of here") Interrupt the patient as gently as possible Use the patient's name to register attention
The patient consistently wants lengthy encounters.	Realize the patient's need for attention State clear limits on consultation (e.g., "I can only discuss this medication now with you")
The patient interrupts your daily routine.	Realize the patient's need for attention Set a time period for your availability (e.g., "I can meet with you for no more than 5 minutes after lunch")
The patient continues to discuss issues that cannot be resolved.	Realize the patient is frustrated, wants attention, or desires control Acknowledge the differences (e.g., "We disagree on whether you should keep taking this medication") Use diverting tactics, switch to discussing something else State need to move on to next task

- Do not expect to know everything.
  - A pharmacist must read, research, and ask for help when needed.
- Do not be afraid to make mistakes.
  - Just learn from them.
  - Often, apologizing to the patient for the mistake can go a long way to building the patient–pharmacist relationship.
- Do not second-guess the prescriber in front of the patient.
  - Comments such as "I'm not sure why you're getting this drug when we usually use (another therapy)" should be avoided. This creates confusion and doubt in the patient's mind and can lead to conflict between medical and pharmacy staff. If the pharmacist has doubts about a prescribed drug or therapy, the physician should be consulted in a private and professional manner for clarification.
- Do not leave the patient without hope.
  - Pharmacists will counsel patients whose diseases are progressing despite maximal therapeutic efforts. These patients may be looking for answers that are not there. Statements such as "You're getting all the prescribed medications available for X condition" are

TABLE 4.3 Dealing with Resistance with Reflective Listening[7]

Type of Reflection	Example
Simple reflection (repeating, rephrasing, and paraphrasing)	Patient: I do not want to start using insulin. Pharmacist: You do not believe starting insulin will start working for you right now.
Amplified reflection	Patient: I don't know why my wife is pushing me to use insulin. Pharmacist: So your wife is concerned for no reason.
Double-sided reflection	Patient: I know you want me to start insulin, but I am not going to do that! Pharmacist: You can see that there are some real problems with your glucose control, but you are not willing to think about starting insulin.
Agreement with a twist	Patient: I don't know why my wife wants me to take insulin. She wouldn't like it much if she had to poke herself so many times. Pharmacists: That's right I don't think injections would be much fun either, but it is important to have your blood sugar controlled.
Reframing	Patient: My wife bringing up insulin and nagging me about food and my blood sugars. Pharmacist: I can see how you might think your wife is nagging you about your insulin, but she must really care about you to do it.
Emphasizing personal choice	Patient: I am just not ready to start insulin. Pharmacist: Ultimately it is your decision to take your insulin. I cannot make you do it, but I am here to help you when you are ready. I can offer several resources and tips which may help you.
Shifting focus	Patient: I do have diabetes, but I still feel fine. Pharmacist: I am glad you still feel good, and I want to keep you feeling that way.

not helpful and should be avoided. What patients need is support. Pharmacists should use reflecting responses such as "It must be very frustrating to feel like you're not getting any better."

- Do not judge the patient who does not adhere to the care plan.
  - Examples include the patient with lung cancer who still smokes or a patient with diabetes who had a recent myocardial infarction but still does not take his insulin to maintain his blood sugar. Dealing with such patients can be frustrating to the health care provider, because the provider and the patient do not share the same goals.

A health care practitioner should never give up on a patient. An open, honest, and sincere presence should be maintained, and information should be provided that is appropriate to the patient's level of readiness to accept responsibility for his or her health care or readiness for change. Use of a readiness scale is a great way to identify stage of readiness and also can lead to a discussion on barriers and strengths.

- Do not negate positive steps with judgment or attempts to encourage further actions. For example: "Great job with the recent diet and weight loss, but we still need to get you down to your goal weight." The negative comment at the end of the conversation leaves the patient feeling that he or she is not good enough or not able to meet your goals. Remember that small goals need to be encouraged and eventually, the patient will meet larger goals.
- Do not belittle the problem or the diagnosis. For example saying: "Your blood sugar is only a little elevated." Stating the laboratory level is only a "little high" will make patients feel that problem is not something that they should worry about it.
- Resist the righting reflex. Solving the patients' problems for them can make you feel better but isn't always good for the patient. The patient may not believe the solutions are acceptable and potentially may not make the change.[8]

Medication Therapy Management Patient Consultation

MTM is a method for providing patients with coordinated health care that is efficient, cost-effective, quality driven, and patient centered. Currently, many Americans lack access to primary care providers, and as the population continues to age, there will be a need for more care associated with the management of chronic disease. A large portion of chronic disease is managed through medication use; thus, MTM delivered by pharmacists is an ideal solution for the identified need.[9] The core elements an MTM service model are

- Medication therapy review (MTR)
  - Patient and pharmacist consultation in which a systematic review of the patient health information and assessment for medication-related problems

- Personal medication record (PMR)
- Medication-related action plan (MAP)
- Intervention and/or referral
- Documentation and follow-up[10]

Performance of an MTR should be conducted in conjunction with the patient to include patient-specific goals and patient-specific medication-related problems. The MTR can be targeted to a single disease state, medication regimen, or comprehensive pharmacist's delivered patient care. The problems should be prioritized, and then a plan is developed to resolve the identified problem.[10] Potential medication-related problems that should be reviewed:

- Medication without an indication
- Indication without a medication
- Adverse drug effects
- Wrong medication
- Wrong dose
- Adherence to therapy
- Drug–drug, drug–food, and drug–herbal interaction[11]
- Drug causing illness
- Clinical appropriateness
- Therapeutic duplication or unnecessary medications
- Medication cost decisions[10]

Integrate Effective Communication Skills into Patient Consultation

The specific verbal communication skills that may be incorporated into medication counseling and MTM encounters are described in the following sections.

Elements to include in the patient care session:

- Open-ended questions to discover patient needs and knowledge deficiencies
- Active and reflective listening
- Demonstration techniques on the part of the patient and the pharmacist
- Did learning occur? Verify and summarize what the patient knows through teachback.
- Responses that are sensitive to patient needs

- Adherence investigation
  - Is medication being taken correctly?
  - Is the care plan being followed?
  - Identify causes of problems.
- Work toward solutions of problems identified.
- Assess pharmacist/patient encounters: Strive for continual improvement.

Motivational interviewing is a tool that has been useful as pharmacists identify ways to encourage and empower patients to adopt change. This change could be a lifestyle modification such as increasing exercise or improving food choices or the action of taking a medication correctly every single day. This technique creates a tension or dissonance in a patient. The patient realizes that there is a conflict between personal goals and his or her behavior. An example is the patient who states that his grandkids mean everything to him and he wants to see them graduate from college, yet he continues to smoke. The pharmacist interviews the patient to help him or her recognize and resolve ambivalence in behavior. Components of motivational interviewing include steps associated with the OARS acronym:

- Ask *O*pen-ended questions to gather information.
  - What do you think about the changes we have discussed?
  - Tell me about what kinds of exercise you enjoy.
  - How much do you exercise?
  - Describe what kinds of activities you work into a typical week.
  - What is your view about the exercise you engage in? Do you get as much exercise as you need?
  - What questions do you have?
- *A*ffirm the patient's willingness and ability to implement the care plan that has been developed. Also always affirm achievements and steps toward the goal. Congratulate the patient.
  - What is your understanding of the consequences of not getting adequate exercise?
  - What are the positive things associated with incorporating more exercise and movement into your week? Negative?
  - Describe your goal for increasing movement and exercise.
  - How does this goal line up with where you currently are with regard to exercise?
  - How might you address this discrepancy between where you are and where you want to be in the future?

- Reflective listening during the patient encounter.
  - Reflect back what you have heard through techniques in Table 4.3.
  - Offer encouragement.
  - Strategize with patients for solutions to identified problems.
  - Create dissonance with current actions and goals.
- Summarize the patient's views, strategies, goals, questions, and concerns.
  - Reiterate the pros and cons discussed.
  - Restate where the gap is between the current behavior and the target goal.
  - Reaffirm the patient's action plan and timeline.

Adherence is an arena to which the pharmacist must pay attention. Recognition of problems with adherence should be under the purview of the pharmacist. Strategies to address and improve adherence include the following:

- Use a universal statement to open the conversation. Examples include the following:
  - "Mrs J., a lot of patients have trouble fitting taking medication into their daily schedule. What's been your experience?"
  - "Many patients have trouble remembering when to take this medication, especially since it's only changed once a week. What's been your experience, Mr. K.?"
- Use a probing statement following the "I noticed/I'm concerned" formula. Examples include the following:
  - "Mr. K, I noticed this clonidine patch prescription was due to be refilled 3 weeks ago. I'm a little concerned about that."
- Listen for clues that may indicate the patient is reluctant to take the prescription. Examples include the following:
  - "Why do I have to keep taking this medicine?"
  - "My doctor *says* I should take it…,"
  - "My doctor *wants* me to…,"
  - "I'm *supposed* to be taking it."
- Link medication taking to a daily activity.
  - Have the patient describe a typical day. Then work with the patient to identify an appropriate time to take the medication.
- Suggest the use of pill boxes, calendars, and cell phone applications.
- Suggest that medication be kept where it is easily seen.

- Do not assume that when a patient is doing well and has no complaints, it must be because the medication is working and not causing problems.
- Do not assume that the patient adheres to prescribed therapy.[12]
  - One-third of patients do not get their original prescription filled.
  - One-third of patients take the medication incorrectly.
  - One-third take the medication as prescribed.

Empowering the patient is key to a successful care plan implementation or an effective medication regimen to which the patient is to adhere.

- The *patient's acceptance* that a problem exists and his or her acceptance of the value of treatment forms the essential foundation for successful treatment.
  - The *patient* controls the outcome of his or her disease by taking or not taking prescribed medications and/or implementing lifestyle changes.
    - The empowerment model shifts patients from *receiving* health care to *managing* health.
      - The practitioner's role is to facilitate the patient using medications and managing lifestyle changes to the best benefit; the pharmacist and patient form a partnership.
      - Work with the patient to identify barriers to care plan implementation, which can include the following:
    - Knowledge deficits that may prevent adherence[13]
      - Insufficient information
      - Insufficient skills
      - Misinformation
    - Practical limitations, including but not limited to the following:
      - Transportation
      - Multiple daily doses
      - Manual dexterity
      - Vision and hearing difficulties
- Medication complexity
    - Attitudinal barriers
      - Perceived severity of risk compared with perceived benefit of treatment[14]
      - Patient's desire to be in control
      - Patient's belief that he or she can or cannot successfully implement the recommended treatment[15]

- » Incorrect or inappropriate pervasive patient ideas such as the following:
  a. "I can develop immunity to a medication's effects."
  b. "If one pill helps, then two must be twice as good."
  c. "If I feel good, then I don't need medication."
- Work with the patient to prioritize barriers.
- Work with the patient to overcome and/or manage barriers.

The National Community Pharmacists Association and American Association of Colleges of Pharmacy developed a teaching supplement on teaching medication adherence called "Medication Adherence: Educators Toolkit." The toolkit provides exercises for instruction in the topic as well as several excellent resources for pharmacists to implement in patient encounters. The toolkit is available at https://www.ncpanet.org/educators.

Summary

The techniques and issues discussed in this chapter contribute to good rapport with patients and success in helping patients manage chronic illnesses. Pharmacists should seek out model practitioners, observe their skills and techniques, and then practice these skills and techniques during pharmacy practice experiences.

Acknowledgment

The author would like to acknowledge Linda Garrelts MacLean on whose third edition and Marie Gardner on whose second edition work on which this current fourth edition has been based.

References

1. Pfizer, Inc. *Pharmacist-Patient Consultation Program, Unit 2: Counseling Patients in Challenging Situations*. New York: Pfizer Inc.; 1993.
2. Schnipper J, Kirwin J, Cotugno M, et al. Role of pharmacist counseling in preventing adverse drug events after hospitalization. *Arch Intern Med*. 2006;166:565–571.
3. http://www.hcahpsonline.org. Baltimore, MD: Centers for Medicare & Medicaid Services. Accessed April 29, 2013.

4. Prochaska JO, Velicer WF. The transtheoretical model of health behavior change. *Am J Health Promot.* 1997;12(1):38–48.
5. Boyce RW, Herrier RN, Gardner ME. *Pharmacist-Patient Consultation Program, Unit 1: An Interactive Approach to Verify Patient Understanding.* New York: Pfizer Inc.; 1991.
6. Bolton R. *People Skills.* New York: Simon & Schuster; 1979.
7. Miller WR, Rollnick S. *Motivational Interviewing: Preparing People to Change Addictive Behavior.* New York: The Guilford Press; 1991.
8. Rollnick S, Miller WR, Butler CC. *Motivational Interviewing in Healthcare: Helping Patients Change Behavior.* New York: The Guilford Press; 2008.
9. McInnis T. Pharmacist can become the single most important transformative force in improving health care and reducing health care cost—but will they? Available at http://pharmacists4knowledge.org/cips/blog/view/Pharmacist_Can_Become_The_Single_Most_Important_Transformative_Force_In_Improving_Health_Care_And_Reducing_Health_Care_Costs_But_Will_They_Terry_McInnis_MD_MPH. Accessed May 10, 2013.
10. American Pharmacists Association and National Association of Chain Drug Stores Foundation. Medication therapy management in pharmacy practice: core elements of an MTM service model (version 2.0). *J Am Pharm Assoc.* 2008;48:341–351.
11. Lemay G. Medication therapy management in community pharmacy practice. *Med Health.* 2012;95(9):281–282.
12. *Pharmacist–Patient Consultation Program, Unit 3: Counseling to Enhance Compliance.* New York: Pfizer Inc.; 1995.
13. Powell MF, Burkhart VD, Lamy PP. Diabetic patient compliance as a function of patient counseling. *Ann Pharmacother.* 2006;40:747–752.
14. Eraker SA, Kirscht JP, Becker MH. Understanding and improving patient compliance. *Ann Intern Med.* 1984;100:258–268.
15. Viinamaki H. The patient–doctor relationship and metabolic control in patients with type 1 (insulin-dependent) diabetes mellitus. *Int J Psychiatry Med.* 1993;23:265–274.

5

Providing Drug Information

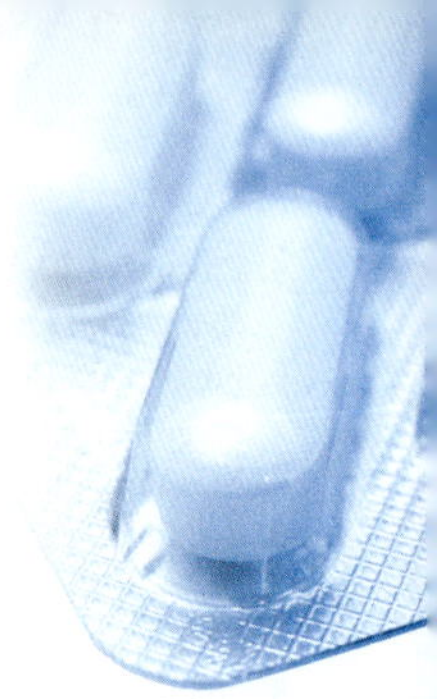

Brad S. Fujisaki, Kristine B. Marcus, and Kate Farthing

Preparing to Provide Drug Information

Regardless of which experiential rotation you are scheduled for, it is common for all pharmacy students to provide drug information as part of their patient care and non–patient care activities. When orienting to your experiential rotation, gain a clear understanding of your preceptor's expectations concerning your role as a provider of drug information. To get at the information you need quickly, you need to learn what resources are available to you through your experiential site, as well as any library access and resources available to you remotely through your pharmacy program. Spending 30 minutes with your preceptor, reference librarian, or drug information specialist at your site at the beginning of your rotation will pay off in efficiency later. Be sure to note any passwords or constraints to the use of that resource (e.g., single-user license, on campus only). If you are unfamiliar with an available reference, spend some time learning to use it so you are comfortable with its contents and organization.

To assist you in orienting to your available drug information holdings, we have created a Providing Drug Information Questionnaire in Appendix 5A. Identifying your available resources ahead of time will allow you to use our drug information question tables to find your answer more quickly.

Improvements in technology have allowed many drug information references to become available in various media formats. Within the last decade, content from traditional print resources have become available as e-books or electronic databases. Also, companies such as Lexicomp have partnered with American Society of Health System Pharmacists (ASHP) to have American Hospital Formulary Service (AHFS) Drug Information incorporated into the Lexicomp Online suite of products.

Similarly, some monograph content from Clinical Pharmacology (Gold Standard) can be found in other vendors' products such as MD Consult (Elsevier) and McGraw-Hill's AccessMedicine and AccessPharmacy online sites. What this means is that you may have access to content from a traditional source of drug information via a nontraditional route that your school or site has subscribed to (e.g., Drug Prescribing in Renal Failure: Dosing Guidelines for Adults and Children via STAT!Ref electronic book collection). Refer to the crosswalk of print and electronic resources in Appendix 5B to help you navigate to these alternative resources.

Finding Useful Drug Information

Traditionally, student pharmacists are trained to answer drug information questions using a systematic approach. An example of a stepwise approach is outlined in Table 5.1.[1] The goal of using a systematic approach is to instill a consistent process to provide useful drug information to the requestor. This stepwise approach is traditionally taught to pharmacy students during introductory drug information coursework when they have not yet fully acquired the content knowledge and clinical judgment they will apply when answering questions as practicing pharmacists. More recently, a structured approach that incorporates the principles of the stepwise approach but places more focus on understanding the context of the question, improving communication with the requestor, and elucidating and assessing the factors critical to providing a patient-specific response has been

TABLE 5.1 Modified Systematic Approach to Drug Information

Step I	Secure demographics of requestor
Step II	Obtain background information
Step III	Determine and classify the ultimate question
Step IV	Develop strategy and conduct search
Step V	Perform evaluation, analysis, and synthesis
Step VI	Formulate and provide response
Step VII	Conduct follow-up and documentation

advocated.[2] This framework is more likely to be used by pharmacy students during their Advanced Pharmacy Practice Experiences (APPEs).

The usefulness of medical information has been described as a function of validity, relevance, and the time it takes to find the information.[3] With this in mind, pharmacy students can maximize the usefulness of drug information by the following:

1. Locating information that is valid
2. Locating information that is relevant to the posed question
3. Locating information efficiently in the least amount of time

Locating Information That Is Valid and Relevant

Table 5.2 provides a list of resources to serve as a review in evaluating the validity and relevancy of literature in answering drug information questions. Finding valid and relevant information often requires a search of the primary literature. As the volume of published journal articles continues to increase, the utility of indexing and abstracting services (also known as secondary resources) has become that much more important. MEDLINE is the primary electronic indexing system for medical journals and is available as a free searchable database through the National Library of Medicine's PubMed. A comprehensive tutorial is available for

TABLE 5.2 List of Resources to Assist in Literature Evaluation

Resource in Print	Resource on Internet
The Evidence-Based Medicine Working Group. Users' Guide to the Medical Literature. American Medical Association (AMA) Press	Available online by subscription at the JAMA Evidence Web site: http://www.jamaevidence.com/
Greenhalgh T. How to read a paper—the basics of evidence based medicine. BMJ Books	Similar information available online at British Medical Journal (BMJ) Web site: http://www.bmj.com/about-bmj/resources-readers/publications/how-read-paper

Sources: Centre for Evidence Based Medicine. EBM Tools for literature evaluation including Critical Appraisal Sheets. Available from www.cebm.net
MedlinePlus Web site. Evaluating Internet health information: a tutorial from the National Library of Medicine. Available from www.nlm.nih.gov/medlineplus/webeval/webeval.html

PubMed: www.nlm.nih.gov/bsd/disted/pubmedtutorial/. In addition, a review of your drug information course notes or textbook on basic search techniques such as the use of Boolean operators (e.g., AND, OR, NOT) may be useful.

Locating Information Efficiently

Finding valid and relevant drug information is important; however, efficiently finding this information is equally critical—providing information after the point that it is needed clearly decreases its overall usefulness. Therefore, the remainder of this chapter is designed to assist you in efficiently locating the most likely resources that will answer a particular type of drug information question. We have focused our efforts on the types of questions that pharmacists often face in practice. Certain types of questions are best answered using specialized resources. However, pharmacists do not always have easy access to these specialized resources, so we have taken into consideration the most common information resources that you will likely have access to. From there, we have recommended resources that are most likely to provide you, and subsequently the requestor, with useful information. In our tables, we designate specific resources when needed or whether any General Drug Information Compendia is likely to answer your question. Familiarize yourself with the bibliographic list in Appendix 5C that is organized by the resource types referred to in our tables.

Published drug information resource matrices or pathfinders[4,5] are available by type of request. We have tried to improve on these excellent resources by incorporating the element of time and limiting the scope of our recommendations to the most common scenarios where pharmacy students are asked to provide drug information. Our time frames reflect both the usual expected turnaround time for a given scenario and the amount of research time that is generally required to use the cited references and synthesize a response for that question type. We used the following standard time estimates in the tables:

- Minutes (e.g., question asked on rounds for an immediate patient need)
- Minutes to hours (e.g., question on a patient to be seen in clinic later that same day)
- Hours to days (e.g., preparing a 5-minute in-service for tomorrow)

Answering the Most Common Question Types

Knowing the frame of reference of your requestors and how they plan to use the drug information you give them is fundamental to providing a targeted response that will be put into action. Obtaining adequate background material and defining the ultimate question the requestor is asking require practice, and your approach needs to vary for different question types. Until this skill is second nature, it is not uncommon to need to contact the requestor after the initial question is received to gain further clarification. Standard questions to elicit background information by question type can be found in Appendix 5D.

The remainder of this section of the chapter is organized by drug information question type so that you can quickly find the resources that are most likely to be useful in answering your question. Asking yourself, "What question type is this?" and "How much time do I have to answer this question?" will facilitate the use of the following tables. The tables are organized from the most common question type you are likely to encounter to the least common question type (Table 5.3). As part of your preparation for providing drug information, you may find it helpful to practice using the references associated with the higher-frequency question types.

Adverse Drug Reactions

Requestors seeking information on side effects or adverse drugs reactions often have two basic questions:

1. Has this adverse reaction been previously associated with this drug?
2. How do you prevent or manage this adverse drug reaction (ADR)?

Questions related to accidental or intentional ingestion of drugs or chemicals should be immediately triaged to a poison center (1-800-222-1222).

General tertiary resources will often provide information on ADRs that are common, serious, or classic. Information on the clinical presentation, time course, risk factors, and management of specific ADRs are often described in textbooks and review articles. There are also a handful of specialized tertiary references focused around drug-induced disease such as *Meyler's Side Effects of Drugs and Drug-Induced Diseases*. Conversely, information in handbook-type

TABLE 5.3 Common Drug Information Question Types Asked of Pharmacy Students

Frequency of Question Type Encountered by Students	Corresponding Table in This Chapter
Highest Frequency	
• ADRs	Table 5.4, page 92
• Dosing or administration	Table 5.6, page 96
• Drug interactions	Table 5.7, page 99
• Indication or therapeutic use	Table 5.8, page 102
• Product information or identification	Table 5.9, page 104
Moderate Frequency	
• Safety in pregnancy and lactation	Table 5.10, page 106
• IV compatibility stability	Table 5.11, page 109
Lowest Frequency	
• Natural products and dietary supplements	Table 5.12, page 112
• Nonsterile compounded formulations	Table 5.13, page 114

drug compendia is less detailed, often limited to a list of ADRs with approximated frequency of occurrence. Therefore, a more comprehensive search of the primary literature is often required for finding information on reactions associated with drugs. Drug-focused secondary indexing references may be useful for finding information on ADRs. These include subscription indexing databases such as EMBASE, International Pharmaceutical Abstracts (IPA), and Iowa Drug Information Service (IDIS).

Pharmacists, as health care providers in the United States, are not currently required to report ADRs to the Food and Drug Administration (FDA). However, voluntary reporting of ADRs via the MedWatch program is strongly encouraged, particularly for drugs that have been marketed for <3 years (www.fda.gov/Safety/MedWatch). Adverse reactions from vaccines are currently reported through the Vaccine Adverse Event Reporting System (VAERS) program (www.vaers.hhs.gov/index). Many health care systems and hospitals use a centralized reporting system for ADRs or medication errors; therefore, it is prudent to determine the practice setting's standard procedure for reporting to minimize duplication of effort. Table 5.4 describes common ADR questions with resources for information given an amount of time to research the response.

A slight variation on the ADR question may be posed as "Is this reaction associated with any of the medications my patient is taking?" Some electronic drug information databases allow you to query by a specific adverse reaction and provide results in the form of drug lists

TABLE 5.4 Questions on Adverse Drug Reactions

	How Much Time Do You Have?			
Question Type	**Minutes**	**Minutes to Hours**	**Hours to Days**	**Comments**
Has this adverse reaction been previously associated with this drug?	• General print DI compendia • General electronic DI compendia • Product information/ package insert	• Therapeutics textbooks and databases • Gilman, Goodman and Gilman's Pharmacologic Basis of Therapeutics • Katzung, Basic and Clinical Pharmacology • MEDLINE	• Aronson, Meyler's Side Effects of Drugs • Davies, Textbook of Adverse Drug Reactions • Tilsdale, Drug-Induced Diseases • Pharmacy-focused primary literature indexing databases	–Information on common and classic ADRs are often covered in most General DI compendia. –Specialized resources and a search of the primary literature are usually required to find information on specifics such as time course, clinical presentation, proposed mechanism, risk factors, and management strategies of less common ADRs –General DI compendia provide variable depth of information with regard to ADRs
How do you prevent or manage this ADR?	• Electronic resources • Micromedex DRUGDEX • Clinical Pharmacology • Electronic/Print resources • Drug Facts and Comparisons or Facts & Comparisons eAnswers • AHFS drug information • Product information/ package insert	• Therapeutics textbooks and databases • MEDLINE	• Aronson, Meyler's Side Effects of Drugs • Davies, Textbook of Adverse Drug Reactions • Tilsdale, Drug-Induced Diseases • Pharmacy-focused primary literature indexing databases	–Package insert information may include specifics on the management of an ADR in the cautions, warnings, or Black Box Sections rather than the adverse reactions section

Is this reaction associated with any of the medications my patient is taking?	• Micromedex DRUGDEX • Clinical Pharmacology • Lexicomp Online • Facts & Comparisons eAnswers	• General print DI compendia • General electronic DI compendia • Therapeutics textbooks and databases • Gilman, Goodman and Gilman's Pharmacologic Basis of Therapeutics • Katzung, Basic and Clinical Pharmacology • MEDLINE • Aronson, Meyler's Side Effects of Drugs • Davies, Textbook of Adverse Drug Reactions • Tilsdale, Drug-Induced Diseases • Pharmacy-focused primary literature indexing databases	–Electronic databases that allow you to query by adverse reaction will be the most efficient means to evaluate a patient's medication list for likely offenders

- General print DI compendia: AHFS drug information; Lexicomp Drug Information Handbook; Drug Facts and Comparisons
- General electronic DI compendia: Micromedex Healthcare Series; Clinical Pharmacology; Lexicomp Online; Facts & Comparisons eAnswers
- Therapeutics textbooks and databases: Chisholm-Burns, Pharmacotherapy Principles & Practice; DiPiro, Pharmacotherapy; Helms, Textbook of Therapeutics; Koda-Kimble, Applied Therapeutics; MD Consult or First Consult; UpToDate
- Pharmacy-focused primary literature indexing and abstracting databases: EMBASE, IDIS/Web, IPA

See Appendix 5C for bibliography of cited resources

DI, drug information.

associated with that reaction—Micromedex DRUGDEX, Lexicomp Online, and Clinical Pharmacology allow you to search by reaction. Additionally, some niche textbooks are also designed in this way.

Dosing or Administration

The entire medical team and the patient rely on the pharmacist to be the expert on the dosing of medicines. One of the pharmacist's key functions is to review medication orders for appropriate dosing given the patient's age, weight, organ function, other medical conditions, and current treatments. When responding to questions regarding "What is the dose of drug X?" your recommendation must also consider the treatment indication and the route of administration.

Pharmacy students are often also consulted by nurses and prescribers regarding switching patients' medications from one route to another when there is a change in the patient's status (e.g., scheduled for surgery and now unable to take anything by mouth). Due to differences in bioavailability or drug release characteristics, dosing conversions may be necessary when a route of administration or dosage formulation is changed. Dose conversions are also common when interchanging patients from one formulary agent to another in the same therapeutic class.

For parenteral medications, nurses often also consult the pharmacy regarding how to prepare and administer a drug and how quickly it can be given. Pharmacy students need to be familiar with common language used by nurses and in drug administration texts (Table 5.5). Questions dealing with the compatibility of coadministering parenteral drugs are included elsewhere in this chapter.

Your general drug information compendia are initial resources for all of these types of questions but usually are most useful for adult patients. For pediatric patients, additional specialized references are frequently checked. Table 5.6 summarizes questions on dosing or administration while listing resources for information.

Drug Interactions

Medications on a patient's profile change frequently, especially during a hospital stay. To complicate this even further, drug interactions include not just drug–drug interactions, but drug–food, drug–lab, and drug–disease interactions. When a patient experiences a new side effect or unexpected change in laboratory value, the medical team frequently cites the patient's drug therapy as the cause for the change. Understanding the time course of drug interactions, along with the mechanism of the interaction, is

TABLE 5.5 Intravenous Administration Language

Phrase	Usual Meaning
Direct IV injection or infusion	May be administered as provided. Does not require further dilution
IV bolus or IV push	May be administered as fast as desired
Slow IV push	Should be administered no more quickly than over 3–5 minutes
Intermittent injection or infusion	Administered intermittently according to ordered schedule. During the time between administrations, no drug is given. Nurse should follow instructions for "Administer over X minutes or hours" as labeled
Continuous injection or infusion	Administered continuously over 24 hours

important in providing helpful information in determining whether the patient should continue to receive both drugs or whether a change in drug therapy is needed. For a comprehensive review of the principles of drug interactions, consider reading the introductory chapter of one of the major drug interactions textbooks (*Drug Interactions Analysis and Management* or *Drug Interaction Facts*). Other books also contain a review of the principles of drug interactions (e.g., Goodman & Gilman's *The Pharmacological Basis of Therapeutics; Pharmacotherapy; Applied Therapeutics*; Lexicomp). These references typically include lists of known CYP450 and P-glycoprotein inducers, inhibitors, and substrates. Similar lists or tables are available online (for CYP 450, http://medicine.iupui.edu/clinpharm/ddis/; drugs known to prolong the QT interval, www.azcert.org/medical-pros/drug-lists/drug-lists.cfm). Table 5.7 lists drug interaction questions frequently received by pharmacists and pharmacy students.

Indication for Therapeutic Use

Pharmacy students may need to research these types of questions either from the drug or disease perspective. When reviewing a patient's medication profile, your preceptor and medical team will expect you to be able to state the associated treatment indication for each drug the patient is currently receiving or has received recently. You may also be asked to recommend a therapy or review the available pharmacologic treatment options given a stated disease, treatment indication, or need for prophylaxis.

Although drugs are approved by the FDA based on evidence submitted with their New Drug Application (NDA), prescribers are not

(*Text continued on page 101*)

TABLE 5.6 Questions on Dosing or Administration

	How Much Time Do You Have?			
Question Type	**Minutes**	**Minutes to Hours**	**Hours to Days**	**Comments**
What is the dose of drug X?	• General print DI compendia • General electronic DI compendia • Product information/package insert	• Therapeutics textbooks and databases • MEDLINE	• Pharmacy-focused primary literature indexing databases • Contact drug manufacturer	–It is important to know what indication the drug is intended for as most DI resources list dosing by specific indication –Certain indications such as oncology regimens will need specialized references or review of the primary literature
Do you need to taper drug X when discontinuing therapy?	• General print DI compendia • General electronic DI compendia • Product information/package insert	• Therapeutics textbooks and databases • MEDLINE	• Pharmacy-focused primary literature indexing databases • Contact drug manufacturer	–Dosing tapers for discontinuing therapy is often recommended to avoid a withdrawal syndrome with specific drugs. The dosing information may be listed in the adverse effects or warnings section under "withdrawal syndrome"
How do I adjust the dose for a patient with organ dysfunction (e.g., renal dysfunction; liver failure)?	• General print DI compendia (AHFS often helpful for liver dosing) • General electronic DI compendia • Product information/package insert • Institution-specific protocols or guidelines for dosage adjustment	• Aranoff, Drug Dosing in Renal Failure	• Pharmacy-focused primary literature indexing databases • Contact drug manufacturer	–When clinical data are not available, evaluation of pharmacokinetic parameters may be helpful in guiding dosing changes. Some of these data will be included in the pharmacokinetics section of drug monographs –Some institutions also have renal dosing protocols in place

What is the dose for patients in this special population (e.g., pediatrics, geriatrics, obesity)?	• General print DI compendia • General electronic DI compendia • Product information/package insert • Institution-specific dose standardization or dose rounding protocols or guidelines	• Semla, Geriatric Dosage Handbook • Taketomo, Pediatric Dosage Handbook • Robertson, Harriet Lane Handbook • Young, NeoFax • Phelps, Pediatric Injectable Drugs (Teddy Bear Book) • MEDLINE	• Pharmacy-focused primary literature indexing databases • Contact drug manufacturer	–Many institutions that specialize in care of these populations often have drug dosing guidelines for commonly used medications. This guidance may be searchable via the Internet or may be restricted to the site's intranet
How do I adjust the dosage regimen for a patient receiving renal replacement therapy (e.g., hemodialysis, peritoneal dialysis, continuous venovenous hemodiafiltration)	• General print DI compendia • General electronic DI compendia • Product information/package insert	• Aranoff, Drug Dosing in Renal Failure • MEDLINE	• Pharmacy-focused primary literature indexing databases • Contact drug manufacturer	–Removal of drug via renal replacement therapy is related to many factors including the rate of filtration, the size of the molecule, the filter type, and other physiochemical properties of the drug

(continued)

TABLE 5.6 Questions on Dosing or Administration *(continued)*

Question Type	How Much Time Do You Have? Minutes	Minutes to Hours	Hours to Days	Comments
How do I administer this parenteral drug?	• Gahart, Intravenous Medications Handbook for Nurses • General print DI compendia • General electronic DI compendia • Product information/package insert • Institution-specific policies for IV administration	• Trissel, Handbook on Injectable Drugs • King, King Guide to Parenteral Admixture	• Pharmacy-focused primary literature indexing databases • CINAHL • Contact drug manufacturer	–Many institutions will have policies regarding administration of high-alert medications and required monitoring for certain IV medications. This guidance may be searchable via the Internet or may be restricted to the site's intranet

- General print DI compendia: AHFS drug information; Lexicomp Drug Information Handbook; Drug Facts and Comparisons
- General electronic DI compendia: Micromedex Healthcare Series; Clinical Pharmacology; Lexicomp Online; Facts & Comparisons eAnswers
- Therapeutics textbooks and databases: Chisholm-Burns, Pharmacotherapy Principles & Practice; DiPiro, Pharmacotherapy; Helms, Textbook of Therapeutics; Koda-Kimble, Applied Therapeutics; MD Consult or First Consult; UpToDate
- Pharmacy-focused primary literature indexing and abstracting databases: EMBASE, IDIS/Web, IPA

See Appendix 5C for bibliography of cited resources

DI, drug information; CINAHL, Cumulative Index to Nursing & Allied Health Literature; IV, intravenous

TABLE 5.7 Questions on Drug Interactions

Question Type	How Much Time Do You Have? Minutes	Minutes to Hours	Hours to Days	Comments
Do these drugs interact?	• Lexicomp online (Lexi-Interact) • Facts & Comparisons eAnswers (Interactions interactive tool) • Clinical Pharmacology • Hansten, Drug Interactions Analysis and Management • Tatro, Drug Interaction Facts • Lexicomp Drug Interactions Handbook	• Micromedex (Interactions tab to build a list of drugs to evaluate for interactions) • General electronic DI compendia • General print DI compendia	• MEDLINE • Pharmacy-focused primary literature indexing databases	–The general electronic DI compendia have drug interaction checking databases; create a list of products for the database to analyze and evaluate the potential or documented interactions –The general DI compendia also have drug interaction listings in the individual drug monograph
Does this herb–herb or herb–drug combination interact?	• Facts & Comparisons eAnswers (Interaction Resources: Herbal Interaction Facts) • Jellin, Natural Medicines Comprehensive Review (Natural product/drug interaction checker)	• Micromedex (AltMedDex) • General DI compendia may be helpful for more common herbal products	• MEDLINE • Pharmacy-focused primary literature indexing databases • CINAHL	

(continued)

TABLE 5.7 Questions on Drug Interactions *(continued)*

Question Type	How Much Time Do You Have?			Comments
	Minutes	Minutes to Hours	Hours to Days	
Does this drug interact with foods my patient may be taking?	• Start in general drug–drug interaction references for specific foods • Tatro, Drug Interaction Facts: Herbal Supplements and Food • Drug–food interactions: GlobalRPh.com, www.globalrph.com/drugfoodrxn.htm • Beers, Merck Manual of Diagnosis and Therapy (Nutrient–drug interactions)		• MEDLINE • Pharmacy-focused primary literature indexing databases • CINAHL	
Does this drug interact with or affect laboratory values?	• Young, Effects of Drugs on Clinical Laboratory Tests		• MEDLINE • Pharmacy-focused primary literature indexing databases	
Is this drug impacted by my patient's disease state? Or, can this drug alter my patient's disease state?	• General electronic DI compendia • General print DI compendia • Tilsdale, Drug-Induced Diseases		• MEDLINE • Pharmacy-focused primary literature indexing databases • CINAHL	

- General print DI compendia: AHFS drug information; Lexicomp Drug Information Handbook; Drug Facts and Comparisons
- General electronic DI compendia: Micromedex Healthcare Series; Clinical Pharmacology; Lexicomp Online; Facts & Comparisons eAnswers
- Pharmacy-focused primary literature indexing and abstracting databases: EMBASE, IDIS/Web, IPA

See Appendix 5C for bibliography of cited resources

DI, drug information; CINAHL, Cumulative Index to Nursing & Allied Health Literature

limited to prescribing marketed drugs in these doses, by these routes, or only for the tested indications. Although the FDA does not regulate the prescribing of drugs, the pharmacist still has the duty to assess the safety and likely effectiveness of the unlabeled use before recommending or dispensing it. Manufacturers may be pursuing obtaining a labeled use for a drug by conducting clinical trials to gather evidence to submit to the FDA. New drugs, new uses for old drugs, and new formulations of old drugs being studied in these ways are considered investigational new drugs (INDs). Until the manufacturer submits an NDA, these data are proprietary and largely unavailable. Patients may be eligible to have access to these INDs before they receive market approval by enrolling in a clinical trial or through a Treatment IND (formerly called compassionate use). Treatment INDs are reserved for individual patients with no other treatment options. Navigating the pathways to these drugs in the pipeline will require the assistance of preceptors and their understanding of applicable rules and site policies and procedures.

Orphan drugs are FDA-approved drugs that came to market to serve patients with rare diseases. In exchange for pursuing licensing of these drugs that are not likely to make the company a lot of money, manufacturers are rewarded with tax breaks and extended market exclusivity. Because these are unique drugs, they may be available only through specialty distributors and not through normal wholesale channels. Table 5.8 describes common questions on indications for therapeutic use with resources for information given an amount of time to research the response.

Product Information or Identification

Simply identifying a product (what it is and what it is used for) is possible with most of the readily available pharmacy references. Go to your favorite general drug information compendia and look up the information. With a few more steps or clicks, these same resources provide additional depth of product information to prepare you for the inevitable next questions (What is the dose? What else do I need to know before prescribing or dispensing this drug?). Accurate spelling of the drug in question is always a challenge when hearing the product name for the first time, especially from a patient or consumer. Ask the requestor to write it down, if possible, or to sound it out as he or she has interpreted the product name. Knowing its intended use or manufacturer can often help you to narrow the field of similar-sounding products.

If the product is a tablet or capsule to identify, collect the imprint code, shape, size, and color of the product. For foreign drug identification,

TABLE 5.8 Questions on Indication for Therapeutic Use

Question Type	How Much Time Do You Have? Minutes	Minutes to Hours	Hours to Days	Comments
Why was this drug prescribed? What can be used for prophylaxis or treatment of X?	• General print DI compendia • General electronic DI compendia • Product information/ package insert	• Therapeutics textbooks and databases • Gilman, Goodman and Gilman's Pharmacologic Basis of Therapeutics • Katzung, Basic and Clinical Pharmacology	• MEDLINE • Pharmacy-focused primary literature indexing databases • All EBM Reviews • CINAHL • www.guidelines.gov	–General DI compendia often designate whether FDA approved or unlabeled use
Is the use of drug X for this purpose: • FDA approved? • Unlabeled use? • Investigational use? • Compassionate use? • Orphan drug designation?	• General electronic DI compendia • Facts & Comparisons eAnswers (References: Off-Label Drug Facts, Orphan Drugs)	• MEDLINE • Pharmacy-focused primary literature indexing • Government-funded clinical trials enrolling, in progress, or recently completed: www.clinicaltrials.gov • Orphan drug by drug: http://www.accessdata.fda.gov/scripts/opdlisting/oopd/index.cfm • Orphan drug by disease: http://www.rarediseases.org/rare-disease-information/rare-diseases • Contact drug manufacturer		–Manufacturers' medical services divisions are often helpful in providing unlabeled use information and may have a standard letter on the topic if it is common. In contrast, medical product representatives are not allowed to discuss unlabeled uses –Manufacturers may be unable to provide detailed information on investigational drugs they are studying due to proprietary restrictions

- General print DI compendia: AHFS drug information; Lexicomp Drug Information Handbook; Drug Facts and Comparisons
- General electronic DI compendia: Micromedex Healthcare Series; Clinical Pharmacology; Lexicomp Online; Facts & Comparisons eAnswers
- Therapeutics textbooks and databases: Chisholm-Burns, Pharmacotherapy Principles & Practice; DiPiro, Pharmacotherapy; Helms, Textbook of Therapeutics; Koda-Kimble, Applied Therapeutics; MD Consult or First Consult; UpToDate
- Pharmacy-focused primary literature indexing and abstracting databases: EMBASE, IDIS/Web, IPA

See Appendix 5C for bibliography of cited resources

DI, drug information; CINAHL, Cumulative Index to Nursing & Allied Health Literature

request information on the country of origin, the indication or anticipated use of the product, the dose of the product, and if the patient has been using the drug while abroad. Be prepared that foreign drug identifications often become adverse reaction, dosing, or therapeutic use questions once the drug is identified. Table 5.9 summarizes questions on product information or identification while listing resources for information.

Safety in Pregnancy and Lactation

Drug information questions regarding safety of medication use in pregnancy and lactation fall into two categories: questions about the potential risk *before* exposure of the mother and fetus/infant to the drug and questions about the potential risk to the fetus/infant *after* exposure to the drug. When assessing the potential risk to the fetus, it is important to determine the mother's stage or weeks of pregnancy since timing of the drug exposure is important when linking a defect with an exposure. The stages of fetal development and associated organogenesis are available at www.cerebral-palsy.net/update2001/fetal.html (click on Critical Periods of Fetal Development link). Also understanding the mother's indication for a medication or therapy along with the anticipated duration of therapy will be helpful in assessing the situation.

Useful information for questions about breast-feeding or lactation includes the current age of the infant, the frequency and exclusivity of breast-feeding, the drugs or products the mother is taking (or considering taking), the indication for therapy, and the anticipated duration of therapy. Table 5.10 lists drug safety in pregnancy and lactation questions received by pharmacists and pharmacy students.

IV Compatibility/Stability

Pharmacists often have need to research information on the preparation and stability of intravenous (IV) admixtures that they provide for patients or that are administered at the bedside by other caregivers. To establish the institution's standard concentrations and policies on IV admixture production, pharmacies rely heavily on specialized textbooks and published literature. They also must consider applicable rules and standards of practice. Stability, sterility, preparation conditions, and anticipated storage must be considered when determining what fluid, drug concentration, and beyond-use dating will be assigned to a sterile compounded product. Chapter 797 in the United States Pharmacopeia (USP <797>, Pharmaceutical Compounding: Sterile Preparations) provides guidance for establishing acceptable beyond-use dating.[6]

(*Text continued on page 108*)

TABLE 5.9 Questions on Product Information or Identification

Question Type	How Much Time Do You Have?			Comments
	Minutes	**Minutes to Hours**	**Hours to Days**	
What is this drug (assume commercially available in the United States)?	• General print DI compendia • General electronic DI compendia	• Product information/ package insert • General Internet search (Google or MetaCrawler search) • Billups, American Drug Index • USP Dictionary of USAN and International Drug Names	• MEDLINE • Pharmacy-focused primary literature indexing databases	–Basic product information is covered in most general DI compendia. These provide variable depth of information with regard to the logical next questions –Searching the primary literature is the least efficient but may provide information on a little-used product
What is this drug (unknown origin or known foreign product)?	• Micromedex (integrated index to search Index Nominum, Martindale—the complete drug reference, additional subscription may be needed to access these subreferences) • Facts & Comparisons eAnswers (Canadian drug index)	• Textbooks: foreign drug formularies or compendia; USP Dictionary of USAN and International Drug Names • Web sites: Farmamondo, international drug wholesaler: www.farmamondo.com • Pharmaceutical Journal, index of foreign third-party Web sites with lists of products available by country: http://www.rpharms.com/support-resources-a-z/identification-of-foreign-medicines-resources.asp (subscription only) • General Internet search (Google or MetaCrawler search)		–Both Index Nominum and Martindale have a synonym section, linking products with common generic names

What is this drug (imprint code or product physical description)	• Micromedex (drug identification) • Facts & Comparisons eAnswers (drug identifier) • Lexicomp online (Lexi-Drug ID) • Jellin, Ident-a-Drug • Clinical Pharmacology	• Drugs.com Pill Identification Wizard: www.drugs.com/imprints.php	–Check with your preceptor prior to identifying tablets for consumers or the general public regarding site policies on doing this; other factors may need to be considered

- General print DI compendia: AHFS drug information; Lexicomp Drug Information Handbook; Drug Facts and Comparisons
- General electronic DI compendia: Micromedex Healthcare Series; Clinical Pharmacology; Lexicomp Online; Facts & Comparisons eAnswers
- Pharmacy-focused primary literature indexing and abstracting databases: EMBASE, IDIS/Web, IPA

See Appendix 5C for bibliography of cited resources
DI, drug information.

TABLE 5.10 Questions on Safety in Pregnancy and Lactation

	How Much Time Do You Have?			
Question Type	**Minutes**	**Minutes to Hours**	**Hours to Days**	**Comments**
What is the risk (or potential risk) to the fetus when exposed to this drug?	• Briggs GG, Drugs in Pregnancy and Lactation	• Micromedex (DRUGDEX and REPRORISK Databases: TERIS, Shepards, Reprotox, and Reprotext) • Contact drug manufacturer	• MEDLINE • Pharmacy-focused primary literature indexing databases • CINAHL	–Briggs is the gold standard text reference; includes useful appendices with drugs grouped by use category and associated pregnancy risk categories –It is important to review the material in each of the Micromedex REPRORISK databases—each has a different style for presenting the information and with limited published information, reviewing all available material to generate an appropriate assessment of the patient's potential risk is important
What is the risk (or potential risk) to the fetus when exposed to this vaccine or biologic drug?	• Grabenstein, ImmunoFacts	• MEDLINE • Pharmacy-focused primary literature indexing databases • CINAHL • Contact product manufacturer		
For risk questions involving natural products, herbal or dietary supplements	• Jellin, Natural Medicines Comprehensive Database	• Facts & Comparisons eAnswers (Reference: Review of Natural Products) • Micromedex (AltMedDex) • MEDLINE • Pharmacy-focused primary literature indexing databases • CINAHL		

What is the risk (or potential risk) to the breast-feeding infant when exposed to this drug (taken by mother)?	• Hale, Medications and Mothers Milk • NIH's LactMed	• Micromedex (DRUGDEX and REPRORISK: TERIS, Shepards, Reprotox, and Reprotext) • American Academy of Pediatrics policy statement on transfer of drugs and other chemicals into human breast milk (aap-policy.aappublications.org, then search by title of article). • Lactation: Thomas Hale Breastfeeding Pharmacology page and information center, http://www.infantrisk.com/ • MEDLINE • Pharmacy-focused primary literature indexing databases • CINAHL • Contact drug manufacturer	–The Hale book is the best print reference available; the information in the front of the text is a helpful review of the pharmacokinetics of lactation
For lactation questions involving a vaccine or biologic drug	• Grabenstein, ImmunoFacts	• MEDLINE • Pharmacy-focused primary literature indexing databases • CINAHL • Contact product manufacturer	
For lactation questions involving natural products, herbal or dietary supplements	• Jellin, Natural Medicines Comprehensive Database	• Facts & Comparisons eAnswers (Reference: Review of Natural Products) • MEDLINE • Pharmacy-focused primary literature indexing databases • CINAHL	

- General print DI compendia: AHFS drug information; Lexicomp Drug Information Handbook; Drug Facts and Comparisons
- General electronic DI compendia: Micromedex Healthcare Series; Clinical Pharmacology; Lexicomp Online; Facts & Comparisons eAnswers
- Pharmacy-focused primary literature indexing and abstracting databases: EMBASE, IDIS/Web, IPA

See Appendix 5C for bibliography of cited resources

DI, drug information; CINAHL, Cumulative Index to Nursing & Allied Health Literature

Pharmacies often also receive questions from nurses administering these prepared doses. Nurses' questions often have to do with the practicality of administering the IV medication given how many IV administration ports the nurse has access to and the patient's other IV medications or maintenance fluids that are already running through those available ports. Pharmacy students need to be familiar with terms used in interpreting compatibility data in published references: additive syringe compatibility (drawn up in the same syringe), Y-site compatibility ("piggybacking" into the same administration line as a maintenance fluid or other IV medication that is already running), and in-solution compatibility (admixed in the same bag). Other common IV questions from nurses, especially in the intensive care setting, concern the ability to concentrate drips to deliver more medication in less volume or to change to another fluid based on the patient's clinical condition. Table 5.11 describes common questions on IV compatibility and stability with resources for information.

Natural Products and Dietary Supplements

Finding information on these products requires the use of specialized references. Students need to be aware that double-blind, placebo-controlled trials are not widely available to evaluate the safety and effectiveness of these agents. Even when clinical trials are found, dosing standardization remains an issue. A number of groups such as the National Center for Complementary and Alternative Medicine (www.nccam.nih.gov/) are continuing to add to the body of available literature for these products, which should improve our ability to apply evidence-based medicine (EBM) principles to clinical decision making concerning these therapies.

Since these products are regulated under the Dietary Supplement Health and Education Act of 1994 (DSHEA), they are not required to meet the same burden of proof of efficacy as are drugs regulated by the FDA. Unsafe products are not allowed for human use, but premarketing safety testing is not required. The FDA must prove that a product is unsafe before its removal from the market can be mandated.[7] Even if adequate information on the clinical utility and potential harm of a product has satisfied the practitioner caring for the patient, the next issue that must be addressed is whether a reliable, quality product is available for patient use. Manufacturing standards for identity, strength, quality, purity, packaging, and labeling that are expected with drug

TABLE 5.11 Questions on Intravenous Compatibility/Stability

Question Type	How Much Time Do You Have? Minutes	Minutes to Hours	Hours to Days	Comments
What concentration can an IV drug be admixed?	• General electronic DI compendia • AHFS drug information • Product information/package insert • Institution-specific guidance on standard concentrations of IV admixtures	• Trissel, Handbook on Injectable Drugs • King, King Guide to Parenteral Admixture • Contact drug manufacturer • MEDLINE	• MEDLINE • Pharmacy-focused primary literature indexing databases • CINAHL	
What IV fluid can the drug be prepared in?	• General electronic DI compendia • AHFS drug information • Product information/package insert • Institution-specific guidance on standard IV admixtures	• Trissel, Handbook on Injectable Drugs • King, King Guide to Parenteral Admixture • Contact drug manufacturer • MEDLINE	• MEDLINE • Pharmacy-focused primary literature indexing databases • CINAHL	–This information is sometimes located in the narrative section rather than the tables of the print resources
Can the following drugs be administered simultaneously in the same IV line? (Are these drugs y-site compatible?)	• Product information/package insert • Electronic IV compatibility checking • Micromedex (IV Index with Trissel's 2 compatibility tool) • Lexicomp Online (King Guide) • Facts & Comparisons eAnswers (Trissel's IV-Chek)	• Trissel, Handbook on Injectable Drugs • King, King Guide to Parenteral Admixture • Gahart, Intravenous Medications A Handbook for Nurses • Contact drug manufacturer • MEDLINE	• Pharmacy-focused primary literature indexing databases • CINAHL	–Verify what each symbol/abbreviation/code means in the reference source you are using –It is also important to note the concentrations of drugs that are being used and how these compare to published compatibility data –Some references include compatibility as a sub-type of drug–drug interaction

(continued)

TABLE 5.11 Questions on Intravenous Compatibility/Stability *(continued)*

	How Much Time Do You Have?			
Question Type	**Minutes**	**Minutes to Hours**	**Hours to Days**	**Comments**
What expiration date should be used on the prepared IV medication?	• General electronic DI compendia • AHFS drug information • Product information/package insert • Institution-specific policies for beyond-use dating of products	• Trissel, Handbook on Injectable Drugs • King, King Guide to Parenteral Admixture • Contact drug manufacturer • MEDLINE	• Pharmacy-focused primary literature indexing databases • CINAHL • USP Chapter <797>	–Most studies evaluate stability of drug. Sterility is also a concern and largely dependent on the sterile technique of the person preparing the admixture and the conditions under which it was prepared –USP <797> specifies maximal beyond-use dating based on risk level of sterile preparation

- General print DI compendia: AHFS drug information; Lexicomp Drug Information Handbook; Drug Facts and Comparisons
- General electronic DI compendia: Micromedex Healthcare Series; Clinical Pharmacology; Lexicomp Online; Facts & Comparisons eAnswers
- Pharmacy-focused primary literature indexing and abstracting databases: EMBASE, IDIS/Web, and IPA

See Appendix 5C for bibliography of cited resources

DI, drug information; CINAHL, Cumulative Index to Nursing & Allied Health Literature

therapies are not standardized or regulated by a single authority for products covered by the DSHEA. Voluntary good manufacturing practices (GMPs) are used by some manufacturers, but there is not a single GMP standard that is recognized industrywide. Products bearing a trade association (e.g., National Nutritional Foods Association), independent testing group (e.g., National Safety Foundation International, ConsumerLab), or quasi-public institution (e.g., USP) Seal of Approval certify that the product has met that group's published standards. Certificates of Analysis may also be requested from reputable manufacturers detailing the assayed contents of their product.

The common question types asked of the pharmacy student concerning the use of these nondrug products are as follows:

- What is this product, what is it used for, and how is it used?
- Is there medical evidence to support the product's efficacy?
- Is the product safe for continued use in my patient given their medication regimens and disease states?
- What is the quality of the product?

Your frontline specialty references are available in several formats and should be helpful in quickly answering the first three questions. All cover a broad range of natural products, including herbs, nutritional supplements (vitamins, minerals, amino acids, essential fatty acids, antioxidants, and nutraceuticals), and glandular extracts. Information on Ayurvedic, Chinese, or homeopathic medicines is more difficult to find and may require you to first identify the active ingredients in the product and then proceed with looking up information on each component. Questions concerning drug interactions or safety in pregnancy and lactation of these products can be found under those question types published elsewhere in this chapter. Table 5.12 summarizes questions on natural products and dietary supplements with resources for information.

Compounded Formulations: Recipes and Stability

Certain patient populations such as children or those with enteral feeding tubes may require extemporaneously prepared pharmaceutical products. These scenarios often form the background for drug information questions regarding compounding recipes and stability/beyond-use dating (expiration dating) of these products. Lexicomp Online as well as the *Drug Information Handbook*, *Pediatric and Neonatal Dosage Handbook*, and Micromedex contain referenced information on common extemporaneous recipes and beyond-use

TABLE 5.12 Questions on Natural Products and Dietary Supplements

	How Much Time Do You Have?			
Question Type	**Minutes**	**Minutes to Hours**	**Hours to Days**	**Comments**
What is its use, pharmacologic action, dosing, safety, or efficacy?	• Jellin, Natural Medicines Comprehensive Database • Facts & Comparisons eAnswers (Review of Natural Products) • Lexicomp Online (Lexi-Natural Products) • Micromedex (AltMedDex)	• Blumental, Herbal Medicine Expanded Commission E Monographs • Brendler, Physicians' Desk Reference (PDR) for Herbal Medicine	• MEDLINE • Pharmacy-focused primary literature indexing databases • All EBM reviews • CINAHL	–The Natural Medicines Comprehensive Database uses a safety and efficacy rating system and contains detailed summaries of available studies. Look up by natural product name, disease or condition –Lexicomp Natural Products has useful charts and lists, patient information leaflets on the top products, monographs, and disease decisions trees with incorporated product recommendations –The Review of Natural Products has particularly useful sections on botany, uses and pharmacology, chemistry, and toxicology
What is the quality of the product?	• Jellin, Natural Medicines Comprehensive Database • Look for Seal of Approval from reputable certifying body		• Request Certificate of Analysis from manufacturer	–Seals of Approval and Certificates of Analysis can be used to identify high-quality dietary supplements, but these do not ensure safety and effectiveness –The Natural Medicines Comprehensive Database has quick links to USP-verified products and will mention specific brands used in clinical trials in the Dosage/Administration section

• Pharmacy-focused primary literature indexing and abstracting databases: EMBASE, IDIS/Web, and IPA.
See Appendix 5C for bibliography of cited resources.
DI, drug information; CINAHL, Cumulative Index to Nursing & Allied Health Literature.

dating. Specialized textbooks may also be available in the pharmacy. A search of specialized indexing systems such as IDIS or IPA may also be necessary for more difficult-to-find recipes and stability data. Chapter 795 in the USP <795>[8] provides additional guidance for establishing beyond-use dating when published data are not available. Table 5.13 lists questions on recipes and stability of nonsterile compounded formulations with resources for obtaining information.

Writing Responses to Drug Information Requests

While many drug information responses are provided verbally, it is common for a follow-up email or chart note to be requested of the pharmacy student. Drug information consultations should be guided by examples of acceptable responses from prior students and any institutional standards or templates. Since providing drug information is part of the pharmacist's delivery of care, student work must be approved by the preceptor before sending. A written response often follows this "friendly letter" structure:

- Month, Date, Year
- Salutation
- Restatement of Question being Answered
- Summarize Information Resources/Data Sources Used in Search Strategy
- Literature Review
- Applicability of Literature to Patient/Scenario
- Summary/Recommendations
- Closing
- References

An example patient-specific drug interaction response prepared by a summer IPPE pharmacy intern:

Month, Date, Year

Dear Requestor,
This letter is in response to your question regarding the presence of any clinically significant drug interactions between clopidogrel and omeprazole. Specifically, the patient is a 62-year-old male who is allergic to aspirin

TABLE 5.13 Questions on Recipes and Stability of Nonsterile Compounded Formulations

	How Much Time Do You Have?			
Question Type	**Minutes**	**Minutes to Hours**	**Hours to Days**	**Comments**
Is there a recipe and stability information for compounding this drug formulation?	• Lexicomp Online • Drug Information Handbook • Pediatric Dosage Handbook • Micromedex (Found under Storage and Stability: Extemporaneous Formulation in DRUGDEX)	• Allen, Allen's Compounded Formulations • Jew, Children's Hospital of Philadelphia: Extemporaneous Formulations • Trissel, Trissel's Stability of Compounded Formulations • US Pharmacist Web site • Pharmacy Times Web site • Secundum Artem Web site • International Journal of Pharmaceutical Compounding (search by formulation—requires paid subscription) • Professional Compounding Centers of America Formulations (paid subscribers only can access over 8,000 proprietary formulas)	• Pharmacy-focused primary literature indexing databases MEDLINE • Local compounding pharmacy • USP Chapter <795>	–General DI compendia/resources do not extensively contain compounding recipes –USP Chapter <795> provides guidance on beyond-use dating for situations where stability data cannot be obtained

- General print DI compendia: AHFS drug information; Lexicomp Drug Information Handbook; Drug Facts and Comparisons
- General electronic DI compendia: Micromedex Healthcare Series; Clinical Pharmacology; Lexicomp Online; Facts & Comparisons eAnswers
- Pharmacy-focused primary literature indexing and abstracting databases: EMBASE, IDIS/Web, and IPA

See Appendix 5C for bibliography of cited resources

DI, drug information

and is prescribed clopidogrel for his recent stroke. He is also currently taking OTC Prilosec (omeprazole) for his upset stomach. The patient is otherwise in good health and is not taking any other medications.

To evaluate any potential drug–drug interactions, the online databases Lexi-Comp, Drug Facts & Comparisons, and Micromedex were searched using the terms "omeprazole" and "clopidogrel" in the drug interaction tool for each site.

All three databases displayed a significant interaction between the drugs that could result in a decrease in the efficacy of clopidogrel and a resulting increased risk of cardiovascular events. Clopidogrel is a prodrug that must be activated by the CYP2C19 isoenzyme before it can potentiate its antiplatelet effects.[1] Omeprazole is a CYP2C19 competitive inhibitor and therefore would diminish the therapeutic effect of clopidogrel if concurrently administered.[2] Maximum serum concentrations of the active metabolite of clopidogrel dropped by almost half with combined use.[3] Simply separating the time of administration by 12 hours did not reduce this interaction.[1] Various small, prospective, randomized, crossover trials have found statistically diminished inhibition of platelet aggregation when clopidogrel is used with omeprazole.[3] This does not appear to be a proton pump inhibitor (PPI) class effect, since the effect appears to be limited to omeprazole.[1]

The drug interaction between omeprazole and clopidogrel was given a severity rating of major with fair documentation. There is disagreement in the clinical literature about whether or not the concurrent use of clopidogrel with omeprazole should be avoided. While one retrospective cohort study suggested that the concurrent use of the medications showed an increased risk of 6% to 18% for negative cardiovascular complications and increased mortality of 3% to 9%, other clinical studies have shown minor to no complications.[3] Despite the disagreement in findings, the FDA has continued to advise against their concurrent use.

In summary, concomitant use of clopidogrel and omeprazole may reduce the effectiveness of clopidogrel by decreasing serum concentrations of its active metabolite. This increases the risk of cardiovascular events, stroke, and death. Due to the potential for mortality, the FDA advises to avoid coadministration despite the conflicting data. The risk of gastrointestinal (GI) bleeds should be weighed against the potential for cardiovascular events when omitting a PPI. I recommend avoiding this combination or altering the therapy that the patient uses to control his dyspepsia. An alternate PPI with less CYP2C19 inhibitory effect, such as lansoprazole, pantoprazole, or rabeprazole that does not interact with the activation of clopidogrel, may be considered.

I hope this information is helpful in the care of your patient. Please do not hesitate to contact me if you have any questions regarding the information provided.

Sincerely,
Student Name,
PharmD candidate 20XX, Your School of Pharmacy
IPPEsummerintern@yoursite.org

References

1. Omeprazole/clopidogrel. Micromedex 2.0: Drug Interactions. Truven Health Analytics Inc.; 2013 [cited June 8, 2013]. Available from http://www.micromedexsolutions.com with subscription.
2. Proton-Pump Inhibitors/clopidogrel. Facts and Comparisons 4.0. St Louis, MO: Facts and Comparisons (Wolters Kluwer); 2013 [cited June 8, 2013]. Available from http://online.factsandcomparisons.com with subscription.
3. Clopidogrel/omeprazole. In: *Interactions Online*. Hudson, OH: Lexi-Comp; 1978–2013 [cited June 8, 2013]. Available from http://online.lexi.com with subscription.

Example non–patient-specific product information response prepared by an APPE student:

Month, Date, Year

Dear Requestor,

This information is in response to your inquiry regarding whether or not Lifestyles® Skyn™ brand condoms protect against human immunodeficiency virus (HIV) and sexually transmitted diseases/infections (STDs/STIs).

To research this question, tertiary drug compendia and product information from the manufacturers and FDA were consulted. The terms "latex," "nonlatex," "polyurethane," "polyisoprene," "lambskin," "natural," and "synthetic" combined with "condom" were searched.

Male condoms are used globally for contraception and disease protection. Typically, condoms are made out of latex, lambskin, or synthetic material such as polyurethane or, more recently, polyisoprene. In the United States, the majority of condoms are made out of latex. Latex condoms protect from pregnancy, STDs, and HIV. However, people with an allergy to latex can have anaphylaxis, and therefore, other alternative condom materials should be used. Lambskin is one alternative to latex, but it only protects from pregnancy since the material is porous enough to let through viral particles.[1–2]

Another option for those with a latex allergy is a synthetic product. Polyurethane and polyisoprene are different types of synthetic material used to make nonlatex condoms. Polyurethane can protect from pregnancy, STDs, and HIV like latex condoms. Polyurethane condoms are not as flexible or malleable as latex and may be more likely to break during sexual intercourse.[1–2] An improvement on polyurethane condoms is a softer and suppler synthetic material, polyisoprene.

Currently, Durex® Avanti Bare condoms and LifeStyles® SKYN™ condoms are polyisoprene condoms that have been clinically tested and FDA approved for pregnancy protection and reducing the risk of transmission of HIV (AIDS) infection and many other STDs.[3] Cis-1, 4 polyisoprene is a type of natural rubber from the rubber tree *Hevea brasiliensis*.[4] In 2008, the FDA approved polyisoprene, a synthetic nonlatex material, for condom use. According to Durex®'s proposed product submission to the FDA, "condoms made from synthetic polyisoprene have been shown to have similar performance properties as natural rubber latex condoms and conform to the relevant physical test requirements of national and international voluntary standards for natural rubber latex male condoms ISO 4073:2002, and ASTM D3492-03 and of the synthetic condom standard ASTM D6324-05."[5]

In summary, polyisoprene condoms are as effective as latex and polyurethane nonlatex condoms for prevention of pregnancy and STD's/HIV transmission. They are another option for people or partners who are allergic to latex.

I hope you find this information helpful. Please do not hesitate to contact me with any further questions.

Sincerely,
Student Name,
PharmD candidate 20XX, Your School of Pharmacy
APPEstudent@yourschool.edu

References

1. Pray WS. Recent developments in birth control and STD prevention for men. *US Pharm*. 2009;34(8):12–15. Available from http://www.uspharmacist.com/content/d/consult%20your%20pharmacist/c/14459/.
2. Shrader SP, Diaz VA. Chapter 88. Contraception. In: Talbert RL, DiPiro JT, Matzke GR, et al., eds. *Pharmacotherapy: A Pathophysiologic Approach*. 8th ed. New York: McGraw-Hill; 2011. Available from http://www.accesspharmacy.com/content.aspx?aID=7993297. Accessed April 30, 2012.
3. Lifestyles® Skyn™ condoms [package labeling]. Red bank, NJ: Ansell Healthcare Products, LLC; 2008.
4. Partridge EG, Leucken JJ. "Rubber," in AccessScience, ©McGraw-Hill Companies, 2008. [cited April 30, 2012]. Available with subscription from http://www.accessscience.com/content.aspx?searchStr=polyisoprene&id=594800#594800s014.
5. US Food and Drug Administration. Durex Synthetic Polyisoprene Male Condom Pre-market Notification 510(k) submission. July 7, 2007. [cited April 30, 2012]. Available from http://www.accessdata.fda.gov/cdrh_docs/pdf7/K072169.pdf?utm_campaign=Google2&utm_source=fdaSearch&utm_medium=website&utm_term=polyisoprene%20condom&utm_content=3.

Citation Style and Resources

Referencing your written drug information response adds to its credibility and allows the requestor to identify and review the same source material you used to make your assessment or recommendation. In medical writing, a commonly recognized standard format for reference citation is the National Library of Medicine's Style Guide[9]: www.nlm.nih.gov/citingmedicine.

These uniform requirements contain detailed explanations and examples of citing the various types of materials found in a physical or virtual medical library. A few referencing sources are often encountered in responding to drug information questions that are not covered in the NLM's guidance: package inserts and personal communications with experts such as drug manufacturers or specialty practitioners (Table 5.14).

TABLE 5.14 Referencing Special Sources of Drug Information

Type	Example
Package insert (Note: date is the date of publication of package insert and not the date cited)	Lexapro (escitalopram oxalate) tablets [product information]. St. Louis, MO: Forest Pharmaceuticals, December 2012
Personal communication	Personal communication with Jane Doe (Eisai Medical Information, Eisai, Inc., Woodcliff Lake, NJ), July 15, 2013

In providing drug information based on the question-type tables we have provided, the citation formats you will use repeatedly are more limited than the NLM's extensive list. We have cited our recommended resources in the NLM format in the Bibliography in Appendix 5C. If you need further guidance, the NLM's online style guide is very easy to navigate and allows you to quickly see the citation rules and examples for the type of material you are citing. Close attention must be paid to the use of capitalization, punctuation, spacing, and title source abbreviations to meet the NLM standards. According to NLM standards, all authors should be listed if there are six or fewer; otherwise the first three are listed followed by "et al."

References

1. Kirkwood CF, Kier KL. Modified systematic approach to answering questions. In: Malone PM, Kier KL, Stanovich JE, eds. *Drug Information: A Guide for Pharmacists*. 3rd ed. New York: McGraw-Hill; 2006:29–37.
2. Calis KA, Sheehan AH. Formulating effective responses and recommendations: a structured approach. In: Malone PM, Kier KL, Stanovich JE, eds. *Drug Information: A Guide for Pharmacists*. 4th ed. New York: McGraw-Hill; 2012:35–58.
3. Slawson DC, Shaughnessy AF, Bennett JH. Becoming a medical information master: feeling good about not knowing everything. *J Fam Pract*. 1994; 38:505–513.
4. Galt KA. Gathering drug information and evidence. In: *Developing Clinical Practice Skills for Pharmacists*. Bethesda, MD: American Society of Health-System Pharmacists; 2006:114–162.
5. Shields KM, Blythe E. Drug information resources. In: Malone PM, Kier KL, Stanovich JE, eds. *Drug Information: A Guide for Pharmacists*. 4th ed. New York: McGraw-Hill; 2012:59–110.

6. United States Pharmacopeial Convention. *USP on Compounding: A Guide for the Compounding Practitioner* [12 month electronic subscription]. June, 2012 (cited July, 2013). Available from http://www.usp.org/store/products-services/usp-compounding.
7. American Society of Health-System Pharmacists. ASHP statement on the use of dietary supplements. *Am J Health Syst Pharm.* 2004;61:1707–1711.
8. Allen LV. USP chapter <795> pharmaceutical compounding—non-sterile preparations. Secundum Artem [serial on the internet]. Date Unknown (cited July, 2013);13(4): 6 p. Available from http://www.perrigo.com/business/education.aspx.
9. Patrias K. Citing medicine: the NLM style guide for authors, editors, and publishers [Internet]. 2nd ed. Wendling DL, technical ed. Bethesda, MD: National Library of Medicine (US); 2007. (cited July, 2013). Available from www.nlm.nih.gov/citingmedicine.

APPENDIX 5A

Providing Drug Information Questionnaire

- Discuss with your preceptor his or her expectation of your role in providing drug information.
  - Will both verbal and written drug information be provided?
  - May any type of drug information be provided to the requestor without prior approval of the preceptor?
  - What documentation format is to be followed for written drug information responses?
  - Is there an expectation of the number or types of questions that should be responded to during the learning experience?
- Discuss with your preceptor any resources that are available to students.
  - Is a medical library available on site or remotely? How is it accessed?
  - Build yourself a Drug Information Resource Finder (Appendix 5A.1) following the format below and note any constraints on use (e.g., on-site access only, log-in and password required, limited user access).

APPENDIX 5A.1

Examples of Drug Information Resource Finder

Resource	Format	Through Site (✔)	Through School (✔)	Access Constraints
General drug information compendia				
Example: Lexicomp Drug Information Handbook	Online and print	✔	✔	• Site: via UpToDate, on-site access only • School: access via Library page, student log-in/password (PW) • Own: print 2013–2014 edition

(continued)

Resource	Format	Through Site (✔)	Through School (✔)	Access Constraints
Specialty references				
Example: Briggs Drugs in Pregnancy and Lactation	Online and print	✔	✔	• Site: print copies in Drug Information and pharmacy satellites • School: access via Facts & Comparisons eAnswers on Library page, student log-in/password (PW)
Primary literature indexing services				
Example: All EBM reviews	Via Ovid		✔	Ovid: on-site and off-site access with log-in and password
CINAHL	Via Ovid	✔	✔	
EMBASE	Via Ovid	✔	✔	
IDIS	Via Web	✔		Site: Single-user license at Drug Info only
IPA	Via Ovid		✔	Ovid: on-site and off-site access with log-in and password
MEDLINE	Via Ovid or PubMed	✔	✔	Ovid: on-site and off-site access with log-in and password; PubMed: on-site and off-site access via NLM Web site

- Use the bibliography of resources in Appendix 5C to check for on-site General DI Compendia and Specialty Reference titles that may be useful.
- Review the list again to see if you may have access remotely through your school if the resource is not available on site.
- Use the crosswalk in Appendix 5B for any unavailable resources to see if you may have access via an alternative pathway.

- Discuss with your preceptor any resources that he or she consults frequently and why the preceptor finds them useful.

APPENDIX 5B

Crosswalk to Locating Alternative Sources of Drug Information

If you are looking for information from...	...the same content may also be available from these sources
A to Z Facts	Facts & Comparisons eAnswers www.drugs.com
AHFS Drug Information	STAT!Ref (e-book collection) Lexicomp Online
Basic and Clinical Pharmacology (Katzung)	AccessPharmacy (McGraw-Hill) Books@OVID
Cecil Medicine (Textbook of Medicine)	MD Consult (Elsevier)
Clinical Pharmacology (Gold Standard/Elsevier)	MD Consult (Elsevier) AccessPharmacy (McGraw-Hill)
Drug Facts and Comparisons	Facts & Comparisons eAnswers
Drug Information Handbook	Lexicomp Online UpToDate
Drug Interaction Facts	Facts & Comparisons eAnswers
Drug Prescribing in Renal Failure	R2 Library (e-book collection) STAT!Ref (e-book collection)
Drugs in Pregnancy and Lactation (Briggs)	Books@OVID Facts & Comparisons eAnswers
Geriatric Dosage Handbook	Lexicomp Online UpToDate
Goldfrank's Toxicologic Emergencies	AccessPharmacy (McGraw-Hill) STAT!Ref (e-book collection)
Goodman & Gilman's The Pharmacologic Basis of Therapeutics	AccessPharmacy (McGraw-Hill) STAT!Ref (e-book collection)
Handbook of Injectable Drugs (Trissel)	STAT!Ref (e-book collection) Some data available via Micromedex IV Index (Trissel's 2 Clinical Pharmaceutics Database)
Harriet Lane Handbook	MD Consult (Elsevier)
Harrison's Principles of Internal Medicine	AccessPharmacy or AccessMedicine (McGraw-Hill) STAT!Ref (e-book collection)
Index Nominum: International Drug Directory	Micromedex 2.0 (additional subscription)
King Guide to Parenteral Admixture	Lexicomp Online

(continued)

If you are looking for information from...	...the same content may also be available from these sources
Laboratory Test Handbook	Lexicomp Online
Martindale: The Complete Drug Reference	Micromedex 2.0 (additional subscription)
Merck Manual of Diagnosis and Therapy	STAT!Ref (e-book collection)
Pediatric Dosage Handbook	Lexicomp Online UpToDate
Pharmacotherapy: A Pathophysiologic Approach (Dipiro)	AccessPharmacy (McGraw-Hill)
Physicians' Desk Reference (PDR)	Alternate Sources for Package Insert information: NLM DailyMed: http://dailymed.nlm.nih.gov Drugs @ FDA: http://www.accessdata.fda.gov/scripts/cder/drugsatfda
Pocket Guide To Diagnostic Tests	AccessPharmacy (McGraw-Hill)
Review of Natural Products (Lawrence Review)	Facts & Comparisons eAnswers
Stedman's Medical Dictionary	STAT!Ref (e-book collection) www.drugs.com
Trissel's Stability of Compounded Formulations	R2 Library (e-book collection) STAT!Ref (e-book collection)
USP DI Volume 2—Advice for the Patient (renamed Detailed Drug Information for the Consumer)	Micromedex 2.0 STAT!Ref (e-book collection) www.drugs.com
Washington Manual of Therapeutics	Books@OVID

APPENDIX 5C

Bibliography of Resources in Drug Information Question Tables

General print drug information compendia:

- American Society of Health-System Pharmacists. *AHFS Drug Information 2013* (AHFS Drug Information). Bethesda, MD: American Society of Health-System Pharmacists; 2013.
- *Drug Facts and Comparisons* [looseleaf]. 2013 ed. St. Louis, MO: Wolters Kluwer Health; updated monthly.
- Lacey CF, Armstrong LL, Goldman MP, et al. *Drug Information Handbook 2013–2014.* 22nd ed. Hudson, OH: Lexicomp, Inc.; 2013.

General electronic drug information compendia:

- Clinical Pharmacology [database online]. Tampa, FL: Gold Standard, Inc.; 2013. Available from www.clinicalpharmacology.com. Updated periodically.
- Facts & Comparisons eAnswers [database online]. St. Louis, MO: Wolters Kluwer Health, Inc.; 2013. Available from http://www.factsandcomparisons.com/facts-comparisons-online.aspx. Updated periodically.
- Lexicomp Online [database online]. Hudson, OH: Lexicomp, Inc.; 2013. Available from http://www.lexi.com/institutions/products/online/. Updated periodically.
- Micromedex 2.0 [database online]. Greenwood Village, CO: Truven Health Analytics Inc.; 2013. Available from http://www.micromedex.com/2/home.html. Updated periodically.

Therapeutics textbooks and databases:

- Alldredge BK, Corelli RL, Ernst ME, et al. *Koda-Kimble and Young's Applied Therapeutics: The Clinical Use of Drugs*. 10th ed. Philadelphia, PA: Lippincott Williams & Wilkins; 2012.
- Chisholm-Burns MA, Wells BG, Schwinghammer TL, et al., eds. *Pharmacotherapy Principles and Practice*. 3rd ed. New York, NY: McGraw-Hill; 2013.
- Dipiro JT, Talbert RL, Yee GC, et al., eds. *Pharmacotherapy: A Pathophysiologic Approach*. 8th ed. New York, NY: McGraw-Hill; 2011.
- Helms RA, Herfindal ET, Gourley DR, et al., eds. *Textbook of Therapeutics: Drug and Disease Management*. 8th ed. Philadelphia, PA: Lippincott Williams & Wilkins; 2006.
- MD Consult [database online]. Maryland Heights, MO: MD Consult LLC. 1997–2013 (cited July, 2013). Available from www.mdconsult.com.
- UpToDate online [database online]. Waltham, MA: UpToDate. 2001–2013 (cited July, 2013). Available from www.uptodate.com.

Other drug information references:

- Allen LV. *Allen's Compounded Formulations: The Complete US Pharmacist Collection*. Washington, DC: American Pharmaceutical Association; 2003.
- Allen LV. USP chapter <795> pharmaceutical compounding—non-sterile preparations. Secundum Artem [serial on the internet]. Date unknown (cited July, 2013);13(4):6 p. Available from http://www.perrigo.com/business/education.aspx.

- Aranoff GR, Bennett WM. *Drug Prescribing in Renal Failure: Dosing Guidelines for Adults and Children*. 5th ed. Philadelphia, PA: American College of Physicians; 2007.
- Aronson JK, ed. *Meyler's Side Effects of Drugs—The International Encyclopedia of Adverse Drug Reactions and Interactions*. 15th ed. Amsterdam, the Netherlands: Elsevier; 2006.
- Billups NF, Billups SM. *American Drug Index*. 57th ed. St. Louis, MO: Wolters Kluwer Health; 2013.
- Blumental M, Goldberg A, Brinckmann J, eds. *Herbal Medicine: Expanded Commission E monographs*. 1st ed. Newton, MA: Integrative Medicine Communications; 2000.
- Brendler T, Jaenicke C, eds. *PDR for Herbal Medicines*. 4th ed. Montvale, NJ: Thomson PDR; 2007.
- Briggs GG, Freeman RK, Yaffe SJ. *Drugs in Pregnancy and Lactation*. 9th ed. Philadelphia, PA: Lippincott Williams & Wilkins; 2011.
- Brunton LL, Chabner BA, Knollmann BC, eds. *Goodman and Gilman's: The Pharmacological Basis of Therapeutics*. 12th ed. New York, NY: McGraw Hill; 2011.
- Davies DM, Ferner RE, de Glanville H, eds. *Davies's Textbook of Adverse Drug Reactions*. 5th ed. London: Lippincott-Raven; 1999.
- Department of Medicine, Washington University School of Medicine. *The Washington Manual of Medical Therapeutics*. 34th ed. Philadelphia, PA: Lippincott Williams & Wilkins; 2013.
- Gahart BL. *2014 Intravenous Medications: A Handbook for Nurses and Other Allied Health Personnel*. 30th ed. St. Louis, MO: Mosby; 2013.
- Goldman L, Schafer AI, eds. *Goldman's Cecil Medicine*. 24th ed. Philadelphia, PA: Elsevier/Saunders; 2012.
- Grabenstein JD. *Immunofacts 2013: Vaccines and Immunologic Drugs*. St. Louis, MO: Wolters Kluwer Health; 2012.
- Hale TW. *Medications and Mothers' Milk 2012: A Manual of Lactational Pharmacology*. 15th ed. Amarillo, TX: Hale Publishing; 2012.
- Hansten PD, Horn JR. *Drug Interactions Analysis and Management 2013*. 8th ed. St. Louis, MO: Wolters Kluwer Health; 2013.
- International Journal of Pharmaceutical Compounding [serial on the internet]. Available from www.ijpc.com.
- Jellin JM, ed. Ident-a-Drug [database online]. Stockton, CA: Therapeutic Research Center; annual, 1997–2013 ed. Available from http://identadrug.therapeuticresearch.com.

- Jellin JM, ed. Pharmacist's letter/prescriber's letter natural medicines comprehensive database [database online]. Stockton, CA: Therapeutic Research Faculty; annual, 1999–2013 ed. Available from http://pharmacistsletter.therapeuticresearch.com.
- Jew RK, Mullen RJ, Soo-Hoo W. *Children's Hospital of Philadelphia: Extemporaneous Formulations*. Bethesda, MD: American Society of Health-System Pharmacists; 2003.
- Katzung BG, Masters SB, Trevor AJ, eds. *Basic and Clinical Pharmacology*. 12th ed. New York, NY: McGraw-Hill; 2012.
- King JC, Catania PN. *King Guide to Parenteral Admixtures*. 35th ed. Napa, CA: King Guide Publications, Inc.; 2010.
- Longo DL, Fauci AS, Kasper DL, eds. *Harrison's Principles of Internal Medicine*. 18th ed. New York, NY: McGraw-Hill; 2012.
- National Library of Medicine. LactMed [database online]. Bethesda, MD: ToxNet, National Library of Medicine; 2013 (cited July, 2013). Available from http://toxnet.nlm.nih.gov/cgi-bin/sis/htmlgen?LACT.
- Pharmacy Times [serial on the internet]. Plainsboro, NJ: Intellisphere LLC; c2006–2013 (cited July, 2013). Available from www.pharmacytimes.com.
- Phelps SJ, Thompson AJ, Hagemann TM. *Pediatric Injectable Drugs* (The Teddy Bear Book). 10th ed. Bethesda, MD: American Society of Health-System Pharmacists; 2013.
- Porter RS, Kaplan JL, eds. *The Merck Manual of Diagnosis and Therapy* [electronic book]. 19th ed. Whitehouse Station, NJ: Merck Research Laboratories; 2004–2012 (cited July, 2013). Available from www.merckmanuals.com/professional/index.html.
- Professional Compounding Centers of America Formulations Team. PCCA Member Formulary Database [database online]. Available from www.pccarx.com/pcca-services/pcca-formulations-team.
- Tschudy MM, Arcara KM. *The Johns Hopkins Hospital. The Harriet Lane Handbook: A Manual for Pediatric House Officers*. 19th ed. Philadelphia, PA: Elsevier/Mosby; 2012.
- Secundum Artem [homepage on the internet]. Allegan, MI: Perrigo Company; c2011–2013 (cited July, 2013). Available from http://www.perrigo.com/business/education.aspx.
- Semla TP, Belzer JL, Higbee MD. *Geriatric Dosage Handbook*. 18th ed. Hudson, OH: Lexicomp, Inc.; 2012.
- Taketomo CK, Hodding JH, Kraus DM. *Pediatric and Neonatal Dosage Handbook*. 19th ed. Hudson, OH: Lexicomp, Inc.; 2012.

- Tatro DS, ed. *Drug Interaction Facts: Herbal Supplements and Food* [looseleaf]. 2003 ed. St. Louis, MO: Wolters Kluwer Health; updated quarterly.
- Thomson-Reuters Clinical Editorial Staff. *Neofax 2011*. 24th ed. Montvale, NJ: Thomson Reuters Healthcare; 2012.
- Tilsdale JE, Miller DA, eds. *Drug-Induced Diseases: Prevention, Detection, and Management*. 2nd ed. Bethesda, MD: American Society of Health-System Pharmacists; 2010.
- Trissel LA, ed. *Handbook on Injectable Drugs*. 17th ed. Bethesda, MD: American Society of Health-System Pharmacists; 2013.
- Trissel LA. *Trissel's Stability of Compounded Formulations*. 5th ed. Washington, DC: American Pharmacists Association; 2012.
- U.S. Pharmacist [serial on the internet]. East Rutherford, NJ: Jobson Medical Information LLC; c2000–2013 (cited July, 2013). Available from www.uspharmacist.com.
- United States Pharmacopeial Convention. *USP Dictionary of USAN and International Drug Names*. Rockville, MD: United States Pharmacopeial Convention; 2012.
- United States Pharmacopeial Convention. USP on Compounding: A Guide for the Compounding Practitioner [12 month electronic subscription]. 2012 June (cited July, 2013). Available from http://www.usp.org/store/products-services/usp-compounding.
- Young DS, ed. *Effects of Drugs on Clinical Laboratory Tests*. 5th ed. Washington, DC: American Association for Clinical Chemistry; 2000.

Primary literature indexing and abstracting services:

- CINAHL—Cumulative Index to Nursing & Allied Health Literature [database on Ovid SP]. New York, NY: Ovid Technologies; 2000–2012. 1982 to July Week 2 2013 (cited July, 2013). Available from www.ovid.com.
- EMBASE Drugs & Pharmacology [database on Ovid SP]. New York, NY: Ovid Technologies; 2000–2012. 1974 to 2nd Quarter 2013 (cited July, 2013). Available from www.ovid.com.
- Evidence-Based Medicine Reviews—Cochrane DSR, ACP Journal Club, DARE, CCTR, CMR, HTA, and NHSEED [database on Ovid SP]. New York, NY: Ovid Technologies; 2000–2012. Through 2nd Quarter 2013 (cited July, 2013). Available from www.ovid.com.

- IDIS/Web [database on Internet]. Iowa City, IA: Iowa Drug Information Service. 1966 to June 2013 (cited July, 2013). Available from http://itsnt14.its.uiowa.edu/.
- International Pharmaceutical Abstracts [database on Ovid SP]. New York, NY: Ovid Technologies; 2000–2012. 1970 to June 2013 (cited July, 2013). Available from www.ovid.com.
- Ovid MEDLINE [database on Ovid SP]. New York, NY: Ovid Technologies; 2000–2012. 1946 to July Week 2, 2013 (cited July, 2013). Available from www.ovid.com.
- PubMed [database on the Internet]. Bethesda, MD: National Library of Medicine. 2013 (cited July, 2013). Available from www.ncbi.nlm.nih.gov/PubMed/.

APPENDIX 5D

Standard Questions for Obtaining Background Information from Requestors

General information to gather for all question types:

- Requestor's name, title/profession, contact information, and affiliation
- Resources already consulted by requestor
- How will the requestor use the information provided (e.g., patient-specific decision, research, presentation, or academic interest)?
- If patient-specific, is information concerning an inpatient, outpatient, or private patient (gather patient identifiers and location)?
- Urgency of the request (negotiate time of response)
- Format of response (verbal or written or both)

Adverse drug reactions:

- What are the names, dosages, and routes for all drugs currently and recently prescribed?
- What are the patient's specifics (age, gender, height, weight, organ dysfunction, and indication for drug use)?
- Does the patient have any food intolerance?
- What were the events/findings that characterize this ADR (include onset and duration)?
- What is the temporal relationship with the drug?

- Was the suspected drug ever administered before? Why was it discontinued then?
- Has the patient experienced this adverse relationship (or similar event) with this drug (or similar agent) previously?
- Is there a family history for this ADR and/or drug allergy?
- Has any intervention been initiated at this time?
- What is the patient's current condition?

Dosing or administration:

- What disease is being treated? What is the extent/severity of the illness? What is the clinical status of the patient?
- What are the drugs being prescribed? What dosage form or preparation is to be used? What drugs has the patient received to date?
- What is the patient's age, gender, height, and weight?
- Does the patient have any insufficiency of the renal, hepatic, or cardiac system?
- For drugs with renal elimination, what are the serum creatinine/creatinine clearance, blood urea nitrogen (BUN), and/or urine output? Is the patient receiving a renal replacement therapy (peritoneal or hemodialysis, continuous venovenous hemofiltration [CVVH])?
- For drugs with hepatic elimination, what are the liver function tests (LFTs), bilirubin (direct and indirect), and/or albumin? Does the patient have liver disease (Child-Pugh score)?
- Are these lab values recent? Is the patient's condition stable?
- Does this patient have a known factor that could affect drug absorption or metabolism?
- For drugs with serum level monitoring utility, characterize the most recent levels per timing relative to dose, reported results, and clinical monitoring parameters.

Drug interactions:

- What event(s) suggest that an interaction occurred? Please describe.
- For the drugs in question, what are the doses, volumes, concentrations, rate of administration, administration schedule, indication, and length of therapies?
- What is the temporal relationship between the drugs in question?
- Has the patient received this combination or a similar combination in the past?

- Other than the drugs in question, what other drugs is the patient receiving currently? When were these started?
- What other disease states does the patient have?
- Has Clinical Chemistry (or the appropriate laboratory) been contacted about the abnormal result? Are they aware of any known nonpharmacologic interference similar to this event?
- Was this one isolated test abnormality or a trend in results?

Indication for therapeutic use:

- What medications, including doses and routes of administration, is the patient receiving? Has the patient been compliant?
- What are we treating and what is the severity of illness?
- What are the patient's other pathology(ies) and disease(s) severity?
- What are the patient's specifics: age, weight, height, gender, organ dysfunction?
- Has the patient received the drug previously? What was the prior response?
- What alternative approved or accepted therapies has the patient received? Was therapy maximized for each of these before discontinuation? What other therapies are being considered?
- What monitoring parameters have been followed (serum concentrations/levels, clinical status, other clinical lab results, objective measurements, and subjective assessment)?

Product information or identification:

- What is the generic or trade name of the product? What is the dosage form, shape, color, markings, size, coating, etc.?
- Who is the manufacturer? What is the country of origin?
- What is the suspected reason for use of this product? How is the patient taking it?
- How long will the patient be staying in the USA (for foreign product identifications)?
- What is the source of your information about the product?

Safety in pregnancy and lactation:

- What was the drug the patient received and what was the dose? What was the duration of therapy? Was the patient compliant?
- Is the patient pregnant or planning to become pregnant?
- When during pregnancy was the exposure (trimester or weeks)?

- What are the patient's specifics (age, height, weight, organ dysfunction, other medical conditions including prior gynecologic/obstetric history)?
- What event(s) suggest that a safety concern has arisen? Please describe.
- What was the indication for prescribing the drug? Was this initial or alternate therapy?
- What is the source of the case information?
- How long has the infant been breast-feeding?
- What is the frequency of breast-feeding? What is the milk volume consumed?
- How old is the infant and what is his or her health status?
- Has the infant ever received feedings other than breast milk? Is bottle or cup feeding a plausible alternative?
- Has the mother breast-fed previously while on the drug?

IV compatibility/stability:

- What are the routes for the patient's medications?
- What are the dose amounts, concentrations, and volumes for all pertinent medications?
- What are the infusion times/rates expected or desired?
- What is the base solution or diluent used?
- Does the patient have water, sodium, dextrose, or volume restriction?
- Was the product stored in the refrigerator or at room temperature? For how long?
- Was the product exposed to sunlight? For how long?
- Was the product frozen? For how long?
- When was the product compounded/prepared?
- Under what conditions was the product compounded/prepared?

Natural products and dietary supplements:

- Is there a particular concern about this product?
- Why was the patient receiving the product or what is the intended use?
- What drugs is the patient currently receiving? What alternative therapies were tried before?
- What is the product's name and manufacturer?
- What is the dosage form, strength, and how does the patient use it?

Recipes and nonsterile compounded formulations:

- What is the dosage form desired?
- What administration routes are feasible with this patient?
- Does the patient have a feeding tube in place that will be used to administer the drug? What type of feeding tube is it? Anatomically, where does it begin and end?
- What other special factors regarding drug administration should be considered?

Adapted from Kirkwood CF, Kier KL. Modified systematic approach to answering questions. In: Malone PM, Kier KL, Stanovich JE, eds. *Drug Information: A Guide for Pharmacists.* 3rd ed. New York, NY: McGraw-Hill; 2006:29–37, with permission

6

Physical Examination

Kam L. Capoccia

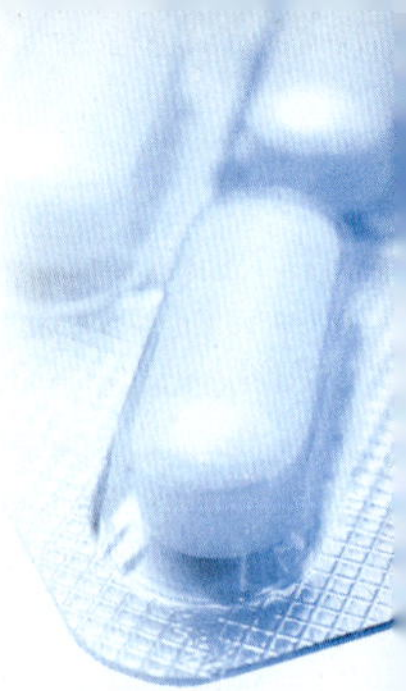

Entire books are dedicated to the topic of physical examination. The goal of this chapter is not to provide a thorough explanation of how to perform an adult physical examination but rather to describe and highlight some common physical exam techniques and assessments that a pharmacist may perform when evaluating a patient's drug therapy. It is not comprehensive. Basic knowledge and understanding of anatomy and physiology are assumed. For further explanation and details, refer to Bates' *Guide to Physical Examination and History Taking*, 11th edition, 2012.[1]

Medical History

When a patient is admitted to the hospital or undergoes a detailed medical evaluation, the clinician typically obtains a thorough medical history before physically examining the patient. The history describes the events in the life of the patient that are relevant to the patient's mental and physical health. Although this chapter concentrates on physical examination, it should be noted that the history itself contributes the most to understanding a patient's problem or monitoring a drug's effects. The components of the medical history usually follow a standardized format (Table 6.1).

Subjective and objective information obtained from the history and physical examinations are crucial to the assessment of drug efficacy and toxicity. Both positive and negative findings may be noted. Pertinent positive findings can rule in a diagnosis while pertinent negative findings can rule out a diagnosis. Please see Table 6.2 for common abbreviations used in a patient history and physical exam.

TABLE 6.1 The Medical History

Section	Contents
Patient profile	Age, race, sex, date of birth, marital status
Chief complaint (CC)	The reason for seeking medical attention
History of present illness (HPI)	A chronologic account of events and symptoms of the chief complaint; laboratory/diagnostic procedures and negative findings
Past medical history (PMH)	General state of health Childhood illnesses Immunizations Medical illnesses Psychiatric illnesses Surgical procedures Hospitalizations Injuries Medications Allergies
Family history (FH)	Age and health of living relatives Age and cause of death of relatives Occurrence and relation of family members with diabetes mellitus, high BP, cancer, mental illnesses, tuberculosis, and other serious or hereditary illnesses
Social history (SH)	Financial situation, health habits (sleeping, diet, recreation, use of tobacco, alcohol, or other drugs of abuse), education, religion, and family dynamics
Review of systems (ROS)	Common symptoms by body system; the body areas reviewed are skin, head, eyes, ears, nose, and sinuses, mouth and throat, neck, breasts, chest and lungs, heart, vascular, gastrointestinal, urinary, reproductive, musculoskeletal, neurologic, psychiatric, endocrine, and hematologic

Techniques of the Physical Exam

Physical examination uses four main techniques: inspection, palpation, percussion, and auscultation. Inspection is visual observation of the patient with unaided eyes (e.g., examination of the skin), although instruments (e.g., an ophthalmoscope) are often used. Palpation is the use of touch to detect normal and abnormal physical findings (e.g., palpating enlarged lymph nodes). Percussion

TABLE 6.2 Common Abbreviations in a History and Physical Exam

System	Physical Exam Documentation	Explanation of Abbreviation
General (Gen)	NAD, WDWN, WF, WM, AAF, AAM, A&Ox3	No acute distress, well-developed well-nourished, white female, white male, African American female, African American male, alert and oriented times 3 (person, place, and time)
Vital signs (VS)	T, HR, BP, P, RR, SPO_2, Ht, Wt, BMI, BSA, IBW, AdjBW	Temperature, heart rate, blood pressure, pulse, respiratory rate, oxygen saturation measured by pulse oximetry, height, weight, body mass index, body surface area, ideal body weight, actual body weight
Skin, hair, and nails	CR	Capillary refill
Head and neck	HEENT, NCAT, MMM, PERRLA, EOMI, AV, TM, BC, AC, CN I-XII, JVD, LAD	Head eyes ears nose and throat, normocephalic atraumatic, mucous membranes moist, pupils are equal round reactive to light and accomodation, extraocular muscles intact, atriovenous, tympanic membrane, bone conduction, air conduction, jugular venous distention, lymphadenopathy
Thorax and lungs	CTA, CTAB, ICS	Clear to auscultation, clear to auscultation bilaterally, intercostal space
Cardiovascular system (CV or CVS)	RRR, m/r/g, PMI, HJR, LLSB	Regular rate and rhythm, murmurs/rubs/or gallops, point of maximal impulse, hepatojugular reflux, lower left sternal border
Breasts and axillae	MCL	Midclavicular line
Abdomen (Abd)	NT/ND, BS, CVA, HSM	Nontender/Nondistended, bowel sounds, costovertebral angle, hepatosplenomegaly
Peripheral vascular system	UE, LE, CCE, ABI, DP, PT	Upper extremities, lower extremities, clubbing cyanosis edema, ankle brachial index, dorsalis pedis, posterior tibial
GU and rectal system	GU, CMT, BRBPR, LAD	Genitourinary, cervical motion tenderness, bright red blood per rectum, lymphadenopathy
Musculoskeletal system	MS, UE, LE, ROM, DTR	Musculoskeletal, upper extremities, lower extremities, range of motion, deep tendon reflexes
Nervous system	CN I-XII, MMSE	Cranial nerves 1–12, mini mental state exam

is the tapping of a body surface with a fingertip to produce sounds that help determine whether underlying structures are air filled, fluid filled, or solid (e.g., percussion of the chest). During percussion, the examiner strikes the body surface to sense the vibrations and sounds generated with each tap. Pitch and tone of the generated sounds help categorize the status of the underlying structures (see "General" under "Thorax and Lungs" section for a more detailed description of findings on percussion). Auscultation, with the aid of a stethoscope, is listening for normal and abnormal sounds (e.g., heart tones, breath sounds, blood pressure [BP] measurement). There are numerous Web sites and videos for learning physical exam techniques and for listening to heart and lung sounds. Here are a few I have found to be helpful:

- http://acousticheart.com/learning_heart_and_lung_sounds.html
- www.easyauscultation.com/
- www.wilkes.med.ucla.edu/inex.htm

Signs and Symptoms

When interpreting a history and physical examination, clinical signs and symptoms are often described. A sign refers to objective information gathered by the examiner during the physical examination (e.g., heart murmur, ankle edema, rales). Signs can be a result of any part of the physical exam (inspection, palpation, percussion, auscultation) but do not include anything reported by the patient.

A symptom refers to subjective information gathered from the patient while obtaining the history (e.g., nausea, pain). The patient's descriptions of symptoms may be scrutinized further, clarified, and quantified by the examiner's additional questioning.

Approach and Organization to Adult Physical Examination

An outline of a comprehensive physical exam is provided below. Following the outline is a description of each system with abbreviated physical examination instructions. For a more complete explanation and additional information, please see *Bates' Guide to Physical Examination and History Taking*, 11th edition, 2012.

- General survey
- Vital signs (VS)
- Skin, hair, and nails
- Head, eyes, ears, nose, throat (HEENT)
- Neck
- Thorax and lungs
- Cardiovascular system
- Breasts and axillae
- Abdomen
- Peripheral vascular system
- Genitourinary (GU) and rectal system
- Musculoskeletal system
- Nervous system

General Survey

Observe the patient's general state of health (acute or chronically ill, frail, etc.) and overall appearance, paying particular attention to the following:

- Level of consciousness (awake, alert, unresponsive, etc.)
- Note orientation to person, place, and thing; if normal, it is often documented as A & O × 3 (alert and oriented to (i) person, (ii) place, and (iii) time).
- Signs of distress (cardiac, respiratory, pain, anxiety, fear, shock, etc.)
- Height (tall or short), build (muscular, slender, stocky), weight (overweight, obese, emaciated, thin)
- Skin color (jaundice, cyanosis, rashes or bruises)
- Dress (appropriate for the temperature and weather, clean, dirty, fit properly)
- Grooming and personal hygiene (appropriate for age, lifestyle, etc.)
- Facial expression (eye contact, change or reaction to certain topics during physical exam, interaction with others, flat or sad affect, etc.)
- Odor of body or breath (fruity odor of diabetes, scent of alcohol, etc.)

- Posture (sitting up, leaning forward, etc.)
- Gait (walking smoothly, with or without assistance, etc.)
- Motor activity (tremor, involuntary movements, paralyses)

The above observations are typically made throughout the interview and physical exam. An observation example might include the following: "This is a thin, elderly man who looks jaundiced and chronically ill. He is leaning forward in the chair, alert, and making good eye contact."

Vital Signs

VS are important because they are coarse objective measurements for a patient's physical state. The four VS are temperature, pulse, BP, and respiratory rate (RR).

Temperature

Body temperature can be measured orally, rectally, in the axilla, or by using an infrared beam aimed at the tympanic membrane. Documentation of the route is essential for interpretation of the measured result.

Normal adult body temperatures are as follows:

- Oral: 35.8°C to 37.3°C (96.4 to 99.1°F)
- Axillary: 35.3°C to 36.8°C (95.9 to 99.6°F)
- Rectal: 36.3°C to 37.8°C (94.9 to 99.6°F)

Fever is an oral temperature >37.9°C (100.9°F). Hypothermia is a core body temperature (confirmed rectally) of <35.0°C (95°F)

Pulse

Pulse or heart rate is the number of palpable transmitted heartbeats in 1 minute.

- Palpate the radial pulse at the wrist (do not use your thumb).
- Count the beats for 15 seconds (or 30 seconds) and multiply by four (or two).
- Note the rhythm of the pulse during palpation: regular, irregular, regularly irregular, or irregularly irregular.

Normal adult sinus rhythm is 60 to 100 beats per minute (bpm). Bradycardia is <60 bpm. Tachycardia is >100 bpm.

Atrial fibrillation is the most common adult arrhythmia. It produces an irregularly irregular rhythm. In this setting, palpating the radial pulse will underestimate the actual ventricular response rate. Auscultate the cardiac apex to determine the heart rate.

Blood Pressure

- The patient should be seated still for at least 5 minutes (when possible) with feet resting comfortably on the floor.
- The bare upper arm should be at heart level.
- The bladder of the BP cuff should encircle at least 80% of the upper arm.
- The middle of the cuff should align with the brachial artery that was palpated just proximal to the antecubital fossa.
- The cuff should fit snugly and firmly around the bare upper arm.
- The lower edge of the cuff should be 2 to 3 cm proximal to the antecubital fossa.

Palpate

- Determine the level for maximal inflation by observing the pressure at which the radial pulse is no longer palpable as the cuff is rapidly inflated.
- Add 30 mm Hg to the measurement when the radial pulse disappears.
- Rapidly and steadily deflate the cuff.
- Wait at least 15 to 30 seconds before reinflating.

Auscultate

- Position the diaphragm of the stethoscope over the palpated brachial artery distal to the BP cuff at the antecubital fossa, making sure it is not underneath the cuff to prevent any extraneous sounds.
- Apply light pressure to the stethoscope, ensuring skin contact at all points.
- Heavy pressure may distort sounds.
- Sound generated over the vessels is relatively low in frequency; use of the bell (instead of the diaphragm) may enhance sound detection.
- Rapidly and steadily inflate the cuff 20 to 30 mm Hg above the pressure determined by palpation.
- Release the air in the cuff so that the pressure falls at a rate of 2 to 3 mm/s while auscultating the Korotkoff sounds.

- The first appearance of two consecutive faint, repetitive, tapping sounds is the systolic BP (phase I Korotkoff sounds).
- Disappearance of repetitive sounds is the diastolic BP (phase V Korotkoff sounds).
- Measure and record to the nearest 2 mm Hg.
  - Normal adult BP is <120/80 mm Hg. Prehypertension is 120 to 139/80 to 89 mm Hg.
- Hypertension is ≥140/90 mm Hg.

Orthostatic BP and pulse are defined as a systolic BP drop of >20 mm Hg or a pulse rise of >20 bpm when the patient changes from a sitting to a standing position (after waiting for at least 3 minutes on position change).

In some patients, the Korotkoff sounds temporarily disappear and then reappear as the cuff is deflated to the level below phase I. The area of disappearance is called an auscultatory gap. This may occur in 10% to 20% of the elderly hypertensive population. The cause is unknown. To avoid underestimating the systolic BP, palpate the radial pulse for the level of maximal inflation.

If the bladder of the BP cuff is too small, the BP may be falsely elevated.

Respiratory Rate

Observe the patient breathing and count the respirations for 15 seconds (or 30 seconds) and multiply by four (or two).

Normal adult RR is 8 to 20 breaths per minute. Bradypnea is RR <8. Tachypnea is RR >20. Apnea is the cessation of breath for ≥20 seconds.

Height, Weight, Body Mass Index

Although not classic VS, height and weight are typically recorded in this section. Height and weight can be used together to calculate body surface area (BSA), ideal body weight (IBW), and adjusted body weight (AdjBW).

BSA

$$\text{BSA}\ (\text{m}^2) = ((\text{height in in.} \times \text{weight in lb})/3,131)^{1/2}\ \textit{or}$$
$$((\text{height in cm} \times \text{weight in kg})/3,600)^{1/2}$$

IBW

IBW is the estimated ideal body weight in kilograms (kg):

$$\text{Males: IBW} = 50 \text{ kg} + 2.3 \text{ kg for each inch over 5 ft}$$

$$\text{Females: IBW} = 45.5 \text{ kg} + 2.3 \text{ kg for each inch over 5 ft}$$

AdjBW

AdjBW is the estimated adjusted body weight (kg).

If the actual body weight is >30% of the calculated IBW, calculate the AdjBW as follows:

$$\text{AdjBW} = \text{IBW} + 0.4\,(\text{actual weight} - \text{IBW})$$

Body Mass Index

Body mass index (BMI) is a calculation based on the height and weight of the patient.

$$\text{BMI} = \text{weight in kg/height in m}^2 \textit{ or } \text{weight in lb/height in in.}^2 \times 703$$

BMI Categories

Healthy	18.5–24.9 kg/m^2
Overweight	25–29.9 kg/m^2
Obese	≥30 kg/m^2

Pain

Assess the patient's level of pain or discomfort. Traditionally, a scale of 1 to 10 (10 being the worst imaginable pain) is used.

Skin

The integumentary system is perhaps one of the most assessable organ systems for examination. See Table 6.3 and Figure 6.1 for information on descriptive dermatologic terms and examples.

Inspect

- Color (e.g., brownness, cyanosis, yellowness or jaundice)
- Vascularity (including ecchymoses such as petechiae or purpura)
- Edema
- Temperature (use the backs of the fingers to make this relative assessment)

TABLE 6.3 Descriptive Dermatologic Terms and Examples

Lesion	Description	Example
Acneiform	Erythematous pustules	Acne
Annular	Ring shaped	Ringworm
Confluent	Lesions run together	Viral exanthems
Discoid	Disc shaped without central clearing	Lupus erythematosus
Eczematoid	An inflammation with a tendency to vesiculate and crust	Eczema
Erythroderma	Diffuse red color	Sunburn
Exfoliative	Sloughing of skin layers	Toxic epidermal necrolysis
Grouped	Clustered lesions	Vesicles of herpes simplex
Iris	Bull's-eye or target-type lesions	Erythema multiforme
Keratotic	Thickening	Psoriasis
Linear	In lines	Poison ivy
Papulosquamous	Raised papules or plaques with scaling	Psoriasis
Urticarial	Raised local edema of the skin (wheal)	Hives
Zosteriform	Linear arrangement along a dermatome	Herpes zoster

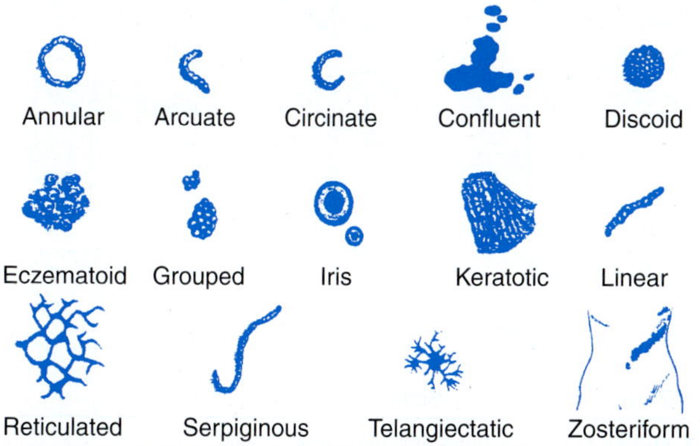

FIGURE 6.1 Descriptive dermatologic terms.

- Texture (roughness or smoothness)
- Moisture (dryness, sweating, and oiliness)
- Mobility
- Turgor (the speed with which the skin returns into place when a fold is lifted)
- Lesions

Skin lesions are described in terms of primary and secondary lesions (Fig. 6.2). Primary lesions may arise from previously normal skin and can be divided into three categories:

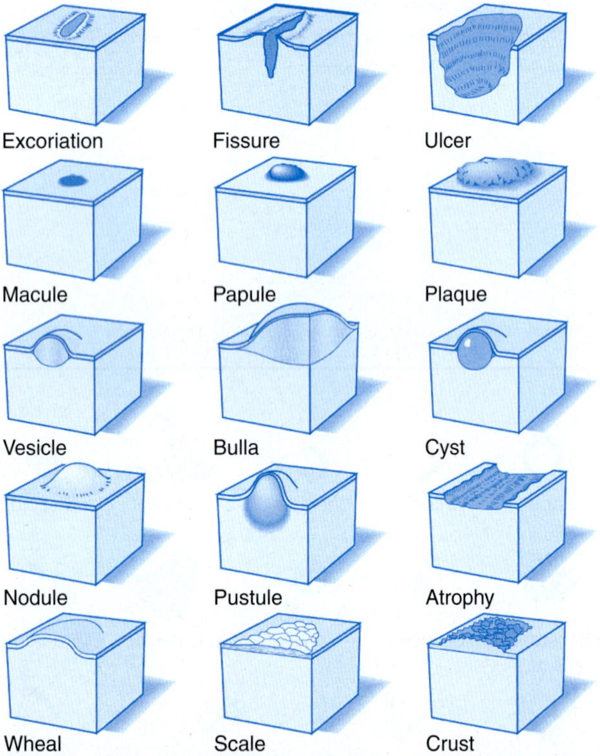

FIGURE 6.2 Basic types of skin lesions.

1. Circumscribed, flat, nonpalpable changes in skin color (macules and patches)
2. Palpable solid elevations in the skin (nodules, plaques, papules, cysts, and wheals)
3. Circumscribed superficial elevations of the skin formed by free fluid within the skin layers (vesicles, bulla, and pustules)

Secondary lesions result from changes in a primary lesion and include the development of erosions, ulcers, fissures, crusts, and scales.

Examples of skin lesions (with their potential drug culprits in parentheses) include the following:

- Acneiform or pustular (corticosteroids)
- Erythroderma (vancomycin-induced red man's syndrome)
- Exfoliation (Stevens-Johnson syndrome from sulfonamides)
- Maculopapular (beta-lactams)
- Lupus-like (procainamide, hydralazine)
- Photosensitivity (sulfonamides, fluoroquinolones, methotrexate)
- Urticaria (aspirin sensitivity)
- Hyperpigmentation (phenothiazines, hydroxychloroquine, amiodarone, oral contraceptives)

Hair

Hair is considered a skin appendage.

Inspect

- Quantity
  - Alopecia or hair loss can be total, sparse, or patchy.
    - A result of drug therapy (during or after chemotherapy), infection (fungal such as tinea capitis or ringworm), or trichotillomania (pulling, plucking, or twisting one's hair)
  - Hirsutism is the growth of hair in women in a characteristically male pattern.
  - A result of androgen excess syndromes, corticosteroids and Cushing syndrome, oral contraceptives, and androgenic medications
- Distribution
  - Hypertrichosis is increased hair growth, particularly on the face.
    - A result of an adverse effect of medications such as minoxidil and cyclosporine

Palpate

- Texture
  - Dry or coarse as seen in hypothyroidism
  - Fine and silky as seen in hyperthyroidism

Nails

Nails are considered a skin appendage. The fingernails and toenails should be examined.

Inspect

- Color
- Shape
- Lesions

Palpate

- Nail beds
  - Pitting and ridging of the nails is another common finding and is characteristic of psoriasis.
  - Beau lines (horizontal ridges on the nails) can occur during chemotherapy.

Clubbing of the fingers is the selective bullous enlargement of the distal segment of the digit due to an increase in soft tissue and is associated with flattening of the angle between the nail and nail base from 160 to 180 degrees or more (Fig. 6.3). The proximal nail bed feels spongy or floating. Clubbing can be hereditary or idiopathic and is associated with various conditions, including cyanotic heart disease and pulmonary disorders (such as chronic obstructive pulmonary disease [COPD], cystic fibrosis, tuberculosis, and lung cancer).

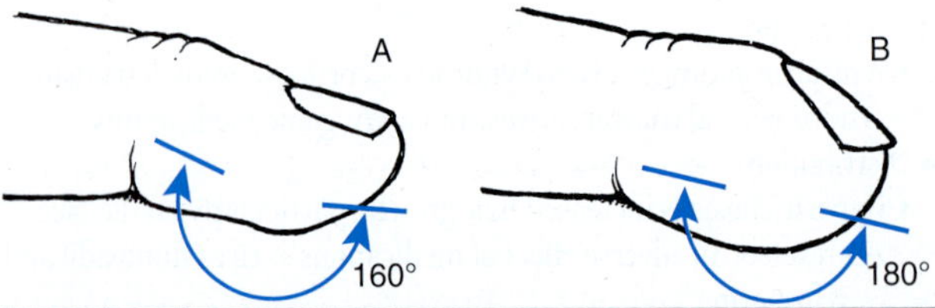

FIGURE 6.3 Clubbing of the finger. **A:** Normal angle of the nail. **B:** Abnormal angle of the nail seen in late clubbing.

Head, Eyes, Ears, Nose, Throat

Head

Inspect

- Shape (normocephalic, hydrocephalic, or microcephalic)
- Hair (described above)
- Scalp (erythema, scales, lumps, evidence of trauma)
- Skull (size, contour, deformities, lumps, or tenderness)
- Face (expression, contour, asymmetry, involuntary movements, edema, masses)
- Skin (described above)

Several disorders have characteristic facial features, including the moon facies of Cushing syndrome (or corticosteroid use), exophthalmos of Graves disease, and the masked facies of scleroderma or parkinsonism. Several skin disorders and rashes affect the face, including acne vulgaris, acne rosacea, the butterfly-pattern (malar) rash over the cheeks in systemic lupus erythematosus (SLE), and the zosteriform rash of herpes zoster.

Eyes

The anatomy of the external and internal eye is depicted in Figures 6.4 and 6.5. Physical exam on the eye involves testing the vision, inspecting the eye, assessing the pupils and ocular motility, and an ophthalmoscopic exam.

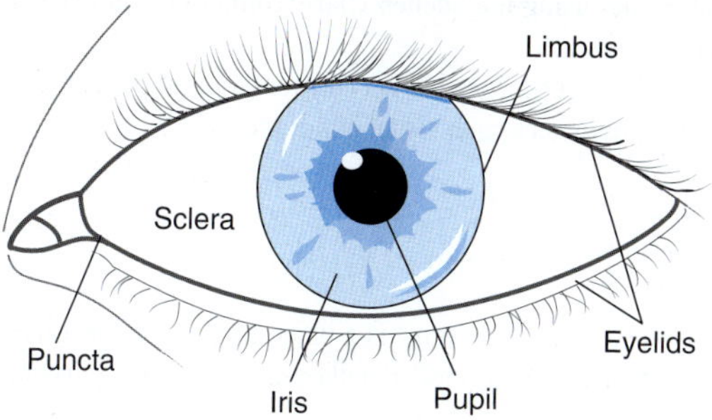

FIGURE 6.4 External anatomy of the eye. Note how the upper lid normally covers the upper rim of the iris and limbus. (Reprinted from Longe RL, Calvert JC. *Physical Assessment: A Guide for Evaluating Drug Therapy*. Vancouver, WA: Lippincott Williams & Wilkins; 1994, with permission.)

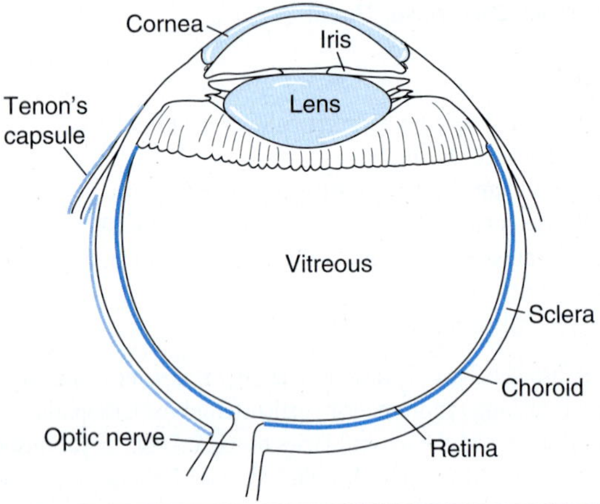

FIGURE 6.5 Internal eye and optic nerve. Diagram of the internal eye with its three layers (the retina, the choroids, and sclera) and the optic nerve, with its posterior chamber containing the lens and retina. (Reprinted from Longe RL, Calvert JC. *Physical Assessment: A Guide for Evaluating Drug Therapy*. Vancouver, WA: Lippincott Williams & Wilkins; 1994, with permission.)

Vision

- Visual acuity using the Snellen chart (commonly known as the "E" chart).
- Visual fields can be assessed via confrontation; if patient complains of blind spots, check each visual quadrant.

Inspection

- Eyebrows
- Eyelids
  - A stye (external hordeolum) is a painful tender nodule caused by a virus or bacteria; the gland/hair follicle of the eyelid margin is inflamed.
- Lashes
- Conjunctiva
  - Inflammation, mattering, or exudates (conjunctivitis or conjunctival infection).
  - Scleral icterus (a yellowish pigmentation of the sclera) signifies jaundice in a patient with a bilirubin serum concentration >2 to 3 mg/dL.

- Cornea
- Interior chamber
- Iris

Pupillary Assessment

- Reactivity to light
  - PERRLA (pupils equal, round, reactive to light and accommodation) is a typical mnemonic description.
- Pupil size
  - Anticholinergics and stimulants (cocaine and methamphetamines) may cause mydriasis or pupillary dilation.
  - Opiates may cause miosis or pinpoint pupils.
- Pupil symmetry
  - Anisocoria (a difference in the size of the pupils).
- Alignment of corneal light reflex with penlight

Ocular Motility Assessment

- Cranial nerves III, IV, and VI and the muscles they innervate
  - Muscle palsy or a cranial nerve problem could be detected if the patient is unable to follow the examiner's finger when directed up-down or left-right.
  - *Strabismus* is the lack of parallelism of the eyes' visual axes.
  - *Nystagmus* is an abnormal rapid rhythmic spontaneous movement of the eyes (i.e., under conditions of fixation, the eyes drift slowly vertically or horizontally and are corrected by a quick movement to the original position); it may be congenital or a sign of drug toxicity (phenytoin, lithium).

Direct Ophthalmoscopy

- Red reflex (a reddish-orange reflection of light from the retina)
- Optic cup/disc
  - Papilledema is reversible inflammation of the optic disc.
- Retinal blood vessels
  - Hypertension can cause extensive changes in the eye including arteriovenous (AV) nicking, hemorrhaging, exudates, and papilledema.
  - Diabetic retinopathy is characterized by early microaneurysm and exudates that can progress to proliferation of blood vessels, retinal detachment, and vitreal hemorrhage.

- Retinal background
- Macula
  - Macular edema (localized swelling or thickening of the macula) can be seen in diabetes mellitus.

Ears

The normal anatomy of the external and middle ear is depicted in Figures 6.6 and 6.7.

Inspect for deformities, lumps, or skin lesions. Inspect the normal or noninfected ear first for easier comparison.

- External ear
- Auricle
- Surrounding tissue

Palpate the pinna and tragus for tenderness:

- Suspect otitis externa (infection of the external ear) if pulling on the pinna or pressing on the tragus causes pain.

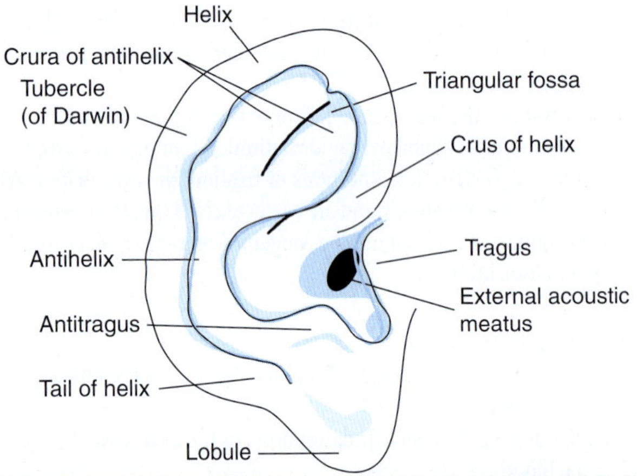

FIGURE 6.6 External ear (auricle or pinna). The helix, lobule, tragus, and external acoustic meatus (opening into the external auditory canal) are frequently used during physical examination to evaluate deeper structures. (Reprinted from Longe RL, Calvert JC. *Physical Assessment: A Guide for Evaluating Drug Therapy*. Vancouver, WA: Lippincott Williams & Wilkins; 1994, with permission.)

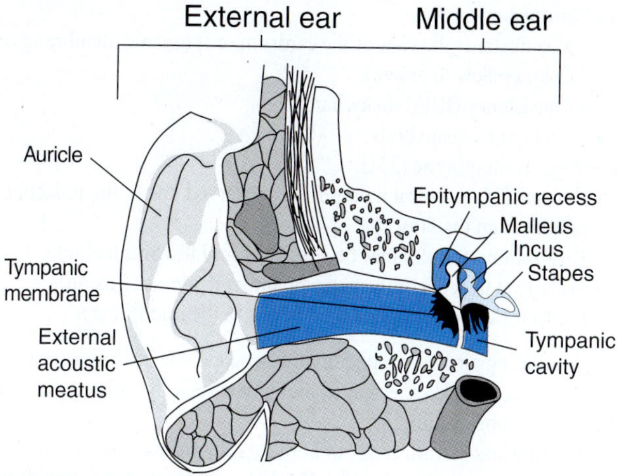

FIGURE 6.7 Three compartments of the ear. The three compartments of the ear include the external ear (auricle to tympanic membrane), middle ear (tympanic membrane to round window of inner ear), and inner ear. (Reprinted from Longe RL, Calvert JC. *Physical Assessment: A Guide for Evaluating Drug Therapy*. Vancouver, WA: Lippincott Williams & Wilkins; 1994, with permission.)

- Suspect otitis media (infection of the middle ear) if pressing firmly behind the ear causes pain or is tender.

Before inserting the otoscope, gently pull the auricle upward, backward, and away from the head so the ear canal is straightened. Holding the otoscope between the thumb and index finger, brace your hand against the patient's face to ensure your hand and instrument will move with the patient and any unexpected movements. Insert the speculum gently into the ear canal, moving it through any hair and in a downward and forward direction. Move the speculum so you can see as much of the tympanic membrane or drum as possible.

Inspect

- External auditory canal
  - Redness
  - Inflammation
  - Discharge

- Cerumen or ear wax
  - May obstruct the view of the eardrum or tympanic membrane
  - Color (yellow to brown)
  - Consistency (flaky, sticky, hard)
- Presence of foreign body

- Tympanic membrane (TM)
  - Normal TM: a conical light reflex is observed due to the reflection of light from the otoscope.
  - Perforations or holes may be a result of middle ear infection.
  - Color (red in acute otitis media or amber if serous effusion).
  - Contour (bulging suggests fluid or pus in the middle ear).

By insufflating air using a pneumatic otoscope, the TM's ease of mobility can be assessed. Decreased mobility is seen in otitis media and eustachian tube dysfunction.

Hearing loss can affect one or both ears. To estimate hearing or auditory acuity, test one ear at a time. Occlude one ear at a time, stand 1 to 2 ft away from the patient and whisper a word or number of two equally accented syllables ("baseball" or "three-four") toward the unoccluded ear. You may need to increase the intensity of the whisper, possibly to a soft, medium, or loud voice. Cover your lips or ask the patient to close the eyes to avoid lip reading. If hearing is decreased, it is important to distinguish between conductive or sensorineural hearing loss. See Table 6.4 for an explanation of the differences and instructions on how to perform the physical exam to assess these patterns of hearing loss. A tuning fork (512 or 1,024 Hz) and a quiet room are needed.

Nose and Sinuses

Inspect

- Nose
  - Asymmetry or deformities
  - Swelling
  - Septal defects
  - Discharge
- Nasal mucosa: A penlight or an otoscope may be used to view inside the nostrils or nasal vestibules. The nasal mucosa is normally a bit redder than the oral mucosa.
  - Swelling
  - Bleeding
  - Exudates (clear, purulent, or mucopurulent)

TABLE 6.4 Conductive Hearing Loss Versus Sensorineural Hearing Loss

	Conductive Loss	Sensorineural Loss
	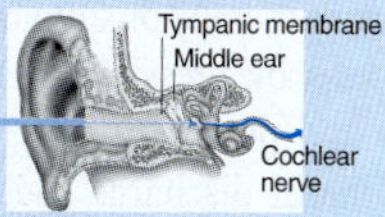	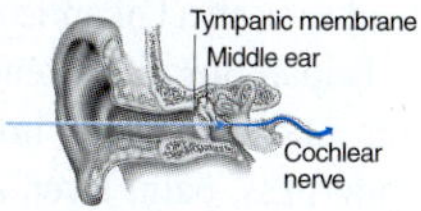
Pathophysiology	External or middle ear disorder impairs sound conduction to inner ear. Causes include foreign body, otitis media, perforated eardrum, and otosclerosis ossicles	Inner ear disorder involves cochlear nerve and neuronal impulse transmission to the brain. Causes include loud noise exposure, inner ear infections, trauma, tremors, congenital and familial disorders, and aging
Usual age of onset	Childhood and young adulthood, up to 40 years of age	Middle or later years
Ear canal and drum	Abnormality usually visible, except in otosclerosis	Problem not visible
Effects	• Little effect on sound • Hearing seems to improve in noisy environment • Voice becomes soft because inner ear and cochlear nerve are intact	• Higher registers are lost, so sound may be distorted • Hearing worsens in noisy environment • Voice may be loud because hearing is difficult
Weber test (in unilateral hearing loss)	• Tuning fork at vertex • Sound lateralizes to impaired ear—room noise not well heard, so detection of vibrations improves	• Tuning fork at vertex • Sound lateralizes to good ear—inner ear or cochlear nerve damage impairs transmission to affected ear
Rinne test	• Tuning fork at external auditory meatus and then on mastoid bone • Bone conduction longer than or equal to air conduction (BC ≥ AC). While air conduction through the external or middle ear is impaired, vibrations through bone bypass the problem to reach the cochlea	• Tuning fork at external auditory meatus and then on mastoid bone • Air conduction longer than bone conduction (AC > BC). The inner ear or cochlear nerve is less able to transmit impulses regardless of how the vibrations reach the cochlea. The normal pattern prevails

Reprinted from Bickley LS, Szilagyi PG. *Bates' Guide to Physical Examination and History Taking*. 9th ed. Philadelphia, PA: Lippincott Williams & Wilkins; 2007, with permission.

In allergic rhinitis, the mucosa may be pale, bluish, or red. In viral rhinitis, the mucosa may be reddened and swollen. *Rhinitis medicamentosa*, a side effect of prolonged nasal vasoconstrictor therapy, may manifest as mucosal swelling and edema. *Epistaxis*, a nosebleed, may represent an adverse effect of anticoagulant therapy or steroid nasal spray.

Palpate for sinus tenderness by pressing on the frontal sinuses from under the bony brows and pressing on the maxillary sinuses. Tenderness, pain, fever, and nasal discharge suggest acute sinusitis involving the respective sinuses.

Throat (or Mouth and Pharynx)

Inspect

- Lips (color, moisture, ulcers, lumps, cracking)
- Oral mucosa (color, ulcers, white patches, nodules)
- Gums (color)
- Teeth (missing, discolored, loose)
- Roof of the mouth (color and architecture)
- Tongue (symmetry, color, texture, sides, undersides)
- Floor of the mouth (color, ulcerations)
- Pharynx (color, symmetry, exudates, swelling, ulcerations, and tonsillar enlargement)
    - Ask the patient to open the mouth very wide and say "ah." A tongue blade placed firmly down the midpoint of the tongue may help to see the pharynx better. Be careful not to place the tongue blade too far back or you may cause gagging.

Visual examination of the mouth and oropharynx can identify a number of diseases and adverse drug manifestations. Cyanosis of the lips might indicate hypoxemia. Gingival hyperplasia can be caused by phenytoin. *Stomatitis* (mouth sores) is a common complication of cytotoxic drugs. *Xerostomia* (dry mouth) is observed as a lack of saliva and can be caused by various connective tissue diseases (e.g., SLE, rheumatoid arthritis [RA], Sjögren syndrome) and medications (e.g., anticholinergics). Infectious disease manifestations include pharyngitis, erythema (with or without exudates), oral thrush/candidiasis (e.g., in immunocompromised patients or infants), and herpetic lesions. Aphthous stomatitis is a common nonspecific painful ulceration of the buccal mucosa. Hairy leukoplakia, a common manifestation of acquired immune deficiency syndrome, appears as a white, raised lesion on the lateral margins of the tongue.

Neck

Inspect

- Symmetry
- Masses
- Scars
- Abnormal pulsations
- Enlarged lymph nodes
- Distention of the jugular veins (described below in the "Blood Vessels" section)
- Deviation of the trachea
- Range of motion
- Goiter
  - The normal neck should be soft, supple, and without masses or enlargement of the thyroid gland.

Lymph Nodes

There are many lymph nodes in the face and neck. To palpate the lymph nodes, use the pads on the index and middle fingers to move the skin over the underlying tissues in a gentle circular motion. The patient should be relaxed with the neck flexed slightly forward and toward the side being examined. Both sides can be examined at the same time when the examiner is standing in front of the patient. See Figure 6.8 for locations of the lymph nodes in the face and neck. The cervical, submandibular, and supraclavicular are most commonly examined.

Palpate the nodes and note the following:

- Discrete or matted together
- Size
- Shape (round, oblong, irregular or smooth)
- Mobility
- Consistency (hard, soft, rubbery, fluid filled)
- Tenderness

Normal nodes are nontender, discrete, mobile, and small. Tender nodes suggest inflammation, which may be a result of infection. Hard or fixed nodes suggest malignancy. If nodes are enlarged, it is important to determine between regional or generalized lymphadenopathy.

Blood Vessels

Before palpating the carotid artery, look for carotid pulsations medial to the sternomastoid muscles. Place your index and middle finger on

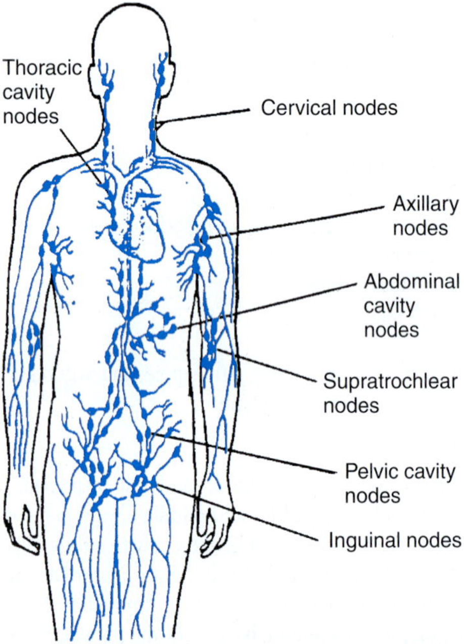

FIGURE 6.8 Location of lymph nodes in the body.

the carotid artery in the lower third of the neck; pressing posteriorly, feel for pulsations. Do not palpate both carotid arteries simultaneously. To assess for amplitude and duration, the patient should be reclined at a 30-degree angle. A delayed upstroke is characteristic of aortic stenosis. A bounding pulse is characteristic of high-stroke volume states such as aortic regurgitation. Auscultation of the carotid arteries can detect bruits (a blowing or turbulent sound caused by blood flowing past an obstruction such as an atherosclerotic narrowing).

Jugular venous distention (JVD) reflects central venous pressure as seen in Figure 6.9. With the patient reclining at a 30-degree angle, apply pressure over the liver and observe subsequent neck vein distention. This is known as the hepatojugular reflux test, and it assesses liver congestion and right ventricular function. The height of distention is measured in centimeters above the sternal angle. JVD >3 cm is

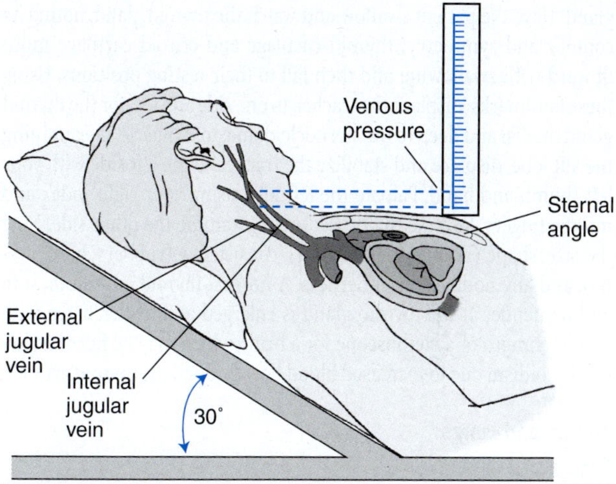

FIGURE 6.9 Assessment of jugular venous pressure. Place the patient supine in bed and gradually raise the head of the bed to 30, 45, 60, and 90 degrees. Using tangential lighting, note the highest level of venous pulsation. Measure the vertical distance between this point and the sternal angle. Record the distance in centimeters and the angle of the head of bed. (Reprinted from Instructors Resource CD-ROM to Accompany *Critical Care Nursing: A Holistic Approach*. 8th ed. Philadelphia, PA: Lippincott Williams & Wilkins; 2005, with permission.)

considered positive for volume overload. JVD is decreased in patients who are hypovolemic. JVD is increased in patients with congestive heart failure (CHF), right ventricular dysfunction, cardiac tamponade, and cor pulmonale. In normal patients, JVD rises temporarily and returns to normal within a few seconds because the body can compensate for the shift in pressure and volume.

Thyroid Gland

The thyroid gland can be palpated from either the front or the back of the patient. With the patient seated comfortably, palpate down the midline of the neck to feel the hyoid bone, thyroid cartilage, cricoid cartilage, and trachea. Diseases or masses in the neck or thorax (mediastinal mass, atelectasis, or pneumothorax) may push the trachea to one side. With the patient's head tilted back a bit, inspect the thyroid gland. Have the patient swallow and watch the thyroid gland, noting its contour and symmetry; thyroid cartilage and cricoid cartilage move upward with swallowing and then fall to their resting positions. Using these landmarks, displace the trachea to one side and feel for the thyroid gland medial and deep to the sternocleidomastoid muscle. If examining the left lobe, displace and stabilize the trachea to the left side with your left thumb and hand. Palpate the left lobe using your right index and middle fingers. Reverse the procedure to examine the other side. Note the size, shape (nodular or irregular), consistency (rubbery, hard, cystic), and any nodules or tenderness. A normal thyroid is smooth, soft, and nontender. If the thyroid gland is enlarged and tender, listen with the diaphragm of a stethoscope for a bruit, which may be heard in hyperthyroidism due to increased blood flow through the thyroid arteries.

Thorax and Lungs

General

Examination of the chest necessitates inspection, percussion, palpation, and auscultation. Because pulmonary and cardiac diseases are commonly associated, it is critical to do a thorough evaluation of both systems (see "Cardiovascular System" on page 161).

Inspection

- Look for any signs of respiratory difficulty.
  - Assess color of patient for cyanosis.
  - Listen to the patient breathing.
  - Inspect the neck for use of accessory muscles to help the patient breathe.
  - Check for symmetry with respiratory efforts.

Note the shape of the chest and any deformities (Fig. 6.10).

Palpation

- Areas of tenderness (pain, lesions, or bruises)
- Masses
- Tactile fremitus (normal vibration that can be felt on the thoracic wall during phonation)

Percussion

Percussion helps to determine whether tissue is air filled, fluid filled, or solid.

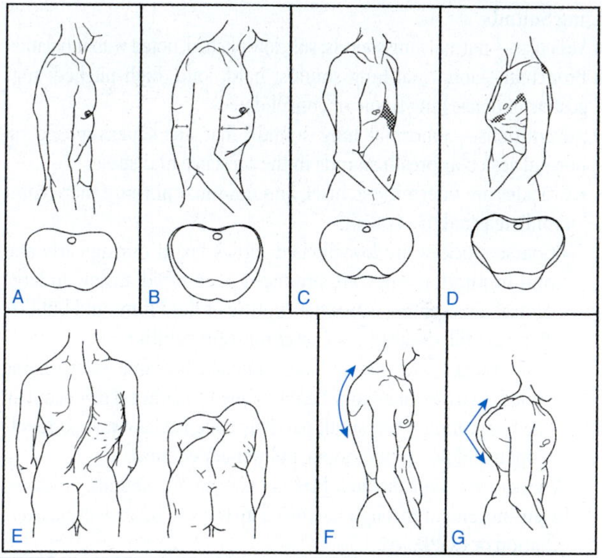

FIGURE 6.10 Chest wall contours. **A:** Normal. **B:** Barrel chest associated with emphysema. **C:** Pectus excavatum (i.e., funnel chest). **D:** Pectus carinatum (i.e., pigeon breast). **E:** Scoliosis. **F:** Kyphosis. **G:** Gibbus (i.e., extreme kyphosis). (Reprinted from Longe RL, Calvert JC. *Physical Assessment: A Guide for Evaluating Drug Therapy*. Vancouver, WA: Lippincott Williams & Wilkins; 1994, with permission.)

- Right and left sides, spine and costovertebral angles (CVAs) for tenderness
  - Resonant (normal)
  - Flat or dull (consolidation, pleural effusion, atelectasis)
  - Hyperresonant or tympanitic (pneumothorax or emphysema)

Lungs

Auscultate the anterior and posterior lung fields using the diaphragm of a stethoscope on the skin of the chest wall (not over clothing). Auscultation involves listening to the sounds generated by breathing and for any added (adventitious) sounds. If abnormalities are detected, listen to the sounds of the patient's spoken or whispered words as they are transmitted through the chest wall.

Lung Sounds

- Vesicular—normal lung sounds; soft, low pitched, noted with inhalation
- Bronchial—abnormal lung sounds; hard, loud, high-pitched, suggestive of dense lung tissue or consolidated
- Adventitious—abnormal lung sounds that are superimposed on normal vesicular breath sounds in the presence of disease
  - Crackles are intermittent, brief, and not musical (once more commonly referred to as rales).
    - Coarse crackles are low-pitched rattles heard during early and mid inspiration. They are produced from rapid airflow in large central airways that cause the rupture of fluid films and bubbles along air-filled walls (acute or chronic bronchitis).
    - Fine crackles are soft and high-pitched like fine Velcro being pulled apart or like hairs being rubbed together. They occur in late inspiration when small partially collapsed airways suddenly reopen and pop (pneumonia, pulmonary edema).
  - Wheezes are high-pitched, hissing, continuous sounds produced by air movement through narrowed airways as in an asthma exacerbation or COPD.
  - Rhonchi are low-pitched, snoring, continuous sounds that are suggestive of secretions in the airways.
  - Rubs are loud and creaky sounds caused by two inflamed pleural areas rubbing together.
- Transmitted voice—normally the sounds transmitted through the chest wall are muffled and indistinct.
  - Bronchophony is an increase in the clarity of spoken voice sounds.
  - Whispered pectoriloquy is an increase in clarity of whispered voice sounds (indicative of lung consolidation).
  - Egophony is a nasal bleating sound detected when the spoken letter "E" sounds more like "A" (indicative of lung consolidation).

Back

Examination of the back discloses any spinal deformities (e.g., scoliosis, kyphosis) or tenderness. Conditions of endogenous or exogenous corticosteroid excess can produce a "buffalo hump" over the upper back. Kyphosis in the elderly can occur due to osteoporosis.

The CVA, the angle formed by the lower border of the 12th rib and the transverse process of the upper lumbar vertebrae, defines the area to assess for kidney tenderness. Tenderness in the posterior flank or CVA tenderness is a classic sign of pyelonephritis.

Cardiovascular System

It is best to have the patient supine and examine from the right of the patient.

Inspect and Palpate

- The point of maximal impulse (PMI) is palpable in only 30% of adults (Fig. 6.11).
  - Palpate at or medial to the midclavicular line between the 4th and 5th intercostal space (ICS).
  - Normal PMI is <2 cm diameter in the supine position and <4 cm in the partial left lateral decubitus position.
- A *heave* or *lift* is a sustained, systolic outward movement of the precordium associated with heart failure.
- A *thrill* is a palpable vibration (like a cat purring) felt when a cardiac murmur is grade IV to VI/VI.

Auscultate

- Listen for several cardiac cycles to determine if there are additional sounds other than S1 and S2 ("lub-dub"). Focus on systole for a few cycles and then on diastole, listening for extra sounds or murmurs.

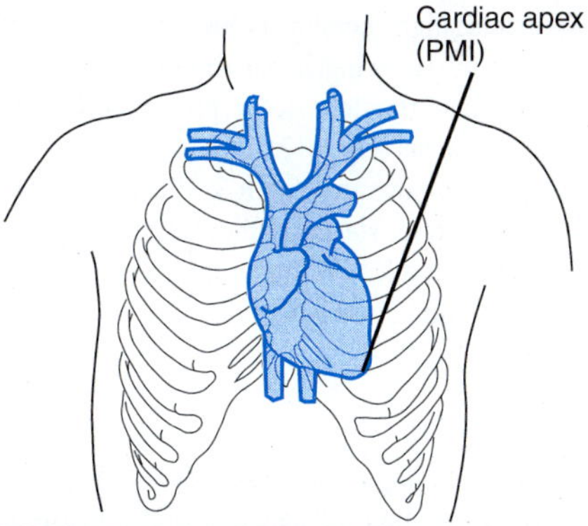

FIGURE 6.11 Surface topography of the heart. PMI, point of maximal impulse. (Reprinted from Longe RL, Calvert JC. *Physical Assessment: A Guide for Evaluating Drug Therapy*. Vancouver, WA: Lippincott Williams & Wilkins; 1994, with permission.)

- S1 is heard the loudest at the apex. It occurs with closure of the mitral and tricuspid valves at the onset of ventricular systole.
- S2 is heard loudest between the 2nd and 3rd ICS. It occurs with closure of the aortic and pulmonic valves at the end of systole.
- S3 is best heard with the bell of the stethoscope at the apex. It occurs during early diastole when blood is flowing into an overfilled noncompliant ventricle and suddenly decelerates. It is normal in young adults; age older than 40 years suggests severe systolic heart failure or valvular regurgitation. S3 occurs after S2 and sounds like "lub-dub-dah."
- S4 is best heard with the bell of the stethoscope at the apex. It occurs in late diastole when the atrial contraction pushes blood into the left ventricle that is stiff as seen in hypertrophy. S4 precedes S1 and sounds like "luh-lub-dub."
- If a murmur is heard (use diaphragm of stethoscope), it should be graded and described:
  - Grades I–III (thrill absent)
    - I: hard to hear, faint
    - II: quiet, but heard immediately with stethoscope
    - III: moderately loud
  - Grades IV–VI (thrill present)
    - IV: loud, heard with stethoscope on chest
    - V: very loud, heard with edge of stethoscope on chest
    - VI: very loud, heard with stethoscope off the chest
  - Pitch of murmur: high, medium, or low
  - Quality of murmur: blowing, harsh, rumbling, musical

- Using the diaphragm of the stethoscope, press firmly on bare skin in a quiet room in four areas (Fig. 6.12).
  - Cardiac apex (mitral valve area, 5th ICS, S1 is louder than S2)
  - Tricuspid area (left lower sternal border [LLSB])
  - Pulmonic area (left 2nd ICS, S2 louder than S1)
  - Aortic area (right 2nd ICS, S2 louder than S1)

Breasts and Axillae

Breasts

Breast examination is an important component of the physical examination and involves inspection and palpation of the breasts and nipples in women and men. Examination of the breasts in women should be completed in four views—arms at sides, arms over head, arms pressed against hips, and leaning forward. These views may reveal dimpling or retraction, which suggests an underlying cancer.

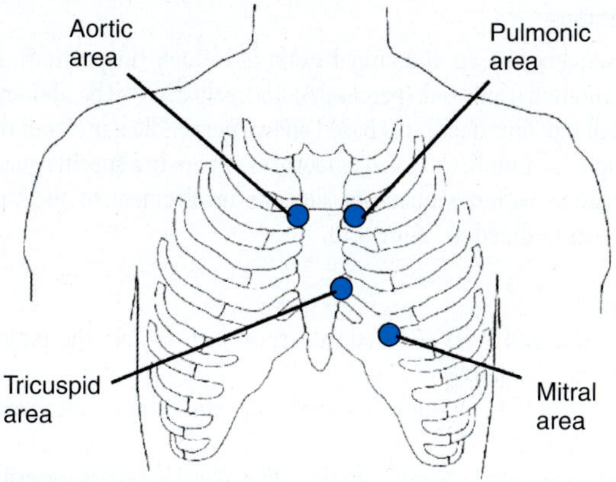

FIGURE 6.12 Location sites for auscultating the heart. (Reprinted from Longe RL, Calvert JC. *Physical Assessment: A Guide for Evaluating Drug Therapy*. Vancouver, WA: Lippincott Williams & Wilkins; 1994, with permission.)

Inspection

- Skin—color; large pores or thickening
- Breasts—size, symmetry, contour (masses, dimpling, or flattening)
- Nipples—size, symmetry, direction in which they point, rashes, ulcerations, discharge

Palpation

- Breast tissue—consistency, tenderness, nodules
- Nipple—elasticity, nodules, swelling, ulcerations

Axillae

Inspection and palpation of the axillae should be performed with the patient in a sitting position.

Inspection

- Skin of each axilla (rash, infection, unusual pigmentation)

Palpation

- Axillary nodes—the central nodes are most often palpable; if the central nodes are tender, large, or hard, palpate the other groups of axillary lymph nodes (pectoral, lateral, and subscapular nodes)

Abdomen

The sequence of an abdominal exam is to look (inspection), listen (auscultation), and feel (percussion and palpation). The abdomen is divided into four quadrants based on two perpendicular planes drawn through the umbilicus. Noted tenderness or pain in a specific quadrant or location within a quadrant suggests involvement of the various organs as outlined in Figure 6.13.

Inspection

- Presence and level of patient distress (does it hurt the patient to move or cough?)
- Contour (flat, rounded, scaphoid, distention—localized or generalized)
- Skin (scars, striae [stretch marks], dilated veins, rashes, or lesions)
- Masses
- Pulsations (normal aortic pulsation is visible in the epigastrium)

Auscultation

Auscultate to listen for bowel sounds and for bruits.

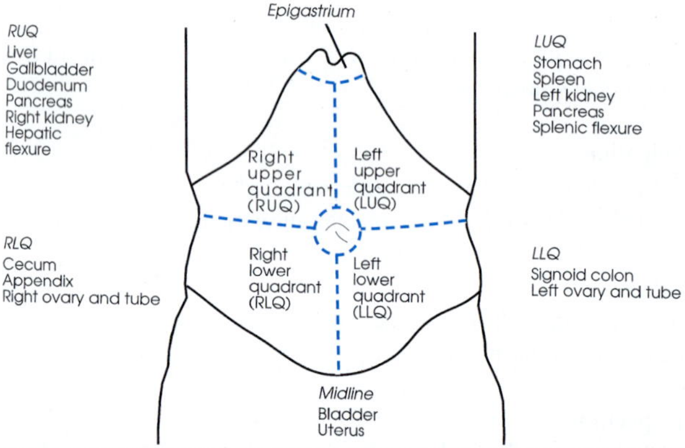

FIGURE 6.13 Location of physical findings in the abdomen are described in terms of the four-quadrant scheme as shown. (Reprinted from Longe RL, Calvert JC. *Physical Assessment: A Guide for Evaluating Drug Therapy*. Vancouver, WA: Lippincott Williams & Wilkins; 1994, with permission.)

- Listen in one place until bowel sounds are heard (normal rate 5–34/minute):
  - Normal bowel sounds (borborygmi) are generally gurgling and relatively low pitched.
  - In bowel obstruction, sounds can be high pitched and tinkling.
  - In complete obstruction, no bowel sounds will be heard (listen for at least 2 minutes).
- Bruits can occur with pathologic arterial stenosis but are also common in normal adults:
  - Midabdominal bruit may suggest atherosclerotic disease in abdominal aorta.
  - Flank bruit may suggest atherosclerotic disease in renal arteries.
  - Hepatic bruit may suggest carcinoma of the liver or alcoholic hepatitis.

Percussion

Percuss all four quadrants and over any suspicious areas of abdominal asymmetry or swelling.

- General
  - Normal abdomen should have tympanitic areas (gas-filled bowel) and dull areas (fluid-filled bowel).
  - Normal pattern is more tympanitic than dull.
- Liver
  - Determine liver span, which is directly correlated to liver size (normal span is 6 to 12 cm).
  - Palpate in all four quadrants once, then again more deeply.
- Abdominal tenderness
  - *Guarding* is voluntary contraction of the abdominal musculature due to fear, the patient's anxiety, the examiner's cold hands, or tenderness.
  - Rebound is abdominal tenderness that is worse when the palpating fingers are quickly removed from the area being palpated.
  - Rigidity is involuntary contraction of the abdominal musculature in response to peritonitis.
- Abdominal mass
- Liver—normal-sized liver generally does not distend more than 1 to 2 cm below the right costal margin
  - Spleen.
  - Descending aorta.
  - Assess for enlargement in people older than 50 years or in those with risk factors for vascular disease.

Peripheral Vascular System

To assess the peripheral vascular system, inspect the arms and legs, palpate pulses, and look for edema. See Figure 6.14 for location of peripheral pulses.

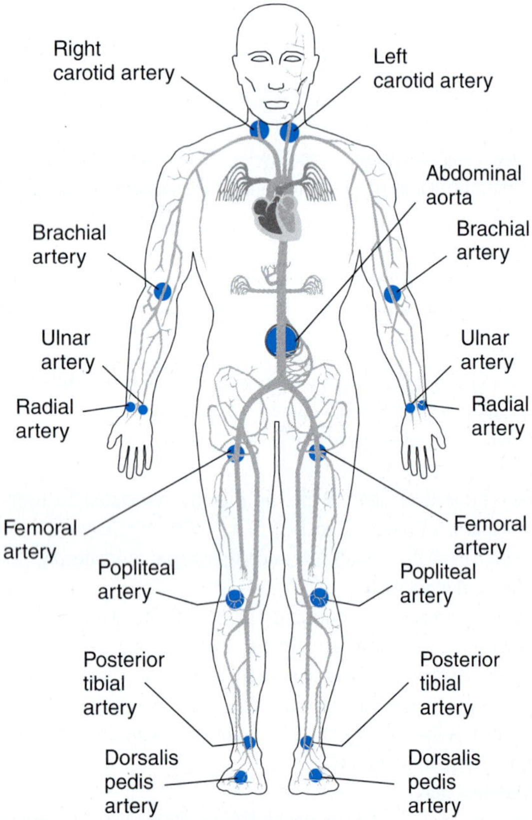

FIGURE 6.14 Locations of peripheral pulses. (Reprinted from Longe RL, Calvert JC. *Physical Assessment: A Guide for Evaluating Drug Therapy*. Vancouver, WA: Lippincott Williams & Wilkins; 1994, with permission.)

Examination of the Arms

- Size, symmetry, edema, color
- Radial and brachial pulses

Examination of the Legs

- Size, symmetry, edema, color
- Femoral, popliteal, dorsal pedis, and posterior tibial pulses
- Peripheral edema

Several different grading systems are used to characterize peripheral pulses. One such system describes a gradation of pulse intensity from 0 to 4+, with 0 being the absence of a pulse, 3+ being normal, and 4+ denoting a bounding (strong and forceful) pulse. See example in Table 6.5.

Edema may be pitting or nonpitting. Pitting refers to a noticeable transient indentation in the tissue subsequent to firm pressure with the fingertips over a bony surface and reflects displacement of the excess interstitial fluid. Pitting is graded depending on severity from trace to 4+. It is also important to note the location of the pitting edema (i.e., foot, ankle, midshin, knee, etc.).

Genitourinary and Rectal System

Male

The male GU examination is performed with the patient in the upright position. The penis is examined for skin lesions (e.g., syphilitic ulcers, chancroid, herpetic lesions, condyloma) and urethral discharge (suggesting a sexually transmitted disease). If the foreskin is present,

TABLE 6.5 Sample Recording System for Peripheral Pulses

Pulse	Right	Left
Carotid	2/4	2/4
Brachial	2+	2+
Radial	3+	3+
Femoral	3+	3+
Popliteal	2+	2+
Dorsalis pedis (DP)	1+	0
Posttibial (PT)	1+	1+

retract it or ask the patient to retract it and look for chancres and carcinomas. Phimosis is the inability to retract the foreskin.

The inguinal area is examined for skin rashes (e.g., tinea cruris, *Candida*). Hernias present as inguinal or scrotal masses. A bulge that appears on straining is suggestive of a hernia. An incarcerated hernia cannot be reduced by pushing the contents back through the defect in the abdominal wall musculature. Other scrotal masses include varicoceles (dilated scrotal veins) and hydroceles (fluid collections are translucent on transillumination with a bright light). Testicular size and masses are noted. Testicular self-examination is important for early diagnosis of cancer. Testicular atrophy can accompany alcoholism. Testicular tenderness is noted in testicular torsion (an acute GU emergency) or orchitis. Epididymal tenderness is present in epididymitis.

Female

The female pelvic examination is typically performed in the dorsal lithotomy (supine with legs in stirrups) position on a specialized examination table. The examination consists of an examination of the external genitalia, a speculum examination, and a bimanual examination of the pelvic organs. The speculum examination allows direct visualization of the vagina and cervix. Appropriate specimens are obtained to evaluate vaginitis or sexually transmitted diseases. The Papanicolaou (Pap) smear is taken to detect cervical cancer. The bimanual examination is so named because both hands are used to examine the pelvic organs (one internally and the other externally, on the abdominal wall). The cervix is examined for cervical motion tenderness, suggesting pelvic inflammatory disease. The uterus and ovaries (adnexa) are examined for size, tenderness, and the presence of masses.

Rectal Examination

The rectal examination includes palpation of the prostate gland in men to screen for malignancy or enlargement. The prostate is examined for nodules (suggesting cancer) and tenderness (suggesting prostatitis). A normal prostate should feel rubbery, for example, as when pushing the thumb tightly to the little finger. Firm areas identified on prostate examination should be referred for further evaluation.

The rectal examination in men and women should include visual inspection for lumps, ulcers, inflammation, rashes, or excoriations and palpation of the rectum in all directions to identify any masses. The tone of the anal sphincter, the presence of hemorrhoids (internal or external), fissures, or masses should be noted. If stool is present, it can be tested for occult blood (as a screen for malignancy or occult gastrointestinal bleeding). Normally the muscles of the anal sphincter close snugly around the finger. Altered anal sphincter tone may be a sign of neurologic dysfunction.

Musculoskeletal System

The musculoskeletal system comprises the supporting structures of the body such as bones, joints, tendons, ligaments, and musculature.

Joint Examination

- Bony deformities, symmetry, alignment
- Swelling or effusions
- Temperature
- Redness
- Tenderness
- Strength and range of motion
- Surrounding tissue for nodules, skin changes, muscle atrophy, crepitus (an audible or palpable crunching during movements of ligaments or tendons over the bone)

Two common types of arthritis, osteoarthritis (OA) and RA, have differing patterns of joint involvement. OA often affects the large weight-bearing joints—the knees, hips, and spine—causing swelling and bony proliferation. In the hands, OA affects the proximal and distal interphalangeal (PIP and DIP) joints due to nodules known as Bouchard and Heberden nodes, respectively. Although RA can also affect weight-bearing joints, it classically causes symmetrical small joint arthritis, particularly of the hands, wrists, elbows, and feet. In contrast to OA, RA affects the metacarpophalangeal joints (MCP) and PIP joints of the hands by causing joint inflammation, swelling, warmth, and pain and spares the DIP joints. A joint's range of motion can become limited by a number of diseases that affect the joint. Improvements in symptoms and examination findings can occur with disease-modifying agents for certain arthritic diseases.

The musculature or motor system is examined for bulk, strength, tone, tenderness, and the presence of abnormal spontaneous movements (e.g., fasciculations). Examination of the motor system is part of the neurologic examination and is discussed in that section.

Nervous System

Mental Status

A detailed neurologic assessment is an important component of a geriatric physical examination. Impairment of cognitive and motor/sensory function in this population may severely affect quality-of-life issues and level of function.

Examine

- Appearance (dress, grooming, personal hygiene)
- Behavior (level of consciousness—alert, awake, obtunded, stupor, coma)
- Speech and language
  - Quantity (talkative, silent, responsive to direct questioning, spontaneous comments)
  - Rate
  - Loudness
  - Articulation (clear, distinct, nasal quality)
  - Fluency (rate, flow, and melody of speech; content; and use of words)
- Mood and affect
- Thoughts and perceptions
  - Thought processes (logic, organization, relevance, coherence, repetition, confabulation)
  - Thought content (compulsions, obsessions, phobias, anxieties, delusions, feelings of unreality or depersonalization)
  - Perceptions (illusions, hallucinations)
  - Insight and judgment
- Cognition: There are many tests available to screen for cognitive dysfunction or dementia such as the Mini Mental State Exam (MMSE).[2]
  - Orientation (time, place, person)
  - Attention (common tests include digit span, serial 7s, spell the word WORLD backward)
  - Remote memory (inquire about past historical events, birthdays, anniversaries, etc.)
  - Recent memory (inquire about the events of the day that you can confirm)
  - Information and vocabulary (e.g., name the last four presidents)
  - Calculations (use simple addition and progress to multiplication)
  - Abstract thinking (ask patient how an apple and an orange are alike)
  - Constructional ability (ask the patient to draw a clock face complete with numbers and hands)

Cranial Nerves

The functions of the 12 cranial nerves (CN I to XII) are described in Table 6.6. A common mnemonic uses the first letter of each word in the following sentence: "*On Old Olympus' Towering Tops, A Finn And German Viewed Some Hops*" to identify the 12 cranial nerves (olfactory, optic, oculomotor, trochlear, trigeminal, abducens, facial, acoustic, glossopharyngeal, vagus, spinal accessory, and hypoglossal).

TABLE 6.6 Cranial Nerves and Their Functions

Cranial Nerves	Function
Olfactory (I)	Sensory: smell reception and interpretation
Optic (II)	Sensory: visual acuity and visual fields
Oculomotor (III)	Motor: raise eyelids, most extraocular movements, changes of lens shape and papillary constriction
Trochlear (IV)	Motor: inward and downward eye movement
Trigeminal (V)	Motor: chewing, mastication, jaw opening and clenching Sensory: sensation to facial skin, ear, tongue, nasal and mouth mucosa, cornea, iris, lacrimal glands, conjunctiva, eyelids, forehead, and nose
Abducens (VI)	Motor: lateral eye movement
Facial (VII)	Motor: movement of facial expression muscles except jaw, close eyes, labial speech sounds (m, b, w, and round vowels) Sensory: taste, anterior two-thirds of tongue, sensation to pharynx Parasympathetic: secretion of tears and saliva
Acoustic (VIII)	Sensory: hearing and balance of equilibrium
Glossopharyngeal (IX)	Motor: voluntary muscles for phonation or swallowing Sensory: sensation of nasopharynx, gag reflex, taste posterior one-third of tongue Parasympathetic: secretion of salivary glands, carotid reflex
Vagus (X)	Motor: voluntary muscles of phonation (guttural speech sounds) and swallowing Sensory: sensation behind ear and part of external ear canal Parasympathetic: secretion of digestive enzymes, peristalsis, carotid reflex, involuntary action of heart, lungs, and digestive tract
Spinal accessory (XI)	Motor: turn head, shrug shoulders, some actions for phonation and swallowing
Hypoglossal (XII)	Motor: tongue movement for speech sound articulation (l, t, n) and swallowing

Motor System

When examining the motor system, pay attention to body position, involuntary movements, coordination, and the characteristics of the muscle (bulk, tone, strength). Use this sequence when examining the arms, legs, and trunk. If an abnormality is discovered, think about its origin (central or peripheral) and what nerves innervate the area.

- Body position (at rest and during movement)
- Involuntary movements (tremors, tics, fasciculations)
- Muscle bulk (compare size and contour)
- Muscle tone (resistance to passive stretching)
- Muscle strength (Table 6.7)
- Coordination (rapid alternating movements, point-to-point movements, gait, stance)

Sensory System

In evaluating a sensory abnormality, the clinician tests whether a deficit fits a dermatomal distribution, indicating dorsal root involvement (Figs. 6.15 and 6.16), or the distribution of a collection of spinal segments, constituting a peripheral nerve (peripheral neuropathy).

- Pain (use a sharp object for a pinprick to assess sharp vs dull).
- Temperature (hot versus cold; may omit if pain sensation is normal)
- Light touch (use soft piece of cotton)
- Vibration (tuning fork of 128 Hz vibrating on pad of large toe, not the bone)
- Position (move digit upward or downward and have the patient verbalize the direction of movement)

TABLE 6.7 Muscle Strength Grading

Grade	Muscle Strength
0	No muscle contraction
1	Flicker or trace of contraction
2	Movement possible, but not against gravity
3	Moves against gravity, but not against resistance
4	Can move against resistance
5	Normal strength

(*Text continued on page 177*)

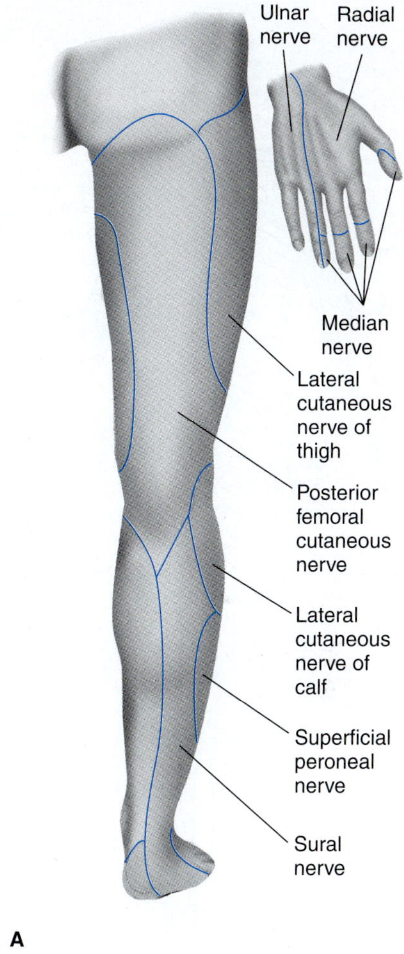

FIGURE 6.15 **A:** Areas innervated by peripheral nerves.

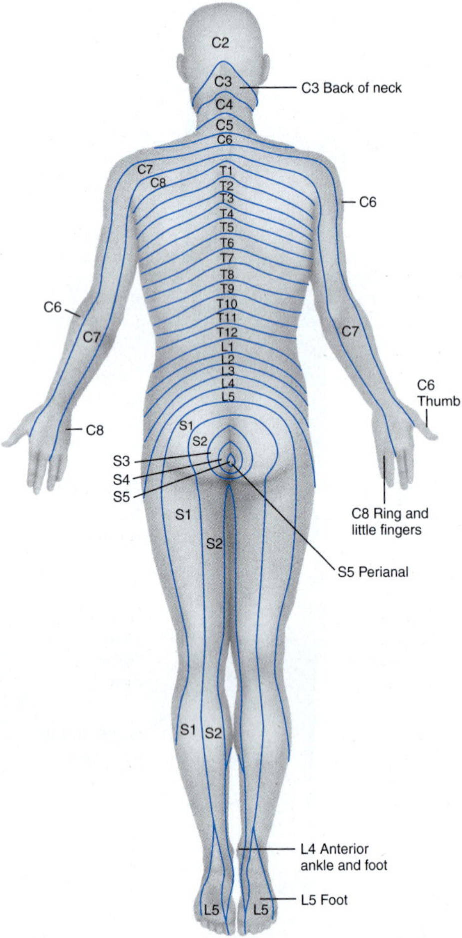

FIGURE 6.15 (*continued*) **B:** Dermatomes innervated by posterior roots. (Reprinted with Bickley LS, Szilagyi PG. *Bates' Guide to Physical Examination and History Taking*. 9th ed. Philadelphia, PA: Lippincott Williams & Wilkins; 2007, with permission.)

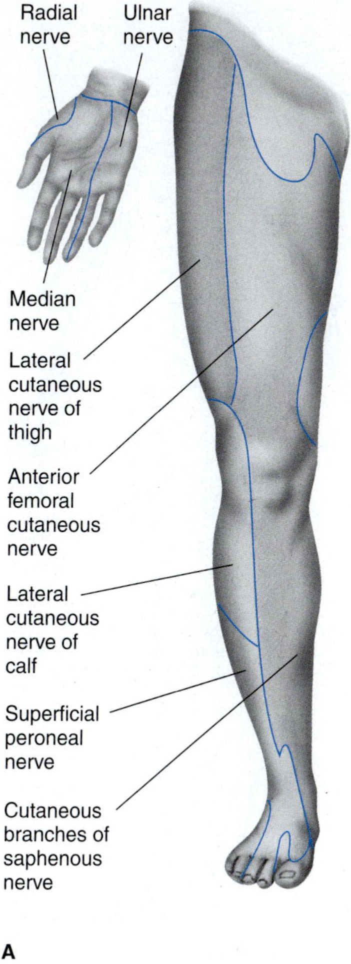

FIGURE 6.16 **A:** Areas innervated by peripheral nerves.

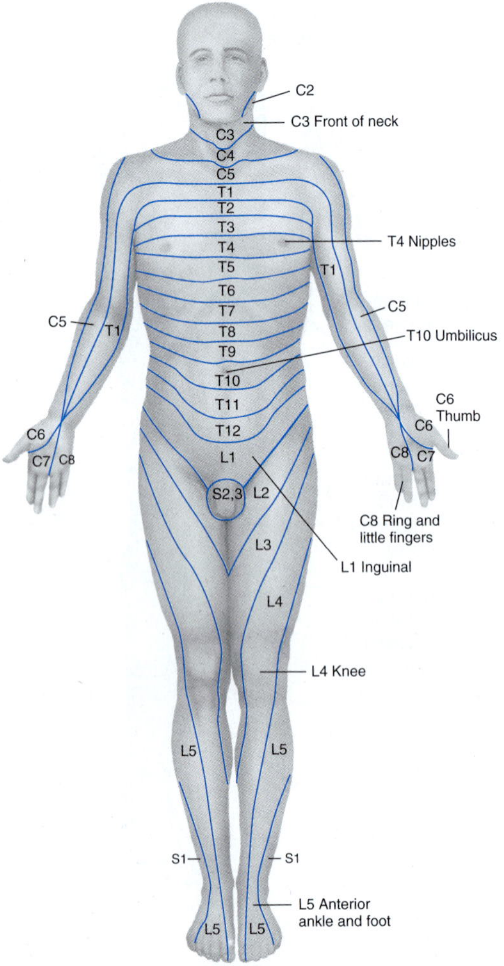

B

FIGURE 6.16 (*continued*) **B:** Dermatomes innervated by posterior roots. (Reprinted from Bickley LS, Szilagyi PG. *Bates' Guide to Physical Examination and History Taking*. 9th ed. Philadelphia, PA: Lippincott Williams & Wilkins; 2007, with permission.)

- Discriminative sensations (useful only if touch and position sense is intact; stereognosis: ability to identify an object by feeling it; the patient's eyes should be closed)

Annual foot exams in a patient with diabetes should include inspection of footwear, inspection for any foot deformity, palpation of DP and PT pulses, and test sensation using a 10-g monofilament and a tuning fork of 128 Hz. The 10-g monofilament is an inexpensive tool used to assess the loss of protective sensation in the feet. It is a single, nylon thread that requires a 10-g force to bend or buckle the monofilament. It is placed on the skin of the patient's foot and is used to assess peripheral neuropathy. The tuning fork is also used to assess peripheral neuropathy by testing its vibratory sensation on the bone of the great toe.

Reflexes

A reflex hammer is needed for evaluation of reflexes, which examines the spinal reflex arc. When an already partially stretched tendon is tapped briskly with a reflex hammer, stretch receptors in the tendon send an impulse to the spinal cord that elicits a contraction of the corresponding muscle. The spinal reflex arc is modified by control from the brain via descending corticospinal tracts. Typically, this often has an inhibitory influence. With damage to those higher centers, as in stroke or descending nerve tracts (i.e., the upper motor neurons), the spinal reflex arc is uninhibited and the reflexes are hyperactive. With damage to the peripheral nerve or particular dorsal roots (i.e., low motor neurons), the reflex arc is interrupted and the reflexes are diminished. Reflexes are graded on a scale from 0 to 4. A stick figure typically appears in the chart to designate the elicited reflexes (Fig. 6.17).

Reflex Response Exam

- Biceps reflex
- Triceps reflex
- Supinator or brachioradialis reflex
- Knee reflex
- Ankle reflex

The plantar reflexes refer to the reflex motion of the great toe after a noxious stimuli is applied to the bottom of the foot. An upgoing toe, the Babinski sign, is suggestive of an upper motor neuron lesion (but

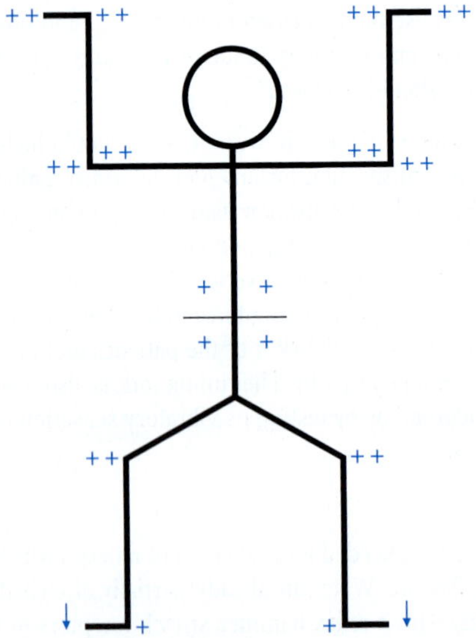

FIGURE 6.17 Example of deep tendons reflex (DTR) recording. Grading scale: 0, no response; +, diminished; ++, normal; +++, hyperactive; ++++, hyperactive, often with clonus. (Reprinted from Longe RL, Calvert JC. *Physical Assessment: A Guide for Evaluating Drug Therapy*. Vancouver, WA: Lippincott Williams & Wilkins; 1994, with permission.)

can be normal in infants). A downgoing toe is normal. It is common but incorrect to say the Babinski sign is positive or negative; it is either present or absent.

References

1. Bickley LS, Szilagyi PG. *Bates' Guide to Physical Examination and History Taking*. 11th ed. Philadelphia, PA: Lippincott Williams & Wilkins; 2012.
2. Folstein MF, Folstein SE, McHugh PR. "Mini-mental state." A practical method for grading the cognitive state of patients for the clinician. *J Psychiatr Res*. 1975;12(3):189–198.

7

Interpretation of Clinical Laboratory Test Results

Kristina L. Butler and Jonathan R. White

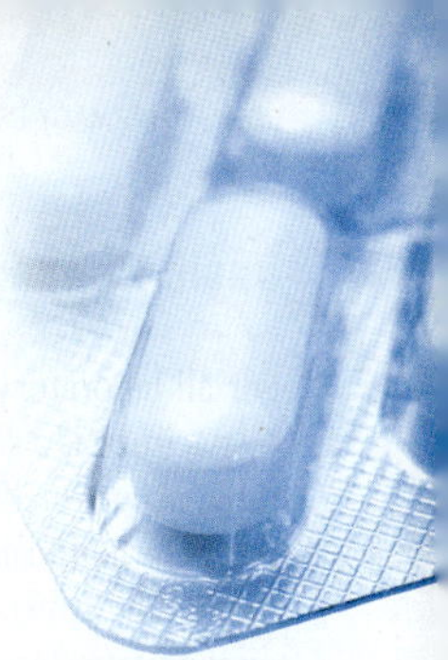

Clinical laboratory tests are valuable tools that may be used to gain additional information about the patient. Although not therapeutic on their own, these tests can be used to differentiate among possible diagnoses, confirm a diagnosis, assess current status, or evaluate response to therapy when history and physical exam alone cannot. Selection of laboratory tests is based on clinical judgment, with evidence-based medicine increasingly used to guide these decisions. This chapter contains many commonly encountered laboratory tests used in clinical medicine and is designed to provide the user with (a) brief descriptions of specific tests, (b) reference ranges in conventional units and International System of Units (SI), and (c) descriptions of the clinical implications of values falling outside of the reference range. Examples of conditions that may be associated with increased or decreased values are also included, but these examples may not be all-inclusive.

If specific tests are not included or if more detailed information is desired, including an overview of the clinician's role in using laboratory tests, the reader is advised to consult the most recent edition of Frances T. Fischbach and Marshall B. Dunning's *A Manual of Laboratory and Diagnostic Tests*, published by Lippincott Williams & Wilkins (Philadelphia, Pennsylvania); Mary Lee's *Basic Skills in Interpreting Laboratory Data,* published by American Society of Health-System Pharmacists (Bethesda, Maryland); Justin Schmidt and Jeffrey Wieczorkiewicz's *Interpreting Laboratory Data: A Point-of-Care Guide*, published by American Society of Health-System Pharmacists (Bethesda, Maryland); or Richard A. McPherson and Matthew R. Pincus's *Henry's Clinical Diagnosis and Management by Laboratory Methods*, published by W.B. Saunders (Philadelphia, Pennsylvania). Before using the information in this chapter, it is important to review the following general principles regarding laboratory tests.

Basic Concepts

For all laboratory tests, a *specimen* is needed for laboratory analysis. A specimen is a sample that may be obtained through *invasive* (needle, tube, scope, or other device used to penetrate the skin or enter the body) or *noninvasive* method. See Table 7.1 for a list of common specimens. The substance measured by the laboratory assay is called the *analyte*. Some analytes exist in different forms (referred to as fractions, subtypes, isoenzymes, subforms, or isoforms), and therefore, each will have a different *reference range* of values considered acceptable.

The reference range is a statistically derived numeric range obtained by testing a sample of individuals assumed to be healthy, usually established as the mean ± 2 standard deviations (SDs). The upper and lower limits reflect points beyond which the probability of clinical significance begins to increase; they are not absolute (i.e., "normal" versus "abnormal"); however, values that fall within the reference range are often referred to as "normal values." Reference ranges may vary between labs and facilities, depending on the analytic technique, reagent, and equipment.[1–5] Reference ranges may also vary between populations and may change as new data are published.

Laboratory tests may be *quantitative* or *qualitative*. The result of a quantitative test is reported as an exact number and assessed in the context of a reference range. A *critical value* is a result that is far enough outside the reference range that it indicates current or impending morbidity. Laboratory test results are reported with

TABLE 7.1 Common Laboratory Specimens

Venous blood
Arterial blood
Plasma (watery acellular portion of blood)
Serum (liquid remaining after fibrin clot is removed from plasma)
Urine
Stool
Sputum
Sweat
Saliva
Gastric secretions
Vaginal fluid
Exhaled air
Cerebrospinal fluid
Tissues (including nails, hair)

various units, which can be confusing. In an attempt to standardize quantitative measurements worldwide, International System (SI) of units was introduced in the 1960s; however, most clinicians and the general public continue to use and understand conventional units. The result of a qualitative test is reported as positive or negative without comment on the degree of positivity or negativity; exact quantities may be measured but are reported qualitatively using predetermined reference ranges. The exception to this is a *semi-quantitative* test, in which the result is reported as either negative or with varying degrees of positivity (e.g., 1+, 2+, 3+) without exact quantification.

Many factors can influence laboratory results (Table 7.2). Patients should be evaluated for endogenous or exogenous factors that may influence the accuracy of laboratory values. Laboratory errors are uncommon but may occur. Such errors should be suspected if one or more of the following occurs:

- Unusual trends develop.
- The magnitude of error is large.
- The result is not in agreement with confirmatory results.
- The result is inconsistent with clinical signs, symptoms, or other patient-specific information.

Abnormal values are not always clinically significant, and on occasion, values within the reference range can be considered abnormal in some diseases or conditions. Therefore, it is important to refer to published data or reference standards used by the laboratory performing the test and to consider potential interferences with the test in question.[1] The reference ranges in this chapter refer primarily to adults unless otherwise indicated and may vary between laboratories.

The clinical value of a laboratory test depends on its *sensitivity*, *specificity*, *accuracy*, *precision*, and the *incidence* of the disease/disorder in a given population. Accuracy and precision are measures of how well the test performs day-to-day in a laboratory, whereas sensitivity and specificity reflect the ability of the test to distinguish disease from absence of disease. The accuracy and precision of each test are preestablished and are frequently monitored by professional laboratory personnel. Sensitivity and specificity data are determined by research studies, are generally published in medical literature, and do not change with different populations. In contrast, the *predictive value*

TABLE 7.2 Factors That May Influence Laboratory Results

Patient-Specific Factors	
Demographics	• Age • Gender • Ethnicity • Genetics (enzyme polymorphisms) • Height, weight, body surface area (BSA)
Food/nutrition	• Type of food ingested/diet and time of consumption (post-prandial or fasting status) • Food–assay interactions • Nutritional and hydration status
Drugs	• Drug–drug, drug–disease, drug–assay interactions • Time of last dose (peak versus trough) • Steady-state status • Nonadherence • Undisclosed drug, tobacco, or alcohol use
Clinical situation	• Disease acuity and severity • Type of illness • Disease–assay interactions • Pregnancy • Organ function • Interfering diagnostic or therapeutic procedures
Other	• Time of day (biologic rhythms) • Nonadherence with instructions and pretest preparation • Incorrect/incomplete patient preparation (position, activity, timing, etc.) • Altitude
Laboratory-Specific Factors	
Specimen Issues	• Specimen type (Table 7.1) • Incorrect order of draw • Wrong/absent preservative, wrong transport medium • Incomplete collection (especially timed samples), insufficient volume, insufficient number of samples • Hemolyzed blood sample, old/deteriorating specimen • Air bubbles in tube
Collector issues	• Improper collection, handling, storage, labeling, or preparation • Incorrect timing of sample (especially for peak/trough levels) • Discrepancy between test ordered and specimen collected
Testing issues	• Different/incorrect method of analysis • Free versus bound analyte • Deteriorated reagents • Calibration errors • Technical/equipment error • Calculation errors • Misreading results • Computer entry/documentation errors

Source: Fischbach F, Dunning MB. *A Manual of Laboratory Diagnostic Tests*. 8th ed. Philadelphia, PA: Lippincott Williams & Wilkins; 2008.

of a single test can vary with age, gender, and geographic location.[4] See Table 7.3 for definitions and formulas to further explain these concepts.

Laboratory tests can be categorized as *screening* or *diagnostic* tests. Screening tests detect disease early when interventions are likely to be effective and are generally fairly simple and highly sensitive tests, performed in individuals without signs or symptoms of common diseases. In comparison, diagnostic tests are performed in patients with signs, symptoms, or history of a specific disease or disorder, or an abnormal screening test. These tests tend to be more complex and highly specific for the associated condition. Related tests may be grouped into a set called a *profile* or a *panel* (Table 7.4); small differences may exist between panels and preferred panels, and their names may vary between laboratories/institutions. Abbreviations for specific laboratory tests and panels are common, and test results may be recorded in a patient's chart using various formats. With experience, clinicians are often able to identify particular laboratory tests by knowing the reference range.

Laboratory testing occurs in many environments, including hospitals, clinics, and the community. *Point-of-care* testing (POC or POCT) refers to tests done at the site of patient care, i.e., at the patient's bedside, clinic, pharmacy, or even home (usually referred to as *home-testing*). POC testing can provide rapid results with increased portability and convenience and may further engage patients in the management of their disease or condition. Other POC advantages include blood conservation, decreased specimen transport/storage/processing error, and overall cost savings. However, POC testing has the potential for misuse or misinterpretation of results, delays in seeking medical advice, loss of epidemiologic data, documentation errors, inappropriate material disposal, and quality assurance issues.[5]

Before obtaining the test specimen, a relevant history and assessment should be performed, with particular attention paid to any conditions that could affect the testing process or test results (e.g., allergies, phobias, pregnancy, diseases, cultural or language diversity, physical or mental impairments). Standard/universal precautions should be observed with every patient, and all patients should be monitored for complications following their specimen procurement, particularly if invasive tests are performed.[4]

(*Text continued on page 187*)

TABLE 7.3 Laboratory Terminology

Term	Definition	Formula
True positive (TP)	Individuals with a given disease or condition who are detected by the test	
True negative (TN)	Individuals without a given disease or condition who are not detected by the test	
False positive (FP)	Individuals without a given disease or condition who test positive	
False negative (FN)	Individuals with a given disease or condition who are not detected by the test	
Sensitivity	The ability of a test to correctly identify those individuals who have a given disease or condition; TP rate	$[TP \div (TP + FN)] \times 100\%$
Specificity	The ability of a test to correctly identify those individuals who do not have a given disease or condition; TN rate	$[TN \div (TN + FP)] \times 100\%$
Accuracy	The ability of a test to produce a result that approaches the absolute true value of the substance being measured	$[(TP + TN) \div (TP + TN + FP + FN)] \times 100\%$
Precision	The reliability of a test to produce similar results on repeated analysis of the same sample, with small amounts of random variation	
Incidence/prevalence	The rate of presence of a disease or condition within a (tested) population or community	$[(TP + FN) \div (TP + TN + FP + FN)] \times 100\%$
Predictive values	The ability of a screening test result to correctly identify the presence or absence of a given disease or condition in a population; predictive values may be positive (PPV) or negative (NPV)	
Positive predictive value (PPV)	The percentage of positive tests with TP results	$[TP \div (TP + FP)] \times 100\%$
Negative predictive value (NPV)	The percentage of negative tests with TN results	$[TN \div (TN + FN)] \times 100\%$

Sources: Fischbach F, Dunning MB. *A Manual of Laboratory Diagnostic Tests*. 8th ed. Philadelphia, PA: Lippincott Williams & Wilkins; 2008; and Lee M. *Basic Skills in Interpreting Laboratory Data*. 5th ed. Bethesda, MD: American Society of Health-System Pharmacists; 2013

TABLE 7.4 Common Laboratory Panels

Panel (Abbreviation)	**Basic Metabolic Panel (BMP)**	**Comprehensive Metabolic Panel (CMP)**	**Electrolytes (Lytes)**	**Renal Function Panel**	**Hepatic Panel**
Elements (abbreviation)	• Sodium (Na^+) • Potassium (K^+) • Chloride (Cl^-) • Carbon dioxide (CO_2) • Blood urea nitrogen (BUN) • Creatinine (Cr or SCr) • Glucose • Calcium (Ca^{2+})	BMP plus • Albumin (Alb) • Total protein (TP, albumin/globulin [A/G] ratio) • Alkaline phosphatase (ALP, Alk phos) • Alanine aminotransferase (ALT) • Aspartate aminotransferase (AST) • Total bilirubin (T Bili, TBIL)	• Na^+ • K^+ • Cl^- • CO_2	BMP plus • Phosphorus • Lactic acid dehydrogenase (LDH) • Creatinine clearance (CrCl) • TP, A/G ratio • Alb	• ALT • AST • ALP • T Bili • Direct bilirubin (D Bili, conjugated bilirubin) • Alb • TP, A/G ratio • Gamma glutamyl-transferase (GGT) • LDH
Panel (Abbreviation)	**Thyroid Function**	**Cardiac Markers**	**Lipid Profile**	**Enzymes**	**Hematology Panel (Hemogram)**
Elements (abbreviation)	• Triiodothyronine (T_3) • T_3 uptake ratio (T_3 UR) • Total thyroxine (T_4) • Free T_4 • Thyroid-stimulating hormone (TSH)	BMP plus • Cardiac troponin (troponin) • Creatine kinase (CK) • Creatine kinase–myoglobin (CK-MB) • Homocysteine • B-Type Natriuretic Peptide (BNP)	• Total cholesterol (TC) • Triglycerides (TG) • High-density lipoprotein (HDL) • Low-density lipoprotein (LDL) May also include: • Very–low-density lipoprotein (VLDL) • Cholesterol/HDL ratio	• ALT • AST • Amylase • Lipase • GGT • LDH • CK	• Red blood cell (RBC) count • Hemoglobin (Hgb) • Hematocrit (Hct) • Platelet count • White blood cell (WBC) count • Mean corpuscular volume (MCV) • Mean corpuscular hemoglobin (MCH) • Mean corpuscular hemoglobin concentration (MCHC) • Red cell distribution width (RDW)

(continued)

TABLE 7.4 Common Laboratory Panels *(continued)*

Panel (Abbreviation)	**Complete Blood Count (CBC) with Differential (diff)**	**Iron Tests**	**Coagulation Panel**	**Arterial Blood Gases (ABG)**	**Urine Electrolytes**
Elements (abbreviation)	Hemogram plus • WBC differential • Segmented neutrophils • Bands • Eosinophils • Basophils • Lymphocytes • Atypical lymphocytes • Monocytes	• Serum iron (Fe) • Total iron-binding capacity (TIBC) • Serum ferritin • Tranferrin	• Prothrombin time (PT)/International normalized ratio (INR) • Activated partial thromboplastin time (aPTT) • Fibrinogen • Hemogram with platelet	• pH • PCO_2 • PO_2 • Base excess • Bicarbonate (HCO_3)	• Na+ • K+

Laboratory Tests

Hematologic Tests

A hemogram consists of a white blood cell (WBC) count, red blood cell (RBC) count, hemoglobin (Hgb or Hb), hematocrit (Hct), RBC indices, and a platelet count. A complete blood count (CBC) consists of a hemogram plus a differential WBC. The tests of a CBC provide information on both the quantity and quality of blood cells. Table 7.5 provides descriptions, reference ranges, and clinical implications of CBC results in adults. The reference ranges of Hgb, Hct, WBC, and other hematologic tests vary for infants, children, and adolescents but are often higher at birth and decrease over several years. However, values may be higher for adults than for older children and adolescents.

Iron is necessary for the production of Hgb, and iron tests measure the body's iron in its several components. Transferrin, serum iron (Fe), and total iron-binding capacity (TIBC) are used together in the differential diagnosis of anemia, assessing treatment of iron deficiency anemia, and evaluating other blood disorders. Table 7.6 provides descriptions, reference ranges, and clinical implications of iron study results in adults. Reference ranges for newborns and children can be found in other resources.

Hemostasis and coagulation tests are used to diagnose, evaluate, and monitor patients with bleeding or clotting disorders or vascular injury or trauma. The common coagulation and hemostasis tests are presented in Table 7.7.

Chemistry Tests

Many chemical blood constituents are available to be tested, including electrolytes, enzymes, blood glucose, lipids, hormones, proteins, vitamins, minerals, and drug levels; other individual tests are available. It is common to need to test several of these over a period of time to be able to establish patterns.

Electrolytes, Minerals, and Trace Elements

Determining serum electrolyte concentrations is one of the most common laboratory tests and is routinely ordered as a basic metabolic panel (BMP). Some components included in metabolic panels are not electrolytes, minerals, or trace elements and are addressed in the section most appropriate for that item. Table 7.8 presents descriptions, reference ranges (for adults), and clinical information for common electrolyte tests.

(*Text continued on page 214*)

TABLE 7.5 Hemogram Reference Ranges for Adults

Test Name (Abbreviation)	Description	Reference Range: Conventional Units	Reference Range: SI Units	Increased With	Decreased With	Other Comments
Hematocrit (Hct)	Measures the volume of blood that is RBCs, indirectly measures RBC mass	Male: 42%–52% Female: 36%–48%	Male: 0.42–0.52 Female: 0.36–0.48	Erythrocytosis, dehydration, chronic obstructive pulmonary disease (COPD), polycythemia, shock, high altitude	Anemia (various causes), hemolytic reactions, leukemia, lymphoma, myeloproliferative disorders, cirrhosis, massive blood loss, hyperthyroidism	• Approximately three times Hgb • Usually parallels the RBC count when erythrocytes are of a normal size • Lacks clinical validity in sickle cell anemia, immediately after moderate blood loss or transfusion; may appear normal after acute hemorrhage • Decreased in iron deficiency anemia because microcytic (small) cells pack into a smaller volume; however, RBC count may appear normal • Critical values: <20% leads to cardiac failure and death; >60% associated with spontaneous clotting
Hemoglobin (Hgb)	Measures amount of Hbg contained in RBCs; indication	Male: 13–18 g/dL Female: 12–16 g/dL	Male: 8.1–11.2 mmol/L Female: 7.4–9.9 mmol/L	Dehydration, hemoconcentration (polycythemia, burns), excess production of RBCs in the bone	Anemia (various causes), myeloproliferative disorders, leukemia, hemorrhage, hemolytic reactions, cirrhosis,	• Consists of globin (four protein subunits), a heme core, iron atom, and porphyrin ring • When Hgb carries O_2, blood is scarlet (arterial); when it loses O_2, the blood becomes dark red (venous)

	of oxygen capacity of blood			marrow, hyperlipidemia, COPD, congestive heart failure (CHF), high altitude, use of erythropoietin-stimulating agents (ESAs)	increased fluid intake, kidney disease, other chronic illnesses, pregnancy	• One gram of Hgb carries 1.34 mL of O_2 • Used to assess anemia severity, response to treatment, or progression of associated disease(s) • A decrease in the protein subtypes A_1, A_2, and F (fetal), and the appearance of type S Hgb is associated with sickle cell anemia • Concentration fluctuates in patients with hemorrhages and burns because of fluid replacement and blood transfusions • Critical values: <7 g/dL increases risk of heart failure and death or <8–9 g/dL if cardiac disease
Red blood cell (RBC, erythrocyte) count	Quantification of RBCs; functional changes usually monitored by Hgb or Hct	Male: 4.4–5.9 $\times 10^6$ cells/μL (or /mm^3) Female: 3.8–5.2 $\times 10^6$ cells/μL (or /mm^3)	Male: 4.4–5.9 $\times 10^{12}$ cells/L Female: 3.8–5.2 $\times 10^{12}$ cells/L	Polycythemia vera, secondary polycythemia (hormone-secreting tumors), diarrhea/dehydration, vigorous exercise, burns, high altitudes	Anemia (various causes), myeloproliferative disorders, systemic lupus erythematosus (SLE)	• Decreased O_2 stimulates RBC production via erythropoietin • Usually released into the circulation as mature cells; if demand is high, immature cells (reticulocytes) will be released • RBCs have a life span ~120 days; older RBCs are removed from circulation by phagocytes in the spleen, hepatic, and bone marrow (reticuloendothelial system [RES])

(continued)

TABLE 7.5 Hemogram Reference Ranges for Adults *(continued)*

Test Name (Abbreviation)	Description	Reference Range: Conventional Units	Reference Range: SI Units	Increased With	Decreased With	Other Comments
Mean corpuscular volume (MCV)	= Hct/RBC Calculates the mean volume/size of RBCs	78–100 μm^3	78–100 fL/cell	(Macrocytic) hepatic disease, alcoholism, folate/B_{12} deficiency, reticulocytosis, hyperglycemia, leukemia, drugs (antimetabolites, zidovudine, valproate, phenytoin, oral contraceptives, primidone, phenobarbital, methotrexate, pentamidine, sulfamethoxazole, triamterene, trimethoprim, colchicine, neomycin)	(Microcytic) iron deficiency, pernicious anemia, thalassemia	• Expressed as normocytic (normal size), microcytic (small size, <75 fL), or macrocytic (large size, >105 fL) • Useful in the diagnosis of anemia. • Questionable value in sickle cell anemia, because the Hct is unreliable due to the abnormal RBC shape • A calculated value; therefore, possible to have a wide variation in macrocytes/microcytes and still have a normal MCV • Anemia of inflammatory disease may present with normal or low MCV
Mean corpuscular hemoglobin (MCH)	= Hgb/RBC Calculates amount of Hgb inside RBCs	25–35 pg/cell	25–35 pg/cell	Folate/B_{12} deficiency, hyperlipidemia	Iron deficiency	• Useful in the diagnosis of anemia • Affected by RBC size

Mean corpuscular hemoglobin concentration (MCHC)	= Hgb/Hct Amount of Hgb in terms of % volume of cell	31–37 g/dL	310–370 g/L	(Hyperchromia) hyperlipidemia, hereditary spherocytosis	(Hypochromia) iron deficiency, thalassemia, microcytic anemia, pyridoxine-responsive anemia, hypochromic anemia	• Expressed as normochromic (normal color), hypochromic (light color), or hyperchromic (dark color) • A better index of RBC Hgb than MCH, because MCHC is not affected by cell size
Reticulocyte (Retic) count	Quantification of immature, nonnucleated cells of the erythrocyte series in circulation	0.5%–2.5% of RBCs	0.005–0.025	Acute blood loss, sickle cell disease, hemolysis; indication that RBC production is accelerated	Untreated iron/vitamin B_{12}/folate deficiency, aplastic anemia, chronic infection, radiation therapy; indication that bone marrow RBC production is reduced	• If demand is high, reticulocytes will be released from the bone marrow into circulation prior to maturation to erythrocytes • If anemia present and reticulocyte count not increased, suggests insufficient production of erythrocytes by bone marrow • An increase in retics (~20%, maximum seen 7–14 days after treatment) reflects the effectiveness of anemia treatment
RBC distribution width (RDW)	Calculation of the variation in RBC size/volume (anisocytosis)	11.5%–15%	0.115–0.150	Iron/B_{12}/folate deficiency, hemolytic anemia, mixed anemias		• The greater the variation in RBC size, the larger the % • In some anemias (e.g., pernicious anemia), the anisocytosis (along with variation in shape, poikilocytosis) causes an increase in the RDW • Normal RDW is seen in thalassemia and in anemia of inflammatory disease

(continued)

TABLE 7.5 Hemogram Reference Ranges for Adults *(continued)*

Test Name (Abbreviation)	Description	Reference Range: Conventional Units	Reference Range: SI Units	Increased With	Decreased With	Other Comments
Platelet (PLT, thrombocytes) count	Quantification of platelets	140–400 × 10^3 cells/μL (or /mm^3)	140–400 × 10^9/L	(Thrombocythemia/ thrombocytosis) cancer, polycythemia vera, splenectomy, trauma, cirrhosis, myelogenous/ granulocytic leukemia, stress, iron deficiency anemia, rapid blood regeneration, acute and chronic infection and inflammatory diseases, renal failure, recovery from bone marrow suppression	(Thrombocytopenia) idiopathic thrombocytopenia purpura (ITP), disseminated intravascular coagulation (DIC), pernicious, aplastic and hemolytic anemias, bone marrow lesions, toxemia or eclampsia in pregnancy, alcohol toxicity/abuse, CHF, inherited syndromes, hypersplenism, renal insufficiency, antiplatelet antibodies, thrombopoietin deficiency, drugs (amrinone, antineoplastic agents, gold salts, heparin, sulfonamides, quinidine, H_2 receptor antagonists, penicillins, penicillamine, valproic acid), radiation, HIV infection	• Necessary for clot formation. During adhesion/aggregation, coagulation is triggered and thrombin is formed. Platelets then become interspersed with RBCs and WBCs to form a clot • Life span of ~7–12 days; 2/3 circulating and 1/3 in the spleen • Spontaneous bleeding, prolonged bleeding time, petechiae, or ecchymosis may occur with values <20,000; the precise number necessary for hemostasis is not established • Aspirin and nonsteroidal anti-inflammatory drugs (NSAIDs) primarily affect platelet function rather than number

Mean platelet volume (MPV)	Measurement of the average size of platelets	6.4–11 μm^3	6.4–11 fL	ITP, septic thrombocytopenia, myeloproliferative disorders, myelogenous leukemia, massive hemorrhage, splenectomy, vasculitis, prosthetic heart valve, megaloblastic anemia	Aplastic anemia, Wiskott–Aldrich syndrome	• Platelet size is larger when the body is producing increased numbers of platelets; results can be used to make inferences about platelet production in bone marrow • Has been positively associated with measures of platelet activity; may be a useful indicator of the risk of vascular events
White blood cell (WBC, leukocyte) count	Quantification of leukocytes (WBCs)	4.4–11 × 10^3 cells/μL (or /mm^3)	4.4–11 × 10^9 cells/L	(Leukocytosis) hemorrhage, trauma, drugs (mercury, epinephrine, corticosteroids), necrosis, toxins (eclampsia), leukemia; mild: food, exercise, emotion, menstruation, stress, seizures, cold baths	(Leukopenia) viral infections, hypersplenism, leukemia, drugs (antimetabolites, antibiotics, anticonvulsants, chemotherapy), pernicious/aplastic anemia	• Main functions are fighting infection, phagocytosis of foreign organisms, and production or transportation/distribution of antibodies. The two major types of WBCs are granulocytes (neutrophils, eosinophils, and basophils) and agranulocytes (lymphocytes and monocytes) • Leukocytosis: WBC increase to 10.5–20 (slight); >30 (moderate); >50 (high); usually due to an increase of only one cell type (e.g., neutrophilia). Absence of anemia helps to distinguish infection from leukemia • Leukopenia: WBC decrease to <4

(continued)

TABLE 7.5 Hemogram Reference Ranges for Adults *(continued)*

Test Name (Abbreviation)	Description	Reference Range: Conventional Units	Reference Range: SI Units	Increased With	Decreased With	Other Comments
Differential WBC count (diff)	Determines the specific patterns of WBCs in circulation					
Neutrophils (polymorphonuclear segmented neutrophils, PMNs, polys, segs)	Most laboratories report neutrophils by combining segs and bands and reporting as an absolute number; also reported as % of WBCs. Absolute neutrophil count (ANC) = WBC × (%segs + %bands)	1.7–7.5 × 10^3 cells/μL (or /mm^3), 45%–74% ANC: 1.5–8 × 10^3 cells/μL (or /mm^3)	1.7–7.5 × 10^9/L, 0.45–0.75	(Neutrophilia) bacterial or parasitic infections, metabolic disturbances, hemorrhage, myeloproliferative disorders; mild/temporary: stress, excitement, exercise; notable increases compared to total WBC count may indicate a severe infection	(Neutropenia) decreased neutrophil production, increased cell disappearance, viral infection, blood diseases, hormonal disorders, toxic agents, massive infection	• Neutrophils fight bacterial infection (phagocytosis) and inflammatory disorders (rheumatoid arthritis [RA], asthma, and inflammatory bowel disease [IBD]) • A "shift to right" (an increase in segs, mature cells) occurs in hepatic disease, megaloblastic anemia due to B_{12}/folate deficiency, hemolysis, tissue breakdown, surgery, certain drugs (corticosteroids) • Degree of neutrophilia is proportionate to the amount of tissue involved in inflammation

Bands	Reported as an absolute number or % of WBCs	0–0.4 × 10^3 cells/μL (or /mm^3), 0%–5%	0–0.4 × 10^9/L, 0–0.05	(Shift to left) infection, chemotherapeutic agents, a cell production disorder (leukemia), hemorrhage		• Bands are neutrophils in early stages of maturity
Eosinophils (EOS)	Reported as an absolute number or % of WBCs	0–0.5 × 10^3 cells/μL (or /mm^3), 0%–8%	0–0.5 × 10^9/L, 0–0.08	(Eosinophilia) neoplasm, Addison disease, allergic reactions, collagen vascular disease, parasitic infections, L-tryptophan (eosinophilic myalgia syndrome)	(Eosinopenia) glucocorticoid excess (endogenous—bodily stress [infectious mononucleosis], Cushing disease—or exogenous)	• Eosinophils fight allergic disorders (ingest antigen–antibody complexes) and parasitic infections (phagocytosis) • EOS disappear early in pyogenic infections • Eosinophilia can be masked by steroid use
Basophils (mast cells)	Reported as an absolute number or % of WBCs	0–0.2 × 10^3 cells/μL (or /mm^3), 0%–3%	0–0.2 × 10^9/L, 0–0.03	(Basophilia) is granulocytic and basophilic leukemia, myeloid metaplasia, allergic reactions with high serum concentration of histamine	(Basopenia) acute infections, stress reactions, after prolonged steroid therapy	• Basophils fight blood dyscrasias and myeloproliferative disease; phagocytic cells that contain heparin, histamine, and serotonin
Monocytes (monomorphonuclear monocytes)	Reported as an absolute number or % of WBCs	0.2–0.9 × 10^3 cells/μL (or /mm^3), 4%–11%	0.2–0.9 × 10^9/L, 0.04–0.11	(Monocytosis) viral, bacterial, and parasitic infections, collagen, vascular, and hematologic disorders	(Monocytopenia) secondary to stress, glucocorticoids, myelotoxic or immunosuppressive drugs	• The largest cells in the blood; serve as the body's second line of defense. Macrophages capable of phagocytosis and scavenger functions • Monocytes fight severe infections • Monocytes also produce interferon

(continued)

TABLE 7.5 Hemogram Reference Ranges for Adults *(continued)*

Test Name (Abbreviation)	Description	Reference Range: Conventional Units	Reference Range: SI Units	Increased With	Decreased With	Other Comments
Lymphocyte (monomorphonuclear lymphocytes)	Reported as an absolute number or % of WBCs	1–3.5 × 10^3 cells/μL (or /mm^3), 16%–46%	1–3.5 × 10^9/L, 0.16–0.46	(Lymphocytosis) viral diseases (mumps, mononucleosis, upper respiratory infections), bacterial diseases, hormonal disorders	(Lymphopenia) Hodgkin disease, SLE, burns, trauma	• Lymphocytes are the second most common WBC; these small, motile cells migrate during early and late stages of inflammation, elaborate immunoglobulins, and are important in cellular immune response. Located in the spleen, lymphatic tissue, and lymph nodes • Virocytes (stress lymphocytes, Downey-type cells, atypical lymphocytes) are atypical cells that can also appear in viral, fungoid, and parasitic infections, after transfusions and as a response to stress • Transformed lymphocytes are used as a measure of histocompatibility

Sources: www.labtestsonline.org. Accessed May 14, 2013; Kratz A, Lewandrowski KB. Case records of the Massachusetts General Hospital. Weekly clinicopathological exercises. Normal reference laboratory values. *N Engl J Med*. 1998;339:1063–1072; Fischbach F, Dunning MB. *A Manual of Laboratory Diagnostic Tests*. 8th ed. Philadelphia, PA: Lippincott Williams & Wilkins; 2008; Schmidt J, Wieczorkiewicz J. *Interpreting Laboratory Data: A Point-of-Care Guide*. 1st ed. Bethesda, MD: American Society of Health-System Pharmacists; 2012; and Lee M. *Basic Skills in Interpreting Laboratory Data*. 5th ed. Bethesda, MD: American Society of Health-System Pharmacists; 2013

TABLE 7.6 Iron Studies and Related Hematologic Tests

Test Name (Abbreviation)	Description	Reference Range: Conventional Units	Reference Range: SI Units	Increased With	Decreased With	Other Comments
Serum iron (Fe)	Measures the amount of iron bound to transferrin	30–175 μg/dL	5.4–31.3 μmol/L	Hemolytic anemia, pernicious anemia, thalassemia, acute hepatitis, acute porphyria, hemochromatosis, pyridoxine deficiency, excessive iron therapy, repeated transfusions, nephritis, lead poisoning, acute leukemia	Iron deficiency anemia, remission of pernicious anemia, chronic blood loss, kwashiorkor, some systemic infections, idiopathic pulmonary hemosiderosis, hypothyroidism, paroxysmal nocturnal hemoglobinuria, pregnancy (third trimester), progesterone oral contraceptives, RA, SLE	• Many patients with iron deficiency anemia have levels in the low-normal range (false-negative results). • Fe alone has limited utility for diagnosis or monitoring, as well as significant (<30%) diurnal and day-to-day variations

(continued)

TABLE 7.6 Iron Studies and Related Hematologic Tests *(continued)*

Test Name (Abbreviation)	Description	Reference Range		Increased With	Decreased With	Other Comments
		Conventional Units	SI Units			
Total iron-binding capacity (TIBC)	Indirect measure of serum transferrin	225–450 µg/dL	40.3–76.1 µmol/L	Iron deficiency anemia, acute and chronic blood loss, acute hepatic damage, pregnancy, oral contraceptives	Hemochromatosis, anemias (of chronic diseases and infections), other non–iron deficiency anemias, nephrosis, thalassemia, hypoproteinemia (malnutrition and burns), cirrhosis, hyperthyroidism	• Less sensitive to changes in iron stores than is serum ferritin
Transferrin	Measures the transport protein that regulates iron absorption	250–425 mg/dL	2.5–4.25 g/L	Iron deficiency anemia, estrogen therapy, pregnancy, hypoxia, oral contraceptives	Anemia of chronic disease, nephrosis, gastrointestinal (GI) losses, severe burns, chronic infections, malnutrition, genetic deficiency (atransferrinemia), kwashiorkor, severe hepatic disease, some inflammatory conditions, iron overdose	• High levels relate to the ability of the body to deal with infections

Transferrin (iron) saturation	% = (100 × Fe) ÷ TIBC	~30% Male: 10%–50% Female: 1%–50%		Hemochromatosis, increased iron intake, thalassemia, hemosiderosis, acute hepatic disease	Iron deficiency anemias, malignancy (standard and small intestine), anemia of infection and chronic disease, iron neoplasms	• Remaining unsaturated % reflects TIBC (though relationship is not linear)
Ferritin	Measure of iron stores; most reliable indicator of total body iron status	Male: 20–322 ng/mL Female: 10–291 ng/mL	Male: 20–322 μg/L Female: 0–291 μg/L	Hemochromatosis, hemosiderosis, iron supplementation, alcoholic hepatic disease, end-stage renal disease (ESRD), some malignancies, hyperthyroidism, non–iron deficiency anemias, chronic inflammation	Iron deficiency anemia	• More specific and sensitive than Fe or TIBC for diagnosing iron deficiency • Decreases seen before anemia and other changes occur • Levels should return to normal within a few days of the start of iron therapy; if they remain low, consider nonadherence or continued iron loss • Increases with age • No value in alcoholic hepatic disease

(continued)

TABLE 7.6 Iron Studies and Related Hematologic Tests *(continued)*

Test Name (Abbreviation)	Description	Reference Range: Conventional Units	Reference Range: SI Units	Increased With	Decreased With	Other Comments
Glucose-6-phosphate dehydrogenase (G6PD) in erythrocytes	Identification of sex-linked disorder, with major variants in specific ethnic groups • Affects 13% of African American men and 3% of African American women (~20% carriers) • Decreased in ~50% of Iraqis, Kurds, Sephardic Jews, and Lebanese (less common in Greeks, Italians, Turks, and North Africans) • Decreased enzyme levels also seen in Southeast Asians	7–20.5 IU/g Hgb	0.11–0.34 nkat/g Hgb	G6PD deficiency, congenital nonspherocytic anemia, nonimmunologic hemolytic disease of the newborn (Asian and Mediterranean)	Untreated pernicious/megaloblastic anemia, thrombocytopenia purpura, hyperthyroidism, viral hepatitis, chronic blood loss, myocardial infarction (MI)	• Deficiencies: ◦ Class I: most severe; presents as chronic hemolysis in the absence of oxidative stress ◦ Class II: G6PD <10% of normal; associated with severe episodic hemolysis ◦ Class III: occasional hemolytic episodes with identifiable precipitating factors ◦ Class IV: normal • Precipitating factors include aspirin, aminoquinoline antimalarials, salicylates, methylene blue, quinine, quinidine, large doses of ascorbic acid, nitrofurantoin, some sulfonamides and sulfones, fava beans, infections, and diabetic ketoacidosis (DKA); hemolysis generally occurs by day 3 of factor exposure • Degree of hemolysis depends on extent of deficiency and dose of precipitating agent

Vitamin B_{12} (VB_{12})	Antipernicious anemia factor	200–950 pg/mL	148–701 pmol/L	Leukemia, chronic renal failure, hepatic disease, cancer with hepatic metastasis, polycythemia vera, CHF, DM, obesity, COPD, pregnancy, blood transfusion, high vitamin A and C doses, smoking	Pernicious/megaloblastic anemia, malabsorption syndromes (IBD, tapeworm, loss of gastric mucosa, Zollinger-Ellison syndrome [ZES], blind loop syndromes), vegetarian diet, folic acid deficiency, hypothyroidism	• Necessary for the production of RBCs • Increases with age • The Schilling test is used to determine whether vitamin B_{12} deficiency is caused by malabsorption
Folic acid (folate)		1.9–20 ng/mL (serum) 140–628 ng/mL (RBC)	4.3–45.3 nmol/L (serum) 317–2,045 nmol/L (RBC)	Blind loop syndrome, vegetarian diet, pernicious anemia, VB_{12} deficiency	Inadequate intake (alcoholism, chronic disease, malnutrition, anorexia, lack of fresh vegetables), malabsorption (small bowel disease), high requirements (pregnancy, hypothyroidism), megaloblastic anemia, hepatic disease, celiac disease, vitamin B_6 deficiency, carcinomas, leukemia, Crohn disease, intestinal resection, drugs (anticonvulsants, methotrexate, antimalarials, alcohol, oral contraceptives, high-dose antiacids)	• Needed for normal RBC and WBC function and production of cellular genes

Sources: www.labtestsonline.org. Accessed May 14, 2013; Kratz A, Lewandrowski KB. Case records of the Massachusetts General Hospital. Weekly clinicopathological exercises. Normal reference laboratory values. *N Engl J Med.* 1998;339:1063–1072; Fischbach F, Dunning MB. *A Manual of Laboratory Diagnostic Tests.* 8th ed. Philadelphia, PA: Lippincott Williams & Wilkins; 2008; Schmidt J, Wieczorkiewicz J. *Interpreting Laboratory Data: A Point-of-Care Guide.* 1st ed. Bethesda, MD: American Society of Health-System Pharmacists; and Lee M. *Basic Skills in Interpreting Laboratory Data.* 5th ed. Bethesda, MD: American Society of Health-System Pharmacists; 2013

TABLE 7.7 Coagulation Tests

Test Name (Abbreviation)	Description	Reference Range: Conventional Units	Reference Range: SI Units	Increased With	Decreased With	Other Comments
Bleeding time	Measures the primary phases of hemostasis; best test to screen for platelet function disorders	2–10 minutes		Platelet function disorders, thrombocytopenia, decreased or abnormal plasma factors (von Willebrand factor, fibrinogen), DIC, abnormalities in small blood vessel walls, vascular disease, leukemia, renal failure, hepatic failure, scurvy, excessive alcohol consumption, drugs (aspirin, dipyridamole, dextran, fibrinolytics)		• Extreme temperatures can alter test results • Edema or cyanosis of the extremity used will invalidate the test
Prothrombin time (Pro time, PT)	Directly measures for potential defects in the extrinsic thromboplastin system (factors 1 [fibrinogen], II [prothrombin], V, VII, and X)	10–15 seconds (can vary significantly by laboratory)		Extrinsic thromboplastin factor deficiencies, vitamin K deficiency, DIC, hemorrhagic disease of the newborn, premature newborns, hepatic disease, biliary obstruction, poor fat absorption, ZES, lupus or other endogenous circulating anticoagulants, salicylate intoxication, drugs (warfarin, heparin)	Increased vitamin K intake (green leafy vegetables)	• Not affected by platelet disorders (ITP), polycythemia vera, hemophilia A (factor VIII deficiency), Christmas disease (factor IX deficiency), von Willebrand disease, or tannin disease • Evaluation of bleeding is necessary if significantly prolonged • Prothrombin time ratio (PTR) = patient's PT ÷ control PT (lab's mean normal); therapeutic levels are 2.0–2.5

International normalized ratio (INR)	Standardizes PT results between laboratories; used for warfarin monitoring	0.8–1.2		Same as PT	Same as PT	• Conversion of PTR to INR requires knowledge of the sensitivity of the thromboplastin reagent used (expressed as an international sensitivity index [ISI]). $INR = PTR^{ISI}$ • Therapeutic range (during warfarin therapy) is usually 2–3.5 (depending on anticoagulation indication) • Evaluation of bleeding is necessary if significantly elevated
Activated partial thromboplastin time (aPTT)	Detects deficiencies in the intrinsic thromboplastin system (factors I, II, V, VIII, IX, X, XI, and XII); used for heparin monitoring	21–45 seconds (varies by laboratory)		von Willebrand disease, hemophilia, congenital deficiency of Fitzgerald/ Fletcher factor, hepatic disease, DIC, drugs (heparin, streptokinase, urokinase, warfarin), vitamin K deficiency	Very early DIC, extensive cancer (except when hepatic involved), immediately after acute hemorrhage	• Therapeutic range (during heparin therapy) is usually 1.5–2.5 times normal (varies between laboratories) • Can be used to identify circulating anticoagulants (antibodies induced in hemophiliacs by plasma transfusions)
Fibrinogen	Investigates abnormal PT, aPTT, and thrombin time (TT); screens for DIC and fibrin–fibrinogenolysis	200–450 mg/dL	2.0–4.5 g/L	Inflammatory diseases (RA), infections, acute MI (AMI), cerebral accidents/disease, cancer, nephrotic syndrome, pregnancy, eclampsia	DIC, hepatic disease, cancer, primary fibrinolysis, dysfibrinogenemia, hypofibrinogenemia, high FDP/FSP levels (fibrin degradation/ split levels), elevated antithrombin III (AT III)	• High heparin levels interfere with test results • Critical values: ≤50 or ≥700 mg/dL

(continued)

TABLE 7.7 Coagulation Tests *(continued)*

Test Name (Abbreviation)	Description	Reference Range: Conventional Units	Reference Range: SI Units	Increased With	Decreased With	Other Comments
Fibrin degradation products (FDP), fibrin split products (FSP)	Identifies products (X, Y, D, and E) of fibrin when split by plasmin	Negative at 1:4 dilution or <2.5 μg/mL	<2.5 mg/L	DIC, primary fibrinolysis, venous thrombosis, thoracic and cardiac surgery, renal transplant, AMI, pulmonary embolism (PE), carcinoma, hepatic disease	Normal	• Used to diagnose DIC and other thromboembolic disorders • In DIC, FDPs usually begin to fall within 1 day; if very high at baseline, it may take ≥1 week to return to normal • Elevated urine levels suggest renal disease or rejection crisis following renal transplant • False elevations with exercise, stress, and traumatic venipuncture
D-Dimer	Assesses for one FDP; consists of various size pieces of cross-linked fibrin	Negative or <0.5 μg/mL	<0.5 mg/L	DIC, arterial or venous thrombosis (deep vein thrombosis [DVT]), PE, renal or hepatic failure, late in pregnancy, preeclampsia, MI, malignancy, inflammation, severe infection, surgery, trauma	Normal	• False elevations with high titers of rheumatoid factor, tumor marker CA-125, estrogen therapy, and normal pregnancy

Thrombin time (TT)	A sensitive test for fibrinogen deficiency	Within 3 seconds of control value (control range 16–24 seconds, varies widely by laboratory and method used)		DIC, fibrinolysis, hypofibrinogenemia, multiple myeloma, high levels of FDPs, uremia, severe hepatic disease, drugs (heparin, low molecular weight heparins [LMWH])	Hct >55%, hyperfibrinogenemia	• Tests the fibrinogen-to-fibrin conversion; affected by the concentration of fibrinogen and plasmin, and the presence of FDPs and antithrombotic agents • Elevated in ~60% of DIC cases; less sensitive and specific test for DIC than other tests • Most methods of measuring will give elevated results with heparin, urokinase, streptokinase, and asparaginase therapy • When assayed by the reptilase method, heparin does not elevate
Antithrombin III (At III)	Heparin cofactor	Functional assay: 80%–130% normal pooled plasma (NPP); 0.8–1.3	Immunologic assay: 17–39 mg/dL; 170–390 mg/L	Acute hepatitis, vitamin K deficiency (warfarin), renal transplant, inflammation, menstruation, hyperglobulinemia	Congenital deficiency, DIC, DVT, PE, thrombophlebitis, hepatic transplant, partial hepatectomy, cirrhosis/chronic hepatic failure/disease, nephrotic syndrome, AMI, carcinoma, trauma, severe infection, pregnancy (last trimester), early postpartum period,	• Naturally occurring thrombin inhibitor; also inactivates the activated forms of factors II, IX, X, XI, and XII • Heparin's anticoagulant activity is due to accelerating AT III activity • Decreases may predispose patients to thrombus formation and failure of heparin anticoagulation • Test interferences include anabolic steroids, warfarin, heparin, asparaginase, estrogens, and oral contraceptives

(continued)

TABLE 7.7 Coagulation Tests *(continued)*

Test Name (Abbreviation)	Description	Reference Range: Conventional Units	Reference Range: SI Units	Increased With	Decreased With	Other Comments
					midperiod of the menstrual cycle, heparin failure, protein-wasting disease	
Antifactor Xa Activity (Anti-Xa)	Measures ability of plasma to form complex with coagulation factor Xa	0.5–1.1 units/mL (twice daily LMWH at therapeutic doses), 1–2 units/mL (once daily LMWH at therapeutic doses)		Excessive doses of LMWH, renal insufficiency	Insufficient doses of LMWH, incorrect timing of lab draw	• High levels associated with increased bleeding risk • Low levels associated with increased thrombosis risk • Peak level should be drawn 4 hours after administration

Sources: www.labtestsonline.org. Accessed May 14, 2013; Kratz A, Lewandrowski KB. Case records of the Massachusetts General Hospital. Weekly clinicopathological exercises. Normal reference laboratory values. *N Engl J Med*. 1998;339:1063–1072; Fischbach F, Dunning MB. *A Manual of Laboratory Diagnostic Tests*. 8th ed. Philadelphia, PA: Lippincott Williams & Wilkins; 2008; Schmidt J, Wieczorkiewicz J. *Interpreting Laboratory Data: A Point-of-Care Guide*. 1st ed. Bethesda, MD: American Society of Health-System Pharmacists; and Lee M. *Basic Skills in Interpreting Laboratory Data*. 5th ed. Bethesda, MD: American Society of Health-System Pharmacists; 2013

TABLE 7.8 Electrolytes

Test Name (Abbreviation)	Description	Reference Range: Conventional Units	Reference Range: SI Units	Increased With	Decreased With	Other Comments
Sodium (Na^+)	Most abundant cation in extracellular fluid; maintains oncotic pressure and acid–base balance, aids in transmission of nerve impulses	135–145 mEq/L	135–145 mmol/L	(Hypernatremia) dehydration, aldosteronism, diabetes insipidus, osmotic diuretics, Conn syndrome, coma, Cushing disease, tracheobronchitis, drugs (anabolic steroids, corticosteroids, calcium, fluorides, iron)	(Hyponatremia) burns, diarrhea, vomiting, excessive intake of free water, Addison disease, nephritis, diabetic acidosis, cystic fibrosis, malabsorption, edema, hypothyroidism, syndrome of inappropriate antidiuretic hormone (SIADH), drugs (thiazide diuretics, chlorpropamide, carbamazepine, clofibrate, cyclophosphamide, heparin, laxatives, sulfates), some pulmonary disorders (tuberculosis, pneumonias), high TG (false low), low protein (false low)	• Renal system, central nervous system (CNS), and endocrine system regulate Na^+ concentrations • Clinical signs of hyponatremia: nausea, fatigue, cramps, psychosis, seizures, coma • Clinical signs of hypernatremia: cardiovascular and renal symptoms, heart failure • Total body water deficit = ~1 L for each 3 mmol/L of Na^+ greater than normal • Critical values: ≤120 or ≥160

(continued)

TABLE 7.8 Electrolytes *(continued)*

Test Name (Abbreviation)	Description	Reference Range: Conventional Units	Reference Range: SI Units	Increased With	Decreased With	Other Comments
Potassium (K^+)	Principle intracellular fluid cation (with bicarbonate) serves as primary buffer	3.5–5.2 mEq/L	3.5–5.2 mmol/L	(Hyperkalemia) renal failure, dehydration, cell damage (trauma, burns, DIC, chemotherapy, surgery), acidosis, Addison disease, uncontrolled DM, RBC transfusion, pseudohypoaldo-steronism, SLE, sickle cell disease, interstitial nephritis, renal transplant rejection, specimen hemolysis (false elevation)	(Hypokalemia) severe burns, vomiting, diarrhea, severe sweating, starvation, malnutrition, chronic alcoholism, draining wounds, primary aldosteronism, chronic stress, hepatic disease with ascites, renal tubular acidosis, respiratory alkalosis, Bartter syndrome, cystic fibrosis, drugs (diuretics, mineralocorticoids, antibiotics, cisplatin, ticarcillin, amphotericin), glucose tolerance testing or large ingestions of glucose (shifts intercellularly), WBC >50,000/mm^3 (falsely low)	• ~80%–90% excreted in the urine by the kidneys; aldosterone also regulates concentration • ~10% (50 mmol) of total body K^+ is extracellular; therefore, serum levels are a poor measure of total body K^+ but do correlate with physiologic effects. Values do not vary with circulatory volume • Levels rise ~0.6 mEq/L for every 0.1 decrease in blood pH from normal (pH 7.4) • Specific electrocardiogram (ECG) changes are seen with changes in K^+ levels • Hypokalemia clinical issues: enhanced effects of digitalis agents; need to also correct for hypomagnesemia; affects neuro-muscular function • Hyperkalemia clinical issues: treat with insulin (and glucose); affects neuromuscular function

						• Each mmol/L decrease in the serum K^+ represents a total body 200–400 mmol K^+ deficit • Critical values: ≤2.5 or ≥6.0
Chloride (Cl^-)	Major extracellular anion; involved in acid–base and water balance via influence on osmotic pressure	96–108 mEq/L	96–108 mmol/L	Dehydration, metabolic acidosis, hyperventilation, respiratory alkalosis, renal disorders (renal tubular acidosis), diabetes insipidus, Cushing syndrome, diarrhea, eclampsia, hypothalamic damage/ head injury, primary hyperparathyroidism, salicylate intoxication	Vomiting, gastric suctioning, aggressive diuresis, burns, heat exhaustion, acute infection, diabetic acidosis, chronic respiratory acidosis, metabolic alkalosis, CHF, Addison disease, SIADH, overhydration, acute intermittent porphyria, salt-losing nephritis	• Cl^- concentration useful in diagnosis of acid–base disorders • Plasma concentration can be maintained near normal even in the presence of renal failure
Carbon dioxide (CO_2) content	Plasma CO_2 reflects bicarbonate (HCO_3) concentrations	22–32 mEq/L	22–32 mmol/L	Severe vomiting, emphysema, aldosteronism	Acute renal failure, diabetic acidosis, hyperventilation, salicylate toxicity	• Normal plasma CO_2 is ~95% bicarbonate (a base), which is regulated by the renal system; the remaining ~5% is dissolved CO_2 gas (an acid) and carbonic acid (H_2CO_3), which are regulated by the lungs • Critical values: ≤12 or ≥40

(continued)

TABLE 7.8 Electrolytes *(continued)*

Test Name (Abbreviation)	Description	Reference Range: Conventional Units	Reference Range: SI Units	Increased With	Decreased With	Other Comments
Calcium (Ca^{2+})	Measures total (protein-bound and free) serum calcium	8.5–10.5 mg/dL	2.1–2.6 mmol/L	(Hypercalcemia) hyperparathyroidism, neoplasms, parathyroid adenoma, Hodgkin disease, multiple myeloma, leukemia, bone metastasis, hyperplasia (associated with hypophosphatemia), renal failure, Addison disease, Paget disease, respiratory acidosis, immobilization, drugs (thiazide diuretics)	(Hypocalcemia) hyperphosphatemia, alkalosis, osteomalacia, hypomagnesemia, inadequate calcium replacement, sepsis, pancreatitis, renal failure, malnutrition, alcoholism, drugs (laxatives, furosemide, calcitonin, glucocorticoids, excessive thyroid hormone, exacerbated with bisphosphonates if inadequate calcium and vitamin D), pseudohypocalcemia (low protein/albumin may lead to low total serum Ca^{2+}, but with less protein bound, the level of free Ca^{2+} may be appropriate)	• Ca^{2+} plays an essential role in muscle contraction, cardiac function, transmission of nerve impulses, and blood clotting • Parathyroid hormone (PTH) is released when serum Ca^{2+} decreases. PTH increases renal conversion of vitamin D to the active form (stimulates intestinal Ca^{2+} absorption) and stimulates bone resorption (releases Ca^{2+} and PO_4 into the blood and enhances renal Ca^{2+} reabsorption) • Because Ca^{2+} is 50% protein bound, need to correct for abnormal binding (with low albumin) or measure free calcium • Decreases in Alb of 1 g/dL will decrease the total serum Ca^{2+} by ~0.8 mg/dL (see Chapter 13, A Pharmacy Calculations Anthology) • Critical values: ≤7.0 or ≥13.0 mg/dL

Ionized calcium (free calcium)	Measures only active (unbound/free) form of calcium	4.60–5.20 mg/dL	1.14–1.30 mmol/L	Same as calcium	Same as calcium	• Of the ~1%–2% of the body's total calcium that is in the blood, 50% is ionized/free (active form) and the remainder is bound to serum proteins, mainly albumin • When requesting ionized Ca^{2+} levels, blood pH should be measured concurrently
Phosphate (P, inorganic phosphorus, PO_4)	Measures serum phosphate	2.4–4.7 mg/dL	0.77–1.52 mmol/L	(Hyperphosphatemia) renal dysfunction, uremia, excessive phosphate intake, excessive vitamin D intake, hypoparathyroidism, hypocalcemia, bone tumors, respiratory acidosis, lactic acidosis, DKA, drugs (bisphosphonate therapy)	(Hypophosphatemia) hyperparathyroidism, hypercalcemia, rickets, vitamin D deficiency, diabetic coma, hyperinsulinism, continuous IV glucose administration in a person without DM, diuretic phase of severe burns, respiratory alkalosis, alcoholism, malnutrition, hypothyroidism, hypokalemia, drugs (antacids, overuse of diuretics)	• Phosphate (anion form) is required for generation of bony tissue, metabolism of glucose and lipids, maintenance of acid–base balance, and storage and transfer of energy within the body • ~85% of the body's total PO_4 is combined with Ca^{2+}; therefore, serum Ca^{2+} values must also be checked when evaluating phosphate levels • Critical values: ≤0.9 mg/dL
Uric acid	Measures uric acid levels	Male: 3.5–8.5 mg/dL Female: 2.3–6.6 mg/dL	Male: 208–506 μmol/L Female: 137–393 μmol/L	(Hyperuricemia) leukemia, lymphomas, shock, chemotherapy, metabolic acidosis, psoriasis, significant	Drugs (allopurinol, sulfinpyrazone, high-dose salicylates (>3 g/day) (Hypouricemia is not clinically significant)	• Formed from the breakdown of nucleic acids; serum levels are increased with excessive production/destruction of cells or an inability to excrete urate renally

(continued)

TABLE 7.8 Electrolytes *(continued)*

Test Name (Abbreviation)	Description	Reference Range: Conventional Units	Reference Range: SI Units	Increased With	Decreased With	Other Comments
				renal dysfunction, drugs (thiazide diuretics, low/moderate-dose salicylates, ethambutol, niacin, cyclosporine)		• Useful for monitoring gout therapy with allopurinol
Magnesium (Mg^{2+})	Measures serum magnesium levels	1.4–2.5 mg/dL	0.7–1.25 mmol/L	(Hypermagnesemia) renal dysfunction, diabetic acidosis, high-dose Mg^{2+} antacids with renal insufficiency, hypothyroidism, dehydration	(Hypomagnesemia) high PO_4 diets (suppress absorption), diarrhea, hemodialysis, malabsorption syndromes, lactation, acute pancreatitis, chronic alcoholism, drugs (thiazides, amphotericin B, cisplatin)	• Required for the utilization of adenosine triphosphate (ATP) as an energy source. Role in carbohydrate metabolism, protein synthesis, nucleic acid synthesis, and muscle contraction. Regulates neuromuscular irritability, the clotting mechanism, and Ca^{2+} absorption • Hypomagnesemia can cause hypocalcemia and hypokalemia resulting in severe neuromuscular irritability and ventricular arrhythmias • Hypermagnesemia can act as a sedative and can depress cardiac and neuromuscular activity • Critical values: ≤0.9 or ≥5.0 mg/dL

Total serum protein (TSP, total protein [TP], albumin/globulin ratio, A/G ratio)	Commonly included in CMPs, hepatic and nutrition panels	6.0–8.0 g/dL	60–80 g/L	(Hyperproteinemia) hemoconcentration secondary to dehydration (both albumin and globulin increase), collagen diseases, SLE, acute hepatic disease, multiple myeloma	(Hypoproteinemia) increased loss of albumin in the urine, decreased formation in the liver, insufficient protein intake, severe burns	• Three major categories: (i) tissue or organ proteins, (ii) hemoglobin, and (iii) plasma/serum proteins (albumin and globulins), which reflect nutritional status and serve as buffers in the maintenance of acid–base balance • The A/G ratio decreases/is low if the globulin/TSP increases but the Alb concentration is unchanged, or if the globulin/TSP is unchanged but the Alb is low • See Table 7.12 for information on albumin
Zinc, Serum (Zn)	Measures serum zinc levels; often included in nutritional panels	Male: 75–291 µg/dL Female: 65–256 µg/dL	Male: 11.5–44.5 µmol/L Female: 9.95–39.2 µmol/L	(Uncommon) tissue injury, hemolysis, contaminated collection tubes	Abnormal losses (Crohn disease, pregnancy, fistulas, malabsorption), alcoholism, DM, proteinuria, renal disease, hepatic disease, porphyria, sickle cell disease, trauma, infection, stress, hypoalbuminemia, fasting obese patients, prolonged parenteral nutrition	• Cofactor of many enzymes (alkaline phosphatase, lactic dehydrogenase); ~80% of total in whole blood is in RBCs • Primary/normal losses are in pancreatic and intestinal secretions • Signs of deficiency include dermatitis, hair loss, diarrhea, depression, and hypogeusia • Levels affected by circadian variations, with peaks around 9 AM and 6 PM

Sources: www.labtestsonline.org. Accessed May 14, 2013; Kratz A, Lewandrowski KB. Case records of the Massachusetts General Hospital. Weekly clinicopathological exercises. Normal reference laboratory values. *N Engl J Med*. 1998;339:1063–1072; Fischbach F, Dunning MB. *A Manual of Laboratory Diagnostic Tests*. 8th ed. Philadelphia, PA: Lippincott Williams & Wilkins; 2008; Schmidt J, Wieczorkiewicz J. *Interpreting Laboratory Data: A Point-of-Care Guide*. 1st ed. Bethesda, MD: American Society of Health-System Pharmacists; and Lee M. *Basic Skills in Interpreting Laboratory Data*. 5th ed. Bethesda, MD: American Society of Health-System Pharmacists; 2013

Arterial Blood Gases

Arterial blood gas concentrations are analyzed to assess the exchange of oxygen (O_2) and carbon dioxide (CO_2). An imbalance in these gases is also known as an acid–base imbalance. The specimen for arterial blood gases (ABGs) must be an arterial blood sample and can be obtained by either an arterial puncture or from an indwelling arterial line. Table 7.9 describes the components of ABGs. Common indications for ABGs include the following:

Gas exchange abnormalities:

- Acute and chronic pulmonary disease
- Acute respiratory failure
- Cardiac disease
- Pulmonary testing (at rest and with exercise)
- Monitoring O_2 therapy
- Sleep disorder studies

Acid–base disturbances:

- Metabolic acidosis
- Metabolic alkalosis

Laboratory Tests by Organ System

Although some laboratory tests provide information about a wide variety of body systems, others are used to diagnose, assess status, and monitor treatment of patients with organ system–specific diseases and conditions. Tests used for the cardiac system, endocrine system, gastrointestinal and hepatic system, and renal system are presented.

Cardiac System Tests

While electrolytes and ABGs can provide useful information when dealing with a cardiac patient, additional tests, such as cardiac enzymes and lipoprotein panels, are often needed to evaluate cardiac issues more specifically (Table 7.10).

Endocrine System Tests

Diabetes mellitus (DM), thyroid dysfunction, and hypogonadism are common endocrine disorders. Related tests, such as glycosylated hemoglobin, thyroid function tests and testosterone levels, presented in Table 7.11, are commonly used to diagnose and monitor control of these conditions.

(*Text continued on page 232*)

TABLE 7.9 Arterial Blood Gases

Test Name (Abbreviation)	Description	Reference Range		Increased With	Decreased With	Other Comments
		Conventional Units	SI Units			
Oxygen saturation (SaO_2)	The amount of oxygen (O_2) carried by Hgb; expressed as a % of the capacity of O_2 to combine with Hgb	95%–99% O_2				• Used with pO_2 to evaluate the extent of oxygenation of Hgb and the adequacy of tissue oxygenation • RBCs are able to transport 65 times the amount of O_2 dissolved in plasma. This relationship is determined by pH, temperature, the concentration of 2,3 DPG (diphosphoglycerate), and the molecular species of Hgb
Partial pressure of oxygen (PaO_2, pO_2)	Measure of the partial pressure exerted by the amount of O_2 dissolved in the plasma	(Room air, age-dependent) >80 mm Hg	>10.6 kPa	Increased O_2 delivery by arterial means (nasal prongs, mechanical ventilation), hyperventilation by the patient, polycythemia	COPD, restrictive airway disease (RAD, asthma), anemia, hypoventilation due to physical or neuromuscular impairment, compromised cardiac function	• Provides an estimate of the lung's ability to oxygenate blood • The partial pressure of O_2 dissolved in plasma determines the amount of O_2 bound to Hgb • Critical value: ≤50 mm Hg

(continued)

TABLE 7.9 Arterial Blood Gases *(continued)*

Test Name (Abbreviation)	Description	Reference Range: Conventional Units	Reference Range: SI Units	Increased With	Decreased With	Other Comments
Partial pressure of carbon dioxide ($PaCO_2$)	Measure of the pressure exerted by the CO_2 dissolved in the plasma	35–45 mm Hg	4.6–5.9 kPa	COPD, reduced function of the respiratory center, hypoventilation	Hypoxia, anxiety/ nervousness, PE, hyperventilation	• Used to evaluate the effectiveness of alveolar ventilation and to determine the acid–base status of the blood • In general, for each mEq decrease in HCO_3, the $PaCO_2$ will decrease 1.3 mm Hg • Critical values: ≤20 or ≥60–70 mm Hg
pH	Reflects the chemical balance of acids and bases within the body	7.35–7.45 pH units		Acidemia (due to increased formation of acids)	Alkalemia (due to acid loss)	• Hydrogen ion sources within the body include volatile acids and fixed acids (lactic acid, keto acids) • When evaluating a pH value, pCO_2 and HCO_3 should also be obtained to estimate the respiratory or metabolic component contributing to the acid–base status • Critical values: ≤7.25 or ≥7.55–7.65

Anion gap (AG)	Calculated using available electrolyte information to assist in quantifying unmeasured cations (including Ca^{2+} and Mg^{2+}) and anions (protein, PO^{-}_{4}, sulfate, and organic acids)	8–16 mEq/L (if K^+ included in calculation), 12–20 mEq/L (if K^+ not included in calculation)	(+ High pH): extracellular volume contraction, administration of large-dose penicillins (+ low pH): MULEPAK (*m*ethanol ingestion, *u*remia, *l*actic acidosis, *e*thylene glycol ingestion, *p*araldehyde ingestion, *a*spirin intoxication, *k*etoacidosis)	Hypoalbuminemia, multiple myeloma, hyponatremia caused by viscous serum, marked hypercalcemia, lithium toxicity Normal AG: metabolic acidosis from diarrhea, renal tubular acidosis, drugs (potassium-sparing diuretics, carbonic anhydrase inhibitors)	• Used clinically in the diagnosis of metabolic acidosis • Can be calculated using two different approaches: $AG = Na^+ - (Cl^- + HCO^{-}_{3})$ $AG = (Na^+ + K^+) - (Cl^- + HCO^{-}_{3})$ • See Chapter 13, A Pharmacy Calculations Anthology, and Chapter 10, Fluid and Electrolyte Therapy, for further discussions
Bicarbonate buffer system	Consists of carbonic acid (H_2CO_3) and bicarbonate (HCO_3)	22–26 mEq/L	Respiratory acidosis due to decreased ventilation	Respiratory alkalosis due to increased alveolar ventilation and removal of CO_2 and water, metabolic acidosis due to accumulation of body acids, loss of HCO_3 from the extracellular fluid	• The major buffer system in the extracellular body fluid • Calculated by Total CO_2 content = $H_2CO_3 + HCO_3$

Sources: www.labtestsonline.org. Accessed May 14, 2013; Kratz A, Lewandrowski KB. Case records of the Massachusetts General Hospital. Weekly clinicopathological exercises. Normal reference laboratory values. *N Engl J Med.* 1998;339:1063–1072; Fischbach F, Dunning MB. *A Manual of Laboratory Diagnostic Tests.* 8th ed. Philadelphia, PA: Lippincott Williams & Wilkins; 2008; Schmidt J, Wieczorkiewicz J. *Interpreting Laboratory Data: A Point-of-Care Guide.* 1st ed. Bethesda, MD: American Society of Health-System Pharmacists; and Lee M. *Basic Skills in Interpreting Laboratory Data.* 5th ed. Bethesda, MD: American Society of Health-System Pharmacists; 2013

TABLE 7.10 Cardiac System Tests

Test Name (Abbreviation)	Description	Reference Range: Conventional Units	Reference Range: SI Units	Increased With	Decreased With	Other Comments
Creatine kinase (CK)	Measure of muscle enzyme (formerly known as creatine phosphokinase [CPK])	Male: 60–400 U/L Female: 40–175 U/L (higher in African Americans)	Male: 1.00–6.67 μkat/L Female: 0.67–2.91 μkat/L	MI (begins to rise 3–4 hours after myocardial injury, peaking within 15–24 hours and returning to normal within 3–4 days), cerebrovascular disease, muscular dystrophy, rhabdomyolysis, polymyositis, dermatomyositis, delirium tremens (DTs), chronic alcoholism, subarachnoid hemorrhage, CNS trauma		• High concentrations in heart and skeletal muscle • Used as a specific test for the diagnosis of MI and as a reliable measure of skeletal muscle diseases (muscular dystrophy, polymyositis) • Divided into three isoenzymes: BB (= CK1), MB (= CK2), and MM (= CK3) • Normal CK is virtually 100% MM • Commonly measured in workup for statin-associated myopathy
CK isoenzyme BB (= CK1)	Definitive indication of brain injury	0%		Biliary atresia, brain trauma, certain other brain injuries or tumors		• Brain tissue primarily composed of BB
CK isoenzyme MB (= CK2)	Definitive indication of myocardial injury	0%–4% or ≤9 ng/mL	≤9 μg/L	MI, myocardial ischemia, muscular dystrophy		• In cardiac muscle • If negative throughout 48 hours after onset of chest pain, MI usually ruled out

2CK isoenzyme MM (= CK3)	Indication of skeletal muscle injury	96%–100%		MI, muscle trauma, intramuscular (IM) injections, shock, after surgery		• In skeletal and cardiac muscle
Troponin I	High selectivity as a marker of cardiac damage	≤0.6 ng/mL	≤0.6 μg/L	>1.5 ng/mL suggests current myocardial injury = MI (CK elevates within 6 hours of myocardial injury; remains elevated for 7–10 days)	<0.4 ng/mL indicates no myocardial injury within the previous several days 0.4–2.0 ng/mL is borderline and suggests possible MI; repeat testing recommended	• Globular proteins found in cardiac and skeletal muscle; key role in triggering muscle contraction in response to increased cytosolic calcium • Three cardiac troponins: troponin I (cTnI), T (cTnT), and C (cTnC). Subtype I is found specifically in the heart (C is not specific for the heart and T, while most commonly in heart tissue, can also be expressed in noncardiac tissue on injury) • Levels of troponin I and T used to evaluate suspected MI (6 hours–1 week after the incident)
B-Type Natriuretic Peptide (BNP)	Marker of ventricular systolic and diastolic dysfunction	<100 pg/mL	<100 ng/L	Heart failure, PE, pulmonary diseases		• Hormone produced by heart ventricles in response to ventricular volume expansion and pressure overload • Increased levels associated with shortness of breath and edema

(continued)

TABLE 7.10 Cardiac System Tests *(continued)*

Test Name (Abbreviation)	Description	Reference Range: Conventional Units	Reference Range: SI Units	Increased With	Decreased With	Other Comments
Cholesterol (total cholesterol, TC)	Elevated cholesterol is a risk factor for cardiovascular disease (CVD) Borderline: 200–239 mg/dL High risk: ≥240 mg/dL	Desirable: ≤199 mg/dL Borderline: 200–239 mg/dL High risk: ≥240 mg/dL	≤5.17 mmol/L Borderline: 5.17–6.18 mmol/L High risk: ≥6.21 mmol/L	(Hypercholesterolemia) atherosclerosis, coronary artery disease (CAD), familial type II hypercholesterolemia, hypothyroidism, DM, metabolic syndrome, obstructive jaundice, pregnancy, drugs (anabolic steroids, beta-blockers, testosterone, epinephrine, oral contraceptives, vitamin D)	Malabsorption, hepatic disease, cancer, sepsis, hypolipoproteinemia, pernicious anemia, drugs (lipid-lowering agents such as statins, niacin, fibrates, cholesterol absorption inhibitors, bile acid sequestrants)	• Exists in tissues throughout the body; used to form steroid hormones, bile acids, and cell membranes • Levels of >200 mg/dL are considered to be high and require a TG evaluation
Triglycerides (TGs), fasting	Needed for formation of other lipids and fatty acids	10–150 mg/dL	0.11–1.69 mmol/L	Cirrhosis, anorexia nervosa, biliary obstruction, cerebral thrombosis, chronic renal failure, DM, metabolic syndrome, Down syndrome, hypertension (HTN), idiopathic hypercalcemia, hyperlipoproteinemia (types I, IIb, III, IV, and V),	COPD, severe parenchymal hepatic disease, malnutrition, malabsorption, hyperthyroidism, hyperparathyroidism, hypolipoproteinemia, intestinal lymphangiectasia, drugs (some lipid-lowering agents such	• Found in plasma lipids as chylomicrons and VLDLs • Nutritional/fasting status most affects TGs (and therefore calculated LDL); patients should maintain usual diet for 3 days and must fast for 12 hours before test. Alcohol should not be consumed 24 hours before test

				glycogen storage diseases (types I, III, and VI), gout, ischemic heart disease, hypothyroidism, pregnancy, acute intermittent porphyria, respiratory distress syndrome, thalassemia major, viral hepatitis, Werner syndrome, high-carbohydrate diets, excessive alcohol consumption, drugs (bile acid sequestrants, corticosteroids, estrogens, ethanol, oral contraceptives, spironolactone)	as statins, niacin, fibrates)	• Critical value: >500 mg/dL increases risk for pancreatitis
High-density lipoprotein (HDL) cholesterol (HDLc)	Elevated HDLc is beneficial and protects against CHD	Desirable: >60 mg/dL Borderline: 35–60 mg/dL High risk: <35 mg/dL	Desirable: >1.55 mmol/L Borderline: 0.91–1.55 mmol/L High risk: <0.91 mmol/L	Chronic alcoholism, primary biliary cirrhosis, exposure to industrial toxins or polychlorinated hydrocarbons, exercise, moderate alcohol (especially red wine) intake, drugs (niacin, estrogens, oral contraceptives, phenytoin)	Cystic fibrosis, severe cirrhosis, DM, metabolic syndrome, Hodgkin disease, nephrotic syndrome, malaria, some acute infections, drugs (anabolic steroids, β-adrenergic blockers [mild])	• Products of liver and intestinal synthesis and TG catabolism • There is an inverse relationship between HDLc levels and CHD • Levels >60 mg/dL are protective and counted as a negative risk when calculating CHD risk (i.e., can subtract one risk factor)

(continued)

TABLE 7.10 Cardiac System Tests *(continued)*

Test Name (Abbreviation)	Description	Reference Range: Conventional Units	Reference Range: SI Units	Increased With	Decreased With	Other Comments
Low-density lipoprotein (LDL) cholesterol (LDLc)	Usually calculated with Friedewald equation; can be measured directly (may require specific order)	Desirable: <130 mg/dL Borderline: 130–159 mg/dL High: ≥160 mg/dL	Desirable: <3.36 mmol/L Borderline: 3.36–4.11 mmol/L High: ≥4.13 mmol/L	Familial and idiopathic hyperlipidemia coronary vascular disease, nonfasting status (especially if LDL value is calculated rather than measured directly), types IIa and IIb hyperlipoproteinemia, DM, metabolic syndrome, hypothyroidism, obstructive jaundice, nephrotic syndrome	Hypoproteinemia, abetalipoproteinemia, severe illness, drugs (estrogen, lipid-lowering agents such as statins, niacin, fibrates, cholesterol absorption inhibitors, bile acid sequestrants)	• Plays key role in transporting cholesterol to various tissues where it is needed for membrane synthesis and other functions • Goal for patients with CHD or CHD risk equivalents (including DM): <100 mg/dL (2.59 mmol/L); for patients with DM and CHD (or multiple risk factors), optimal goal of <70 mg/dL (1.81 mmol/L) may be considered • Friedewald equation: LDLc = TC – HDL – (TG/5) (only applicable if TG <400); various factors can affect accuracy of Friedewald calculation (may be less accurate if TG >200 or HDL <50 and affected by variable LDL size/type)

Non-HDL cholesterol	= TC − HDL Reflects total of all atherogenic particles (LDL + VLDL + IDL)	Desirable: <160 mg/dL Borderline: 160–189 mg/dL High: ≥190 mg/dL	Desirable: <4.14 mmol/L Borderline: 4.14–4.89 mmol/L High: ≥4.91 mmol/L	See LDL	See LDL	• Goal is 30 mg/dL more than LDL goal • Goal for patients with CHD or CHD risk equivalents (including DM): <130 mg/dL (3.36 mmol/L); for patients with DM and CHD (or multiple risk factors), optimal goal of <100 mg/dL (2.59 mmol/L) may be considered
Apolipoprotein A-1 (Apo A-1)	Main component of HDL	90–240 mg/dL	0.9–2.4 g/L	Familial hyper-α-lipoproteinemia	Tangier disease (hypo-α-lipoproteinemia), β-lipoproteinemia, Apo A-I Melano disease, Apo A-I-C-III deficiency, Apo C-II deficiency, hepatic disease, nephrotic syndrome/renal failure, poorly controlled DM, hypertriglyceridemia (familial), premature CHD, diet high in polyunsaturated fats, smoking	• <90 mg/dL indicates increased CAD risk • Patients must fast for 12 hours before test
Apolipoprotein B (Apo B)	Main component of LDL and VLDL	45–163 mg/dL	0.45–1.63 g/L	Hyperlipoproteinemia types IIa, IIb, and V, hepatic disease/obstruction, nephrotic syndrome/renal failure,	Tangier disease (hypo-α-lipoproteinemia), hypo-β-lipoproteinemia, α-β-lipoproteinemia,	• >110 mg/dL indicates increased CAD risk • Patients must fast for 12 hours before test

(continued)

TABLE 7.10 Cardiac System Tests *(continued)*

Test Name (Abbreviation)	Description	Reference Range		Increased With	Decreased With	Other Comments
		Conventional Units	SI Units			
				Cushing syndrome, Werner syndrome, DM, hypothyroidism, premature CHD Fredrickson type IIa, porphyria, dysglobulinemia, drugs (statins, others)	Apo C-II deficiency, type 1 hyperlipidemia, hypothyroidism, malnutrition/ malabsorption, Reye syndrome, diet high in polyunsaturated fats, low-cholesterol diets	• Important role in LDL catabolism, regulating cholesterol synthesis, and metabolism
Apo A-I/Apo B ratio	Correlates with increased risk for CAD	0.8–2.63				• Lower ratio = higher CAD risk
High-sensitivity C-reactive protein (hs-CRP)	Highly sensitive measure to detect lower levels of CRP	0.02–0.80 mg/dL	0.2–8 mg/L	MI, CAD risk	Drugs (statins, perhaps other lipid-lowering drugs)	• Suggests risk for CAD • See Table 7.14 for general CRP

Sources: www.labtestsonline.org. Accessed May 14, 2013; Kratz A, Lewandrowski KB. Case records of the Massachusetts General Hospital. Weekly clinicopathological exercises. Normal reference laboratory values. *N Engl J Med*. 1998;339:1063–1072; Fischbach F, Dunning MB. *A Manual of Laboratory Diagnostic Tests*. 8th ed. Philadelphia, PA: Lippincott Williams & Wilkins; 2008; Schmidt J, Wieczorkiewicz J. *Interpreting Laboratory Data: A Point-of-Care Guide*. 1st ed. Bethesda, MD: American Society of Health-System Pharmacists; Lee M. *Basic Skills in Interpreting Laboratory Data*. 5th ed. Bethesda, MD: American Society of Health-System Pharmacists; 2013; and Grundy SM, Cleeman JI, Merz CN, et al. Implications of recent clinical trials for the National Cholesterol Education Program Adult Treatment Panel III guidelines. *Circulation*. 2004;110:227–239

TABLE 7.11 Endocrine System Tests

Test Name (Abbreviation)	Description	Reference Range		Increased With	Decreased With	Other Comments
		Conventional Units	SI Units			
Glucose (fasting blood glucose [FBG], fasting blood sugar [FBS])	Primarily a screening procedure to detect abnormalities in glucose utilization or production; included in BMP. Home and POC testing also available for day-to-day casual blood glucose (CBG) monitoring	70–100 mg/dL	3.89–5.55 mmol/L	(Hyperglycemia), impaired fasting glucose (IFG)/prediabetes (FBS >100–125 mg/dL), DM (FBS >126 mg/dL), Cushing disease, chronic hepatic disease, potassium deficiency, chronic illness, pheochromocytoma, bacterial sepsis, acute distress (surgical procedures and anesthesia), parenteral glucose administration, pregnancy (gestational DM), drugs (alcohol, glucocorticoids, thiazide diuretics, estrogen, epinephrine, phenytoin)	(Hypoglycemia) insulin overdose, Addison disease, malnutrition, hepatic damage (alcoholism), alcohol use	• Abnormal values indicate the inability of the islet cells of the pancreas to produce insulin, the intestines to absorb glucose, cells to utilize glucose efficiently, and/or the liver to accumulate and break down glycogen • Critical values: ≤50 or ≥500

(continued)

TABLE 7.11 Endocrine System Tests *(continued)*

Test Name (Abbreviation)	Description	Reference Range: Conventional Units	Reference Range: SI Units	Increased With	Decreased With	Other Comments
Hemoglobin A1c (A_1c, HbA_1c, $HgbA_1c$, glycosylated hemoglobin)	Measures the blood glucose bound to Hgb; reflects the average blood sugar level in the 2–3 months preceding the test	4.0%–6% of total Hgb In patients with DM, American Diabetes Association goal: <7% or <7.5–8% depending on age/risk factors; American Association of Clinical Endocrinologists goal: <6.5%	0.04–0.06 fraction of total Hgb	DM with poor glucose control over the 2–3 months prior to the test, splenectomy, alcohol toxicity, lead toxicity, (falsely high) iron deficiency anemia, sickle cell anemia, thalassemia	Pregnancy, chronic renal failure, (falsely low) hemolysis, hemolytic anemia, significant blood loss, sickle cell anemia, thalassemia	• Hgb has a life span of 120 days, undergoes glycosylation by a slow nonenzymatic process within the RBC and is dependent on available glucose. The more glucose the RBC is exposed to, the higher the % of glycosylated Hgb • Every 1% increase in A1c reflects a 35-mg/dL increase in blood glucose (A_1c 7% = mean plasma glucose 170 mg/dL) • Used to diagnose DM and monitor DM control • Does not fully reflect temporary or new changes in glycemic control, hypoglycemia, or glycemic variability

Fructosamine	Measurement of glycated protein; reflects the average blood sugar level in the 2–3 weeks preceding the test	170–285 μmol/L		DM with poor glucose control over the 2–3 weeks prior to the test	(Falsely low) decreased protein levels, increased protein loss, change in the type of protein produced by the body	• Serum proteins have a shorter life span than RBCs (~14–21 days) • May be useful in situations where the A1c cannot be reliably measured (rapid changes in DM treatment, gestational DM where tight control is essential, RBC loss or abnormalities) • Since fructosamine concentrations in well-controlled DM may overlap with patients without DM, fructosamine is not useful as a screen for DM • High levels of vitamin C, lipemia, hemolysis, and hyperthyroidism can interfere with test results
Insulin, free	Measures insulin levels	2–20 μU/mL	14.35–143.5 pmol/L	Insulinoma, type 2 DM (untreated), obesity, insulin administration, acromegaly, Cushing syndrome, pancreatic islet cell hyperplasia	Type 1 DM (severe), hypopituitarism	• Critical values: >35 *μ*U/mL (243 pmol/L), fasting

(continued)

TABLE 7.11 Endocrine System Tests *(continued)*

Test Name (Abbreviation)	Description	Reference Range: Conventional Units	Reference Range: SI Units	Increased With	Decreased With	Other Comments
Insulin C-peptide (C-peptide)	Monitors insulin production by the pancreatic beta cells and helps determine DM type and cause of hypoglycemia	0.5–2.7 ng/mL (varies by laboratory)	0.17–0.90 mmol/L	High levels of endogenous insulin production, insulin resistance (prediabetes, type 2 DM), insulinomas (insulin-producing tumors), pancreas or β-cell transplantation, hypokalemia, pregnancy, Cushing syndrome, renal failure (oral hypoglycemic drugs)	Insufficient insulin production by beta cells (type 1 DM), production suppressed by exogenous insulin, radical pancreatectomy, production suppressed with somatostatin suppression tests	• C-peptide can be used to help determine how much insulin the pancreas is still producing
Cortisol, plasma	Used primarily to diagnose Cushing or Addison disease	Morning: 6–24 μg/dL Evening: 3–12 μg/dL	Morning: 165–662 nmol/L Evening: 3–331 nmol/L	Hyperthyroidism, stress (circadian variation less apparent in this setting), obesity, Cushing syndrome, pregnancy, drugs (spironolactone, oral contraceptives), extreme increases in the morning and no variation later in the day suggest carcinoma	Hepatic disease, Addison disease, anterior pituitary hyposecretion, hypothyroidism	• Affects the metabolism of proteins, carbohydrates, and lipids and inhibits the effect of insulin; stimulates hepatic gluconeogenesis and decreases the rate of glucose use by the cells • In healthy patients with normal diurnal rhythms, cortisol secretion is higher in the morning (6–8 AM) and lower in the evening (4–6 PM)

Thyroid-stimulating hormone (TSH)	Measures TSH levels	0.5–5.0 μU/mL	0.5–5.0 mU/L	Primary hypothyroidism (T_4 should be low)	Hyperthyroidism *Normal TSH (with low T_3 and T_4): possible hypopituitarism	• Secreted from the anterior pituitary, stimulates thyroid hormone (triiodothyronine [T_3] and thyroxine [T_4]) release from the thyroid gland. Secretion is under negative feedback control from T_3 and T_4 • Best screen for hypothyroidism (can differentiate primary hypothyroidism from pituitary/hypothalamic hypothyroidism) and hyperthyroidism; also used for monitoring thyroid replacement therapy
Thyroxine, total (T_4)	Measures the level of total circulating T_4	4–10.9 μg/dL Females taking estrogen: 6.5–12.5 μg/dL	51–140 nmol/L Females taking estrogen: 84–161 nmol/L	Hyperthyroidism, acute thyroiditis, pregnancy, early hepatitis, idiopathic thyroxine-binding globulin (TBG) elevation, estrogen use	Hypothyroidism, thyroiditis, nephrosis, cirrhosis, hypoproteinemia, malnutrition, idiopathic TBG decrease, drugs (anabolic steroids, salicylates, phenytoin, propranolol)	• >95% of total T_4 is bound to TBG, prealbumin and albumin
Free thyroxine (free T_4)	Can be assessed in two ways: measured via equilibrium dialysis or indirectly	Equilibrium dialysis: 0.8–2.7 ng/dL	0.010–0.035 nmol/L	Same as T_4	Same as T_4	• Only <5% of total T_4 is the free/unbound (biologically active)

(continued)

TABLE 7.11 Endocrine System Tests *(continued)*

Test Name (Abbreviation)	Description	Reference Range: Conventional Units	Reference Range: SI Units	Increased With	Decreased With	Other Comments
	calculated with the free thyroxine index (measure total T_4 and assess TBG-binding capacity; see T_3UR)					form. Assessment of free T_4 (along with total T_4 and TSH) is needed in thyroid disease workups
Triiodothyronine uptake ratio (T_3UR), thyroid hormone–binding ratio (THBI)	Indirect measurement of unsaturated TBG in the blood	25%–35%	0.25–0.35	Hyperthyroidism, nephrosis, severe hepatic disease, metastatic malignancy, pulmonary insufficiency, drugs (thyroxine [T_4] and desiccated thyroid therapy, heparin, androgens, anabolic steroids, phenytoin, large doses of salicylates)	Elevated levels of TBG, hypothyroidism, pregnancy, hyperestrogenic status, drugs (liothyronine [T_3] treatment)	• Main use of T_3UR is to help provide an indirect measure of free T_4, as described above
Triiodothyronine (T_3)	Measures serum levels of T_3	45–181 ng/dL	0.69–2.78 nmol/L	Hyperthyroidism, T_3 thyrotoxicosis, acute thyroiditis, idiopathic TBG elevation, pregnancy, drugs (liothyronine	Hypothyroidism (some clinically hypothyroid patients will have normal levels), starvation, idiopathic	• More metabolically active but shorter half-life than T_4. There is less T_3 than T_4 in the serum

				>25 μg/d, levothyroxine >300 μg/d, estrogen, oral contraceptives)	TBG depression, acute illness, drugs (anabolic steroids, androgens, high-dose salicylates, phenytoin)	• Diagnostic test for hyperthyroidism and T_3 thyrotoxicosis (elevated T_3 levels seen with normal T_4 levels) • Little value in diagnosing hypothyroidism
Testosterone, total (adult males)	Hormone responsible for development of male secondary sexual characteristics	Males (adult): 270–1,100 ng/dL	Males (adult): 9–38 nmol/L	Hyperthyroidism, adrenal tumors, precocious puberty and adrenal hyperplasia in boys, syndromes of androgen resistance, medications (phenytoin, rifampin, dopamine agonists)	Hypogonadism (pituitary failure), hypopituitarism, cirrhosis, Down syndrome, Klinefelter syndrome, delayed puberty, many medications (carbamazepine, dexamethazone, digoxin, spironolactone, ketoconazole, etc.)	• Draw sample at 7:00 AM for highest levels • Little value for urine testosterone levels Alcoholism and high-dose chronic opiate in males decreases testosterone levels
Testosterone, free (adult males)	Unbound testosterone levels	Males (adult): 50–210 pg/mL	Males (adult): 174–729 pmol/L		Hypogonadism, elderly men	See Testosterone, total

Sources: www.labtestsonline.org. Accessed May 14, 2013; Kratz A, Lewandrowski KB. Case records of the Massachusetts General Hospital. Weekly clinicopathological exercises. Normal reference laboratory values. *N Engl J Med.* 1998;339:1063–1072; Fischbach F, Dunning MB. *A Manual of Laboratory Diagnostic Tests.* 8th ed. Philadelphia, PA: Lippincott Williams & Wilkins; 2008; Schmidt J, Wieczorkiewicz J. *Interpreting Laboratory Data: A Point-of-Care Guide.* 1st ed. Bethesda, MD: American Society of Health-System Pharmacists; Lee M. *Basic Skills in Interpreting Laboratory Data.* 5th ed. Bethesda, MD: American Society of Health-System Pharmacists; 2013; American Diabetes Association. Diagnosis and classification of diabetes mellitus. *Diabetes Care.* 2013;36(Suppl 1):S67–S74; and American Association of Clinical Endocrinologists and the American College of Endocrinology. The American Association of Clinical Endocrinologists Medical Guidelines for the Management of Diabetes Mellitus: the AACE system of intensive diabetes self-management—2002 Update. *Endocr Pract.* 2002;8(Suppl 1):40–82

Gastrointestinal and Hepatic System Tests

Tests associated with gastrointestinal and hepatic disease include many enzymes, as well as some proteins, by-products, and nutritional markers. Given the role of the liver in metabolism and clearance of many medications, liver function tests (LFTs)—more accurately described as hepatic enzyme tests—are routinely monitored and included in a comprehensive metabolic panel (CMP). Table 7.12 presents the tests usually associated with this organ system.

Most liver injuries are hepatocellular or cholestatic in nature. Hepatocellular injury is often identified by disproportionately elevated serum transaminase levels (alanine aminotransferase [ALT] and/or aspartate aminotransferase [AST]) compared with γ-glutamyl transferase (GGT) and alkaline phosphatase (alk phos, ALP, AP) levels. The opposite pattern typically signifies cholestatic injury.

Renal System Tests

In addition to electrolytes and hepatic enzyme tests, renal function tests are among the most common clinical laboratory tests used. Numerous factors, diseases, and conditions affect renal function and therefore, potentially impact the clearance of numerous substances/medications and several regulatory functions. See Table 7.13 for laboratory tests pertinent to the renal system.

Other Blood Chemistry Tests

Table 7.14 provides information on other common blood tests, including those used for select immunologic and rheumatologic diseases or conditions.

Tests for infectious diseases, including hepatitis and human immunodeficiency virus (HIV), are numerous and are beyond the scope of a general review such as this. Standard practices in the therapies, goals, and tests used for these diseases are ever-evolving; therefore, specific infectious disease references should be consulted when diagnosing, assessing, or monitoring these patients.

Urinalysis

A urinalysis (UA) provides many pieces of information (Tables 7.15 and 7.16) and can be used to evaluate patients with renal disease, diabetes, infections, and other conditions.[6–8]

(*Text continued on page 249*)

TABLE 7.12 Gastrointestinal and Hepatic Enzyme and Function Tests

Test Name (Abbreviation)	Description	Reference Range		Increased With	Decreased With	Other Comments
		Conventional Units	SI Units			
Amylase, serum	Measures enzyme concentrations in the serum	20–123 U/L	0.33–2.05 μkat/L	Acute pancreatitis, carcinoma (lung, esophagus, ovaries), acute exacerbation of chronic pancreatitis, partial gastrectomy, obstruction of pancreatic duct, perforated peptic ulcer, mumps, obstruction or inflammation of salivary duct or gland, acute cholecystitis, cerebral trauma, burns, traumatic shock, DKA, dissecting aortic aneurysm	Resolving acute pancreatitis, hepatitis, cirrhosis, toxemia of pregnancy	• An enzyme produced in the salivary glands, pancreas, liver, and fallopian tubes that converts starch to sugar
Lipase	Measures enzyme concentrations in the serum; reference values vary with methodology	10–140 U/L (varies widely by method of testing)	0.17–2.3 μkat/L	Pancreatitis, obstruction of the pancreatic duct, pancreatic carcinoma, acute cholecystitis, IBD, cirrhosis, severe renal disease		• Converts TG to fatty acids and monoglyceride • The major source of lipase is the pancreas • With pancreatitis, elevation may not occur until 24–36 hours after onset of illness, lipase may be high when amylase levels are normal; and lipase persists longer in the serum than amylase • Critical value: ≥500 U/L

(continued)

TABLE 7.12 Gastrointestinal and Hepatic Enzyme and Function Tests *(continued)*

Test Name (Abbreviation)	Description	Reference Range: Conventional Units	Reference Range: SI Units	Increased With	Decreased With	Other Comments
Alanine aminotransferase (ALT)	Measures enzyme concentrations in the serum	10–50 U/L	0.17–0.83 µkat/L	Hepatocellular disease, active cirrhosis, obstructive jaundice/biliary obstruction, hepatitis, drugs (many)		• High enzyme concentrations present in the liver; also found in the heart, muscle, and kidney • More liver specific than AST; used in the diagnosis of hepatic disease and to monitor the course of treatment for hepatitis, postnecrotic cirrhosis, and hepatotoxic effects of drugs • An increase more than three times upper limit of normal (ULN) is generally considered clinically significant
Aspartate aminotransferase (AST)	Measures enzyme concentrations in the serum	5–40 U/L	0.08–0.67 µkat/L	MI, hepatic disease, acute pancreatitis, trauma, acute hemolytic anemia, acute renal disease, severe burns, drugs (many)	Acidotic patients with DM	• Enzyme of high metabolic activity found in heart, liver, skeletal muscle, kidney, brain, spleen, pancreas, and lung. Any injury or death of these cells or disease that causes change in these highly metabolic tissues will release the enzyme into circulation
Alkaline phosphatase (Alk Phos, ALP, AP)	Measures enzyme concentrations in the serum	30–130 U/L	0.5–2.17 µkat/L	Obstructive jaundice, hepatic lesions, cirrhosis, Paget disease, metastatic bone disease, osteomalacia, hyperparathyroidism,	Hypophosphatemia, malnutrition, hypothyroidism	• Enzyme mainly from bone, liver, and placenta, with different isoenzymes from different tissues. High concentrations are found in biliary canaliculi; also found in the kidney and intestines

				total parenteral nutrition, hyperphosphatemia, following IV administration of albumin (moderate)		• In hepatic disease, levels rise when excretion is impaired due to biliary tract obstruction • Bone AP is a marker of bone formation • In most clinical instances, routine AP does not distinguish the isoenzymes. It is possible to measure these separately (for research purposes or patients who may have both hepatic and bone disease) to distinguish the source
γ-Glutamyl transferase (GGT)	Beneficial in detecting acute or chronic alcohol consumption, obstructive jaundice, cholangitis, and cholecystitis	Male: ≤94 U/L Female: ≤70 U/L	Male: ≤1.5 μkat/L Female: <1.12 μkat/L	Cholecystitis, cholelithiasis, cirrhosis, biliary obstruction, drugs (barbiturates, hepatotoxic drugs [especially those that induce the cytochrome P450 system])		• Present mainly in the liver, kidney, spleen, and prostate (men have higher levels); liver is considered the source of normal serum activity, even though the kidney has the highest enzyme levels • Believed to function in the transport of amino acids and peptides • If AP and GGT are elevated, then increased AP is likely to be hepatic in origin • GGT is very sensitive but not specific; elevations of just GGT (not AST, ALT) do not necessarily indicate hepatic damage
Bilirubin (Bili, T. Bili)	Important in evaluating hepatic function, hemolytic	Total: <1.4 mg/dL	Total: <23.9 μmol/L	Unconjugated bilirubin: hemolytic anemia, trauma with evidence of a large		• Hgb breaks down into bilirubin (orange-yellow pigment); primarily removed by the liver and excreted into the bile, with a small amount found in the serum

(continued)

TABLE 7.12 Gastrointestinal and Hepatic Enzyme and Function Tests *(continued)*

Test Name (Abbreviation)	Description	Reference Range: Conventional Units	Reference Range: SI Units	Increased With	Decreased With	Other Comments
	anemias, and hyperbilirubinemia (in newborns)	Conjugated/ Direct: <0.4 mg/dL	Conjugated/ Direct: <7 μmol/L	hematoma, pulmonary infarcts; conjugated bilirubin: pancreatic cancer, cholelithiasis; both forms: hepatic metastasis, hepatitis, cirrhosis, cholestasis secondary to drugs; accompanied by jaundice: hepatocellular injury, disease of parenchymal cells, bile duct obstruction, red cell hemolysis; hemolyzed blood samples (falsely elevated)		• Two forms of bilirubin: indirect/unconjugated (protein bound) and direct/ conjugated (circulates freely in the serum) • Increased conjugated bilirubin is usually associated with increased destruction of RBCs; increased unconjugated bilirubin is more likely due to dysfunction or blockage of the liver
Lactate dehydrogenase (LD, LDH)	Levels are nonspecific but aid in confirmation of MI or pulmonary infarction in combination with other findings; may also be helpful in diagnosing	90–210 U/L (values vary considerably)	1.5–3.5 μkat/L	Acute leukemia, skeletal muscle necrosis, skin disorders, shock, megaloblastic anemia, lymphomas, AMI (LD_1:LD_2 ratio usually "flips" to >1; levels increase within 12–24 hours of MI and usually peak 3–4 days after), pulmonary	Reflect a good response to cancer therapy	• Intracellular glycolytic enzyme, widely distributed in the tissues, particularly in the liver, kidney, heart, lungs, and skeletal muscle • Catalyzes the interconversion of lactate and pyruvate • More specific information can be determined if specific isoenzymes are requested

	muscular dystrophy and pernicious anemia			infarction (increased within 24 hours after onset of pain), drugs (various)		
Albumin (Alb)	Measure of nutritional status	3.5–5.0 g/dL	35–50 g/L	(Uncommon) IV infusions, dehydration	Inadequate iron intake, severe hepatic disease, malabsorption, severe burns, starvation states, nephrotic syndrome, DM, SLE may increase free drug (and effect) for agents that are highly protein bound (phenytoin, aspirin, valproate)	• Formed in the liver and helps maintain normal water distribution (colloidal osmotic pressure); aids in the transport of blood constituents (ions, bilirubin, hormones, enzymes, drugs) • Long half-life (21 days); slow to respond to changes in nutritional status
Prealbumin (PAB, transthyretin)	Preferred measure of nutritional status	17–42 mg/dL	170–420 mg/L		0–5 mg/dL = severe protein depletion; 5–10 mg/dL = moderate protein depletion; 10–15 mg/dL = mild protein depletion	• Shorter half-life (2 days) than albumin; responds quickly to changes in nutritional intake and restoration

(continued)

TABLE 7.12 Gastrointestinal and Hepatic Enzyme and Function Tests *(continued)*

Ammonia (NH_3)	Evaluates metabolism as well as the progress of severe hepatic disease and response to treatment	≤48 μmol/L	≤48 μmol/L	Hepatic disease, hepatic coma, pericarditis, severe CHF, acute bronchitis, emphysema, urinary tract obstruction, azotemia, Reye syndrome, exercise		• Formed by bacterial metabolism of proteins in the intestine; levels vary with protein intake. Normally removed from the blood by the liver, converted to urea and excreted by the kidney • Critical value: ≥150
Hemoccult (guaiac or benzidine method)	Used to measure the presence of blood in stools, nasogastric output, and other bodily secretions Negative			Bleeding in gastrointestinal tract, (false positives: large doses of iron, iodides, phenazopyridine, or red meat within 3 days of the test)	(False negative: high doses of ascorbic acid)	• Blood in stools requires further investigation

Sources: www.labtestsonline.org. Accessed May 14, 2013; Kratz A, Lewandrowski KB. Case records of the Massachusetts General Hospital. Weekly clinicopathological exercises. Normal reference laboratory values. *N Engl J Med.* 1998;339:1063–1072; Fischbach F, Dunning MB. *A Manual of Laboratory Diagnostic Tests.* 8th ed. Philadelphia, PA: Lippincott Williams & Wilkins; 2008; American Diabetes Association. Diagnosis and classification of diabetes mellitus. *Diabetes Care.* 2013; 36(Suppl 1):S67–S74; Schmidt J, Wieczorkiewicz J. *Interpreting Laboratory Data: A Point-of-Care Guide.* 1st ed. Bethesda, MD: American Society of Health-System Pharmacists; and Lee M. *Basic Skills in Interpreting Laboratory Data.* 5th ed. Bethesda, MD: American Society of Health-System Pharmacists; 2013

TABLE 7.13 Renal System Tests

Test Name (Abbreviation)	Description	Reference Range: Conventional Units	Reference Range: SI Units	Increased With	Decreased With	Other Comments
Blood urea nitrogen (BUN)	Provides an index of glomerular filtration	7–25 mg/dL	2.5–8.9 mmol/L	(Azotemia) inadequate excretion secondary to renal disease or urinary obstruction, decreased renal function (shock, dehydration, infection, DM, advanced age), major GI bleeding with subsequent catabolism of blood to nitrogen, increased protein intake, nephrotoxic drugs (aminoglycosides, amphotericin B)	End-stage hepatic failure, overhydration (dilutional), impaired absorption disorders (inability to absorb nitrogen or digest protein)	• Urea is a nonprotein, nitrogenous end product of protein catabolism, formed in the liver, carried by the blood to the kidneys, and excreted in urine • BUN can be affected by tissue necrosis, protein catabolism, and hydration status • Not as sensitive an indicator of renal function as creatinine or CrCl • BUN/Cr ratio of >20 indicates prerenal azotemia; ≤20 when BUN is elevated is associated with intrinsic renal disease and azotemia
Creatinine (Cr, serum creatinine, SCr)	Provides an index of glomerular filtration rate (GFR)	0.6–1.3 mg/dL	62–115 μmol/L	Impaired renal function (nephritis, urinary tract obstruction, muscle disease, severe	Muscular dystrophy, atrophy (spinal cord injury), malnutrition, decreased muscle mass of aging	• Cr is a by-product of muscle creatine/phosphocreatine metabolism and is excreted renally. Since Cr is freely filtered by renal glomeruli and is not

(continued)

TABLE 7.13 Renal System Tests *(continued)*

Test Name (Abbreviation)	Description	Reference Range		Increased With	Decreased With	Other Comments
		Conventional Units	SI Units			
				dehydration); drugs (many); may be normal despite impaired renal function in elderly and malnourished patients due to decreased muscle mass		appreciably reabsorbed in the tubules under normal conditions, SCr and CrCl reflect GFR • Several drugs can interfere with the measurement of SCr independent of their effects on renal function (ascorbic acid, cimetidine, levodopa, methyldopa) • Serum half-life is ~1 day; therefore, it can take several days for new steady-state SCr to reflect changes in renal function • Changes in SCr are not a linear representation of renal function; 2 and 3 mg/dL SCr correspond to ~50% and ~30% of normal renal function, respectively
Creatinine clearance (CrCl)	Reflection of GFR	90–140 mL/min/1.73 m^2 body surface area (BSA)		High cardiac output, pregnancy, burns, carbon monoxide poisoning	Impaired renal function, renal disease/infection, shock, dehydration, hemorrhage, COPD, CHF	• Calculated CrCl is a better reflection of renal function and takes into account the age and weight of the patient; measured CrCl is

					Stages of chronic kidney disease (CKD): stage 1 = GFR >90; stage 2 = GFR 60–89; stage 3 = GFR 30–59; stage 4 = GFR 15–29; stage 5 = kidney failure with GFR <15 or dialysis	better still but requires measurement of Cr in a timed urine collection and SCr • Overestimates GFR in severe renal impairment; SCr is more accurate in this situation
Creatinine, urine	Used when measuring CrCl from a timed sample and albumin-to-creatinine ratio (urine microalbumin)	11–26 mg/kg/d	97–230 μmol/kg/d	Same as SCr, acromegaly, gigantism, DM, hypothyroidism, high-protein diet	Same as SCr, hyperthyroidism, anemia, polymyositis, inflammatory muscle disease, leukemia, advanced renal disease, or renal stenosis	• To calculate CrCl, values for SCr and the total amount of creatinine excreted in urine over a fixed time (usually 24 hours) are required (see Chapter 12, A Pharmacy Calculations Anthology) • If the value is lower than expected (see reference values), then it is likely that the urine collection was not complete and will not allow accurate assessment of CrCl
Albumin, urine	Assesses protein in urine	<30 μg/mg creatinine (random)		(Historically "microalbuminuria": 30–299 μg/mg creatinine; "macro (clinical)-albuminuria": >300 μg/mg creatinine) Diabetic nephropathy, ESRD, marker for increased CVD risk		• Preferred method: albumin-to-creatinine ratio in a random spot collection; 24-hour or timed collections are more burdensome and add little to prediction or accuracy • Measuring urine albumin only (immunoassay or dipstick specific for microalbumin), without simultaneously measuring urine Cr, is

(continued)

TABLE 7.13 Renal System Tests *(continued)*

Test Name (Abbreviation)	Description	Reference Range: Conventional Units	Reference Range: SI Units	Increased With	Decreased With	Other Comments
						• not recommended (false negatives and positives due to variations in urine concentration with hydration and other factors) • Albumin excretion can be variable, so 2/3 of specimens collected within 3–6 months should be abnormal before considering new diagnosis • Numerous factors (recent exercise, infection, fever, CHF, pronounced hyperglycemia, or HTN) may elevate urinary albumin excretion over baseline values
Urine sodium (Na^+)	Assesses fluid balance, aldosterone effects, and renal concentrating ability	40–220 mEq/24 hour	40–220 mmol/24 hour	Diuretic use, Addison disease, SIADH, renal tubular acidosis, renal tubular necrosis (>30 mmol/L with oliguria)	Dehydration, CHF, hepatic disease, nephrotic syndrome	• Wide range of reference values reflects variations in diet, posture, stress, and endocrine effects

Urine potassium (K^+)	Used in workup of aldosteronism, renal tubular acidosis, and alkalosis	25–125 mEq/24 hour	25–125 mmol/24 hour	Chronic renal failure, DM, renal tubular acidosis, dehydration, primary aldosteronism, Cushing disease	Acute renal failure, malabsorption/diarrhea syndromes	• Concentration is dependent on diet • Urine pH is decreased in patients who have decreased potassium levels (hydrogen secreted in exchange for potassium) because less potassium is available for exchange
Na^+/K^+ ratio, urine	Evaluates renal function, fluid and electrolyte balance, acid–base balance, and extent of aldosterone effects on electrolyte composition of the urine	0.9–3.88				• Diurnal variation occurs • Timed collection is required for an accurate measurement; a single collection may be used to assess responses to spironolactone therapy (>1 with effective therapy)
Urine chloride (Cl^-)	Used in workup of acid–base status to determine whether metabolic alkalosis is chloride responsive	110–250 mEq/24 hour	110–250 mmol/24 hour			• Normal values are dependent on diet and perspiration • Only has meaning if Na^+/K^+ intake and output are also known • Can serve as a guide in monitoring individuals eating salt-restricted diets

Sources: www.labtestsonline.org. Accessed May 14, 2013; Kratz A, Lewandrowski KB. Case records of the Massachusetts General Hospital. Weekly clinicopathological exercises. Normal reference laboratory values. *N Engl J Med*. 1998;339:1063–1072; Fischbach F, Dunning MB. *A Manual of Laboratory Diagnostic Tests*. 8th ed. Philadelphia, PA: Lippincott Williams & Wilkins; 2008; Schmidt J, Wieczorkiewicz J. *Interpreting Laboratory Data: A Point-of-Care Guide*. 1st ed. Bethesda, MD: American Society of Health-System Pharmacists; and Lee M. *Basic Skills in Interpreting Laboratory Data*. 5th ed. Bethesda, MD: American Society of Health-System Pharmacists; 2013

TABLE 7.14 Miscellaneous Blood Tests

Test Name (Abbreviation)	Description	Reference Range		Increased With	Decreased With	Other Comments
		Conventional Units	SI Units			
Erythrocyte sedimentation rate (ESR, sed rate)	Nonspecific test that is used for monitoring infections and inflammatory diseases	Males: 1–20 mm/h	Females: 1–30 mm/h	Increased plasma fibrinogen, globulin, or cholesterol, infections (tuberculosis [TB]), inflammatory diseases (RA), tissue destruction (AMI, neoplasms), multiple myeloma, advanced age, female sex, macrocytic anemia, normocytic anemia, pregnancy	CHF, microcytic anemia, sickle cell anemia, polycythemia vera, carcinomas, hepatic disease, corticosteroids	• Increases with age • Useful for following certain diseases (MI, rheumatic fever, RA, TB)
C-reactive protein (CRP)	Marker of inflammatory processes	<0.12 mg/dL	<12 mg/L	Severe trauma, infections (rheumatic fever), inflammation (RA), surgery, cancer		• Sensitive acute-phase reactant • Used to assess activity of inflammatory disease, detect infections after surgery, detect transplant rejection, and monitor inflammatory processes

Beta$_2$-microglobulin (B_2M)	Monitoring may allow diagnosis of renal graft rejection before changes in SCr are seen, allowing for earlier treatment	Urine: <120 µg/24 hour Serum: 1.2–2.5 mg/L		Inflammatory reactions, active chronic lymphocytic leukemia, glomerular disease (serum), tubular dysfunction (urine), aminoglycoside toxicity	Glomerular disease (urine), tubular dysfunction (serum), treatment of acute renal graft rejection (serum B_2M decreases faster than SCr)	• Serum B_2M values depend on GFR, whereas urinary B_2M values vary with the functional activity of proximal renal tubular cells • Useful for evaluating kidney allograft rejection in transplant patients; will often change in advance of SCr
Prostate-specific antigen (PSA)	Used for screening and early detection of prostate cancer	0–4.0 ng/mL	0–40 µg/L	Prostate cancer (80% of patients), benign prostatic hypertrophy (benign prostatic hyperplasia [BPH], <8 ng/mL)		• In both normal prostatic epithelial and carcinoma cells • Most prognostically reliable marker for monitoring recurrence or prostatic carcinoma; however, does not have sensitivity or specificity to be an ideal tumor marker

Sources: www.labtestsonline.org. Accessed May 14, 2013; Kratz A, Lewandrowski KB. Case records of the Massachusetts General Hospital. Weekly clinicopathological exercises. Normal reference laboratory values. *N Engl J Med*. 1998;339:1063–1072; Fischbach F, Dunning MB. *A Manual of Laboratory Diagnostic Tests*. 8th ed. Philadelphia, PA: Lippincott Williams & Wilkins; 2008; Schmidt J, Wieczorkiewicz J. *Interpreting Laboratory Data: A Point-of-Care Guide*. 1st ed. Bethesda, MD: American Society of Health-System Pharmacists; and Lee M. *Basic Skills in Interpreting Laboratory Data*. 5th ed. Bethesda, MD: American Society of Health-System Pharmacists; 2013

TABLE 7.15 Urinalysis

Test Name (Abbreviation)	Description	Reference Range		Increased With	Decreased With	Other Comments
		Conventional Units	SI Units			
Specific gravity	Evaluates patients with renal disease	1.001–1.030		Glucosuria, iodinated contrast media, massive proteinuria (>2 g/24 hour)		• >1.025 in the morning indicates good concentrating ability • 1.010–1.012 means the urine is isotonic with plasma (285–295 mOsm)
Appearance		Straw-colored, yellow				
pH		5.0–7.5		(Alkalinized) urea-splitting organisms (*Proteus* sp., *Klebsiella* sp., *Escherichia coli*), renal tubular acidosis caused by amphotericin		
Protein	A 24-hour urine specimen is collected to quantitate the urinary protein	0–trace (Tr)			Renal disease, DM, prolonged standing (trace amounts), alkaline urine (false positive with dipstick method)	• The urinary protein may be normal, indicating increased glomerular permeability or a renal tubular disorder, or abnormal because of multiple myeloma and Bence Jones proteins

Glucose	More commonly found in routine UA; no longer routinely used for DM monitoring	Negative	DM		• The correlation of urine glucose with serum glucose can be helpful in monitoring and adjusting hypoglycemic medications (rarely used for this anymore)
Ketones		Negative	Starvation, poorly controlled DM, alcoholism		
Blood		Negative			
Sediment analysis		Cell count for RBC, WBC (see Table 7.16)			• No particular type of urine cast is pathognomonic for a specific renal disorder. However, the presence of RBC or WBC casts may signal a clinically significant issue (Table 7.2)
Gram stain		Negative			

Sources: www.labtestsonline.org. Accessed May 14, 2013; Kratz A, Lewandrowski KB. Case records of the Massachusetts General Hospital. Weekly clinicopathological exercises. Normal reference laboratory values. *N Engl J Med*. 1998;339:1063–1072; Fischbach F, Dunning MB. *A Manual of Laboratory Diagnostic Tests*. 8th ed. Philadelphia, PA: Lippincott Williams & Wilkins; 2008; Schmidt J, Wieczorkiewicz J. *Interpreting Laboratory Data: A Point-of-Care Guide*. 1st ed. Bethesda, MD: American Society of Health-System Pharmacists; and Lee M. *Basic Skills in Interpreting Laboratory Data*. 5th ed. Bethesda, MD: American Society of Health-System Pharmacists; 2013

TABLE 7.16 Cell Types in the Urine Sediment

Cell Type	Reference Range	Clinical Considerations
RBC	0–2 per high-power field (hpf)	• Cystitis is the most frequent cause of hematuria, although slight hematuria may occur with exertion, trauma, or febrile illness • Yeast cells may be confused with RBCs; to distinguish between the two, adding acetic acid will cause RBCs, but not yeast cells, to lyse
Epithelial	0–2	• Epithelial cells increase with tubular damage or heavy proteinuria • Should be squamous epithelial cells only
Bacteria	0	• Presence of bacteria on Gram stain of unspun specimen correlates well with culture growth of 10^5 organisms (= urinary tract infection) • A culture and sensitivity (C&S) is useful to confirm the presence of bacteria
WBC	0–5/hpf	• Polymorphonuclear leukocytes are the most common form of WBCs observed; if seen, and two routine cultures are negative, the culture should be tested for tubercle bacilli
Casts	0–occasional per low-power field	• Red cell casts usually signify active glomerular disease • Fatty and waxy casts may be seen with inflammatory or degenerative renal disease • Leukocyte casts are usually associated by pyelonephritis • Hyaline or granular casts may also be present normally, ≤0–1 per hpf

Sources: www.labtestsonline.org. Accessed May 14, 2013; Kratz A, Lewandrowski KB. Case records of the Massachusetts General Hospital. Weekly clinicopathological exercises. Normal reference laboratory values. *N Engl J Med*. 1998;339:1063–1072; Fischbach F, Dunning MB. *A Manual of Laboratory Diagnostic Tests*. 8th ed. Philadelphia, PA: Lippincott Williams & Wilkins; 2008; Schmidt J, Wieczorkiewicz J. *Interpreting Laboratory Data: A Point-of-Care Guide*. 1st ed. Bethesda, MD: American Society of Health-System Pharmacists; and Lee M. *Basic Skills in Interpreting Laboratory Data*. 5th ed. Bethesda, MD: American Society of Health-System Pharmacists; 2013

Acknowledgment

The previous authors, Mary B. Elliot, Richard C. Christopherson, and Karen E. Vick Smith, are acknowledged for their work on this chapter in the first three editions.

References

1. www.labtestsonline.org. Accessed May 14, 2013.
2. Kratz A, Lewandrowski KB. Case records of the Massachusetts General Hospital. Weekly clinicopathological exercises. Normal reference laboratory values. *N Engl J Med.* 1998;339:1063–1072.
3. Schmidt J, Wieczorkiewicz J. *Interpreting Laboratory Data: A Point-of-Care Guide.* 1st ed. Bethesda, MD: American Society of Health-System Pharmacists; 2012.
4. Fischbach F, Bunning MB. *A Manual of Laboratory Diagnostic Tests.* 8th ed. Philadelphia, PA: Lippincott Williams & Wilkins; 2008.
5. Lee M. *Basic Skills in Interpreting Laboratory Data.* 5th ed. Bethesda, MD: American Society of Health-System Pharmacists; 2013.
6. Grundy SM, Cleeman JI, Merz CN, et al. Implications of recent clinical trials for the National Cholesterol Education Program Adult Treatment Panel III guidelines. *Circulation.* 2004;110:227–239.
7. American Diabetes Association. Diagnosis and classification of diabetes mellitus. *Diabetes Care.* 2013;36(Suppl 1):S67–S74.
8. American Association of Clinical Endocrinologists and the American College of Endocrinology. The American Association of Clinical Endocrinologists Medical Guidelines for the Management of Diabetes Mellitus: the AACE system of intensive diabetes self-management—2002 Update. *Endocr Pract.* 2002;8(Suppl 1):40–82.

Other Suggested Readings and Resources

Burtis CA, Ashwood ER, Bruns DE, eds. *Tietz Fundamentals of Clinical Chemistry.* 6th ed. Philadelphia, PA: WB Saunders; 2007.

Burtis CA, Ashwood ER, Bruns DE, eds. *Tietz Textbook of Clinical Chemistry and Molecular Diagnostics.* 5th ed. Philadelphia, PA: WB Saunders; 2011.

Howanitz JH, Howanitz PJ, eds. *Laboratory Medicine: Test Selection and Interpretation.* Philadelphia, PA: WB Saunders; 1991.

McPherson RA, Pincus MR, eds. *Henry's Clinical Diagnosis and Management by Laboratory Methods.* 22nd ed. Philadelphia, PA: WB Saunders; 2011.

Pagana KD, Pagana TJ, eds. *Mosby's Diagnostic and Laboratory Test Reference.* 11th ed. St. Louis, MO: Mosby; 2012.

Pagana KD, Pagana TJ, eds. *Mosby's Manual of Diagnostic and Laboratory Tests.* 5th ed. St. Louis, MO: Mosby; 2013.

Papadakis MA, McPhee SJ, Rabow MW, eds. *Current Medical Diagnosis and Treatment*. 52nd ed. New York, NY: McGraw-Hill; 2012.

Porter RS, Kaplan JL, eds. *The Merck Manual of Diagnosis and Therapy*. 19th ed. Whitehouse Station, NJ: Merck & Co., Inc.; 2011.

Ravel R. *Clinical Laboratory Medicine—Clinical Application of Laboratory Data*. 6th ed. St. Louis, MO: Mosby; 1994.

Sacher RA, McPherson RA. *Widmann's Clinical Interpretation of Laboratory Tests*. 11th ed. Philadelphia, PA: FA Davis Co.; 2000.

Wilson DD. *McGraw-Hill's Manual of Laboratory and Diagnostic Tests*. 1st ed. New York, NY: McGraw-Hill; 2008.

Wu AHB, ed. *Tietz Clinical Guide to Laboratory Tests*. 4th ed. Philadelphia, PA: WB Saunders; 2006.

8

Diagnostic Procedures

Katherine E. Rotzenberg, Roberta A. Aulie,
Robert M. Breslow, and
Kathleen A. Skibinski

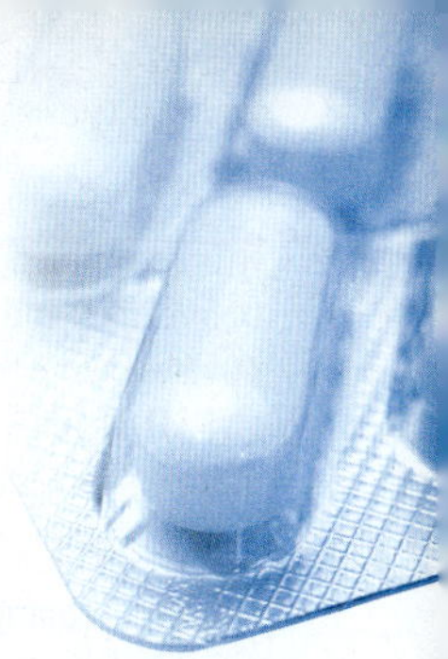

General Procedures

Biopsy[1,2]

Purpose and Description

Biopsies obtain a tissue sample for microscopic analysis (either histologic or cytologic) to determine if the tissue is cancerous, infection is present, or other diagnostic findings are due to inflammation, scarring, or organ rejection. A biopsy is performed by means of an aspiration or cutting needle, fine needle, scalpel, or punch. Biopsies may be closed (i.e., not requiring a surgical incision) or open (i.e., requiring a surgical incision). The technique and equipment used are dependent on the location and type of tissue to be sampled. Diagnostic modalities such as radiographs, computed tomography (CT), and ultrasound (US) are used to guide the needle to the appropriate site.

Findings

Normal and abnormal findings are dependent on the histology or cytology of the specific tissue undergoing biopsy.

Clinical Implications

- Patients may require sedation with a parenteral benzodiazepine (midazolam or diazepam). Patients should be monitored for oversedation and respiratory depression in the recovery period.
- A local anesthetic such as lidocaine or bupivacaine may be used.
- In those patients requiring general anesthesia, an anticholinergic (parenteral atropine or glycopyrrolate), a sedative (diazepam or midazolam), or an analgesic (morphine or meperidine) may be required 15 to 30 minutes before anesthesia.

- It is recommended that antiplatelet agents should be discontinued before open and needle biopsies. Aspirin should be discontinued 7 to 10 days before the procedure. Nonsteroidal anti-inflammatory drugs (NSAIDs) (e.g., ibuprofen, naproxen) should be discontinued 2 to 4 days before the procedure.

Computed Tomography[3–7]

Purpose and Description

Computed tomography (CT or CAT) is a painless, noninvasive method for obtaining a three-dimensional picture of body structures using cross-sectional (transverse) slice x-ray views. A complete scan consists of many pictures. CT scans can confirm the diagnosis of suspected malignancies, assist in determining the staging and extent of neoplastic disease, and determine the effectiveness of therapy. CT scans of the brain and skull (cranial CT) may be performed to define the nature of head trauma, hydrocephalus, increased intracranial pressure, cerebrovascular lesions, degenerative brain diseases, and infections. CT scans of the body (body CT) that examine the neck, thorax, abdomen, and extremities may provide information on the cause of jaundice, inflammatory processes, pleural or chest wall abnormalities, and suspected abnormal collections of blood or fluid. A spinal CT is performed to evaluate disorders of the spine and spinal cord.

Findings

Normal and abnormal findings are dependent on the organs being evaluated.

Clinical Implications

- Sedation with benzodiazepines (e.g., midazolam, diazepam, or lorazepam) or a sedative such as chloral hydrate may be required for the patient to remain still during the scan.
- IV iodine contrast media should be used cautiously in patients with known or suspected hypersensitivity to iodine. Contrast media (e.g., as diatrizoate or iohexol) may be injected intravenously to enhance the images of brain, abdominal structures, and vasculature. Several doses of oral contrast media (diatrizoate) as a 2% solution (4 mL/200 mL H_2O) are administered before abdominal CT scans to provide contrast enhancement of certain abdominal structures.

Gallium Scan[4,6–8]

Purpose and Description

Gallium scans are used to detect or evaluate primary or metastatic neoplasms; inflammatory lesions of bacterial, autoimmune, or other origin; malignant lymphoma or recurrent tumors after chemotherapy or radiation therapy; and lung cancer. In addition, these scans aid in the diagnosis of focal defects in the liver. Radioactive gallium citrate (Ga^{67}) is administered intravenously 24 to 48 hours before the scan. The scanning device measures the radiation emissions of Ga^{67} and shows the distribution or uptake patterns of Ga^{67} throughout the body. The degree of radioactivity Ga^{67} possesses is minimal and not harmful.

Findings

Normal

Ga^{67} uptake is seen in the liver, spleen, bones, and large bowel.

Abnormal

Ga^{67} uptake is seen in abscesses, inflamed tissues, and some tumors.

Clinical Implications

Ga^{67} is excreted into the feces. This could interfere with the detection of inflammatory or neoplastic diseases of the colon. Therefore, a cleansing enema should be administered before the scan.

Magnetic Resonance Imaging[9]

Purpose and Description

Magnetic resonance imaging (MRI) is especially useful for diagnosis of brain and nervous system disorders, cardiovascular disease, and cancer. MRI provides very precise and detailed images of internal organs. With conventional MRI, the patient is placed inside a large circular magnet. This magnet and radiofrequency signals cause hydrogen nuclei to emit their own signal. A computer uses these signals to create detailed, sectional images of the body. Open MRI uses the same technology as conventional MRI but does not have a closed tube into which the patient is placed to perform the imaging. This open technology is advantageous for the patient who experiences claustrophobia in narrow closed spaces.

MRI combines the advantage of anatomic imaging with excellent soft tissue characterization. Although MRI does not use ionizing radiation and does not require a contrast agent to identify vascular structures, a specialized contrast material such as gadolinium is now being used in certain circumstances to enhance MRI images.

Findings

Normal and abnormal findings are dependent on the anatomy being evaluated.

Clinical Implications

- Successful imaging requires patients to lie very still. Uncooperative patients, patients who are claustrophobic, and children should be sedated.
- MRI is contraindicated in patients with cardiac pacemakers, surgically inserted metal hardware such as aneurysm clips, intrauterine devices, and recently inserted metal prostheses.

Ultrasonography[9]

Purpose and Description

US, sonogram, is a noninvasive, nontoxic (without dyes) diagnostic procedure that examines internal structures/soft tissue by recording the reflection of high-frequency sound waves directed into the tissues. Common tissues include the eye, thyroid, breast, heart, liver, lymph nodes, spleen, gallbladder, bile ducts, pancreas, uterus, ovary, bladder, and kidneys. US can detect and evaluate masses, abscess, stones, motion, and fluid. It can determine size, shape, and position of organs and differentiate solid, cystic, and complex masses.

US produces a good image when there are small differences in tissue density of the adjacent structures. However, when there are large differences, as between bone and soft tissue or air-filled spaces and soft tissue, the image is unintelligible because most of the sound waves are reflected back.

Findings

Normal

Absence of masses, obstructions, and abscesses. Normal shape, size, and position of organs.

Abnormal

Presence of masses, obstructions, or abscesses. Abnormal size, shape, or location of organs.

Clinical Implications

None

Allergy/Immunology

Candida, Histoplasmin, and Mumps Skin Test[9]

Purpose and Description

Skin testing is a method of detecting an individual's sensitivity to certain allergens (antigens) or microorganisms responsible for disease. It is used to determine a patient's immunocompetence. Skin testing also assesses the integrity of a person's cell-mediated immune system. Three types of skin tests are generally used: scratch, patch, and intradermal tests. Reaction to a skin test demonstrates a hypersensitivity to the tested antigen. This indicates immunity to a disease or product or can indicate the presence of the active or inactive disease being studied. The antigen is injected (0.1 mL) intradermally as a bleb on the volar (flexor) surface of the forearm by use of a tuberculin syringe and a small (25- to 27-gauge) needle. Evaluate tests within 48 to 72 hours.

These skin tests are referred to as controls because they are used to determine whether a negative response to a skin test (e.g., tuberculin) is the result of negative exposure to the antigen or to incompetent cell-mediated immunity.

Findings

Normal

A positive reaction indicates previous exposure and resistance to the antigen. A positive test is observed when an induration ≥10 mm in diameter appears after injection of the antigen.

Abnormal

A negative reaction indicates that the patient has not been exposed to the antigen or is suggestive (more likely) of a compromised immune system (anergy). No erythema and a lesion <10 mm in diameter indicate a negative test.

Clinical Implications

Skin tests are refrigerated before use. Concurrent or recent use of corticosteroids can produce a false-negative result due to suppression of the cell-mediated (delayed hypersensitivity) immune response.

Antihistamines and H_2-blockers interfere with the cutaneous histamine response of the immunoglobulin E (IgE)–mediated immediate hypersensitivity reaction and can produce false-negative results.

Tuberculin Skin Test (PPD)[9]

Purpose and Description

The tuberculin skin test determines if a patient has tuberculosis. Tuberculin is a protein fraction (purified protein derivative) of the soluble growth product of *Mycobacterium tuberculosis* or *Mycobacterium bovis*. The antigen is administered intradermally (0.1 mL), creating a bleb at the intradermal injection site (usually the volar or dorsal aspect of the forearm). The test is evaluated within 48 to 72 hours.

Findings

Normal

Absence of redness or induration (negative skin test <5 mm wheal diameter)

Abnormal

Induration of the skin, erythema, edema, and central necrosis. The wheal diameter in millimeters is measured around the injection site (5 to 9 mm = doubtful or probable, and positive ≥ 10 mm). A positive skin test indicates prior exposure to the tubercle bacilli (TB) or previous bacille Calmette-Guérin (BCG) vaccination.

Clinical Implications

The skin test does not distinguish between active and dormant tuberculosis. PPD (purified protein derivative of tuberculin) is refrigerated and must be drawn up just before use. The 5-TU concentration is used most frequently; however, the 1-TU concentration is sometimes used as initial screening in patients with suspected tuberculosis to lessen the severity of the reaction. The 250-TU concentration, although rarely used, can be used when tuberculosis is suspected and a state of anergy may be present.

Concurrent or recent use of corticosteroids and other immunosuppressive agents can produce false-negative results. Antihistamines and H_2-blockers interfere with the cutaneous histamine response of the IgE-mediated immediate hypersensitivity reaction and can produce false-negative results. Lymphoid disease can produce a false-positive result. Viral and certain bacterial infections can cause false-negative results due to suppression of the delayed hypersensitivity reaction. Prior administration of BCG vaccine and recent vaccination with attenuated live virus vaccines can result in a false-positive reaction.

Cardiology

Cardiac Catheterization[9]

Purpose and Description

Cardiac catheterization evaluates cardiac valvular disease, heart function, coronary vessels and congenital heart anomalies as well as to determine the need for cardiac surgery. When combined with angiography, the coronary arteries can be evaluated for obstruction (occlusion) to assess patient risk for myocardial infarction (MI). Catheterization can also be used to perform angioplasty and place stents to open up and prevent reocclusion of coronary arteries.

A catheter (a thin, flexible tube) is inserted through a small incision made in an artery or vein in the neck, arm, or groin and threaded into the right or left side of the heart with the assistance of fluoroscopy to help guide the placement of the catheter. Patients are mildly sedated before the test but remain awake throughout the procedure. Cardiac catheterization is usually performed in conjunction with coronary angiography, which uses an IV contrast material to visualize the coronary arteries. Fluoroscopy provides immediate visualization of the coronary circulation.

Findings

Normal

Heart size, motion, thickness, blood supply, and blood pressure within normal limits

Abnormal

Presence of coronary artery disease, valvular heart disease, ventricular aneurysms, or enlargement of the heart

Clinical Implications

- Patients receiving daily digoxin should receive their dose on the day of the procedure.
- Patients will likely receive a benzodiazepine before the procedure.

Echocardiography[9,10]

Purpose and Description

Echocardiography is a noninvasive procedure that examines the heart, providing information about heart size, valve and chamber movements, and blood flow velocity. Echocardiography is done to diagnose or rule out valvular abnormalities or pericardial effusion, measure the size of and evaluate heart chambers, detect atrial tumors and cardiac thrombi, or evaluate cardiac function, wall motion after MI, or blood flow through the heart chambers and valves. Echocardiography is a specialized two-dimensional ultrasonographic technique by which a transducer is placed on the chest where there is no bone or lung tissue. High-frequency sound waves are directed at the heart. The heart reflects these waves (echoes) back to the transducer. These sound waves are then converted to electrical impulses and relayed to an echocardiography machine, which creates a diagram on an oscilloscope.

Conventional (transthoracic echocardiography) is performed by placing the transducer on the exterior chest wall. The problem encountered with this technique is a degraded heart image due to bony structures (sternum and ribs) and an extensive lung interface. Transesophageal echocardiography involves the placement of an echo transducer on the tip of a gastroscope. Following administration of a local anesthetic spray to the back of the throat, a gastroscope is advanced orally into the esophagus, permitting placement of the transducer in closer proximity to the heart. This approach serves to eliminate chest cage and lung interference seen with the conventional technique. Transesophageal echocardiography can use higher-frequency transducers that significantly improve the resolution of the images, due to the transducer being closer to the heart. Three-dimensional Doppler echocardiography gathers hemodynamic information because of its ability to measure the velocity of the red blood cells.

Findings

Normal

No mechanical or gross anatomic abnormalities. Normal cardiac function, blood flow patterns, and blood velocity through the heart chambers and valves.

Abnormal

Abnormal motion, pattern, and structure of the four cardiac valves, left ventricular dysfunction, valve abnormalities, wall thickening, tumors or thrombi in the heart, abnormal size of the heart or chamber, pericardial effusion, or blood flow

Clinical Implications

Conventional Echocardiography

None

Transesophageal Echocardiography

- Patients should be questioned about allergies to topical anesthetic spray.
- Patients will require parenteral sedation (e.g., midazolam) and analgesia (e.g., morphine).

Electrocardiography[4,7,9–13]

Purpose and Description

Electrocardiography (ECG) is a graphic recording of the electrical impulses of the heart that tracks the cardiac cycle from depolarization through repolarization used to diagnose coronary artery disease, MI, pericardial effusion, pericarditis, rhythm disturbances as a result of ischemia or electrolyte abnormalities, and disorders of impulse formation and conduction. It is also helpful for evaluation of the effect of drugs on the heart. Electrodes placed on the patient's limbs and chest detect the electrical current generated by myocardial depolarization, naturally conducted to the surface of the body. To capture the multidirectional electrical activity, 12 ECG leads are used simultaneously to achieve a comprehensive view of the electrical activity of the heart. Leads I, II, III, AVF, AVL, and AVR are attached to the limbs and provide an electrical view of the frontal plane of the heart; leads V1, V2, V3, V4, V5, and V6 are attached to the chest and produce a horizontal view of the heart's electrical activity. The tracing produced by the ECG shows the voltage of the waves, the time duration of waves, and the interval between them.

Findings

Normal

See Table 8.1

Abnormal

Abnormal heart rate, rhythm, axis, or position of the heart; myocardial hypertrophy; or MI

TABLE 8.1 Description of ECG Wave and Normal Findings

Wave/Interval	Explanation	Normal Finding
P wave	Impulse from SA node to atria (atrial depolarization)	Normal size, shape, and deflection
PR interval	P wave to QRS complex	0.1–0.2 seconds
QRS complex	Depolarization of the ventricle	<0.12 seconds
ST segment	Interval between depolarization and repolarization	No elevation or depression
T wave	Recovery phase after contraction (ventricular polarization)	No inversion

SA, sinoatrial

Clinical Implications

Cardioactive drugs (e.g., digoxin, quinidine, beta-blockers) have various specific effects on the ECG tracing.

Electrophysiology Study[9,10]

Purpose and Description

Electrophysiology studies (EPSs) are done via an invasive test for diagnosis and treatment of ventricular and supraventricular arrhythmias. Solid electrode catheters measure cardiac electrical conduction system activity, commonly inserted into the venous system and advanced into the right atrium, across the septal leaflet of the tricuspid valve and into the right ventricle in a fashion similar to cardiac catheterization. As part of the study, ECG leads are attached to the patient's chest. After baseline values have been determined, pacing (electrical stimulation of the heart) is used to induce arrhythmias. When an ectopic site takes over as pacemaker, EPS can help pinpoint its origin. EPS can aid in the diagnosis of disorders of the heart's conduction system, selection of an antiarrhythmic drug, and evaluation of antiarrhythmic drug therapy. Some patients have EPS to assess pacemaker need or as part of a syncope and sick sinus syndrome workup.

Findings

Normal

Normal conduction intervals, refractory periods, recovery times, and absence of arrhythmias. Normal conduction intervals in adults are as follows: H-V interval, 35 to 55 ms; A-H interval, 45 to 150 ms; P-A interval, 20 to 40 ms.

TABLE 8.2 Conduction Intervals and Potential Causes

Interval Prolonged	Possible Cause
H-V	Acute or chronic disease
A-H	Atrial pacing, chronic conduction system disease, carotid sinus pressure, recent MI, and drugs
P-A	Acquired, surgically induced, congenital atrial disease, and atrial pacing

H-V, time from the onset of bundle of His deflection to ventricular activation; A-H, time from atrial activation to onset of His deflection; P-A, time from onset of the p wave on the ECG to atrial deflection; MI, myocardial infarction

Abnormal

Prolonged conduction intervals (Table 8.2), abnormal refractory periods, abnormal recovery times, and induced arrhythmias

Clinical Implications

- Patients are not permitted to have food or fluids for at least 6 hours before the study.
- EPS is contraindicated in patients with severe coagulopathy, recent thrombophlebitis, and acute pulmonary embolism.

Exercise Electrocardiography (Stress Test)[9,10,14]

Purpose and Description

The Stress test measures how efficient the heart is during exercise. Electrical cardiac principles are the same as for the ECG. The chest electrodes are placed according to the lead system selected to provide the desired tracing. A baseline rhythm strip is run and checked for dysrhythmias. The patient then steps onto a treadmill moving at a slow speed. A monitor is continuously observed for any changes in cardiac electrical activity, and a rhythm strip is checked at preset intervals for any abnormalities as the treadmill speed and incline is changed (increased every 2 to 3 minutes). The test is terminated when the maximum (target) heart rate is reached or if unstable changes occur pertaining to the ECG, blood pressure, heart rate, or patient status (i.e., exhaustion or angina). Once the exercise stops, the patient lies down and an ECG tracing is recorded every minute for 5 minutes or until ischemic changes have returned to normal or until the heart rate has returned to normal. Exercise electrocardiography may be used to test cardiac reaction to increased demands for oxygen, help diagnose the source of chest pain or other cardiac pain, determine the functional capacity of the heart after cardiac surgery or MI, screen for coronary artery disease, and identify dysrhythmias.

Findings

Normal

A normal ECG tracing with expected wave forms and intervals (see "Electrocardiography").

Abnormal

The most prominent abnormal findings are a flat or downsloping ST-segment depression and an upsloping but depressed ST segment.

Clinical Implications

- Use of beta-adrenergic blockers may make the stress test difficult to interpret because the heart will be prevented from reaching the maximal target rate. Digoxin may limit the value of the stress test due to its effect on ST waves. The physician may elect to perform stress echocardiography or nuclear imaging instead for patients on these medications.

Holter Monitoring[9,10]

Purpose and Description

Holter monitoring, also known as ambulatory ECG, continuously records heart rate and rhythm for a period of time (24 to 72 hours). Three to five electrodes are placed on the chest, and heart rate and rhythm are recorded on magnetic tape. The tape is analyzed for evidence of cardiac arrhythmias that would normally not have been present during a routine ECG test. Holter monitoring is used to diagnose supraventricular and ventricular cardiac arrhythmias, evaluate therapy (drugs and pacemakers) for cardiac arrhythmias, identify asymptomatic patients at high risk for sudden cardiac death, evaluate syncopal episodes in which arrhythmias are not evident, and detect myocardial ischemia.

Findings

Holter monitoring can demonstrate the relationship between symptoms such as syncope, palpitations, or shortness of breath and a cardiac arrhythmia.

Clinical Implications

Patients keep a diary of all activities and symptoms during the period tested. All medications are recorded at the exact time taken.

MRI of the Heart[9,15,16]

Purpose and Description

MRI of the heart, also referred to as noninvasive cardiac evaluation or cardiac MRI, creates a three-dimensional image of the heart (including valves and coronary vessels) and lungs. The images may be used to estimate left ventricular end-diastolic and end-systolic volumes. These measurements can help calculate stroke volume, ejection fraction, and cardiac output (CO). Cardiac MRI may provide qualitative assessment of left ventricular wall motion and mitral valve function and aid in determination of extent of damage to the myocardium (infarct size and location).

Findings

Normal

No infarct present. All cardiac parameters are within normal limits. No unusual left ventricular wall motion. Mitral valve functioning properly (no regurgitation).

Abnormal

Presence of infarcted tissue or any wall motion abnormalities. Decreased cardiac parameters (ejection fraction < 40%). Cardiomegaly. Prolonged cardiopulmonary transit times.

Clinical Implications

- Many medications affect cardiac parameters and should be assessed.
- Atrial fibrillation may interfere with the accuracy of study results.
- Contrast media may be used to enhance results (allergies and contraindications need to be assessed).

Multiple Gated Acquisition Scan[9]

Purpose and Description

The primary purpose of the multiple gated acquisition (MUGA) is to determine the amount of blood ejected from the ventricle during cardiac cycle (ejection fraction), CO, and left ventricular function. It also is used to evaluate the efficacy of coronary artery disease therapies, differentiate ventricular hypokinesis from left ventricular aneurysms, and detect right ventricular failure and intracardiac shunting in patients with congenital heart disease or septal rupture after MI. Most commonly, radiolabeled erythrocytes are injected into the patient's venous circulation. The distribution of these erythrocytes is imaged by synchronization of the recording of cardiac images with the ECG. This produces sequential images that can be viewed as a motion picture film. The MUGA scan can also be performed after exercise. When compared to the results at rest, changes in ejection fraction and CO can be assessed. The test is also known as cardiac blood pool scanning, because the blood, not the heart itself, is imaged.

Findings

Normal

The left ventricle contracts symmetrically, and the isotope appears evenly distributed in the scans. EF is 50% to 65%.

Abnormal

Asymmetric blood distribution in the myocardium, the presence of coronary artery disease as seen by segmental abnormalities of ventricular motion, the presence of cardiomyopathies as seen by globally reduced EFs, right-to-left shunting as seen by early arrival of activity in the left ventricle or aorta, and the presence of aneurysms in the left ventricle

Clinical Implications

None

Myocardial Biopsy[9]

Purpose and Description

Myocardial biopsy diagnoses cardiac disease (e.g., cardiomyopathy, myocarditis, cardiac amyloid) and assesses suspected rejection of a transplanted heart. It is performed similarly to or as part of cardiac catheterization (see "Cardiac Catheterization"). When myocardial biopsy is performed alone, the jugular vein in the neck is the most common point of insertion for the IV catheter. The catheter is threaded into the right ventricle of the heart, and a cutting instrument is used to remove heart muscle for analysis.

Findings

Normal

Normal pathology and histology

Abnormal

Signs of rejection in a transplanted heart, presence of amyloid protein, or bacterial, viral, or parasitic causes of myocarditis

Clinical Implications

- Antiplatelet agents are discontinued before the procedure. Aspirin should be stopped 7 to 10 days before, and other NSAIDs should be stopped 2 to 4 days before the procedure.

Swan-Ganz Catheterization[7,9]

Purpose and Description

Swan-Ganz catheterization threads a catheter into the patient's right atrium to monitor heart function. The point of insertion can be the internal jugular vein, subclavian vein, femoral vein, or brachial vein. The procedure may be performed with or without the use of fluoroscopy. A chest radiograph is usually obtained after catheter insertion to verify position and to rule out the possibility of pneumothorax if the subclavian or internal jugular approach was used.

Swan-Ganz catheterization is helpful in evaluating severe hypotension, monitoring hemodynamic instability, and diagnosing cardiac tamponade, pulmonary hypertension, and edema. Other indications include monitoring congestive heart failure, patients undergoing open heart surgery, drug overdose, chronic obstructive lung disease exacerbations, and end-stage liver failure with deteriorating renal function.

Findings

See Table 8.3

Clinical Implications

- A benzodiazepine or a parenteral analgesic may be used for sedation.
- Aspirin and NSAIDs should be discontinued in advance of the procedure. However, use of these agents is not an absolute contraindication to performing the procedure.
- The effects of heparin or warfarin should be reversed before catheterization.

Thallium Stress Test/Scan[9]

Purpose and Description

Thallium stress test evaluates regional myocardial perfusion, detect evidence of recent or remote MI, and can identify viable myocardium in

TABLE 8.3 Normal Findings for Swan-Ganz Catheterization

Parameter of Interest	Normal Resting Hemodynamic Value
Right atrium	Mean: 0–8 mm Hg; A wave: 2–10 mm Hg; V wave: 2–10 mm Hg
Right ventricle	Systolic: 15–30 mm Hg; end diastolic: 0–8 mm Hg
Pulmonary artery	Systolic: 15–30 mm Hg; end diastolic: 3–12 mm Hg
Wedge	A wave: 3–15 mm Hg; wave: 3–12 mm Hg; mean: V 5–12 mm Hg
AV_2 difference (mL/L)	30–50
CO (L/min)	4.0–6.5 (varies with patient size)
Cardiac index (L/min/m^2)	2.6–4.6
Pulmonary vascular resistance (dynes/s/cm^2)	20–130
Systemic vascular resistance (dynes/s/cm^2)	700–1,600

a previously infarcted portion of the myocardium. This nuclear medicine study can be performed while the patient is at rest or while exercising on a treadmill. The procedure incorporates the radionuclide thallium,[201] which has biologic properties similar to potassium. These similarities account for its intracellular uptake when administered intravenously. Blood flow then distributes the radionuclide to the myocardium and other organs. A gamma camera measures the radioactivity throughout the myocardium. Healthy myocardium rapidly takes up the thallium, whereas areas of infarcted myocardium show little or no radioactivity. The stress test is performed using a multistage treadmill test and ECG monitoring with thallium[201] being administered at the time of peak exercise. The patient exercises for an additional 30 to 60 minutes with imaging performed immediately after. Three hours later, the myocardium is reimaged, and myocardial perfusion is further assessed following redistribution of the thallium. For those patients unable to exercise, adenosine, dipyridamole, or dobutamine is administered intravenously along with the thallium to simulate the change in cardiac blood flow that would normally occur with exercise.

Findings

Normal

Homogeneous distribution of thallium throughout the myocardium

Abnormal

A thallium defect demonstrates a region of decreased myocardial blood flow. Infarcted areas can be demonstrated on the images immediately after injection and at the time of delayed imaging. Ischemic areas are detected on the early images as defects but disappear with delayed imaging due to thallium redistribution.

Clinical Implications

- Patients should not eat for several hours before the test to prevent increased distribution of the thallium to the gut. Caffeine and theophylline products should be held for 36 to 48 hours before dipyridamole and for 12 hours before adenosine.
- Hold beta-adrenergic blockers, angiotensin-converting enzyme (ACE) inhibitors, and calcium channel blockers 24 to 48 hours before the test if exercise is to be performed.
- Hold nitrates for 6 hours before dobutamine.
- IV aminophylline can be administered (75 to 250 mg) to counteract the systemic adverse effects of IV dipyridamole.

Endocrinology

Adrenocorticotropic Hormone Stimulation Test (Cosyntropin)[9,17]

Purpose and Description

The adrenocorticotropic hormone (ACTH) stimulation test is used to diagnose adrenal insufficiency. A baseline blood cortisol level is drawn, followed by administration of cosyntropin (a synthetic derivative of ACTH) 250 μg IM or IV. Additional cortisol levels are drawn at 30 and 60 minutes.

Findings

Normal

Cortisol >20 μg/dL above baseline. Baseline determinations are affected by the time of day due to diurnal variation. A normal response excludes primary adrenal failure but does not exclude partial secondary adrenocortical insufficiency, further testing is required.

Abnormal

Baseline cortisol will be low and response to cosyntropin will be absent or blunted. This diagnoses adrenal insufficiency, but does not fully differentiate primary from secondary failure, further testing is required.

Clinical Implications

- Fasting is advised prior to the test, but not required. Fasting is required during the test.
- Interfering factors: low albumin levels, prolonged steroid use, estrogens, other drugs that affect cortisol levels

Dexamethasone Suppression Test[9,17]

Purpose and Description

The dexamethasone suppression test (DST) is a screening test to rule out Cushing syndrome. It may be administered as a low-dose test or a high-dose test. Draw baseline blood cortisol levels at 8:00 AM and 4:00 PM, then administer dexamethasone 1 mg (low-dose) or 8 mg (high-dose) orally at 11:00 PM. Draw blood cortisol level the following morning at 8:00 AM. Alternatively, a 2-day test may be used: dexamethasone 2 mg orally every 6 hours for 2 days.

Findings

Normal

Cortisol <5 μg/dL, or <50% of baseline

Abnormal

Cortisol >5 μg/dL (failure to suppress) suggests Cushing syndrome; however, there are many exceptions, and the test must be interpreted with caution.

Clinical Implications

- Patients must fast overnight.
- Ideally, all medications should be discontinued for 24 to 48 hours prior to the test (especially spironolactone, estrogens, cortisol, tetracycline, and phenytoin).
- Drugs that increase metabolism of dexamethasone may cause failure to achieve adequate blood levels and false-negative results.
- Radioisotopes should not be given within the previous week.
- False suppression occurs in pregnancy, high doses of estrogens, alcoholism, uncontrolled diabetes, trauma, high stress, fever, dehydration, and phenytoin.

Oral Glucose Tolerance Test[9,17,18]

Purpose and Description

The oral glucose tolerance test (OGTT) is used to screen for diabetes mellitus in pregnant adults. Fasting plasma glucose (FPG) and HbA_{1C} are the preferred screening methods in nonpregnant adults and children. The OGTT may be considered in these patients if FPG or HbA_{1C} is borderline. FPG is drawn and then the patient consumes a glucose load (ingested over 5 minutes maximum). All adult patients can receive a 75-g glucose dose (some institutions may screen pregnant patients with a 50-g dose and then repeat the test with a higher dose if the screen is positive). Plasma glucose samples are drawn at 30, 60, and 120 minutes. Institutions that use a 100-g dose for pregnant patients may draw a sample at 180 minutes.

Findings

- Nonpregnant adults: At least two measurements must be abnormal to diagnose diabetes mellitus. See Table 8.4.
- Pregnant adults (using 75 g glucose dose): One abnormal measurement meets criteria for gestational diabetes using International Association of Diabetes in Pregnancy Study Groups (IADPSG) criteria. Two abnormal measurements are required for WHO criteria. See Table 8.5.

Clinical Implications

- Patients should eat at least 150 g carbohydrates daily and abstain from alcohol for 3 days before the test. Fasting is recommended for 12 to 16 hours prior to the test.

TABLE 8.4 Diabetes Diagnostic Reference Ranges

	Normal	Prediabetes	Diabetes Mellitus
HbA_{1C}	<5.7%	5.7%–6.4%	≥6.5%
FPG	<100 mg/dL	100–125 mg/dL	≥126 mg/dL
60 minutes after glucose load	<200 mg/dL	>200 mg/dL	≥200 mg/dL
120 minutes after glucose load	<140 mg/dL	≥140–199 mg/dL	≥200 mg/dL

Sources: Fischbach F, Dunning MB. *A Manual of Laboratory and Diagnostic Tests.* 8th ed. Philadelphia, PA: Lippincott Williams & Wilkins; 2009; and Gardner DG, Shoback S. *Greenspan's Basic and Clinical Endocrinology.* 9th ed. New York, NY: The McGraw-Hill Companies; 2011

TABLE 8.5 Comparison of Gestational Diabetes Diagnostic Thresholds

	Gestational Diabetes (IADPSG Criteria)	Gestational Diabetes (WHO Criteria)
FPG	≥92 mg/dL	≥ 126 mg/dL
60 minutes after glucose load	≥180 mg/dL	N/A
120 minutes after glucose load	≥153 mg/dL	≥140 mg/dL

Source: Wendland EM, Torloni MR, Falavigna M, et al. Gestational diabetes and pregnancy outcomes—a systematic review of the World Health Organization (WHO) and the International Association of Diabetes in Pregnancy Study Groups (IADPSG) diagnostic criteria. *BMC Pregnancy Childbirth.* 2012;12:23

- Ideally, the following drugs should be discontinued 3 days before the test: hormones, oral contraceptives, steroids, salicylates, anti-inflammatory drugs, diuretics, hypoglycemic drugs, antihypertensive drugs, and anticonvulsants.
- Prescribed insulin and hypoglycemic drugs may be given after the test. The patient should eat within 30 minutes after these drugs are given.
- Smoking increases glucose levels. No tobacco product may be used during the testing time.
- Allow 2 weeks of recovery after infections, illnesses, or surgery before performing the OGTT. The test has limited value in hospitalized patients.

Radionuclide Thyroid Scan[9,17]

Purpose and Description

A radionuclide thyroid scan is useful in differentiating among causes of thyrotoxicosis by providing information about the size and shape of the thyroid gland and the distribution of tracer activity. It has limited utility in differentiating benign from malignant thyroid nodules. There are two options for type of radionuclide administered.

- ^{123}I (200 to 300 μCi) is given orally, thyroid image obtained 8 to 24 hours later.
- ^{99m}Tc pertechnetate (1 to 10 mCi) is given IV, thyroid image obtained 30 to 60 minutes later.

Images can be obtained via a rectilinear scanner, which produces a life-size picture, or a gamma camera, which records the image on a film or a computer monitor via a fluorescent screen.

Findings

Normal

Evenly distributed concentration of tracer. Normal size, position, shape, site, weight, and function of the thyroid gland with absence of nodules.

Abnormal

- Graves disease: enlarged gland with intense and homogenous concentration of tracer
- Hashimoto disease: mottled areas of decreased tracer
- Toxic nodular goiter: one or more discrete regions of tracer activity, corresponding to palpable nodule
- Hyperthyroidism: diffuse increased tracer
- Hypothyroidism: diffuse decreased tracer

Clinical Implications

- ^{123}I may not be sufficiently absorbed if the patient has severe diarrhea or malabsorptive disorder, and tracer activity may appear falsely low.
- Avoid the following medications starting at least 1 week before the scan: iodine-containing medications (including IV contrast), thyroid hormone, antithyroid medications, weight-control medications, multivitamins, cough medicine, herbal supplements (e.g., kelp), and medications that can lower or enhance iodine uptake.
- Enhanced uptake is seen in cirrhosis, renal failure, and iodine-deficient diets.
- In some situations, the physician may want a small amount of iodine or thyroid hormone present in the body at the time of the scan to test the thyroid's response to these drugs.
- Radionuclide thyroid imaging is contraindicated in pregnancy.

Thyrotropin-Releasing Hormone Test[17]

Purpose and Description

The thyrotropin-releasing hormone (TRH) test is used to diagnose primary hypothyroidism. After a baseline serum thyroid-stimulating hormone (TSH) level is drawn, synthetic TRH (protirelin) is administered as a 200 to 500 μg IV bolus. The TSH level is repeated 30 minutes later (levels should remain elevated for 2 to 3 hours).

Findings

Normal

Three- to fivefold increase in TSH over baseline

Abnormal

- Primary hypothyroidism: elevated basal TSH and exaggerated response to synthetic TRH
- Hyperthyroidism, high-dose thyroxine therapy, or central hypothyroidism: suppressed response to synthetic TRH

Clinical Implications

- Thyroid hormone therapy will affect response to test.

Gastroenterology

Abdominal Radiograph (KUB)[9,19]

Purpose and Description

An abdominal radiograph is often used to evaluate abdominal pain, distention, or clinical signs of an acute abdomen. Other names include abdominal x-ray, plain film, kidney, ureters, bladder (KUB), scout film, flat plate, or abdominal series. X-rays pass through the patient's body and provide an image based on density of the structures within. Both supine and upright radiographs are recommended. Upright radiographs should be centered to include the diaphragm to allow assessment of free intraperitoneal air and air-fluid levels within the bowel. In patients who are unable to stand, a left lateral decubitus view should be obtained instead to detect air between the liver and the right lateral wall.

Findings

Normal

Normal abdominal structures

Abnormal

- Bowel dilation: often caused by obstruction (usually small bowel) or ileus
- Pneumoperitoneum (free intraperitoneal air): indicates a perforated viscus with subsequent peritonitis
- Pneumatosis (gas in the bowel wall): indicates intestinal ischemia or necrosis

- Appendicolithiasis
- Foreign bodies, abnormal fluid or ascites, tumors or masses

Clinical Implications

- Radiographs expose the patient to radiation, avoid unnecessary studies. Staff and patients should be protected from radiation as much as the procedure allows. Pregnant women, and those possibly pregnant, should avoid radiographs of the trunk or pelvis unless absolutely necessary.
- All metallic objects must be removed from the abdominal area. The patient must remain still while the image is obtained.
- Barium may interfere with interpretation; perform barium studies afterward.

Barium Enema[9,19]

Purpose and Description

The barium enema procedure is used to detect colorectal polyps and cancer, diagnose and assess inflammatory bowel disease, diagnose diverticular disease, evaluate lesions in the colon, and evaluate the rectum. The colon must be emptied prior to the procedure; this involves a liquid diet prior to the procedure followed by fasting the night before. Institutional protocols vary in which medications are used to empty the bowel, but a combination of agents is typically required. The patient lies on his back or side while barium is instilled into the large intestine through a rectal tube. Barium serves as the contrast medium in this procedure. Radiographs are obtained after fluoroscopy to record the movement of barium through the large intestine. The barium is then expelled, and a final radiograph is obtained. A variant of this process is the air-contrast or double-contrast examination; air is instilled with the barium. Barium enema with air contrast is more sensitive than barium alone.

Findings

Normal

Normal colon position, contour, filling, movement time, and patency

Abnormal

Lesions or tumors, obstructions, megacolon, fistulas, inflammatory changes, diverticula, chronic ulcerative colitis, stenosis, right-sided colitis, hernias, polyps, intussusception, carcinoma

Clinical Implications

- A poorly cleansed bowel is the most common factor interfering with accurate and complete visualization. The procedure may need to be repeated if the bowel is not thoroughly cleansed.
- Senna, magnesium citrate, and bisacodyl empty the ascending and right to mid-transverse colon. Enemas cleanse the left transverse, descending, and sigmoid colon and the rectum. Suppositories empty the rectum.
- Use of magnesium citrate or magnesium hydroxide cathartics should be avoided in patients with renal failure.
- Radiographs expose the patient to radiation, avoid unnecessary studies. Staff and patients should be protected from radiation as much as the procedure allows. Pregnant women, and those possibly pregnant, should avoid radiographs of the trunk or pelvis unless absolutely necessary.

Barium Swallow (Upper GI with Small Bowel Follow-Through [UGI/SBFT])[9,19]

Purpose and Description

The barium swallow study is used to visualize the form, position, mucosal folds, peristaltic activity, and motility of the stomach and upper gastrointestinal tract. Barium typically serves as the contrast medium in this procedure, but diatrizoate meglumine may be used instead. For a single-contrast study, the patient is positioned in front of the fluoroscopy machine and swallows the barium. Fluoroscopy tracks the gastrointestinal activity in real time. A series of radiographs follow. A biphasic study has the best diagnostic yield—the first phase consists of a double-contrast phase (barium and air) followed by a single-contrast phase (barium alone). Glucagon may be used to induce gastric hypotonia during the double-contrast phase.

Findings

Normal

Normal stomach size, contour, motility, and peristalsis; normal esophagus

Abnormal

Congenital anomalies, gastric ulcer, carcinoma of the stomach, gastric polyps, gastritis, foreign bodies, gastric diverticula, pyloric stenosis, reflux and hiatal hernia, volvulus of the stomach

Clinical Implications

- Any other studies requiring contrast (including barium enema) should be completed 1 to 2 days before the barium swallow study to ensure the contrast has been completely eliminated.
- Fasting from food and fluids is required for 8 hours before the study. Medications other than metformin may be taken with a sip of water.
- The patient should receive a laxative after the study is complete.
- Radiographs expose the patient to radiation, avoid unnecessary studies. Staff and patients should be protected from radiation as much as the procedure allows. Pregnant women, and those possibly pregnant, should avoid radiographs of the trunk or pelvis unless absolutely necessary.

Cholangiography (Percutaneous Transhepatic)[9,19]

Purpose and Description

A cholangiogram visualizes the bile ducts by enhancing them with iodinated contrast. Percutaneous transhepatic cholangiography (PTC) is indicated when additional information is needed about the biliary tree, bile leakage, or intraductal lesions after noninvasive tests are completed. The puncture site is numbed with lidocaine. Using fluoroscopy or *US*, a needle is guided to the liver and iodinated contrast is injected. The contrast behaves differently depending on where it is injected, providing information on structure. Therapeutic bile duct drainage may be performed during the study.

Findings

Normal

Normal-sized ducts and duct anatomy (duct is smooth). Absence of stones or lesions.

Abnormal

Stenosis, obstruction, choledocholithiasis (calculi of the common bile duct)

Clinical Implications

- Prior to the procedure, coagulation tests are performed, and significant abnormalities are corrected with fresh frozen plasma, platelets, or both. PTC is contraindicated in patients with uncorrectable coagulopathy.

- A broad-spectrum antibiotic is administered prior and continued for 48 hours afterward.
- The patient must fast prior to the procedure, follow institutional protocols.
- Iodinated contrast concerns: Assess the patient for iodine allergy and previous reaction to contrast. Metformin should be held for 48 hours following contrast administration.

Cholangiography (T Tube)[9]

Purpose and Description

A cholangiogram visualizes the bile ducts by enhancing them with iodinated contrast. The T tube cholangiogram is performed after cholecystectomy to ensure patency of the common bile duct. Iodinated contrast is injected into the T tube (a self-retaining drainage tube attached to the common bile duct), and a fluoroscopic examination is made. The T tube is then unclamped, and the contrast material drains out.

Findings

Normal

Patent common bile duct with no obstructions

Abnormal

Stenosis, obstruction, choledocholithiasis (calculi of the common bile duct)

Clinical Implications

- Iodinated contrast concerns: Assess the patient for iodine allergy and previous reaction to contrast. Metformin should be held for 48 hours following contrast administration.

CT of the Abdomen

See General Procedures, Computed Tomography

Colonoscopy[9,19]

Purpose and Description

Colonoscopy is examination of the colon and terminal ileum by use of a flexible fiber optic or video colonoscope. This procedure is used to evaluate unexplained gastrointestinal bleeding or treat a known source, screen for colon cancer, evaluate structural abnormalities, assess chronic inflammatory disease, remove foreign bodies, dilation or decompression, and excision of polyps. Following cleansing of the bowel the evening before or morning of the procedure, the patient is placed on his or her left side with knees drawn up toward the abdomen. The colonoscope is lubricated and inserted through the anus and advanced approximately 12 cm to the terminal small bowel. To aid in direct observation of the bowel, air is inserted through the scope. Better views of the bowel occur during withdrawal of the scope, permitting a more careful examination of the bowel during this phase of the procedure. A virtual colonoscopy consists of two- and three-dimensional images generated by CT and is indicated in patients who are unable to undergo optical colonoscopy due to an obstructing mass or spasms.

Findings

Normal

Normal large intestine mucosa

Abnormal

Presence of polyps or tumors, areas of ulceration or inflammation, signs of bleeding, presence of foreign objects, and abnormal anatomy

Clinical Implications

- Patients may need to be on a 48- to 72-hour clear liquid diet prior to the procedure. Fasting for 8 hours before the procedure is recommended. No red or purple liquids are allowed.
- Iron supplements must be discontinued 3 to 4 days before the exam. Aspirin-containing products and other antiplatelets and anticoagulants may be discontinued 1 week before the procedure.
- Different preparation regimens exist, follow institutional protocols. Laxatives may be ordered 1 to 3 days beforehand. An enema may be given the night before.
- To cleanse the bowel, the patient should drink 3 to 6 L (usually 4 L) of a saline iso-osmotic and isotonic laxative over 2 to 3 hours (about 12 ounces every 10 minutes). It is more palatable if refrigerated. The laxative will start to take effect in 30 to 60 minutes. It should be continued until feces are clear liquid. Discard any unused portion after 48 hours.
- The patient may require an IV line for sedatives, narcotics, and potentially an anticholinergic agent or glucagon (for bowel spasms).

Endoscopy[9]

Endoscopy is a general term for visual inspection of any body cavity with an endoscope (a fiber-optic instrument), allowing direct visualization of the interior lumen of the upper gastrointestinal tract. See the following sections for specific types of endoscopic procedures:

- Colonoscopy
- Endoscopic retrograde cholangiopancreatography
- Esophagogastroduodenoscopy (upper endoscopy or EGD)
- Proctoscopy, sigmoidoscopy, and proctosigmoidoscopy

Endoscopic Retrograde Cholangiopancreatography[9,19]

Purpose and Description

Endoscopic retrograde cholangiopancreatography (ERCP) is an examination of the hepatobiliary system to evaluate jaundice, pancreatitis, persistent abdominal pain, pancreatic tumors, common duct stones, and biliary disease. The patient first gargles a topical anesthetic. Then, while lying in the left lateral position with knees flexed, a lubricated side-viewing flexible duodenoscope is passed orally into the duodenum and advanced to the papilla of Vater (the point of junction where the pancreatic duct and the common bile duct enter the duodenum). A cannula is then placed into the papilla, and a radiographic contrast agent is injected. Radiographs are taken of the ducts. Biopsy specimens or cytology brushings may be collected before the duodenoscope is removed.

Findings

Normal

Normal ductal anatomy (pancreatic duct and common bile duct), duodenal papilla, and gallbladder

Abnormal

Stones, stenosis or strictures, tumors, cysts or pseudocysts, pancreatitis, peptic ulcer disease, biliary cirrhosis, primary sclerosing cholangitis, and other structural abnormalities

Clinical Implications

- The patient should fast for 8 to 12 hours prior to the procedure.
- This procedure will require conscious sedation (IV sedatives and narcotics) or general anesthesia.

- Anticholinergics or glucagon may be administered to relax the duodenum when the papilla is cannulated.
- Radiographs expose the patient to radiation, avoid unnecessary studies. Staff and patients should be protected from radiation as much as the procedure allows. Pregnant women, and those possibly pregnant, should avoid radiographs of the trunk or pelvis unless absolutely necessary.

Enteroclysis (Small Bowel Enema)[19]

Purpose and Description

Enteroclysis is a radiographic examination of the small bowel used to evaluate malabsorption, inflammatory bowel disease, small bowel tumors, Meckel diverticulum, and the presence of a small bowel obstruction. First, the patient may ingest metoclopramide to accelerate transit time. A local anesthetic is applied to the throat, and a tube is placed into the distal duodenum or proximal jejunum. Barium, the contrast medium, is delivered through the tube, followed by a methylcellulose solution. The movement of the barium is followed by fluoroscopy and documented by an overhead radiograph. Enteroclysis is the most reliable radiological examination for confirming normal anatomical structure of the small bowel.

Findings

Normal

The presence of normal-appearing bowel mucosa, small bowel wall thickness, and normal fluid transit time. The absence of lesions, obstructions, or fistulas.

Abnormal

Obstruction, adhesions, hernias, malignancy, accumulation of intraluminal fluid, strictures, blind pouch or loop, diverticulosis, fistulae, fold thickening or separation, ulcers

Clinical Implications

- Radiographs expose the patient to radiation, avoid unnecessary studies. Staff and patients should be protected from radiation as much as the procedure allows. Pregnant women, and those possibly pregnant, should avoid radiographs of the trunk or pelvis unless absolutely necessary.

Esophagogastroduodenoscopy (Upper Endoscopy or EGD)[9,19]

Purpose and Description

Esophagogastroduodenoscopy is direct visual examination of the esophagus (esophagoscopy), stomach (gastroscopy), and duodenum (duodenoscopy) using an endoscope. This procedure is used to evaluate patients with dysphagia, reflux symptoms, weight loss, hematemesis, melena, persistent nausea/vomiting, persistent anemia, or persistent pain in the chest or abdomen. EGD can also be used to remove foreign objects, placing a percutaneous feeding tube, or other therapeutic indications. Following the application of a local anesthetic spray to the throat to prevent gagging, a lubricated endoscope is placed through the mouth and throat and passed along the esophagus into the stomach and duodenum. Air is placed into the esophagus and stomach for better visualization. Photographs are taken, and biopsies or cytology brushings may be obtained before the endoscope is withdrawn.

Findings

Normal

Absence of inflammation, lesions, and bleeding. Mucosa and anatomy appear normal.

Abnormal

Hemorrhage, hiatal hernia, inflammation, malignancy, ulcers, varices, strictures

Clinical Implications

- Patients should fast for 6 to 8 hours prior to the procedure.
- This procedure will require conscious sedation (IV sedatives and narcotics).

Hepatobiliary Scintigraphy (Cholescintigraphy, HIDA, PAPIDA, or DISIDA Scan)[9,19]

Purpose and Description

The HIDA scan is used to evaluate acute or chronic cholecystitis, jaundice, biliary obstruction, and biliary leak by visualizing the gallbladder and biliary system. A radionuclide tracer, [^{99m}Tc]HIDA (hepatic iminodiacetic acid-derivative), is injected intravenously (either ^{99m}Tc disofenin or mebrofenin). The tracer undergoes uptake by the liver and is excreted into the biliary tree. Using a scintillation camera, serial images are taken (an image every 5 minutes for 1 hour) following the tracer activity.

Findings

Normal

The gallbladder, bile ducts, liver, and a portion of the small bowel are visualized within 1 hour of radionuclide administration showing normal size, shape, and function of the biliary system.

Abnormal

Nonvisualization of the gallbladder (cystic duct obstruction), reduced bile flow, increased tracer uptake in the liver or gallbladder fossa, tracer activity outside the biliary system

Clinical Implications

- The patient must fast for 3 to 4 hours prior to the procedure (allows time for the gallbladder to relax).
- It is recommended to hold opiate medications for 2 to 6 hours before the study—opiates cause contraction of the sphincter of Oddi, creating a partial biliary obstruction. Morphine may be intentionally given during the procedure for this purpose.
- Administration of cholecystokinin (sincalide) intravenously may be used to stimulate contraction of the gallbladder—the presence of viscous bile can prevent entry of tracer. Phenobarbital may be given to infants.

Laparoscopy

See Gynecology, Laparoscopy

Liver Biopsy[9,19]

Purpose and Description

This invasive bedside procedure is used to diagnose, evaluate severity, and establish etiology of chronic hepatitis, liver cirrhosis, and other diseases of the liver. An anxiolytic may be administered, if deemed necessary. After local anesthesia, a long, large-bore needle is inserted percutaneously to aspirate a core of tissue from the liver. The biopsy may be guided by using US or CT. The tissue is then fixed and sent for histologic analysis.

Findings

Normal

Presence of normal pathology and histology without evidence of inflammation or disease

Abnormal

Presence of tumors or cysts, hepatic cellular changes consistent with cirrhosis or hepatitis, signs of organ rejection, and signs of drug toxicity

Clinical Implications

- Localized disease may be missed, as only a small random sample of the organ is taken.
- The patient must be NPO for 4 to 6 hours prior to the procedure.
- It is recommended that antiplatelet agents be stopped before open and needle biopsies. Aspirin and NSAIDs should be discontinued 7 days before the procedure. Check coagulation labs prior to the procedure, and correct if necessary.

MRI of the Abdomen

See General Procedures, Magnetic Resonance Imaging

Paracentesis[9,19]

Purpose and Description

Paracentesis is the puncture of any cavity for the aspiration of fluid; however, the withdrawal of fluid from the abdomen (abdominal paracentesis) is the most commonly encountered. This procedure is used to evaluate ascites. Prior to the procedure, the patient empties his or her bladder. The patient is placed in Fowler position, and a local anesthetic is applied to the puncture site. A needle is inserted through the abdominal wall into the peritoneum 1 to 2 in. below the umbilicus. For diagnostic purposes, 50 mL of fluid are aspirated and sent to the laboratory for analysis. When performed for therapeutic purposes, fluid volumes of 1.5 to 5 L may be removed.

Findings

Normal

Clear to slightly yellow peritoneal fluid with no abnormal cells

Abnormal

Cloudy or turbid appearance, elevated protein content, elevated glucose, presence of RBCs or bloody fluid, white blood cells (WBCs) > 300/mL, mucin, plasma cells, and cytology positive for malignant cells

Clinical Implications

- There are no medical contraindications to paracentesis, including coagulopathy.

Proctoscopy, Sigmoidoscopy, and Proctosigmoidoscopy[9]

Purpose and Description

These three endoscopic procedures are useful in evaluating rectal bleeding, structural abnormalities (such as diverticula), and detection and diagnosis of malignancy. A flexible fiber-optic endoscope is employed for all three procedures as this is more comfortable for patients than the rigid instrument. The patient is placed in the left lateral position, and the proctoscope or sigmoidoscope is inserted into the rectum.

Findings

Normal

Normal anal, rectal, and sigmoid colon mucosa

Abnormal

Edematous, red, or denuded mucosa. Presence of grainy minute masses. The tissue is easily broken or pulverized. Visible ulcers or pseudomembranes. Spontaneous bleeding on examination.

Clinical Implications

- Fasting is not required; however, clear liquids may be recommended the evening before the exam.
- Laxative suppositories or enemas may be ordered the evening before the procedure; however, 1 to 2 phosphate enemas administered 1 to 2 hours before the exam is sufficient for most patients.

Small Bowel Series

See Gastroenterology, Barium Swallow (Upper GI With Small Bowel Follow-Through [UGI/SBFT]).

Ultrasonography of the Abdomen

See General Procedures, Ultrasonography

Gynecology

Breast Biopsy[9,20]

Purpose and Description

Needle and open breast biopsies are performed to determine if breast tumors are benign or malignant. Receptor assays are done on malignant tissues to determine if the tumor is estrogen receptor (ER) and/or progesterone receptor (PR) positive or negative. ER(+) and PR(+) tumors will respond best to hormonal chemotherapy.

Breast biopsy may be performed by using either needle or open procedures (see "General Procedures, Biopsy"). Diagnostically, needle biopsy is limited by the small tissue sample; it may not be representative of the entire breast mass. There is also an increased risk of seeding the needle tract with potentially malignant cells, thus causing further spread of the disease. Therefore, a needle biopsy is generally reserved for a fluid-filled cyst or an advanced malignant lesion. In an open biopsy of the breast, if the mass is small enough (<2 cm) and looks benign, the mass is excised. For larger masses that look malignant, a representative amount of tissue is excised from the mass (lumpectomy).

Findings

Normal

Results from a breast biopsy will reveal adequate amounts of cellular and noncellular connective tissue with proper development of tissue.

Abnormal

Presence of a benign tumor (such as adenofibroma) or presence of a malignant tumor (such as adenocarcinoma, inflammatory carcinoma, or sarcoma). Plasma cell mastitis or the presence of intraductal papilloma.

Clinical Implications

- Local anesthetics are administered before needle and some open breast biopsies. Some open biopsies require the use of a general anesthetic, in which case, the patient is not to eat or drink after midnight the night before the procedure.

- A penicillinase-resistant antibiotic is sometimes used after an open breast biopsy as prophylaxis against staphylococcal infections.

Colposcopy[9,20]

Purpose and Description

Colposcopy is a visual examination of the cervix and vagina by using a colposcope, an instrument containing a magnifying lens and a light. It is done to observe the vagina and cervix, perform tissue biopsy, evaluate lesions, or monitor antineoplastic therapy.

Findings

Normal

Vaginal and cervical mucosa and epithelium of normal color and appearance

Abnormal

Presence of color tissue changes or lesions

Clinical Implications

The patient may be instructed to take an over-the-counter NSAID (such as ibuprofen, 400 to 600 mg, or naproxen, 125 to 250 mg) the night before the procedure to minimize the cramping that can occur with the colposcopy and biopsy.

Hysterosalpingography[9,20]

Purpose and Description

Hysterosalpingography, also known as a uterogram, is a radiographic examination performed to visualize the outline of the uterine cavity and the fallopian tubes by means of a contrast medium injected through a cannula inserted into the cervix. The uterus and fallopian tubes are viewed under fluoroscopy, and radiographs are taken. It detects abnormalities that can cause infertility.

Findings

Normal

Normal anatomy with no tubal or uterine abnormalities

Abnormal

Tubal adhesions or occlusions. Uterine abnormalities including foreign bodies, fibroid tumors, congenital malformations, or fistulas.

Clinical Implications

- Iodine contrast dye may produce hypersensitivity reactions or anaphylaxis.
- A sedative may be administered before the procedure.

Laparoscopy[9,20]

Purpose and Description

Laparoscopy is the direct visual examination of the pelvic cavity with a laparoscope through the anterior abdominal wall. Indications include performing procedures, such as lysis of adhesions, ovarian biopsy, tubal ligation, removal of foreign bodies, or cholecystectomy, to detect ectopic pregnancy, endometriosis, pelvic inflammatory disease, or appendicitis; to evaluate pelvic masses, ascites, or abdominal trauma; to examine the fallopian tubes for infertile women; to harvest eggs (ovum) for in vitro fertilization; and to diagnosis and stage cancer. In women, the ovaries, uterus, and fallopian tubes are examined. A small incision is made at the level of the umbilicus with the patient under local or general anesthesia.

Findings

Normal

Uterus, ovaries, and fallopian tubes are of normal size and shape without adhesions, cysts, or presence of endometriosis. Normally appearing liver, spleen, and peritoneum.

Abnormal

Presence of cysts, adhesions, fibroids, endometriosis, ectopic pregnancy, infection, abscess, or trauma

Clinical Implications

- The patient should not eat or drink after midnight the night before the procedure.
- The patient should avoid aspirin for 7 to 10 days before the procedure and should avoid NSAIDs 2 to 4 days before the procedure.
- Pelvic or abdominal postoperative discomfort may require analgesics.

Mammography[9,20]

Purpose and Description

A mammogram is a radiograph of the breast. It screens for breast cancer and investigates or detects masses missed during physical examination of the breast. A low-energy x-ray beam (0.1 to 0.8 rads) delineates the breast on mammograms. Frontal and lateral views are taken.

Findings

Normal

No calcification, no abnormal mass, and normal duct contrast with narrowing of ductal branches

Abnormal

A poorly outlined, irregularly shaped, and opaque lesion suggests malignancy. Malignant cysts are usually solitary and unilateral and contain an increased number of blood vessels. Benign cysts are usually round and smooth with definable edges.

Clinical Implications

- No medications/preparations needed

Ultrasonography of Pelvis, Uterus, and Ovaries

See General Procedures, Ultrasound

Hematology

Bone Marrow Aspiration and Biopsy[9,21]

Purpose and Description

Bone marrow specimens may be obtained via aspiration, biopsy, or needle biopsy aspiration. Evaluation of these specimens is used to assess many hematological disorders (e.g., multiple myeloma, acute or chronic leukemia, anemias, agranulocytosis, etc.) and some infectious disease (e.g., histoplasmosis, tuberculosis). An aspiration sample may not contain any hematopoietic cells if activity is sparse or the cells are too tightly packed; in this situation a biopsy would be useful.

Aspiration

The preferred site is the posterior iliac crest in patients older than 12 months. The site is cleansed, shaved, and draped as for a minor surgical procedure, then a local anesthetic is injected. A 3 mm incision is made and a needle-stylet is inserted into the bone cortex. The stylet is removed and 1 to 3 mL of fluid is aspirated.

Biopsy
After the stylet has been removed, the needle is advanced toward the anterosuperior iliac spine using a twisting motion. The needle is rocked in several directions multiple times once the base has been reached in order to "free up" the specimen. The needle is slowly withdrawn containing the bone marrow specimen. Apply pressure to the puncture site until bleeding stops.

Findings

Normal
Normal amounts of the various hematological cells in the appropriate ratios

Abnormal
Detection of malignant cells, atypical amounts or ratios of normal cells (hyper- or hypocellularity), cells with morphological changes, and amyloid deposits.

Clinical Implications

- Patients may require sedation (benzodiazepines) and analgesia (opiates) for this procedure.

Infectious Disease

Gram Stain[9,22]

Purpose and Description

The Gram stain is a simple and inexpensive method used to classify bacteria from a specimen into two groups: gram-positive or gram-negative organisms. First, the specimen smear is stained with gentian or crystal violet. Then, the violet stain is washed off, and the smear is flooded with iodine. After washing off the iodine, the smear is then flooded with 95% alcohol or an acetone–alcohol mixture. Finally, the smear is counterstained with the red dye, safranin O. Bacteria are divided based on their ability to pick up one or both stains. Morphologic features, such as cocci or bacilli, can also be seen with this test.

Findings

- Gram-positive organisms retain the primary dye and appear dark purple.
- Gram-negative organisms will appear pinkish-red following decolorization and counterstaining.

Clinical Implications

The ability to differentiate Gram-positive and Gram-negative organisms and the knowledge of their antibiotic sensitivity patterns aid in the selection of appropriate empiric antibiotic therapy until the final identification of the organism occurs.

Indium-Labeled WBC Scan (Indium-111 Leukocyte Total Body Scan)[9,22]

Purpose and Description

This procedure is used to localize an acute abscess, evaluate osteomyelitis, or investigate potential sources of sepsis symptoms. A 60-mL sample of the patient's blood is taken in order to isolate his or her WBCs. These are labeled with indium oxine (^{111}In) or ^{99m}Tc exametazime and then reinjected intravenously into the patient. The patient returns for imaging either 4 hours later (if ^{99m}Tc exametazime is used) or 24 to 48 hours later (if ^{111}In is used).

Findings

Normal

Normal leukocyte and radiopharmaceutical concentration in liver, spleen, and bone marrow without localization outside the reticuloendothelial system

Abnormal

Collection of labeled leukocytes outside the above areas, signaling an acute abscess

Clinical Implications

- This test cannot be performed in neutropenic patients, as a minimum WBC of 4.0 is required.
- Hyperalimentation, steroid therapy, and long-term antibiotic therapy can produce false-negative results because of their ability to change the chemotactic response of leukocytes.

Nephrology

Renal Biopsy[23]

Purpose and Description

Renal biopsy may be used to diagnose diseases that alter the structure of the glomerulus, evaluate proteinuria of unknown origin, determine the nature of a renal mass or cause of acute renal failure when other etiologic factors have been ruled out, monitor the course of chronic renal disease, evaluate suspected cases of renal dysfunction secondary to inflammatory vasculitides, or evaluate suspected rejection of a transplanted kidney.

See General Procedures, Biopsy. The safest method is percutaneous needle biopsy. The biopsy needle is advanced toward the kidney, where a biopsy core is extracted and the needle is withdrawn. If a tissue sample from a solid lesion is necessary, an open biopsy may need to be performed.

Findings

Normal

Normal pathology and histology

Abnormal

Presence of a tumor, clot, or renal stone. Presence of histologic changes characteristic of lupus erythematosus, amyloid infiltration, glomerulonephritis, renal vein thrombosis, pyelonephritis, and renal transplant rejection.

Clinical Implications

It is recommended that antiplatelet agents be stopped before open and needle biopsies. Aspirin should be discontinued 7 to 10 days before the procedure. NSAIDs (e.g., ibuprofen, naproxen) should be stopped 2 to 4 days before the procedure.

Renal Scan[23]

Purpose and Description

Renal scan is used to detect kidney masses, investigate kidney function, and evaluate kidney transplant viability and renal blood flow. A radioactive tracer, ^{99m}Tc, is injected intravenously. A scanning camera then takes images of the blood flow to and through the kidneys. During the first stage of scanning, images are taken in rapid succession to evaluate renal perfusion. During the second stage, several still images are taken over a 30- to 45-minute period to evaluate renal function.

Findings

Normal

Normal size, shape, position, and function of the kidneys

Abnormal

Tumors (irregular masses) within the kidney, obstructions, decreased renal perfusion, abnormal kidneys (shape or size), and presence of rejection

Clinical Implications

None

Neurology

Brainstem Auditory Evoked Response[9,24]

Purpose and Description

Brainstem auditory evoked response (BAER) is a noninvasive test using electroencephalography (EEG) recordings with specific electrode placements to diagnose cerebral deficiencies of the eighth cranial nerve, brainstem lesions and tumors, multiple sclerosis infarcts, and acoustic neuromas. It can also be used to assess comas and evaluate hearing in newborns, children, and adults.

Findings

Lesions at different sites in a tract along the eighth cranial nerve through the brainstem and into the cerebral cortex will alter electrical waves in different ways, providing a method of locating a suspected brainstem lesion.

Clinical Implications

None

CT of the Head

See General Procedures, Computed Tomography

Electroencephalography[9,24]

Purpose and Description

The EEG records and measures electrical activity from the brain via electrodes that are placed on the scalp. It is used to diagnose seizure disorders in conjunction with simultaneous video monitoring, narcolepsy, Parkinson disease, Alzheimer disease, certain psychoses, and central nervous system (CNS) infections (herpes simplex encephalitis and Creutzfeldt-Jakob disease). It is also used to aid in identifying brain tumors, abscesses, subdural hematomas, cerebral infarcts, and intracranial hemorrhage, among other conditions.

Findings

Normal

The EEG tracing produces a tape that is consistent with normal electrical brain activity in the awake and sleep state.

Abnormal

Brain wave activity consistent with a seizure disorder or other cerebral disease or lesion. A flat EEG results from cerebral hypoxia or ischemia from which there is no neurologic recovery.

Clinical Implications

- Caffeine-containing drinks should be withheld for 8 hours before the test.
- Drugs altering brain wave activity (e.g., anticonvulsants, sedatives, tranquilizers) will interfere with an accurate tracing. A physician may choose to stop anticonvulsant therapy before the EEG.

Electromyography[9,24]

Purpose and Description

Electromyography (EMG) measures nerve conduction and electrical properties of skeletal muscles. The electrical activity of the muscle is measured at three activity levels: rest, mild contraction, and maximal contraction. The muscle is not electrically stimulated during this test. The amplitude, duration, number, and configuration of the muscle action potentials aid in differentiating neurogenic pathology from myogenic involvement. The procedure is used to evaluate the integrity of the nervous system, the neuromuscular junction, and the muscle itself. EMG by itself is not considered diagnostic for any specific disease.

Findings

Normal

A normally relaxed muscle is electrically silent at rest. During voluntary contraction, electrical activity increases significantly.

Abnormal

Waveforms that are different from normal muscle are evaluated to differentiate a muscle disorder from a denervation disorder.

Clinical Implications

Drugs that affect the nerve–muscle junction such as cholinergics, anticholinergics, and skeletal muscle relaxants can interfere with test results.

Lumbar Puncture[9,25]

Purpose and Description

Lumbar puncture (LP) is used to obtain a cerebrospinal fluid (CSF) specimen for diagnostic study. The spinal canal is penetrated with a needle between the third and fourth (or fourth and fifth) lumbar vertebrae to obtain the specimen. CSF study can aid in the diagnosis of suspected meningitis, intracranial hemorrhage, organic CNS disease (e.g., multiple sclerosis and Guillain-Barré syndrome), and CNS involvement from malignant disease (e.g., leukemia, lymphoma). LP can also be used to evaluate electrolyte disturbances, remove blood or exudate from the subarachnoid space, and administer x-ray contrast media or other drugs intrathecally.

Findings

Normal

Normal appearance, consistency, expected cell composition, absence of bacteria, normal chemistry of the fluid, and normal pressure (see the section on CSF examination in Chapter 7, Interpretation of Clinical Laboratory Results).

Abnormal

See Table 8.6

Clinical Implications

Patients may experience a headache after removal of CSF and require treatment with an analgesic.

TABLE 8.6 Abnormal CSF Fluid

Appearance	Cloudy Fluid
Protein content	50 mg/dL
Glucose concentration	<30 mg/dL or >70 mg/dL
WBCs	10/mm^3
pH of fluid	< or >7.3
Bacteria or virus	Present
RBCs	Present

MRI of the Head

See General Procedures, Magnetic Resonance Imaging

Muscle Biopsy[9,24]

Purpose and Description

A muscle biopsy obtains a muscle tissue sample by making a small incision through the skin and into the muscle. A sample of the desired muscle segment is excised (open biopsy). An alternate method is percutaneous by means of a biopsy needle. The needle is inserted into the muscle, and a small plug of muscle tissue is removed when the needle is withdrawn. Muscle biopsy investigates the origin of muscle weakness, evaluates suspected myopathy, and helps diagnose muscle inflammatory, genetic, diffuse vascular, connective tissue, and metabolic diseases.

Findings

Normal

Presence of normal pathology and histology

Abnormal

Presence of myogenic or myopathic changes

Clinical Implications

- Antiplatelet agents should be discontinued before open and needle biopsies. Aspirin should be discontinued 7 to 10 days before the procedure. NSAIDs should be stopped 2 to 4 days before the procedure.
- Preprocedure medications such as parenteral analgesics and parenteral anxiolytics may be administered.
- A local anesthetic such as lidocaine may be necessary.

Myelography[9,24]

Purpose and Description

Myelography visualizes spinal cord abnormalities via radiographic examination of the cervical, thoracic, and/or lumbar spinal cord and the space around the spinal cord. This test is sometimes followed or replaced by CT scanning, which can improve visualization.

Findings

Normal

No evidence of spinal cord abnormalities

Abnormal

Presence of a herniated disc, spinal cord compression, nerve root injury, degenerative spur, vascular abnormalities, CSF leakage, dural tear, traumatic injury, neoplasm, or mass.

Clinical Implications

- The patient should have no food or fluids 4 hours before the examination.
- A local anesthetic, such as lidocaine, is used to anesthetize the area at the site of spinal needle insertion.
- The procedure should not be performed if the patient is receiving anticoagulants.
- Medications that can lower the seizure threshold, such as phenothiazines, monoamine oxidase inhibitors (MAOIs), tricyclic antidepressants, and CNS stimulants, should be discontinued ≥48 hours before and ≥24 hours after myelography.
- The use of phenothiazine antiemetics should be avoided.

Nerve Biopsy[9,24]

Purpose and Description

Nerve biopsy removes nerve tissue for evaluation, diagnoses neuropathic disorders, and distinguishes between demyelinating disease versus axon degeneration disease. The sural nerve (situated in the lower leg near the Achilles tendon), the deep peroneal nerve (located in the area of the calf below the knee), or the superficial radial nerve are the sites most commonly used for nerve biopsy.

Findings

Normal

Presence of normal pathology and histology

Abnormal

Presence of polyarteritis nodosa, amyloidosis, sarcoidosis, vasculitis, various neuropathies, mononeuritis multiplex, specific nerve (radial, distal median, tibial) dysfunction, leprosy, metachromatic leukodystrophy, Krabbe disease, ataxia telangiectasia, giant axonal neuropathy, and genetically determined pediatric neurologic disorders

Clinical Implications

It is recommended that antiplatelet agents be stopped before open and needle biopsies. Aspirin should be stopped 7 to 10 days before the procedure. NSAIDs should be discontinued 2 to 4 days before the procedure.

Nerve Conduction Study[9]

Purpose and Description

Nerve conduction study evaluates peripheral nerve dysfunction. This testing may be done at the same time as EMG to differentiate peripheral nerve disease from myogenic disease. By knowing the time interval between applying the electrical stimulus and the initiation of the action potential along with the maximum nerve conduction velocity, objective information about nerve conduction can be obtained. Nerves commonly tested include the median, ulnar, radial, peroneal, tibial, superficial peroneal, and sural. Nerve conduction studies can evaluate polyneuropathy, assess nerve entrapment (e.g., carpal tunnel syndrome), and confirm sensory deficits and demyelinating diseases.

Findings

Normal

Action potential amplitude, conduction velocity, and latency are within normal ranges

Abnormal

Slowing of conduction velocity, delayed distal latency, and decreased amplitude of the action potential

Clinical Implications

Many medications can cause neuropathy. Review the patient's medication list to identify contributing factors.

Visual Evoked Response[9]

Purpose and Description

Visual evoked response (VER) is a noninvasive test utilizing EEG recordings with specific electrode placements on the scalp over the occipital or visual cortex area to test visual pathway function. It is used to diagnose lesions of the optic nerve or confirming the diagnosis of multiple sclerosis, rule out hysterical blindness, and monitor surgery of the optic nerve.

Findings

Normal

No evidence of optic nerve damage

Abnormal

A difference in the responses between the left and right eyes, with an increased latency and duration in one eye, indicates a lesion in that optic nerve. Both optic nerves can be involved. Presence of optic neuritis, pseudotumor cerebri, toxic amblyopias, nutritional amblyopias, neoplasms interfering with the optic pathway, sarcoidosis, pernicious anemia, and Friedreich ataxia.

Clinical Implications

None

Ophthalmology

Ophthalmoscopy[9,10,26]

Purpose and Description

Ophthalmoscopy examines the eye, including the optic disk, macula, retina, retinal vessels, choroid, and sclera. An ophthalmoscope, an instrument with a special illumination system, is used to view the inner eye. A strong light is directed into the patient's eye by reflection from a small mirror. The light is reflected from the fundus of the eye back through the ophthalmoscope to the examiner.

Findings

Normal

Optic disk is of normal size, color, and vascularity. Macula is devoid of blood vessels and darker than surrounding retina. Retina is attached

TABLE 8.7 Retinal Vascular Grading Systems

Hypertensive Retinopathy (Keith-Wagner Method)	
Grade I	Constriction of retinal arterioles only
Grade II	Constriction and sclerosis of retinal arterioles
Grade III	Hemorrhages and exudates in addition to vascular changes
Grade IV	Papilledema (edema of the optic disk)

Diabetic Retinopathy (Retinal Changes Fall into Two Categories)

Background retinopathy

- Multiple microaneurysms appear
- Veins dilate, multiple dot and blot hemorrhages occur, and hard waxy white and yellow exudates may leak from the retinal vasculature in the area of the macula.
- Cotton-wool patches (microinfarcts of the retinal nerve fiber layer) appear in the superficial retina; hard exudates may form what is described as the macular star.

Proliferative retinopathy

- Neovascularization occurs.
- Neovascularization of the optic disk occurs.
- End stage of retinopathy occurs with organized vitreous hemorrhage, fibrosis, and retinitis proliferans (detached retina) leading to blindness.

and has normal vascularity and color. Choroid and sclera should not be visualized.

Abnormal

Optic disk has abnormal vascularity, elevation (bulging), small hemorrhages, and abnormal color. The macula is edematous and ischemic with degeneration appearing as a round white mass. Blood vessels of the choroid and sclera can be visualized. Malignant melanoma appears as a pigmented elevated mass. Two descriptive approaches for staging or grading of retinopathy are used. The choice of grading methods for retinal vascular changes is influenced by the underlying disease (Table 8.7).

Clinical Implications

- Drugs affecting the retina include chloroquine, hydroxychloroquine, phenothiazines, penicillamine, isoniazid, ethambutol, and indomethacin.
- Dilating eye drops may be used to improve visualization of eye structures.
- Baseline and follow-up ophthalmoscopy is recommended when hypertension or diabetes is present or when certain drugs are being taken.

Slit-Lamp Examination[9,10,26]

Purpose and Description

Slit lamp allows for examination of the lids, cornea, anterior chamber of the eye, and transparent and nearly transparent ocular fluids and tissues. The examination involves the combination of a light and microscopic examination of the eye. Dilation of the pupil, using a mydriatic and cycloplegic agent, facilitates viewing.

Findings

Normal

Clear, avascular vitreous fluid

Abnormal

Vitreous disease including retraction, condensation, shrinkage, and presence of blood, floaters, cataracts, or corneal deposits

Clinical Implications

Slit-lamp examination may be needed to evaluate drug-induced ocular toxicity associated with indomethacin, clofazimine, allopurinol, corticosteroids, gold salts, chloroquine, hydroxychloroquine, griseofulvin, chlorambucil, cytosine arabinoside, mitotane, tamoxifen, amiodarone, quinidine, phenothiazines, phenytoin, and isotretinoin.

Tonometry[9,10,26]

Purpose and Description

Tonometry measures the fluid pressure inside the eye or intraocular pressure (IOP). Increased IOP is a risk factor for glaucoma. The most commonly used contact tonometer is the applanation (Goldman) tonometer. This measures the force needed to flatten an area of the cornea. Noncontact tonometry directs a puff of air at the cornea to determine eye pressure. This method is less reliable when the pressure in the eye is at a higher pressure range, when the cornea is abnormal, or when the patient is unable to establish visual fixation.

Findings

Normal

10 to 20 mm Hg (16 mm average)

Abnormal

Greater than 24 mm Hg is diagnostic for glaucoma.

Clinical Implications

Drugs that may increase IOP include anticholinergics, corticosteroids, and sympathomimetics.

Orthopedics

Arthroscopy[9,27]

Purpose and Description

Arthroscopy is visual examination of a joint (most commonly the knee and less commonly the shoulder or other joints) using an arthroscope, a type of fiberoptic endoscope. This procedure is used to diagnose athletic injuries and acute or chronic joint disorders. It is frequently performed in the ambulatory surgical setting, typically using general or spinal anesthesia. A tourniquet is applied to the appropriate joint and then a small incision is made for the arthroscope. The joint is aspirated and then continuously irrigated. All parts of the joint are examined at various degrees of flexion and extension, and joint washings are examined. A variety of functions may be performed during the procedure, including repair of meniscus tears, removal of loose bodies, and biopsies. Steroids or local anesthetics may be injected into the joint.

Findings

Normal

Normal joint vasculature, color of synovium, ligaments, cartilage, and undamaged suprapatellar pouch

Abnormal

Torn and displaced cartilage and meniscus, trapped synovium, loose fragments of bone or cartilage, torn ligaments, chronic inflammatory arthritis, chondromalacia of bone, secondary osteoarthritis, presence of cysts or foreign bodies, torn rotator cuff, or rotator cuff tendonitis.

Clinical Implications

- The patient should take nothing by mouth starting at midnight the night before the procedure.

- Arthroscopy usually follows arthrography by at least 7 days due to the possibility of chemical synovitis from contrast medium. If earlier arthroscopy is necessary, the joint must be irrigated to remove the contrast agent.
- The patient should not drive or drink alcohol for 24 hours after the procedure due to effects from anesthesia and additive effects from analgesics.

Arthrography[9,27]

Purpose and Description

An arthrogram is a radiograph of a joint following injection of contrast media (air, iodinated contrast, or both) into the synovium. This procedure is performed in patients with persistent, unexplained joint discomfort (most commonly the knee, less commonly other joints) in order to elucidate soft tissue injury in cartilage and ligaments surrounding the joint that cannot be seen with conventional x-ray techniques. A local anesthetic is injected into the tissues around the joint. If fluid is present in the joint space, a sample is aspirated first and sent to the laboratory to detect the presence of bacteria and/or chemicals. Then, contrast is injected into the joint space, and the joint is manipulated to ensure even distribution. Radiographs are taken in several positions. Alternatively, an MRI arthrogram may be performed.

Findings

Normal

Normal filling of encapsulated joint structures, joint space, bursae, ligaments, and cartilage

Abnormal

Ligamentous and cartilaginous tears or injuries, cysts, narrowing of joint space, dislocation

Clinical Implications

- Iodinated contrast may be used. Hypersensitivity reactions to the iodine dye are less likely to occur due to the small amount of iodine present in the synovial space.

Bone Densitometry[9,27]

Purpose and Description

Bone mineral density is the major determinant of fracture risk. Bone density studies are used to identify patients who are at risk for developing osteoporosis, to evaluate fracture risk, and to evaluate the patient's response to osteoporosis therapy. Several noninvasive techniques are used to measure bone density.

- Dual-energy absorptiometry (DEXA or DXA): spine, hip, and forearm density
- Peripheral dual-energy absorptiometry (pDXA): forearm density
- Single-energy x-ray absorptiometry (SXA): heel and forearm density
- Radiographic absorptiometry (RA): phalanges density

DEXA is considered the gold standard for bone mineral density measurement due to its precision and low radiation exposure. The area to be imaged is made immobile through the use of foam blocks under the knees (spine imaging) or a brace (arm or leg imaging). DEXA images take approximately 20 minutes to complete for hip and spine and another 15 minutes for the forearm.

Findings

The T-score (number of standard deviations the bone density is above or below the mean for young, normal subjects) is used to determine fracture risk and the need for treatment. There is approximately a 10% reduction or increase in bone mineral density for each standard deviation below or above zero.

Normal

T-score >-1

Abnormal

T-score of -1 to -2.5 indicates osteopenia. T-score <-2.5 indicates osteoporosis.

Clinical Implications

- Nuclear imaging within the last 72 hours may leave residual emission that can cause misinterpretation.
- Barium imaging within the last 7 to 10 days may interfere with spine imaging.
- Prosthetic or metallic implanted objects may interfere with imaging if in the area of interest.

Bone Scan[9]

Purpose and Description

A bone scan is a radiograph of the whole body to evaluate and monitor patients with known or suspected metastatic cancer, unexplained bone pain, arthritis, osteomyelitis, and fractures and to assess suspected child abuse. A bone-seeking radionuclide, ^{99m}Tc-labeled phosphate, is injected intravenously, followed by imaging 2 to 3 hours later. The patient may drink 4 to 6 glasses of water while waiting for imaging and then void his bladder just prior in order to better visualize the pelvic bones. The patient lies still for 30 to 60 minutes while imaging is completed.

Findings

Normal

The radionuclide is distributed evenly throughout the bone. No "hot spots" (concentrated areas of uptake) are noted.

Abnormal

Presence of "hot spots" indicating increased concentration of radionuclide at sites of abnormal metabolism (e.g., infection, fracture, degenerative bone disease, failing bone grafts, or healing)

Clinical Implications

- A sedative may be required for patients unable to lie still for the procedure.

Otolaryngology

Laryngoscopy[28,29]

Purpose and Description

Laryngoscopy is used to examine vocal fold structure and gross function and to diagnose voice and laryngeal disorders.

- *Rigid endoscope*: With the patient standing, the examiner advances the endoscope just under the uvula while holding the tongue out of the way. Topical anesthesia is not usually required. The endoscope is tilted, and the angle varied to view all areas. Phonation is limited with a rigid endoscope.

- *Flexible endoscope*: A topical anesthetic and vasoconstrictor are applied and then the flexible endoscope is advanced through the nose. Magnification is inferior compared to the rigid endoscope, but the natural function of the larynx can be better observed.

A common therapeutic usage of laryngoscopy is during intubation. The patient may be awake or unconscious, but should be lying supine. Either a curved (Macintosh) or straight (Miller) laryngoscope blade may be used, attached to a laryngoscope handle. Once the laryngoscope is in position, an airway can be placed.

Findings

Normal

Normal position, color, and anatomy of the examined area. Absence of lesions, strictures, inflammation, and foreign bodies.

Abnormal

Abnormal or asymmetrical laryngeal structure, edema, erythema, lesions, surface irregularities, impaired motion, thick mucus, dilated or tortuous vessels

Clinical Implications

None

Pulmonology

Bronchoscopy and Bronchial Alveolar Lavage (BAL)[9,30]

Purpose and Description

Bronchoscopy is the examination of the inside of the tracheobronchial tree by direct visualization. This procedure is used to diagnose tumors and lesions, evaluate pneumonia, find sources of hemorrhage, obtain biopsies, take brushings for evaluation, improve drainage of secretions, lavage, or remove foreign bodies. A topical anesthetic is applied to the throat, and possibly the nasal passage, and an antisialagogue (atropine) is administered to reduce secretions. A bronchodilator may be administered to patients with a history of bronchospasm. Analgesics and/or sedatives may be administered as needed to achieve conscious sedation. Then, a flexible fiberoptic bronchoscope is inserted through the mouth or nose (or endotracheal tube or tracheostomy) and advanced into the tracheobronchial tree. The right lung is examined, followed by the left lung. Bronchial alveolar lavage is performed by instilling normal saline into the lung through the bronchoscope and then aspirating. The aspirated fluid is assessed for gross appearance and sent for a variety of tests that may include cytologic, microbiologic, and cell count analysis. This may be performed safely when biopsy or brushings are not recommended due to bleeding risk.

Findings

Normal

Normal anatomy without malignancies, lesions, source of bleeding, or infection

Abnormal

Presence of malignancies, infections, inflammation, fibrosis, or trauma

Clinical Implications

- The patient should fast 6 hours before and 2 hours after the procedure to reduce risk of aspiration.
- Coagulation status should be evaluated and corrected if needed prior to the procedure.

Chest Radiograph[9,30]

Purpose and Description

A chest radiograph is taken from the front (posteroanterior), side (left lateral), and sometimes back. It is best performed with the patient in the standing position as this demonstrates the presence of fluid levels. Chest radiographs are useful in the diagnosis of pulmonary, mediastinal, and bony thorax disease.

Findings

Normal

Absence of fluids, masses, and infection. Air-filled spaces appear black.

Abnormal

The film will have opacities (shadowy or white areas) suggestive of the presence of fluid, tumors and other lesions, infectious processes, unusual air in the lungs, or a collapsed lung. Spinal deformities, bone destruction, and trauma can be observed.

Clinical Implications

- Radiographs expose the patient to radiation, avoid unnecessary studies. Staff and patients should be protected from radiation as much as the procedure allows. Pregnant women, and those possibly pregnant, should avoid radiographs of the trunk or pelvis unless absolutely necessary.

CT of the Chest

See General Procedures, Computed Tomography

Pulmonary Function Tests (PFTs)[31,32]

Purpose and Description

The respiratory system is responsible for the exchange of carbon dioxide (CO_2) and oxygen (O_2). Together with the circulatory system, body tissues can exchange CO_2 and receive adequate O_2. Various disease processes alter the exchanges of these gases between the alveoli and the bloodstream. Pulmonary function tests are performed to provide an objective measurement of the respiratory system. Pulmonary disorders are often classified as restrictive or obstructive. Typical airflow and volume curves can assist in classifying a disorder, as shown in Figure 8.1.

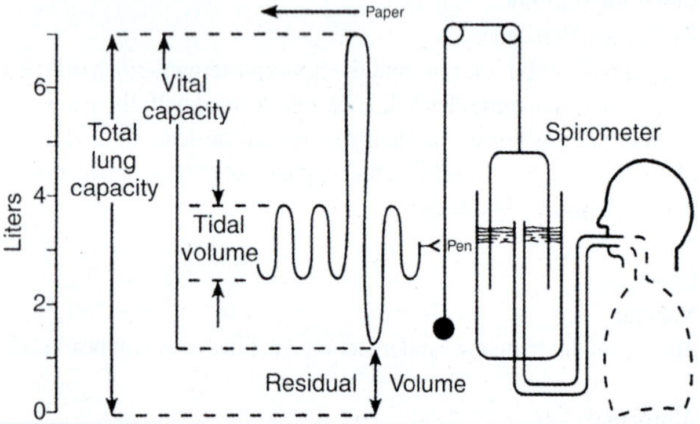

FIGURE 8.1 Flow/volume curve showing a typical pattern for obstructive and restrictive diseases. (Adapted from Young LY, Koda-Kimble MA. *Applied Therapeutics: The Clinical Use of Drugs*. 6th ed. Vancouver, WA: Applied Therapeutics, Inc.; 1995, with permission.)

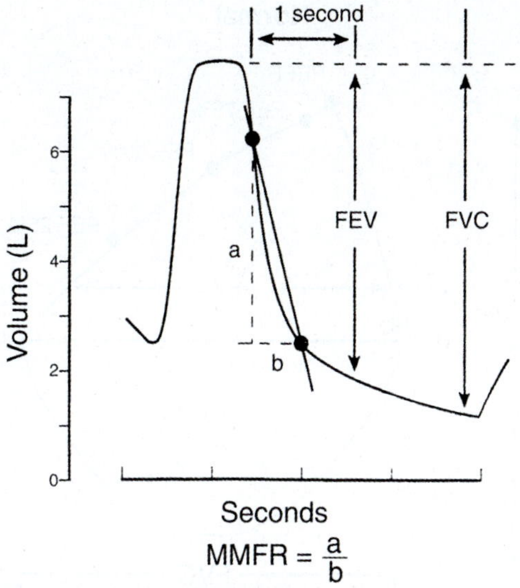

FIGURE 8.2 Spirometric graphics during quiet breathing and maximal breathing. (Reprinted from Alldredge BK, et al. *Koda-Kimble and Young's Applied Therapeutics: The Clinical Use of Drugs*. 10th ed. Philadelphia, PA: Lippincott Williams & Wilkins; 2012, with permission.)

Using spirometry, a patient is instructed to inhale and then exhale as rapidly as possible. As the patient exhales into the spirometer, he or she displaces a bell and the pen deflection records the volume of air entering or exiting the lung (Fig. 8.2).

The tidal volume or the volume of air being inhaled and exhaled during normal breathing can be recorded. The vital capacity (VC) is the amount of air being moved during maximal inhalation and exhalation. Residual volume (RV) reflects the volume of air left in the lung after maximal expiration. Total lung capacity (TLC) is the sum of the VC and the RV. Patients with restrictive lung disease often display a decrease in all lung volumes, whereas those individuals with obstructive disease often have normal TLC but decreased VC and increased RV.

In evaluating the performance of the lung, forced expiration techniques together with a spirometer can measure lung volumes and airflow, providing useful information in graphic form (Figs. 8.3 and 8.4).

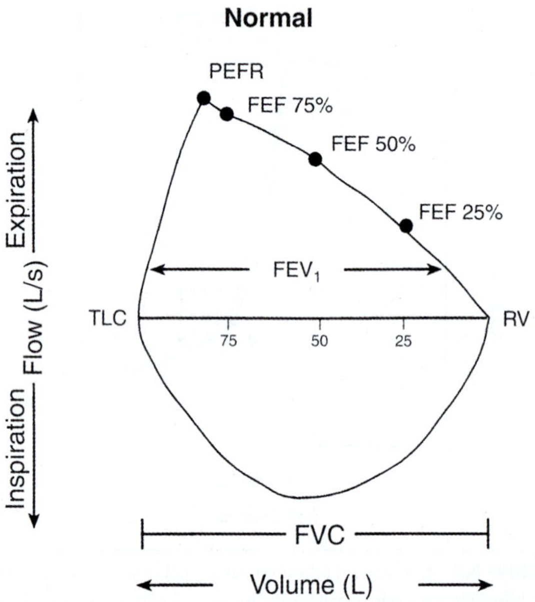

FIGURE 8.3 Volume versus time curve resulting from a forced expiratory volume (FEV) maneuver. FVC, forced vital capacity; MMFR, maximal midexpiratory flow rate. (Reprinted from Alldredge BK, et al. *Koda-Kimble and Young's Applied Therapeutics: The Clinical Use of Drugs*. 10th ed. Philadelphia, PA: Lippincott Williams & Wilkins; 2012.)

The forced expiratory volume (FEV) measures the amount of air the patient can exhale after a maximal inhalation, often over a set period such as 1 second (FEV_1). Together with the forced vital capacity (FVC), which measures the maximum volume of air exhaled with maximally forced effort after a maximal inhalation effort, these values can provide important performance measures of the lung. The peak expiratory flow rate (PEFR) measures the maximal flow that can be produced during the forced expiration. Generally, this measurement provides similar information as the FEV_1 but is less reproducible. Portable peak flow meters are in common use by patients with reactive airway disease to assist patients and medical providers in following variations in airway tone throughout the day. Another measurement

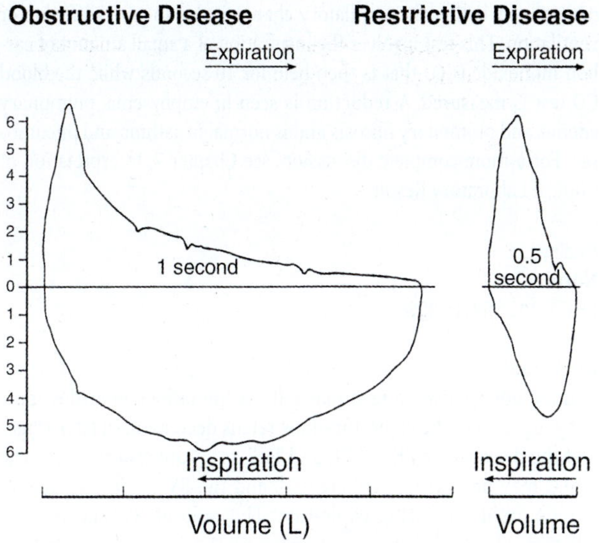

FIGURE 8.4 A normal flow/volume curve resulting from a forced expiratory maneuver. FEF, forced expiratory flow; FEV, forced expiratory volume; FVC, forced vital capacity; PEFR, peak expiratory flow rate; RV, residual volume; TLC, total lung capacity. (Adapted from Young LY, Koda-Kimble MA. *Applied Therapeutics: The Clinical Use of Drugs*. 6th ed. Vancouver, WA: Applied Therapeutics, Inc.; 1995, with permission.)

is the forced expiratory flow, which occurs during the middle 50% of the expiratory curve ($FEF_{25\%-75\%}$, $FEF_{50\%}$, or maximal midexpiratory flow rate [MEFR]). This measure is helpful for patients with emphysema, because it represents the elastic recoil force of the lung and is less dependent on the patient's expiratory effort.

Spirometry can also be used to establish the reversibility of airway disease. The use of bronchodilators can be administered after baseline pulmonary function tests to determine the degree of reversibility. Generally, a significant clinical reversibility is defined as a 15% to 20% improvement in the FEV_1 after administration of the bronchodilator.

Arterial blood gases ($PaCO_2$, pH, PaO_2) are often measured at the same time as spirometry to assess the degree of blood oxygenation. The use of the carbon monoxide diffusing capacity (D_{co}) can help determine whether the ventilatory change is due to poor diffusion or ventilation. This test involves the inspiration of a small amount of carbon monoxide (CO) that is then held for 10 seconds while the blood CO test is measured. A reduction is seen in emphysema, pulmonary edema, and pulmonary fibrosis and is normal in asthma and pneumonia. For a more complete discussion, see Chapter 7, Interpretation of Clinical Laboratory Results.

Findings

Normal

FEV_1/FVC, 75% to 80%

Abnormal

- In the obstructive pattern that reflects limitations to airflow during expiration, the expiratory flow rate is decreased. In later stages of the disease, the FEV_1/FVC and $FEF_{25\%-75\%}$, are also reduced. The TLC may be normal or increased, and the RV is elevated due to trapping of air during expiration. The ratio of RV/TLC is often increased.
- A restrictive pattern of lung disease that closely corresponds to impairment in inhalation (e.g., bronchitis, asthma) will present as a decrease in lung volumes, primarily TLC and VC.

Clinical Implications

- Bronchodilators should be administered before the procedure to evaluate the degree of reversibility.
- No preparation is needed before or after the procedure, unless bronchodilators are used.

Pulse Oximetry[7]

Purpose and Description

Pulse oximetry is used to measure the level of arterial oxygenation at rest, during exercise, when undergoing a surgical procedure, during bronchoscopy, when providing ventilator support, and when evaluating the need for and flow rate of supplemental oxygen therapy.

A spectrophotometric sensor is placed (clipped) on the fingernail, toenail, or earlobe. Light at two different wavelengths is passed through the pulsing capillary bed. The light sensed on the other side of the site is proportional to the amount of oxyhemoglobin present in the arterial capillary bed relative to the amount of hemoglobin available for binding with oxygen. The test may not be as sensitive as arterial blood gas because it does not take into consideration total hemoglobin, carboxyhemoglobin, or methemoglobin. Consequently, pulse oximetry may overestimate the oxygen content of the blood. Advantages of the test include noninvasiveness, portability, and an immediate result.

Findings

Normal

Oxyhemoglobin saturation ≥ 95%

Abnormal

Oxyhemoglobin saturation < 93%. Lower values may be acceptable in patients with chronic obstructive pulmonary disease.

Clinical Implications

- Poor circulation to the tested area will produce an inaccurate result.
- Skin pigmentation can also affect the measurement.

Sweat Test (Quantitative Pilocarpine Iontophoresis Test)[33,34]

Purpose and Description

The sweat test is used to diagnose cystic fibrosis (CF) in conjunction with one or more other symptoms (i.e., pancreatic exocrine deficiency, chronic pulmonary disease, MI, or a positive family history). This test evaluates the concentration of chloride in the patient's sweat, which can be elevated in a number of other disorders. A positive result should be repeated on a different day for confirmation.

Pilocarpine solution is applied topically to the forearm. Iontophoresis causes the pilocarpine to penetrate into the skin, thus stimulating the sweat glands. Sweat is collected with gauze, filter paper, or Macroduct coils and then analyzed for chloride content. A minimum of 75 mg (or 15 μL) of sweat must be collected for an accurate result.

Findings

Normal

Chloride <40 mEq/L in patients older than 3 months, <30 mEq/L in patients <3 months

Abnormal

Chloride >60 mEq/L is diagnostic for CF. Chloride >40 mEq/L is suggestive of CF in patients <3 months old.

Clinical Implications

None

Thoracentesis[9,35]

Purpose and Description

Thoracentesis can be performed for diagnostic purposes (50- to 100-mL sample) or for therapeutic purposes (1,000- to 1,500-mL sample). For diagnosis, thoracentesis is performed to determine the cause of a pleural effusion (abnormal fluid around the lungs).

The patient should be seated and leaning forward, with arms crossed in front and resting on an object such as a bedside table or back of a chair. If unable to sit and lean, the patient may lay supine in bed with the affected side elevated. The site of aspiration is usually 2 in. Below the highest point of dullness, as determined by chest percussion. The skin is prepared with an antiseptic, and then a local anesthetic is applied. A long thoracentesis needle with syringe attached is inserted. The appropriate amount of fluid is removed, as described above, and sent for analysis.

Findings

Normal

No pleural fluid

Abnormal

Malodorous fluid, milky appearance, blood, infectious organisms, cytology characteristic of malignancy

Clinical Implications

- Coagulation status should be assessed and corrected, if needed, prior to the procedure.
- Patients may require a sedative and/or an opiate analgesic before the procedure.

Ventilation-Perfusion Scintigraphy (V-Q Scan)[9,30]

Purpose and Description

The V-Q scan is used to diagnose and locate pulmonary emboli, detect the percentage of the lung that is still functioning normally, and assess the pulmonary vascular supply.

- *Ventilation* (*V*): The ventilation portion of the study demonstrates movement of lack of air in the lungs. The patient breathes in a small amount of radioactive gas (^{99m}Tc DTPA or xenon-133) without swallowing. Images of the first inspiration show regional ventilation in the major airway systems, and images over the following several minutes yield equilibrium information. The patient then breathes room air as a washout; poor ventilation is detected as focal areas of radioactive gas retention.
- *Perfusion* (*Q*): The perfusion portion of the study evaluates blood flow to the lungs. Macroaggregated albumin (MAA) labeled with technetium is injected intravenously. These particles follow the vasculature to the heart and become lodged in the precapillary arterioles in the lungs. Imaging of the pulmonary vasculature follows, including at least six views.

Findings

Normal

Normal perfusion and normal ventilation

Abnormal

Normal areas of regional ventilation combined with abnormal segmental perfusion defects (ventilation–perfusion mismatch) indicate pulmonary embolus. Other abnormal patterns may indicate tumors, pneumonia, atelectasis, bronchitis, asthma, or other inflammatory conditions.

Clinical Implications

- Findings consistent with a diagnosis of pulmonary embolism will generally necessitate initiation of anticoagulants or fibrinolytic agents if no contraindications are present.

Urology

Cystometrography (CMG)[9,36]

Purpose and Description

A cystometrogram is performed to evaluate bladder function, identify abnormal voiding patterns, and assess neuroanatomic connectivity between the brain, spinal cord, and bladder. After the patient voids, a double-lumen catheter is placed into the bladder. Adhesive electrodes are attached on each side of the anus. RV of urine is measured and then the catheter is connected to the cystometer. The cystometer measures the bladder capacity and pressure. Gradually, the bladder is filled with sterile saline, sterile water, or carbon dioxide gas while pressure readings are taken at specified increments. The patient provides observations about temperature sensation, bladder fullness, and bladder urges. When the bladder is completely empty, the catheter and electrodes are removed. The entire study above is repeated 20 to 30 minutes after injection of an anticholinergic or cholinergic drug to evaluate the bladder's response.

Findings

Normal

Bladder wall activity demonstrates appropriate motor and sensory function with a normal bladder filling pattern.

Abnormal

Motor or sensory defects, altered pressures or bladder capacity

Clinical Implications

- Sedation is not administered prior to the procedure because the patient must be alert to provide sensory information.
- Drugs that affect bladder function may affect the outcomes of the test.

Cystoscopy and Cystourethroscopy[9,36]

Purpose and Description

This procedure is used to diagnose and treat lower urinary tract disorders. General anesthesia is required for children; however, adults may undergo this procedure in a clinic if they are healthy enough. An antiseptic is applied to the external genitalia and then a local anesthetic jelly is instilled into the urethra at least 5 to 10 minutes before introducing the cystoscope. The cystoscope is a tubular, lighted, telescopic lens instrument that permits visualization of the interior bladder, urethra, prostatic urethra, and ureteral orifices. Fluid is infused into the bladder through the scope for the duration of the procedure to both distend the bladder and provide clearer images.

Findings

Normal

Normal anatomy; absence of strictures, stones, and tumors

Abnormal

Presence of stones, obstruction, stricture, tumors, signs of inflammation and infection, and sites of bleeding

Clinical Implications

- When general anesthesia is not used, benzodiazepines and/or narcotics may be administered to achieve conscious sedation.
- Prophylactic antibiotics may be given before or after the procedure.
- Rectal opium suppositories may be administered after the procedure.

Intravenous Pyelography or Urography (IVP or IVU)[9,36]

Purpose and Description

IVP is used to visualize urinary tract lesions in patients with suspected renal disease or urinary tract dysfunction. A contrast agent is injected intravenously and concentrates in the urine. A series of radiographs are taken at prespecified increments over 20 to 30 minutes. After the bladder is emptied, a last radiograph is taken.

Findings

Normal

No anatomic defects, obstructions, or masses, and a functional collecting system

Abnormal

Presence of obstruction, masses, stones, signs of trauma to the kidney, or compromised function of the collecting system. A time delay in contrast visualization indicates renal dysfunction.

Clinical Implications

- Feces, intestinal gas, or retained barium can obscure images. Perform this test prior to barium procedures if possible. The patient should take a laxative the evening before the procedure and may receive an enema the morning of the test.
- A serum creatinine may be required for older patients before the procedure to rule out renal insufficiency (due to relative dehydration and use of intravenous contrast).

- The patient must be NPO (food, liquid, and medication) for 12 hours before the procedure.
- Iodinated contrast concerns: Assess the patient for iodine allergy and previous reaction to contrast. Metformin should be held for 48 hours following contrast administration.
- Radiographs expose the patient to radiation, avoid unnecessary studies. Staff and patients should be protected from radiation as much as the procedure allows. Pregnant women, and those possibly pregnant, should avoid radiographs of the trunk or pelvis unless absolutely necessary.

Kidneys, Ureters, Bladder

See Gastroenterology, Abdominal Radiograph (KUB)

Retrograde Pyelography[9,36]

Purpose and Description

Retrograde pyelography allows visualization of the collecting structures of the kidney (renal pelvis) and ureters, which together compose the upper urinary tract. It is used to confirm IVP findings and when IVP provides insufficient results. A ureter is catheterized by means of a cystoscope (See "Cystoscopy and Cystourethroscopy"), and a contrast agent is injected in a retrograde direction (opposite the normal flow of urine). A radiograph is taken to visualize the ureters.

Findings

Normal

Normal anatomy of the ureters and kidney pelvis

Abnormal

Intrinsic disease of ureters and kidney pelvis. Diseases of the ureters including obstructive tumors or stones.

Clinical Implications

- Residual barium from other procedures may interfere with results. Perform this test prior to barium procedures if possible.
- See Cystoscopy and Cystourethroscopy

Voiding Cystourethrography[9,36]

Purpose and Description

The voiding cystourethrogram provides information about bladder position, urethral mobility, stress incontinence, and postvoid residual. Contrast medium is instilled into the bladder via a catheter until the bladder is filled. Radiographs of the full bladder are taken in several different positions. The catheter is removed, and more radiographs are taken during voiding.

Findings

Normal

Appropriate bladder and urethra structure and function

Abnormal

Urethral strictures and diverticula, ureteroceles, prostatic enlargement, vesicoureteral reflux, or neurogenic bladder

Clinical Implications

- Radiographs expose the patient to radiation, avoid unnecessary studies. Staff and patients should be protected from radiation as much as the procedure allows. Pregnant women, and those possibly pregnant, should avoid radiographs of the trunk or pelvis unless absolutely necessary.

Vascular

Arteriography/Venography[9,10]

Purpose and Description

In order to examine and evaluate the flow into or out of the arterial or venous system, an iodine contrast dye is injected into an artery (arteriogram) or a vein (venogram) by means of a needle or catheter to outline and view a portion of the arterial or venous system. The arteries or veins are then observed using fluoroscopy and x-ray studies. This allows for the detection of lesions and abnormalities of flow. It can also allow for surgical correction if possible. Fluoroscopy is used to guide the catheter to the desired location for dye administration.

Findings

Normal

No flow abnormalities

Abnormal

Presence of clots, strictures, obstructions, lesions, incompetent valves, aneurysms, embolism, thrombosis, fistulas, atherosclerosis, trauma, vasculitis, or congenital abnormalities

Clinical Implications

- Iodine contrast dye may produce hypersensitivity reactions or anaphylaxis. Special precautions should be taken in patients with known hypersensitivities to iodine compounds. When necessary, diphenhydramine, ranitidine, and prednisone may be started ≥12 hours before the procedure to prevent or reduce the severity of the hypersensitivity reaction.
- A local anesthetic is used to anesthetize the area of the puncture site.
- Adequate IV hydration should be provided to reduce the risk of renal injury from the contrast media.

Doppler Studies[4,7,9–12,37,38]

Purpose and Description

Doppler Ultrasound

Doppler studies allow the detection of arterial or venous obstruction or thrombi using high-frequency sound waves to create a graphic recording of blood flow. They are also used to monitor patients who have had reconstructive or peripheral artery bypass surgery.

Duplex Doppler Ultrasound

The technique is the same as standard Doppler US. However, with the duplex method, the sound waves may be used to create an image that is recorded on x-ray film.

Colorflow Doppler Ultrasound

Colorflow Doppler enhances standard Doppler US by providing flow data from the studied vessel. Various colors displayed on a screen represent different velocities and direction of blood flow. Red signals indicate flow toward the transducer, and blue signals indicate blood flow away from the transducer.

Findings

Normal

No evidence of narrowing, flow is spontaneous and phasic with respiration (venous). Arterial blood pressure is normal and has a multiphasic signal with prominent systolic sound and one or more diastolic sounds. Signals should fluctuate with respiration, not heart beat. The ankle–arm pressure index (API), the ratio between ankle systolic pressure and brachial systolic pressure, is >1. Proximal thigh pressure is greater than arm pressure by 20 to 30 mm Hg. There is increased flow velocity with compression of vessels.

TABLE 8.8 Relationship of API and Disease Severity

API	Severity of Disease
1–0.7	Mild ischemia
0.75–0.5	Claudication
0.5–0.25	Pain at rest
0.25–0	Pregangrene

Abnormal

Evidence of arterial or venous occlusion or blood clots. API is <1 (see Table 8.8 for severity ranking). Arm pressure is changed. Diminished or absent blood flow velocity signal. Calcified and noncompressible vessels produce unreliable measurements.

Clinical Implications

None

Impedance Plethysmography (Occlusive Cuff)[10]

Purpose and Description

Impedance plethysmography is commonly used to detect thrombi that produce obstruction to venous outflow. The test is sensitive and specific for occlusive thrombosis of the popliteal, femoral, or iliac veins. Diagnostic accuracy nears 90%.

Plethysmography is a noninvasive test that detects blood volume changes in the leg. A pneumatic cuff is placed around the midthigh and inflated to occlude venous return. Occlusion is maintained for a minimum of 45 seconds, and the cuff is then rapidly deflated. Electrodes placed around the calf detect changes in electrical resistance (impedance) due to alteration in blood volume distal to the cuff. The impedance changes occurring during inflation and deflation of the cuff are recorded on an ECG paper strip. The changes in impedance during cuff inflation and deflation are compared against a discriminant line that separates the normal from the abnormal graph.

Findings

Normal

The graph for the patient will fall above the discriminant line (i.e., the test will be negative for proximal vein thrombi). However, false-negative results can occur in patients with extensive collateral circulation, which allows for adequate venous outflow, and in patients in whom proximal vein thrombosis is not occlusive.

Abnormal

The graph will fall below the discriminant line (i.e., positive for proximal vein thrombosis). False-positive results can occur when nonthrombotic occlusion (mechanical) is present and when arterial inflow disease limits the amount of venous filling, decreasing venous return.

Clinical Implications

None

Lymphangiography (Lymphography)[10]

Purpose and Description

Lymphangiography may be used for the following:

- Detecting obstruction, disease, or neoplasm in the lymphatic system
- Staging lymphoma
- Distinguishing between primary and secondary lymph edema
- Evaluating the need for surgical treatment
- Assessing the results of previous chemotherapy or radiation therapy

Lymphography is the radiographic examination of the lymphatic system after radioactive material is injected into a lymphatic vessel in each foot (alternately, the hand, mastoid area, or spermatic cord can be used). Fluoroscopy is used to monitor the spread of the contrast media through the lymphatic system of the legs, groin, and the back of the abdominal cavity. Radiographs are taken of the legs, pelvis, abdomen, and chest. Twenty-four hours later, additional radiographs are taken to compare and evaluate contrast distribution.

Findings

Normal

Homogeneous and complete filling of the lymphatic system with the radioactive contrast material on the initial films

Abnormal

Presence of enlarged, foamy-looking nodes indicates lymphoma. Filling defects or lack of opacification of vessels indicate metastatic involvement of nodes by neoplasm. The number of nodes, the unilateral versus bilateral location of the nodes, and the extent of extranodal involvement determine staging of neoplastic disease.

Clinical Implications

The patient should be evaluated for hypersensitivity to iodine or other contrast media.

Magnetic Resonance Angiography (MRA)[10]

Purpose and Description

MRA uses the same hardware technology as standard MRI (see Magnetic Resonance Imaging) to diagnose vascular abnormalities such as vascular malformations, aneurysms, vertebrovascular and carotid atherosclerosis, thrombosis, and evidence of peripheral vascular disease. Large magnets and radio waves are used to create an image of the vascular anatomy being investigated. This noninvasive test can produce information about the vascular system (head and neck, abdomen, chest, and peripheral) comparable to the information provided by standard angiography. Although MRA can generally be performed without the use of a contrast agent, gadolinium may need to be administered to increase the accuracy of the test. The patient must remain very still during MRA and is placed in a narrow tube to perform the test. Certain implanted metallic objects are absolute or relative contraindications for performing MRA.

Findings

Normal

Absence of atherosclerosis, aneurysm, AV malformation, or occlusive disease

Abnormal

Presence of vascular malformation, occlusive vascular disease, aneurysm, and atherosclerosis

Clinical Implications

Use of a sedating benzodiazepine such as midazolam, lorazepam, or diazepam may be required to keep the patient still and to manage claustrophobia. Patients receiving gadolinium should be monitored for hypersensitivity reactions.

References

1. Kline TS, ed. *Handbook of Fine Needle Aspiration Biopsy Cytology*. 2nd ed. New York: Churchill Livingstone; 1988:9–16.
2. Teplick SK, Haskin PK. Imaging modalities. In: Kline TS, ed. *Handbook of Fine Needle Aspiration Biopsy Cytology*. 2nd ed. New York: Churchill Livingstone; 1988:17–48.
3. Michaels D, ed. Procedures requiring the use of contrast media. In: *Diagnostic Procedures: The Patient and the Health Care Team*. New York: John Wiley and Sons; 1983:274–279.
4. Ford RD, ed. *Diagnostic Tests Handbook*. Springhouse, PA: Springhouse Corporation; 1987.
5. Taub WH. Relative strengths and limitations of diagnostic imaging studies. In: Straub WH, ed. *Manual of Diagnostic Imaging*. Boston, MA: Little, Brown and Company; 1989:13–15.
6. Grossman ZD, et al., eds. *The Clinicians Guide to Diagnostic Imaging Cost Effective Pathways*. 2nd ed. New York: Raven Press; 1987.
7. Golish JA, ed. *Diagnostic Procedures Handbook*. Hudson (Cleveland), OH: Lexi-Comp, Inc.; 1994. Available at www.healthgate.com/dph/html. Accessed February 27, 2000.
8. Hamilton HK, Cahill M, eds. *Diagnostics*. Springhouse, PA: Springhouse Corporation; 1986.
9. Fischbach F, Dunning MB. *A Manual of Laboratory and Diagnostic Tests*. 8th ed. Philadelphia, PA: Lippincott Williams & Wilkins; 2009.
10. Pfenninger JL, Fowler GC. *Pfenninger and Fowler's Procedures for Primary Care*. 3rd ed. Philadelphia, PA: Elsevier; 2011.
11. Adam.com. *Encyclopedia*. Available at www.adam.com/dir/Tests/Tests.htm. Accessed March 6, 2000.
12. Zaret BL, ed. *The Yale University School of Medicine Patient's Guide to Medical Tests*. Boston, MA: Houghton Mifflin; 1997. Available at health.excite.com/yale_books_a_to_z/asset/yale_books_a_to_z/a_to_z/A. Accessed March 6, 2000.
13. Conover MB. *Understanding Electrocardiography*. 3rd ed. St. Louis, MO: Mosby; 1980.
14. Zipe DP, Libby P, Bonow RO, et al., eds. *Branunwald's Heart Disease: A Textbook of Cardiovascular Medicine*. 7th ed. Philadelphia, PA: Elsevier Saunders; 2005:153–186.
15. Shors S, Cotts WG, Pavlovic-Surjancev B, et al. Non-invasive cardiac evaluation in heart failure patients using magnetic resonance imaging: a feasibility study. *Heart Fail Rev*. 2005;10(4):265–273.
16. Myerson SG, Bellenger NG, Pennell DJ. Assessment of left ventricular mass by cardiovascular magnetic resonance. *Hypertension*. 2002;39:750–755.

17. Gardner DG, Shoback S. *Greenspan's Basic and Clinical Endocrinology*. 9th ed. New York: The McGraw-Hill Companies; 2011.
18. Wendland EM, Torloni MR, Falavigna M, et al. Gestational diabetes and pregnancy outcomes—a systematic review of the World Health Organization (WHO) and the International Association of Diabetes in Pregnancy Study Groups (IADPSG) diagnostic criteria. *BMC Pregnancy Childbirth*. 2012; 12:23.
19. Yamada T. *Textbook of Gastroenterology*. 5th ed. West Sussex, UK: Wiley-Blackwell; 2009.
20. Rock JA, Jones HW III. *TeLinde's Operative Gynecology*. 10th ed. Philadelphia, PA: Lippincott Williams & Wilkins; 2008.
21. Hoffman R, Benz EJ, Shattil SJ, et al. *Hematology: Basic Principles and Practice*. 5th ed. Philadelphia, PA: Churchill Livingstone Elsevier; 2009.
22. Mandell GL, Bennett JE, Dolin R. *Mandell, Douglas, and Bennett's Principles and Practice of Infectious Diseases*. 7th ed. Philadelphia, PA: Churchill Livingstone Elsevier; 2010.
23. Brenner BM, et al. *Brenner and Rector's The Kidney*. 9th ed. Philadelphia, PA: Elsevier; 2011.
24. Daroff RB, et al. *Bradley's Neurology in Clinical Practice*. 6th ed. Philadelphia, PA: Elsevier; 2012.
25. Rotschafer JC, Humphrey ZZ, Steinberg I. Central nervous system infection. In: Dipiro JT, et al., eds. *Pharmacotherapy: A Pathophysiologic Approach*. New York: Elsevier Science Publishing Co.; 1989:1074–1088.
26. Bickley LS. *Bates' Guide to Physical Examination and History Taking*. 11th ed. Philadelphia, PA: Elsevier; 2012.
27. Mercier LR. *Practical Orthopedics*. 6th ed. Philadelphia, PA: Mosby Elsevier; 2008.
28. Flint PW, Haughey BH, Lund VJ, et al. *Cummings Otolaryngology Head and Neck Surgery*. 5th ed. Philadelphia, PA: Mosby Elsevier; 2010.
29. Barash PG, Cullen BF, Stoelting RK, et al. *Clinical Anesthesia*. 6th ed. Philadelphia, PA: Lippincott Williams & Wilkins; 2009.
30. Fishman AP, Elias JA, Fishman JA, et al. *Fishman's Pulmonary Diseases and Disorders*. 4th ed. New York: The McGraw-Hill Companies; 2008.
31. Menendez R, Kelly HW. Pulmonary-function testing in the evaluation of bronchodilator agents. *Clin Pharm*. 1983;2:120–128.
32. Kelly HW. Asthma. In: Koda-Kimble MA, Young LY, eds. *Applied Therapeutics: The Clinical Use of Drugs*. 5th ed. Vancouver, BC: Applied Therapeutics; 1992;15:1–4.
33. McMillan JA. *Oski's Pediatrics*. 4th ed. Philadelphia, PA: Lippincott Williams & Wilkins; 2006.
34. Williamson MA, Snyder LM. *Wallach's Interpretation of Diagnostic Tests*. 9th ed. Philadelphia, PA: Lippincott Williams & Wilkins; 2011.

35. Shields TW, LoCicero J, Reed CE, et al. *General Thoracic Surgery*. 7th ed. Philadelphia, PA: Lippincott Williams & Wilkins; 2009.
36. Tanagho EA, McAninch JW. *Smith's General Urology*. 17th ed. New York: The McGraw-Hill Companies; 2008.
37. Berkow R, ed. The Merck Manual of Diagnosis and Therapy. 14th ed. Rahway, NJ: Merck Sharp & Dohme Research Laboratories; 1982.
38. Bastarche MM, et al. Assessing peripheral vascular disease: noninvasive testing. *Am J Nurs.* 1983;85:1552–1556.

9

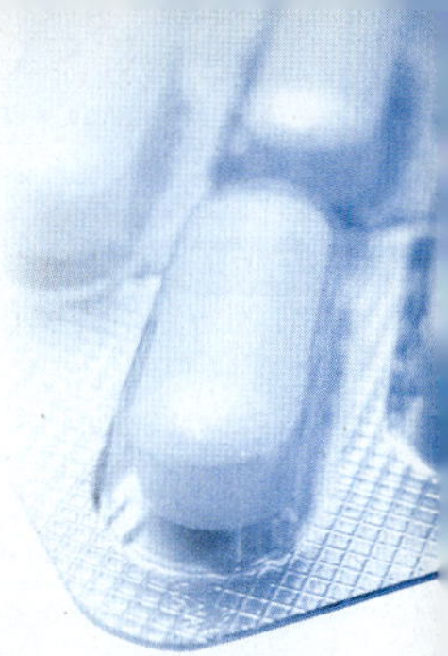

Drug Administration

Susan M. Stein and Breanne Chipman

Advances in technology continually provide a greater variety for administration of drugs. New delivery systems can expand therapeutic indications or decrease adverse effects. This chapter presents various routes of drug administration and provides a selection process to determine the most appropriate drug/dosage formulation and route.

Common routes of drug administration are oral and parenteral. Topical, inhalation, and rectal administration routes are used less often. Site-specific routes also exist, such as ophthalmic and otic administration. Drug characteristics often dictate the dosage form and route available. For example, a drug will initially be available parenterally to avoid complications involving metabolism or may only be available orally as a tablet due to solubility complications.

Patient Assessment

When determining an appropriate route of administration, assessing the patient's clinical health status provides valuable information. The seriousness of the condition being treated can assist in selection of the most effective route of administration. Examples of patient conditions and recommended administration routes are described in Table 9.1.

Routes of Administration

When selecting an appropriate route of administration, available forms of the desired drug should be reviewed. Various references may be used, including Drug Facts and Comparisons, Lexi-Comp, Micromedex, and American Hospital Formulary Service (AHFS). In

TABLE 9.1 Examples of Recommended Routes of Administration for Various Patient Conditions

Patient Status	Recommended Route
Oral intake	Oral, topical
Nothing by mouth (NPO)	Parenteral, enteral, rectal, topical
Critical condition	Parenteral
Chronic condition	Oral, inhalation, rectal, topical
Severe hypokalemia (potassium level <3 mEq/L)	Parenteral
Nausea, vomiting	Parenteral, rectal

addition, a commercially unavailable formulation may be prepared. A literature review is useful to locate compounded drug formulations. Maintaining this information for future reference is advised. Issues relating to various dosage formulations are described in Table 9.2.

Other limitations should be considered when determining the most appropriate dosage form. Factors involving these choices are shown in Table 9.3.

Monitoring Parameters

Clinicians routinely monitor the patient's condition to evaluate the effectiveness of drug therapy (see Chapter 15, for a more detailed discussion). Parameters include signs of an infection (redness, warmth, fever) and the appearance of an allergic reaction to the medication (rash). Table 9.4 contains a sample of monitoring parameters that relate to routes of administration.

Oral and Inhaled Medications

Oral administration is often the most desired route of administration despite limitations. Additional considerations involving oral medications pertain to the ability to crush or divide a tablet to increase dosing flexibility. Due to continually changing formulations, it is vital to clarify this information for each manufacturer and formulation. Box 9.1 and Table 9.5 provide information regarding these issues.[1,2] Inhalation administration provides effective localized drug delivery for the treatment of pulmonary diseases and also achieves rapid systemic effects of anesthetic gases. Correct administration technique is necessary to achieve adequate drug delivery with this form of administration.

TABLE 9.2 Issues Relating to Various Dosage Formulations

Route	Dosage Form	Comments
Oral	Solid—capsule, tablet, powder packet, lozenge, troche, pastille	Limited dose selection
	Solution	Titratable dose
	Suspension	Titratable dose; shake well to resuspend
	Emulsion	Oil-in-water more palatable
Parenteral	Solution (drug source)	Fewer stability issues, sterility issues
	Lyophilized (drug source)	Reconstitution, diluent, stability issues, sterility issues
	Dispersion (liposomal)	Limited availability, sterility issues
Topical	Bulk—cream, lotion, ointment, emulsion, gel, powder	Compounding flexibility
	Transdermal	Controlled release, adhesive irritation
Inhalation	Metered-dose inhaler Dry-powder inhaler, nebulizer	Aerochamber improves delivery of the metered dose; extended stability
Rectal/vaginal	Suppositories	Good absorption, compounding flexibility, temperature dependent
	Cream	Applicator for administration
Ophthalmic	Solution	Sterility issues
	Suspension	Shake well to resuspend, sterility issues
	Ointment	Difficult to apply
Otic	Solution	Sterility issues
	Suspension	Shake well to resuspend, sterility issues

Parenteral Administration

Parenteral delivery of medications is a common form of drug administration in hospitals, long-term care facilities, and the patient's home. Solutions delivered vascularly replenish fluid requirements, deliver medications, and supplement nutritional needs. Direct access, whether by bloodstream, spinal fluid, or peritoneal fluid, eliminates one of the human body's primary defense mechanisms. Therefore, sterility is of utmost importance when dealing with parenteral administration.

Medications intended for parenteral administration are most often delivered via subcutaneous (SC or SQ), intramuscular (IM), or

(Text continued on page 347)

TABLE 9.3 Comparison of Advantages and Disadvantages of Various Dosage Formulations

Route	Advantages	Disadvantages
Oral	Functional gastrointestinal tract maintained Ease of administration Less expensive	Slower to effect First-pass metabolism Bioavailability issues
Parenteral	Rapid time to effect No bioavailability issues Ability to titrate the dose	Expensive preparation Expensive administration Sterility and stability issues Compatibility issues Safety issues (related to administration) Painful administration
Topical	Localized effect Little systemic absorption Few adverse reactions Controlled absorption (transdermal) No first-pass metabolism	Inaccurate dosing Irritation at the application site Response altered with physiologic changes (blood pressure, fever) Drug diversion (transdermal) Increased absorption (elderly patients, exposed skin) May stain clothing
Inhalation	Localized drug delivery Fewer bioavailability issues Combination drugs Decreased systemic side effects	Correct technique for adequate dosing Inspiratory flow necessary to administer Variable drug deposition and absorption based on inspiration
Rectal/vaginal	Well absorbed No first-pass metabolism Generally inexpensive	Socially unacceptable Limited availability May stain clothing Indication/route potentially unrelated
Ophthalmic	Localized effect Little systemic absorption	Difficult self-administration Contamination possible
Otic	Localized effect Little systemic absorption	Difficult self-administration

TABLE 9.4 Examples of Monitoring Parameters Pertaining to Major Routes of Administration

Route	Monitoring Parameters	Examples
Oral	Nausea, pain relief, respiratory rate	Acetaminophen with codeine
Parenteral	Redness at the site, line infiltration	Azithromycin infusion
Topical	Skin irritation, blood pressure	Clonidine transdermal patch

BOX 9.1 Types of Medications That Should Not Be Divided or Crushed

Extended release or enteric coated tablets: examples long-acting (LA), sustained-release (SR), controlled-release (CR), extended-release (XL or XR), sustained action (SA), time delay (TD), time release (TR).

Sublingual tablets

Buccal tablets

Sources: McPherson ML. Don't crush that tablet! Am Pharm. 1994;NS34: 57–58 and Mitchell JF. Oral Dosage Forms That Should Not Be Crushed. 2013. Retrieved from http://www.ismp.org/tools/DoNotCrush.pdf on October 14, 2013.

TABLE 9.5 Oral Dosage Forms That Should Not Be Crushed

Drug Product	Active Ingredient(s)[a]	Dosage Form(s)	Reasons/Comments[b]
AcipHex	**RABE**prazole	Tablet	Extended release
Actiq	fenta**NYL**	Lozenge	Slow release **Note**: This lollipop delivery system requires the patient to slowly dissolve in mouth
Actonel	risedronate	Tablet	Irritant **Note**: Chewed, crushed, or sucked tablets may cause oropharyngeal irritation
Adalat CC	**NIFE**dipine	Tablet	Extended release
Adderall XR	amphetamine salts	Capsule	Extended release[c]
AeroHist Plus	combination	Tablet	Slow release[d]
Afeditab CR	**NIFE**dipine	Tablet	Extended release
Afinitor	everolimus	Tablet	Mucous membrane irritant
Aggrenox	combination	Capsule	Extended release

(continued)

TABLE 9.5 Oral Dosage Forms That Should Not Be Crushed *(continued)*

Drug Product	Active Ingredient(s)[a]	Dosage Form(s)	Reasons/Comments[b]
Alavert allergy (sinus 12 hour)	combination	Tablet	Extended release
Allegra-D	combination	Tablet	Extended release
ALPRAZolam ER	**ALPRAZ**olam	Tablet	Extended release
Altoprev	lovastatin	Tablet	Extended release
Ambien CR	zolpidem	Tablet	Extended release
Amibid DM	combination	Tablet	Extended release
Ampyra	dalfampridine	Tablet	Extended release **Note**: Formerly Fampridine-SR
Amrix	cyclobenzaprine	Capsule	Extended release
Aplenzin	bu**PROP**ion	Tablet	Extended release
Apriso	mesalamine	Capsule	Extended release[c] **Note**: Maintain pH at ≤6.0
Aptivus	tipranavir	Capsule	**Note**: Oil emulsion within spheres; taste
Aquatab C	combination	Tablet	Slow release[d]
Aquatab D	combination	Tablet	Slow release[e]
Aricept 23 mg	donepezil	Tablet	**Note**: Crushing the 25-mg tablet may significantly increase the rate of absorption; the 5-and 10-mg tablet are not affected
Arthrotec	diclofenac	Tablet	Delayed release; enteric coated
Asacol	mesalamine	Tablet	Slow release
Aspirin enteric coated	aspirin	Tablet, caplet	Delayed release; enteric coated
Atelvia	risedronate	Tablet	Extended release **Note**: Tablet coating is an important part of the delayed release
Azulfidine EN	sulfa**SALA**zine	Tablet	Delayed release
Augmentin XR	combination	Tablet	Extended release[d,e]

TABLE 9.5 Oral Dosage Forms That Should Not Be Crushed *(continued)*

Drug Product	Active Ingredient(s)[a]	Dosage Form(s)	Reasons/Comments[b]
AVINza	morphine	Capsule	Enteric coated (not pudding)[c]
Avodart	dutasteride	Capsule	**Note**: The drug may cause fetal abnormalities; women who are, or may become, pregnant should not handle capsules; all women should use caution in handling capsules, especially leaking capsules
Bayer Regular	aspirin	Caplet	Enteric coated
Biaxin-XL	clarithromycin	Tablet	Extended release
Bidex A	combination	Tablet	Extended release
Bidhist-D	combination	Tablet	Extended release
Biltricide	praziquantel	Tablet	Taste[d]
Biohist LA	combination	Tablet	Extended release[d]
Bisa-Lax	combination	Tablet	Enteric coated[f]
Bisac-Evac	bisacodyl	Tablet	Enteric coated[f]
Bisacodyl	combination	Tablet	Enteric coated[f]
Boniva	ibandronate	Tablet	**Note**: Chewed, crushed, or sucked tablets may cause oropharyngeal irritation
Bromfed PD	combination	Capsule	Extended release[e]
Budeprion SR	combination	Tablet	Extended release
Calan SR	verapamil	Tablet	Extended release[d]
Carbatrol	car**BAM**azepine	Capsule	Extended release[c]
Cardene SR	ni**CAR**dipine	Capsule	Extended release
Cardizem	diltiazem	Tablet	**Note**: Although not in the PI, the drug has a coating that is intended to release the drug over ~3 hours

(continued)

TABLE 9.5 Oral Dosage Forms That Should Not Be Crushed *(continued)*

Drug Product	Active Ingredient(s)[a]	Dosage Form(s)	Reasons/Comments[b]
Cardizem CD	diltiazem	Capsule	Extended release
Cardizem LA	diltiazem	Tablet	Extended release
Cardura XL	doxazosin	Tablet	Extended release
Cartia XT	diltiazem	Capsule	Extended release
Cefaclor ER	combination	Tablet	Extended-release
Ceftin	cefuroxime	Tablet	Taste[e] **Note**: Use suspension for children
Cefuroxime	combination	Tablet	Taste[e] **Note**: Use suspension for children
CellCept	mycophenolate	Capsule, Tablet	Teratogenic potential[g]
Charcoal Plus	charcoal, activated	Tablet	Enteric coated
Chlor-Trimeton	combination	Tablet	Extended release[e]
Cipro XR	ciprofloxacin	Tablet	Extended release[e]
Claritin-D	combination	Tablet	Extended release[e]
Claritin-D 24 Hour	combination	Tablet	Extended-release
Colace	docusate	Capsule	Taste[e]
Colestid	colestipol	Tablet	Slow release
Concerta	methylphenidate	Tablet	Extended release
Commit	Nicotine	Lozenge	**Note**: Integrity compromised by chewing or crushing
Coreg CR	carvedilol	Capsule	Extended release[c] **Note**: May add contents of the capsule to chilled, *not warm*, applesauce and consume immediately
Cotazym-S	pancrelipase	Capsule	Enteric coated[c]
Creon	pancrelipase	Capsule	Extended release[c]

TABLE 9.5 Oral Dosage Forms That Should Not Be Crushed *(continued)*

Drug Product	Active Ingredient(s)[a]	Dosage Form(s)	Reasons/Comments[b]
Crixivan	indinavir	Capsule	Taste **Note**: The capsule may be opened and mixed with fruit puree (e.g., banana)
Cymbalta	**DUL**oxetine	Capsule	Extended release[c] **Note**: May add contents of the capsule to apple juice or applesauce but *not* chocolate
Cytoxan	cyclophosphamide	Tablet	**Note**: The drug may be crushed, but company recommends using injection
Cytovene	ganciclovir	Capsule	Skin irritant
Depakene	divalproex	Capsule	Slow release; mucous membrane irritant[e]
Depakote	divalproex	Tablet	Delayed release
Depakote ER	divalproex	Tablet	Extended release
Depakote Sprinkles	divalproex	Capsule	Extended release[c]
Detrol LA	tolterodine	Capsule	Extended release
Dexilant	dexlansoprazole	Capsule	Delayed release[c]
Diclegis	doxylamine / pyridoxine	Tablet	Delayed release
Dilacor XR	diltiazem	Capsule	Extended release
Dilatrate-SR	isosorbide	Capsule	Extended release
Dilt-CD	diltiazem	Capsule	Extended release
Diltia XT	diltiazem	Capsule	Extended release
Ditropan XL	oxybutynin	Tablet	Extended release
Divalproex ER	combination	Tablet	Extended release
Doxidan	bisacodyl	Tablet	Enteric coated[f]
Drisdol	ergocalciferol	Capsule	Liquid filled[h]

(continued)

TABLE 9.5 Oral Dosage Forms That Should Not Be Crushed *(continued)*

Drug Product	Active Ingredient(s)[a]	Dosage Form(s)	Reasons/Comments[b]
Droxia	hydroxyurea	Capsule	**Note**: Exposure to the powder may cause serious skin toxicities; health care workers should wear gloves to administer
Dulcolax	bisacodyl	Tablet; Capsule	Enteric coated[f]; liquid filled
DynaCirc CR	isradipine	Tablet	Extended release
EC-Naprosyn	combination	Tablet	Delayed release; enteric coated
Ecotrin (all)	aspirin	Tablet	Enteric coated
E.E.S. 400	erythromycin	Tablet	Enteric coated[e]
Effer-K	potassium bicarbonate	Tablet	Effervescent tablet[i]
Effervescent Potassium	—	Tablet	Effervescent tablet[i]
Effexor XR	venlafaxine	Capsule	Extended release
Embeda	morphine sulfate	Capsule	Extended release[c]; do *not* give via an NG tube
E-Mycin	erythromycin	Tablet	Enteric coated
Enablex	darifenacin	Tablet	Slow release
Entocort EC	budesonide	Capsule	Extended release; enteric coated[c]
Equetro	car**BAM**azepine	Capsule	Extended release[c]
Ergomar	ergotamine	Tablet	Sublingual form[j]
Erivedge	vismodegib	Capsule	**Note**: PI indicates potential teratogenic; MSDS warns against skin contact; health care workers should take appropriate cautions
Ery-Tab	erythromycin	Tablet	Delayed release; enteric coated
Erythromycin Stearate	—	Tablet	Enteric coated

TABLE 9.5 Oral Dosage Forms That Should Not Be Crushed *(continued)*

Drug Product	Active Ingredient(s)[a]	Dosage Form(s)	Reasons/Comments[b]
Erythromycin Base	—	Tablet	Enteric coated
Erythromycin Delayed Release	—	Capsule	Enteric-coated pellets[c]
Evista	raloxifene	Tablet	Taste; teratogenic potential[g]
Exalgo	**HYDRO**morphone	Tablet	Extended release **Note**: Breaking, chewing, crushing, dissolving before swallowing or injecting could result in overdose
Exjade	deferasirox	Tablet	**Note**: Do *not* give as tablet; tablets are meant to be given as a liquid; see company insert.
Extendryl (all)	combination	Capsule	Extended-release[e]
Feen-a-mint	bisacodyl	Tablet	Enteric coated[f]
Feldene	piroxicam	Capsule	Mucous membrane irritant
Fenta**NYL**	—	Lozenge	Slow release **Note**: This lollipop delivery system requires the patient to slowly dissolve in mouth
Fentora	fenta**NYL**	Tablet	**Note**: Buccal tablet; swallowing the tablet whole or crushing may reduce effectiveness
Feosol	ferrous sulfate	Tablet	Enteric coated[e]
Feratab	ferrous sulfate	Tablet	Enteric coated[e]
Fergon	ferrous gluconate	Tablet	Enteric coated
Fero-Grad 500 mg	combination	Tablet	Slow release
Ferro-Sequels	combination	Tablet	Slow release

(continued)

TABLE 9.5 Oral Dosage Forms That Should Not Be Crushed *(continued)*

Drug Product	Active Ingredient(s)[a]	Dosage Form(s)	Reasons/Comments[b]
Flagyl ER	metro**NIDAZOLE**	Tablet	Extended release.
Fleet Laxative	bisacodyl	Tablet	Enteric coated[f]
Flomax	tamsulosin	Capsule	Slow release
Focalin XR	dexmethylphenidate	Capsule	Extended release[c]
Fortamet	met**FORMIN**	Tablet	Extended release
Fosamax	alendronate	Tablet	Mucous membrane irritant
Gleevec	imatinib	Tablet	Taste[d] **Note**: May be dissolved in water or apple juice
Glucophage XR	met**FORMIN**	Tablet	Extended release
Glucotrol XL	glipi**ZIDE**	Tablet	Extended release
Glumetza	met**FORMIN**	Tablet	Extended release
Gralise	gabapentin	Tablet	Extended release
Guaifed	combination	Capsule	Extended release
Guaifed-PD	combination	Capsule	Extended release
Guai**FEN**esin/ Pseudoephedrine	—	Tablet	Extended release
Guaifenex DM	combination	Tablet	Extended release[d]
Guaifenex GP	combination	Tablet	Extended release
Guaifenex PSE	combination	Tablet	Extended release[d]
Guaimax-D	combination	Tablet	Extended release
Halfprin 81	aspirin	Tablet	Enteric coated
Horizant	gabapentin	Tablet	Extended release
Hista-Vent DA	combination	Tablet	Extended release[d]
Hydrea	hydroxyurea	Capsule	**Note**: Exposure to the powder may cause serious skin toxicities; health care workers should wear gloves to administer
Imdur	isosorbide	Tablet	Extended release[d]
Inderal LA	propranolol	Capsule	Extended release

TABLE 9.5 Oral Dosage Forms That Should Not Be Crushed *(continued)*

Drug Product	Active Ingredient(s)[a]	Dosage Form(s)	Reasons/Comments[b]
Indomethacin SR	indomethacin	Capsule	Extended release[c,e]
InnoPran XL	propranolol	Capsule	Extended release
Intelence	etravirine	Tablet	**Note**: The tablet should be swallowed whole and not crushed; the tablet may be dispersed in water
Intermezzo	zolpidem	Tablet (sublingual)	[j]
Intuniv	guan**FACINE**	Tablet	Extended release
Invega	paliperidone	Tablet	Extended release
Isoptin SR	verapamil	Tablet	Extended release[d]
Isordil Sublingual	isosorbide	Tablet (sublingual)	[j]
Isosorbide Dinitrate Sublingual	isosorbide	Tablet (sublingual)	[j]
Isosorbide SR	isosorbide	Tablet	Extended release
ISOtretinoin	**ISO**tretinoin	Capsule	Mucous membrane irritant
Jakafi	ruxolitinib	Tablet	**Note**: See PI for making a suspension
Jalyn	dutasteride/ tamsulosin	Capsule	**Note**: Women who are, or may become, pregnant should not handle crushed or broken tablets[g]
Janumet XR	sita**GLIP**tin/ met**FORMIN**	Tablet	Extended release
Kadian	morphine	Capsule	Extended release[c] **Note**: May add contents of the capsule to applesauce without crushing

(continued)

TABLE 9.5 Oral Dosage Forms That Should Not Be Crushed *(continued)*

Drug Product	Active Ingredient(s)[a]	Dosage Form(s)	Reasons/Comments[b]
Kaletra	lopinavir/ritoavir	Tablet	Film coated[e] **Note**: Active ingredients are surrounded by a wax matrix to prevent health care exposure; women who are, or may become, pregnant should not handle crushed or broken tablets
Kapidex	dexlansoprazole	Capsule	Delayed release[c]
Kapvay	clo**NID**ine	Tablet	Extended release
Kazano	alogliptin/ met**FORMIN**	Tablet	**Note**: Not scored; no studies available from the company
Keppra XR	lev**ETIRA**cetam	Tablet	Extended release[e]
Ketek	telithromycin	Tablet	Slow release[e]
Klor-Con	potassium	Tablet	Extended release[e]
Klor-Con M	potassium	Tablet	Extended release[d,e] **Note**: To make a liquid, place the tablet in 120 mL of water; disperse for 2 minutes; stir
Kombiglyze XR	combination	Tablet	Extended release **Note**: The tablet matrix may remain in stool
K-Dur	potassium	Tablet	Extended release **Note**: To make a liquid, break the tablet in half and disperse in 120 mL of water for 2 minutes; stir
K-Lyte	potassium	Tablet	Effervescent tablet[i]
K-Lyte CL	potassium	Tablet	Effervescent tablet[i]
K-Lyte DS	potassium	Tablet	Effervescent tablet[i]
K-Tab	potassium	Tablet	Extended release[e]
La**MIC**tal XR	lamo**TRI**gine	Tablet	Extended release

TABLE 9.5 Oral Dosage Forms That Should Not Be Crushed *(continued)*

Drug Product	Active Ingredient(s)[a]	Dosage Form(s)	Reasons/Comments[b]
Lescol XL	fluvastatin	Tablet	Extended release
Letairis	ambrisentan	Tablet	Slow release
Levbid	hyoscyamine	Tablet	Extended release[d]
Levsinex	hyoscyamine	Capsule	Extended release
Lialda	mesalamine	Tablet	Delayed release
Liquibid	combination	Tablet	Extended release[d]
Lithobid	lithium	Tablet	Extended release
Lodrane 24	brompheniramine	Capsule	Extended release
Lodrane 24D	combination	Capsule	Extended release
LoHist 12 Hour	brompheniramine	Tablet	Extended release
Lovaza	combination	Capsule	**Note**: The contents of capsule may erode walls of styrofoam or plastic materials
Luvox CR	fluvoxa**MINE**	Capsule	Extended release
Maxifed DM	combination	Tablet	Slow release[d]
Maxifed DMX	combination	Tablet	Slow release[d]
Maxiphen DM	combination	Tablet	Slow release[d]
Mestinon ER	pyridostigmine	Tablet	Extended release[e]
Metadate ER	methylphenidate	Tablet	Extended release
Metadate CD	methylphenidate	Capsule	Extended release[c]
Methylin ER	methylphenidate	Tablet	Extended release
Metoprolol ER	—	Tablet	Extended release
Micro K Extencaps	potassium chloride	Capsule	Extended release[c,e]
Mirapex ER	pramipexole	Tablet	Extended release
Moxatag	amoxicillin	Tablet	Extended release
Morphine sulfate extended release	—	Tablet	Extended release
Motrin	ibuprofen	Tablet	Taste[k]
MS Contin	morphine	Tablet	Extended release[e]
Mucinex	guia**FEN**esin	Tablet	Slow release

(continued)

TABLE 9.5 Oral Dosage Forms That Should Not Be Crushed *(continued)*

Drug Product	Active Ingredient(s)[a]	Dosage Form(s)	Reasons/Comments[b]
Mucinex DM	combination	Tablet	Slow release
Myfortic	mycophenolate	Tablet	Delayed release
Myrbetriq	mirabegron	Tablet	Extended release
Namenda XR	memantine	Capsule	Extended release[c]
Naprelan	naproxen	Tablet	Extended release
Nex**IUM**	esomeprazole	Capsule	Delayed release[c]
Niaspan	nicotinic acid	Tablet	Extended release
Nicotinic acid	—	Capsule; tablet	Slow release[d]
Nifediac CC	**NIFED**ipine	Tablet	Extended release
Nifediac XL	**NIFED**ipine	Tablet	Extended release
Nitrostat	nitroglycerin	Tablet	Sublingual route[f]
Norflex ER	orphenadrine	Tablet	Extended release
Norpace CR	disopyramide	Capsule	Extended-release form within a special capsule
Norvir	ritonavir	Tablet	**Note**: Crushing tablets has resulted in decreased bioavailability of the drug[e]
Nucynta ER	tapentadone	Tablet	Extended release **Note**: A toxic dose may occur if the tablet is split or crushed
Oleptro	tra**ZOD**one	Tablet	Extended release
Oracea	doxycycline	Capsule	Delayed release
Oramorph SR	morphine	Tablet	Extended release[e]
Orphenadrine citrate ER	—	Tablet	Extended release
Oxy**CONTIN**	oxy**CODONE**	Tablet	Extended release **Note**: Tablet disruption may cause a potentially fatal overdose of oxy**CODONE**

TABLE 9.5 Oral Dosage Forms That Should Not Be Crushed *(continued)*

Drug Product	Active Ingredient(s)[a]	Dosage Form(s)	Reasons/Comments[b]
Oxymorphone ER	—	Tablet	Extended release
Pancrease delayed release	pancrealipase	Capsule	Extended release
Pancrease MT	pancrealipase	Capsule	Enteric coated[c]
Pancrecarb	pancrealipase	Capsule	Enteric coated[c]
Pancrelipase	—	Capsule	Enteric coated[c]
Paxil CR	**PAR**oxetine	Tablet	Extended release
Pentasa	mesalamine	Capsule	Slow release
Pradaxa	dabigatran	Capsule	**Note**: Bioavailability increases by 75% when the pellets are taken without the capsule shell
Pre-Hist-D	combination	Tablet	Extended release[d]
Plendil	felodipide	Tablet	Extended release
Prevacid	lansoprazole	Capsule	Delayed release
Prevacid Solu Tab	lansoprazole	Tablet	**Note**: Orally disintegrating; do not swallow; dissolve in water only and dispense via a dosing syringe or NG tube
Prevacid Suspension	lansoprazole	Suspension	Slow release **Note**: Contains enteric-coated granules; mix with water only; not for NG use
Pri**LOSEC**	omeprazole	Capsule	Delayed release[c]
Pri**LOSEC** OTC	omeprazole	Tablet	Delayed release
Pristiq	desvenlafaxine	Tablet	Extended release
Procardia XL	**NIFED**ipine	Tablet	Extended release
Propecia	finasteride	Tablet	**Note**: Women who are, or may become, pregnant should not handle crushed or broken tablets

(continued)

TABLE 9.5 Oral Dosage Forms That Should Not Be Crushed *(continued)*

Drug Product	Active Ingredient(s)[a]	Dosage Form(s)	Reasons/Comments[b]
Proquin XR	ciprofloxacin	Tablet	Extended release
Proscar	finasteride	Tablet	**Note**: Women who are, or may become, pregnant should not handle crushed or broken tablets
Protonix	pantoprazole	Tablet	Slow release
PROzac Weekly	**FLU**oxetine	Tablet	Enteric coated
Qdall	combination	Capsule	Extended release
Qdall AR	combination	Capsule	Extended release
Ranexa	ranolazine	Tablet	Slow release
Rapamune	sirolimus	Tablet	**Note**: Pharmacokinetic NanoCrystal technology may be affected[e]
Rayos	predni**SONE**	Tablet	Delayed release **Note**: Release is dependent upon intact coating
Razadyne ER	galantamine	Capsule	Extended release
Renagel	sevelamer	Tablet	**Note**: The tablets expand in liquid if broken or crushed
Renvela	sevelamer carbonate	Tablet	**Note**: The tablets expand in liquid if broken or crushed[e]
Requip XL	r**OPINIR**ole	Tablet	Extended release
Rescon	combination	Tablet	Slow release[d]
Rescon JR	combination	Tablet	Slow release[d]
Rescon MX	combination	Tablet	Slow release[d]
Respahist	combination	Capsule	Extended release[c]
Respaire SR	combination	Capsule	Extended release
Revlimid	lenalidomide	Capsule	**Note**: Teratogenic potential; health care workers should avoid contact with capsule contents/body fluids

TABLE 9.5 Oral Dosage Forms That Should Not Be Crushed *(continued)*

Drug Product	Active Ingredient(s)[a]	Dosage Form(s)	Reasons/Comments[b]
Ritalin La	methylphenidate	Capsule	Extended release[c]
Ritalin SR	methylphenidate	Tablet	Extended release
R-Tanna	combination	Tablet	Slow release
Rythmol SR	propafenone	Capsule	Extended release
Ryzolt	tra**MAD**ol	Tablet	Extended release **Note**: Crushing may cause overdose
Sensipar	cinacalcet	Tablet	**Note**: The tablets are not scored, and cutting may cause variable dosage accuracy
SEROquel XR	**QUE**tiapine	Tablet	Extended release
Sinemet CR	levo/carbidopa	Tablet	Extended release[d]
Sinuvent PE	combination	Tablet	Extended release[d]
Slo-Niacin	nicotinic acid	Tablet	Slow release[d]
Solodyn	minocycline	Tablet	Extended release
Somnote	chloral hydrate	Capsule	Liquid filled
Sprycel	dasatinib	Tablet	Film coated **Note**: Active ingredients are surrounded by a wax matrix to prevent health care exposure; women who are, or may become, pregnant should not handle crushed or broken tablets
Strattera	atomoxetine	Capsule	**Note**: The capsule content can cause ocular irritation
Sudafed 12 hour	combination	Capsule	Extended release[e]
Sudafed 24 hour	combination	Tablet	Extended release[e]
Sular	nisoldipine	Tablet	Extended release
Symax Duotab	hyoscyamine	Tablets	Controlled release
Symax SR	hyoscyamine	Tablet	Extended release

(continued)

TABLE 9.5 Oral Dosage Forms That Should Not Be Crushed *(continued)*

Drug Product	Active Ingredient(s)[a]	Dosage Form(s)	Reasons/Comments[b]
Tasigna	nilotinib	Capsule	**Note**: Disruption of capsule may yield blood levels causing enhanced toxicity
Taztia XT	diltiazem	Capsule	Extended release
Tecfidera	dimethyl fumarate	Capsule	Delayed release
TEGretol-XR	car**BAM**azepine	Tablet	Extended release[e]
Temodar	temozolomide	Capsule	**Note**: Accidentally opened or damaged capsules require rigorous precautions to avoid inhalation or contact with the skin or mucous membranes[g]
Tessalon Perles	benzonatate	Capsule	**Note**: Swallow whole; local anesthesia of the oral mucosa; choking could occur
Theo-24	theophylline	Capsule	Extended release **Note**: Contains beads that dissolve throughout the GI tract
Theochron	theophylline	Tablet	Extended release
Tiazac	diltiazem	Capsule	Extended release[c]
Topamax	topiramate	Tablet; Capsule	Taste; taste[c]
Toprol XL	metoprolol	Tablet	Extended release[d]
Touro CC-LD	combination	Tablet	Extended release[d]
Touro LA-LD	combination	Tablet	Extended release[d]
Toviaz	fesoterodine	Tablet	Extended release
Tracleer	bosentan	Tablet	**Note**: Women who are, or may become, pregnant should not handle crushed or broken tablets
TRENtal	pentoxifylline	Tablet	Extended release

TABLE 9.5 Oral Dosage Forms That Should Not Be Crushed *(continued)*

Drug Product	Active Ingredient(s)[a]	Dosage Form(s)	Reasons/Comments[b]
Treximet	combination	Tablet	**Note**: Unique drug matrix enhances rapid drug absorption
Trilpix	fenofibric	Capsule	Extended release
Tylenol Arthritis	acetaminophen	Tablet	Controlled release
Uceris	budesonide	Tablet	**Note**: Coating on tablet is designed to break down at pH of 7.0 or above
Ultram ER	tra**MAD**ol	Tablet	Extended release **Note**: Tablet disruption may cause a potentially fatal overdose of drug
Ultrase	pancrealipase	Capsule	Enteric coated
Uniphyl	theophylline	Tablet	Slow release
Urocit-K	potassium citrate	Tablet	Wax coated; prevents upper GI release
Uroxatral	alfuzosin	Tablet	Extended release
Valcyte	val**GANC**iclovir	Tablet	Teratogenic and irritant potential[e,g]
Verapamil SR	—	Tablet	Extended release[d]
Verelan	verapamil	Capsule	Sustained release[c]
Verelan PM	verapamil	Capsule	Extended release[c]
Videx EC	didanosine	Capsule	Delayed release
Vimovo	naproxen/ esomeprazole	Tablet`	Delayed release
Viramune XR	nevirapine	Tablet	Extended release[e]
Voltaren XR	diclofenac	Tablet	Extended release
VoSpire ER	albuterol	Tablet	Extended release
Votrient	pazopanib	Tablet	**Note**: Crushing significantly increases the AUC and T_{max}; crushed or broken tablets may cause dangerous skin problems

(continued)

TABLE 9.5 Oral Dosage Forms That Should Not Be Crushed *(continued)*

Drug Product	Active Ingredient(s)[a]	Dosage Form(s)	Reasons/Comments[b]
Wellbutrin SR, XL	bu**PROP**ion	Tablet	Extended release
Xanax XR	**ALPRAZ**olam	Tablet	Extended release
Zegerid OTC	omeprazole/ $NaHCO_3$	Capsule	Delayed release[e]
Zenpep	pancrealipase	Capsule	Delayed release[c]
Zolinza	vorinostat	Capsule	**Note**: Irritant; avoid contact with the skin or mucous membranes; avoid contact with crushed or broken tablets
Zortress	everolimus	Tablet	**Note**: Crushed powder may cause dangerous effects to mucous membranes
Zyban	bu**PROP**ion	Tablet	Slow release
Zyflo CR	zileuton	Tablet	Extended release

Disclaimer: This listing is not meant to represent all products, either by a generic or trade name. The author encourages manufacturers, pharmacists, nurses, and other health professionals to notify him of any change or updates.

Correspondence regarding this list may be addressed to John F. Mitchell, PharmD, FASHP; Email: rxmitchell@att.net.

[a] The generic name is provided merely as a reference point and is only listed for single-ingredient medications; it should not be assumed that drugs with the same generic are equivalent to the specific brand name listed relative to crushing or chewing. If questions arise, please check with your pharmacist.

[b] Two official USP terms are used to designate the special-release medication form: "extended release" and "delayed release." Others such as "sustained release" and "controlled release" are commonly used on package labeling. The term "slow release" is being used here to signify all such drugs with a special-release mechanism.

[c] The capsule may be opened and the contents taken without crushing or chewing; soft food such as applesauce or pudding may facilitate administration; contents may generally be administered via a nasogastric tube using an appropriate fluid, provided entire contents are washed down the tube.

[d] The tablet is scored and may be broken in half without affecting release characteristics.

[e] Liquid dosage forms of the product are available; however, dose, frequency of administration, and manufactures may differ from those of the solid dosage form.

[f] Antacids and/or milk may prematurely dissolve the coating of the tablet.

[g] Skin contact may enhance tumor production; avoid direct contact.

[h] The capsule may be opened and the liquid contents removed for administration.

[i] Effervescent tablets must be dissolved in the amount of diluent recommended by the manufacturer.

[j] Tablets are made to disintegrate under the tongue.

[k] The taste of this product form would likely be unacceptable to the patient; administration via nasogastric tube should be acceptable.

Reprinted with permission from Dr. John Mitchell. *Oral Dosage Forms That Should Not Be Crushed.* http://www.ismp.org/tools/DoNotCrush.pdf

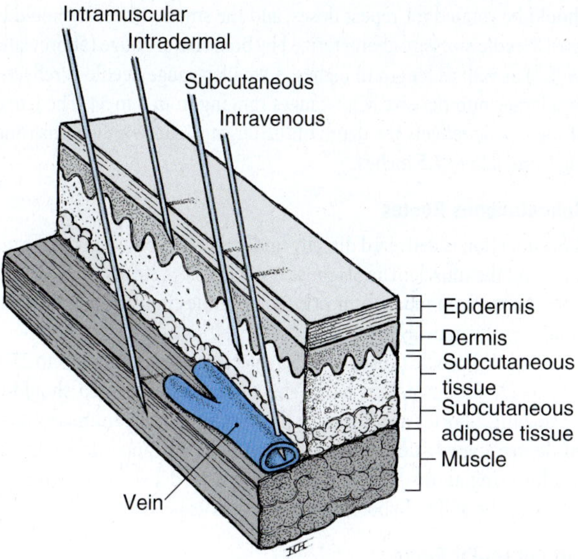

FIGURE 9.1 Diagram of various routes of drug administration.

intravenous (IV) route. Other less common methods of administration are also available. The following discussion describes these routes in more detail, and Figure 9.1 provides a visual display.

Not all parenteral drugs may be given by SQ, IM, and IV routes. Table 9.6 lists examples of route limitations.

When using the SQ or IM route of administration, it is important to alleviate patient discomfort when possible. The site of administration

TABLE 9.6 Examples of Drugs Restricted to Specific Routes of Administration

Drug	SQ	IM	IV
Insulin	Yes	Yes	Yes
Midazolam	No	Yes	Yes
Erythropoietin	Yes	No	Yes
Heparin	Yes	No	Yes
Bleomycin	Yes	Yes	Yes

should be rotated for repeat doses, and the smallest needle should be used. Needle sizes are characterized by bore size or gauge (abbreviated as "G") as well as length in inches. A smaller-gauge needle is reflected by a larger number size, with gauges ranging from 6 to 34. The length of the needle reflects the depth of the target tissue, with lengths ranging from 0.25 to 3.5 inches.

Subcutaneous Routes

A SQ injection is delivered directly under the skin, between the dermal layer and the muscle. The SQ route results in slow, steady drug absorption.[3] Absorption must occur prior to systemic circulation of the drug, which results in delayed effect.[4]

A shorter needle is used for a SQ injection. Generally, a 24- to 27-G, 5/8- to 1/2-inch needle is used. The volume administered should be <1 to 2 mL. Shorter needles allow the injection to be administered at a 90-degree angle.[3] Additionally, continuous SQ infusion is possible with insulin using an insulin pump. Insulin can be delivered at a constant rate with the ability to bolus prior to a meal as needed.[5]

Intramuscular Route

An IM injection delivered directly into the muscle produces rapid drug absorption. IM injections require a longer needle to access the muscle tissue. Again, patient comfort is of utmost importance. A typical needle used is 21 to 23 G, 1.5 inches.[6] The volume of medication is determined by the age of the patient and the muscle selected. Table 9.7 specifies these limitations.[7,8]

When administering an IM injection, the needle should enter the muscle at a 90-degree angle.[3,9] If the bone is contacted, the needle should be withdrawn a small distance. Another concern regarding IM administration involves the possibility of aspiration. This can be avoided by pulling the plunger of the syringe back slightly, piercing the tissue. If no blood is present, the needle is not in a vein and the medication may be administered. The typical rate of IM administration is approximately 1 mL every 10 seconds.[3]

A highly recommended method of IM administration is the Z-track method. Before injection, the skin is displaced downward approximately 1 to 2 cm. The injection is then given. After 10 seconds, the needle is removed and the skin is released. The skin movement allows the tissue to close over the site of entry after administration to decrease drug loss. This method decreases pain for the patient as well.[3]

TABLE 9.7 Volume Limitations of Intramuscular Administration

Muscle Group	Birth–1.5 Year (mL)	1.5–3 Year (mL)	3–6 Year (mL)	6–15 Year (mL)	Adult (mL)
Deltoid	Not recommended	Not recommended; if no other sites, 0.5	0.5	0.5	1
Gluteus maximus	Not recommended	Not recommended; if no other sites, 1	1.5	1.5–2	2–2.5
Ventrogluteal	Not recommended	Not recommended; if no other sites, 1	1.5	1.5–2	2–2.5
Vastus lateralis	0.5–1	1	1.5	1.5–2	2–2.5

Sources: Howry LV, Bindler RM, Tso Y. *Pediatric Medications*. Philadelphia, PA: JB Lippincott; 1981:62 and Losek JD, Gyuro J. Pediatric intramuscular injections: do you know the procedure and complications? *Pediatr Emerg Care*. 1992;8(2):79–81.

IV Administration

Administration of a medication directly into a vein is an IV infusion. Drug administered by rapid infusion will mix with the blood and reach a maximum concentration in 4 minutes.[4]

IV administration delivers the medication into the bloodstream through direct push, intermittent, or continuous infusion methods. Direct push, or bolus, administration is a very short infusion, lasting a few seconds to minutes, with the intent of producing a high drug concentration rapidly. The drug is concentrated and often removed from the vial immediately before administration. Intermittent infusions, or IV piggybacks, involve dilute drug solutions, which are given periodically throughout the day. These solutions may be infused over 30 to 120 minutes. Continuous infusion generally refers to large-volume (250 to 1,000 mL) solutions, with or without drug, running uninterrupted.[10] Table 9.8 shows examples of various IV delivery systems available.

Multiple factors influence the most suitable method of infusion for a particular medication. Table 9.9 presents some examples of each method of IV infusion.[11]

TABLE 9.8 Comparison of Intravenous Delivery Systems

Type	Diagram	Details	Comments
Large volume administration	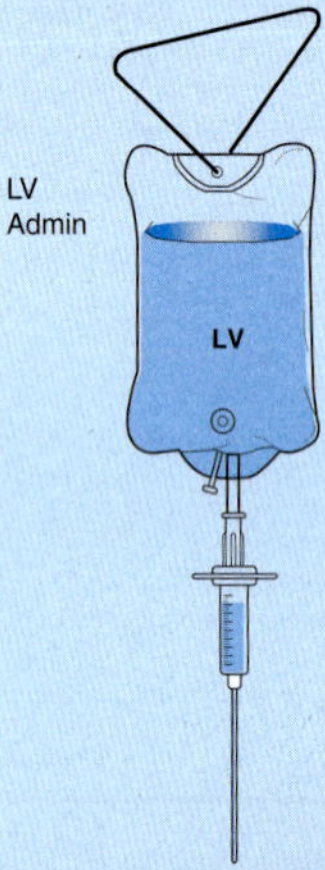	500–1,000 mL, gravity drip set or pump administration	Safest, drug not concentrated
Mini-infusion administration	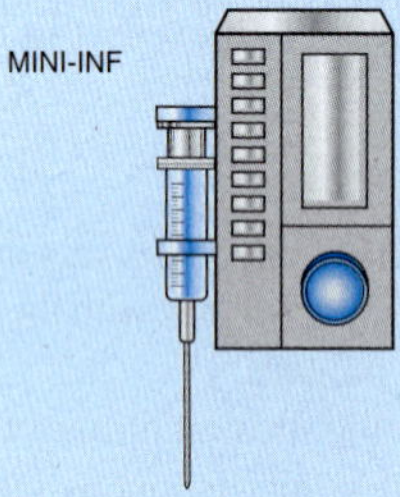	Prefilled syringe placed in pump, connects to the primary infusion line	Program pump for the rate of delivery
Piggyback	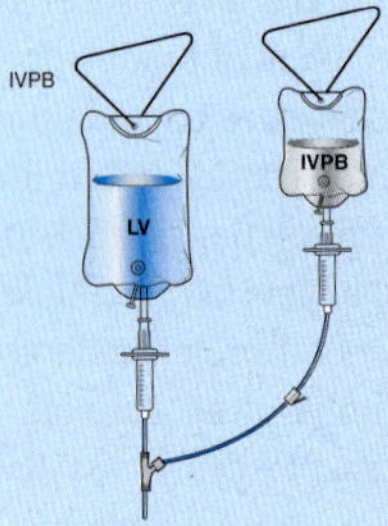	25–250 mL, short tubing connects to the Y-port of the primary infusion line	Separate from the primary fluid, hang above the primary fluid (height affects rate), premix available (frozen and precipitated)

TABLE 9.8 Comparison of Intravenous Delivery Systems *(continued)*

Type	Diagram	Details	Comments
Volume control administration: for example, buretrol	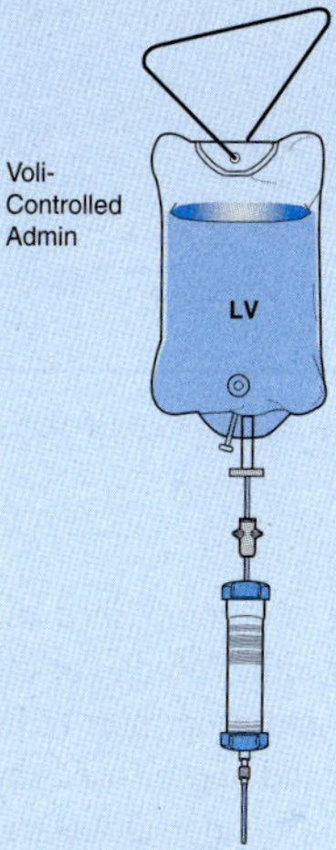	Small container (50–150 mL) connects to the primary infusion bag	Allows small volumes (5–60 mL) for drug administration
Intermittent venous access: for example, saline lock	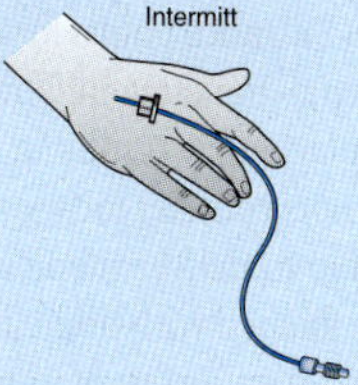	IV catheter injection port (peripheral or central), administered directly into circulation	Flush to keep line patent (usually saline, may use heparin)
IV bolus	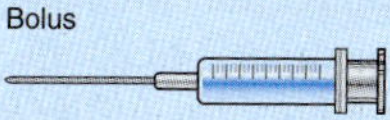	Drug only in needle, directly into the patient	Concentrated, may be irritating, confirm the rate of administration (volume per time, e.g., mL/min)

TABLE 9.9 Examples of Various Methods of IV Infusion

Drug IV	Infusion	Concentration	Indication
Epinephrine	Push (1–2 minutes)	1 mg/mL	Cardiac emergency
Magnesium sulfate	Push (150 mg/min)	10%	Hypomagnesemia
Sodium chloride	Continuous	0.9%	Hydration
Vancomycin	Intermittent (over 1 hour)	≤5 mg/mL	Antibiotic
Rituximab	Intermittent (50–400 mg/h)	1–4 mg/mL	Chemotherapy

Source: Gahart BL, Nazareno AR. *Intravenous Medications.* 24th ed. St. Louis, MO: Mosby Elsevier; 2008.

Vascular Access

Vascular access for IV infusion is accomplished by using vascular access devices (VADs). Generally, either needles or catheters are used. Needles are placed peripherally and used short term. Catheters provide peripheral or central access and may be used short or long term. Peripheral catheters are placed in the dorsal metacarpal or cephalic vein in the arm, whereas central catheters span a small distance from the skin to the intravascular space. Entrance points for central catheters are usually the subclavian or external jugular vein. This additional distance from the point of entry to placement results in lower infections and longer patency. Figure 9.2 depicts catheter locations. Various types of catheters are available, each able to deliver medications and fluids to specific targets. These lines are flushed with dilute heparin or saline (0.9% sodium chloride sterile for injection) to maintain patency. The frequency of flushing catheters ranges from twice daily to once weekly, and volumes administered range from 5 to 20 mL. Supplementary information regarding catheters is provided in Table 9.10.[6,12,13] Various catheter placements are shown in Figure 9.3.

Extravasation, which is unintentional leakage of IV fluid into interstitial tissue, is a major concern when dealing with IV administration of particular drugs. Box 9.2 lists common drugs considered vesicants. Vesicants require close monitoring due to their tendency to produce serious consequences such as necrosis and severe irritation on extravasation.[10,12,14] The risk of extravasation can be reduced by administering drugs at the proper dilution and IV administration rate. For example, it is now recommended to administer IV promethazine

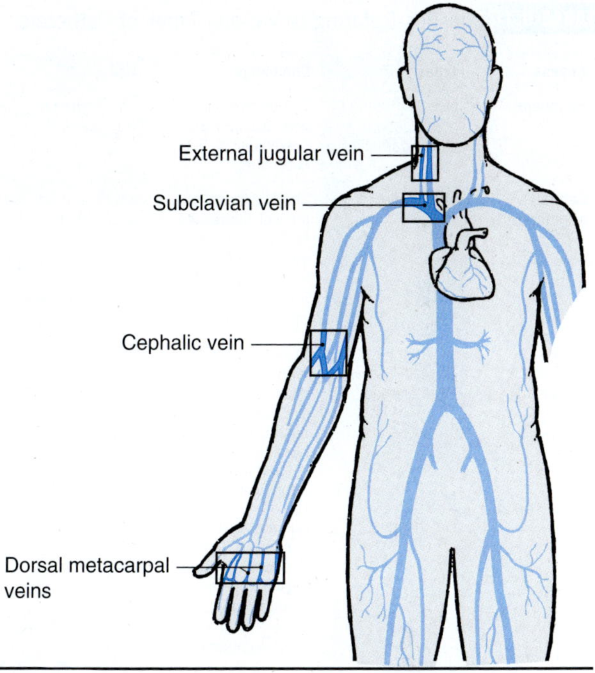

FIGURE 9.2 Possible catheter access and location.

in at least 10 to 20 mL of normal saline and administer over 10 to 15 minutes to prevent extravasation and serious complications seen with undiluted, slow IV push administration.[15]

Unconventional Routes

Available routes for parenteral administration of medications have evolved. In many cases, the drug can be delivered directly to the target tissue or organ. Table 9.11 describes some of these alternative routes of administration.[16,17]

Flow Rate

When drugs are given by intermittent or continuous infusion, the flow of the solution is regulated. The rate at which the solution is administered to the patient is considered the flow rate. Flow rates vary

TABLE 9.10 Issues Relating to Various Types of Catheters

Access	Types	Comments	Use
Peripheral	Needle, butterfly needle, short plastic catheters	Catheters more comfortable than needles; flush every 6–8 hours	Short-term IVs (<60 days)
Central—nontunneled	Subclavian	Short distance to the exit site results in higher risk of infections; flush heparin every 12 hours; single or multiple lumen	Short-term IVs (<60 days)
Central—tunneled (indwelling)	Hickman, Broviac, Corcath, Raaf, Hemed	Inserted centrally (surgically); long distance to the exit site, lower infection; flush biweekly with heparin when not using daily; single or multiple lumina	Long-term IVs (1–2 years), total parenteral nutrition, chemotherapy
	Groshong	See above; also contains a three-position valve and closed tip; infrequent flushing; single or double lumina; flexible catheter	Infusions and blood draws
Central—PICC	Intrasil, C-PICs, Per-Q-Cath	Inserted peripherally (no surgery); increased phlebitis risk; flush every 12 hours; single or multiple lumina	Long-term IVs (weeks to months)
Implantable (port)	Port-A-Cath, Infus-A-Port, Medtronic, Cath Link	Implanted SC (surgically—usually the chest wall); low risk of infection; flush monthly or after draws	Long-term IVs

PICC, peripherally inserted central catheter.
Sources: Lindley CM, Deloatch KH. *Infusion Technology Manual: A Self-Instructional Approach*. Bethesda, MD: ASHP Special Projects Division; 1993:37–50; LaRocca JC, Otto SF. *Mosby's Pocket Guide to Intravenous Therapy*. 3rd ed. St. Louis, MO: Mosby; 1997:42–60; and Abeloff MD, Armitage JO, Niederhuber JE, et al. *Clinical Oncology*. 3rd ed. Orlando, FL: Churchill Livingstone; 2004.

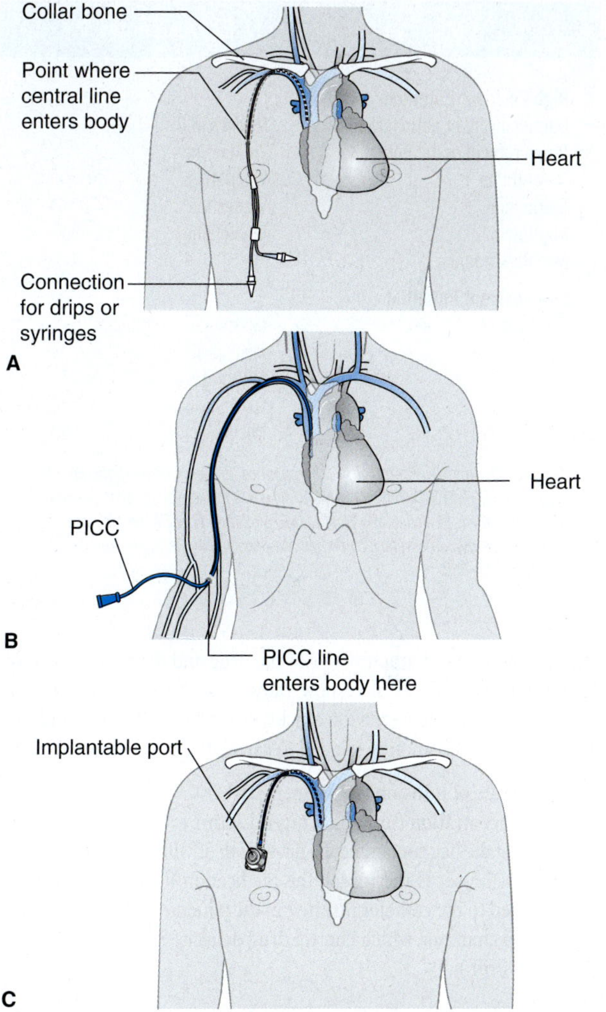

FIGURE 9.3 **A:** Diagram showing a central line. **B:** Diagram showing a PICC line. **C:** Diagram showing an implantable port. (From the patient information Web site of Cancer Research UK: http://www.cancerresearchuk.org/cancerhelp)

BOX 9.2 Medications Known to Be Vesicants

High Vesicant Potential

Dactinomycin or actinomycin D
Daunorubicin or daunomycin
Doxorubicin
Epirubicin
Idarubicin
Mechlorethamine
Mitomycin C
Vinblastine
Vincristine
Vindestine
Vinorelbine

Low Vesicant Potential

Cisplatin
Dacarbazine
Docetaxel
Etoposide
Fluorouracil
Liposomal doxorubicin
Menogaril
Mitoxantrone
Oxaliplatin
Paclitaxel

Sources: Phillips LD. Manual of I.V. Therapeutics. 2nd ed. Philadelphia, PA: FA Davis Co; 1997:513; LaRocca JC, Otto SF. Mosby's Pocket Guide to Intravenous Therapy. 3rd ed. St. Louis, MO: Mosby; 1997:252; and Ener RA, Meglathery SB, Styler M. Extravasation of systemic hemato-oncological therapies. Ann Oncol. 2004;15:858–862.

depending on the characteristics of the drug and drug concentration. It is imperative to calculate flow rates correctly to ensure that the medication is not delivered too quickly (see Chapter 13 for calculation tips). Specific information needed to calculate the flow rate includes

- Desired rate of infusion (mL/min, mL/h)
- Drug concentration (units/mL, mg/mL, g/mL)
- Volume of the bag containing the drug (with or without overfill volume)
- Set size (the set is the tubing the medication flows through that is connected to the catheter inserted in the patient. It has a roller clamp and drip chamber, which control drug delivery. Set sizes are defined by drops/mL)

Pumps or Infusion-Controlled Devices

Parenteral infusion flow rates may be controlled by gravity or by an infusion-controlled device (pump).

TABLE 9.11 Examples of Unconventional Routes of Administration

Route	Location	Drug Treatment
Iontophoresis	Via electrical current into tissue	Corticosteroids
Intradermal	Superficial skin layer	Diagnostic test, vaccines (<0.5 mL)
Intra-arterial catheter	Hepatic, celiac, or carotid artery	Chemotherapy
Intraosseous needle	Bone marrow	Emergency administration of IV drug
Intraperitoneal catheter	Peritoneal cavity	Chemotherapy
Intraspinal catheter	Epidural or intrathecal	Pain management, chemotherapy
Intraventricular catheter	Lateral ventricle of the brain	Chemotherapy, antifungal, antibacterial

Sources: West VL. Alternate routes of administration. *J Intraven Nurs.* 1998;21(4): 221–231; and CDER Data Standard Manual, Route of Administration. Available at http://www.fda.gov/ForIndustry/DataStandards/StructuredProductLabeling/ucm162034.htm. Accessed May 10, 2013.

- Gravity (without a controller)
  - System based on hydrostatic pressure, controlled by clamps
  - Used for peripheral sites only
  - Requires frequent monitoring to check the drip rate
- Infusion-controlled device
  - Measured by various types of sensors
  - Used for central or peripheral infusion
  - Programmable, little monitoring

Multiple forms of infusion-controlled devices are currently available. Recent technology has developed smaller, more accurate devices. Table 9.12 explains in further detail characteristics of each type of device.[6,18,19]

Summary

As technology increases, the availability of more effective and efficient dosage formulations and administration devices to deliver the right drug to the patient will expand. It is imperative to maintain a working

TABLE 9.12 Characteristics of Various Infusion-Controlled Devices or Pumps

Pump Type	Mechanism	Comments	Volume	Variance
Gravity				
Controller	Gravity driven	Electronically measures and compensates the drip rate; good for nonviscous solutions	No volume limits	5%–10%
Positive pressure				
Peristaltic	Tubing undergoes micropulses or constant massaging; linear or rotary pump	Inexpensive; use special sets to avoid tubing distortion	No volume limits	5%–10%
Cassette—piston	Piston actuated	Dual piston available also; special tubing required	50–100 mL	2%–5%
Cassette—syringe	Mechanical or electric	Programmable; special tubing required	≤60 mL	2%–5%
Syringe	Programmable; good for slow flow rates, small volumes	≤60 mL	≤2%	
Elastomeric	Nonelectric; constant elastic pressure; flow-restricted rate	Limited pump volumes; small and portable; disposable	50–500 mL	10%–20%
Vacuum pressure	Nonelectric; constant vacuum pressure; flow-restricted rate	Specific flow rates; disposable	0.5–200 mL	Not available

Sources: Lindley CM, Deloatch KH. *Infusion Technology Manual: A Self-Instructional Approach.* Bethesda, MD: ASHP Special Projects Division; 1993:37–50, 82–91; Capes DF, Asiimwe D. Performance of selected flow-restricting infusion devices. *Am J Health Syst Pharm.* 1998;55:351–59; and Schleis TG, Tice AD. Selecting infusion devices for use in ambulatory care. *Am J Health Syst Pharm.* 1996;53:868–877.

knowledge of this area of pharmacy to ensure that patients receive appropriate, safe, and high-quality care.

References

1. McPherson ML. Don't crush that tablet! *Am Pharm*. 1994;34:57–58.
2. Mitchell JF. Oral Dosage Forms That Should Not Be Crushed. 2013. Retrieved from http://www.ismp.org/tools/DoNotCrush.pdf on October 14, 2013.
3. Workman B. Safe injection techniques. *Nurs Stand*. 1999;13(39):47–53.
4. Turco SJ. *Sterile Dosage Forms: Their Preparation and Clinical Applications*. 4th ed. Philadelphia, PA: Lea & Febiger; 1994:7, 105.
5. Wallymahmed M. Insulin therapy in the management of type 1 and type 2 diabetes. *Nurs Stand*. 2006;21(6):50–56; quiz 58.
6. Lindley CM, Deloatch KH. *Infusion Technology Manual: A Self-Instructional Approach*. Bethesda, MD: ASHP Special Projects Division; 1993:37–50:82–91.
7. Howry LV, Bindler RM, Tso Y. *Pediatric Medications*. Philadelphia, PA: JB Lippincott; 1981:62.
8. Losek JD, Gyuro J. Pediatric intramuscular injections: do you know the procedure and complications? *Pediatr Emerg Care*. 1992;8(2):79–81.
9. Burden M. A practical guide to insulin injections. *Nurs Stand*. 1994;8(29): 25–29.
10. Phillips LD. *Manual of I. V. Therapeutics*. 2nd ed. Philadelphia, PA: FA Davis; 1997:199–204, 208–213, 398–420, 513.
11. Gahart BL, Nazareno AR. *Intravenous Medications*. 24th ed. St. Louis, MO: Mosby Elsevier; 2008.
12. LaRocca JC, Otto SF. *Mosby's Pocket Guide to Intravenous Therapy*. 3rd ed. St. Louis, MO: Mosby; 1997:42–60, 252.
13. Abeloff MD, Armitage JO, Niederhuber JE, et al. *Clinical Oncology*. 3rd ed. Orlando, FL: Churchill Livingstone; 2004.
14. Ener RA, Meglathery SB, Styler M. Extravasation of systemic hemato-oncological therapies. *Ann Oncol*. 2004;15:858–862.
15. Institute for Safe Medication Practices. Action needed to prevent serious tissue injury with IV promethazine. ISMP Medication Safety Alert! August, 2006.
16. West VL. Alternate routes of administration. *J Intraven Nurs*. 1998;21(4): 221–231.
17. CDER Data Standard Manual, Route of Administration. Available at www.fda.gov/CDER/dsm/DRG/drg00301.htm. Accessed January 10, 2008.
18. Capes DF, Asiimwe D. Performance of selected flow-restricting infusion devices. *Am J Health Syst Pharm*. 1998;55:351–359.
19. Schleis TG, Tice AD. Selecting infusion devices for use in ambulatory care. *Am J Health Syst Pharm*. 1996;53:868–877.

10

Fluid and Electrolyte Therapy

Pauline A. Low

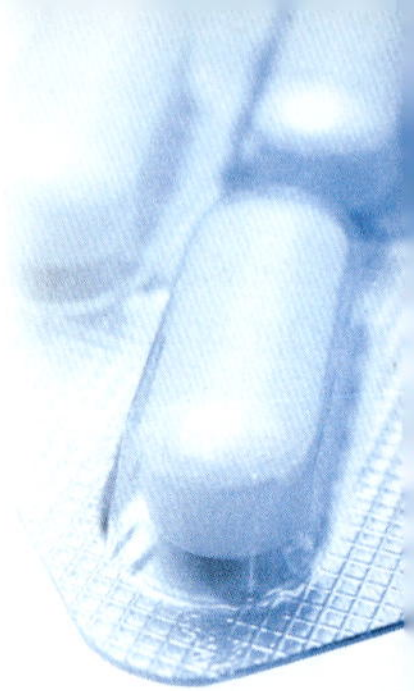

This chapter provides reference information to assess each of the general approach elements to intravenous (IV) fluid and electrolyte therapy included in Box 10.1. The information in this chapter must be used in the context of good clinical judgment.

Fluid Distribution Within the Body

Total Body Water

- The amount of water present within the body is described as total body water (TBW). TBW for adults is estimated by using Equation 10.1.

$$\text{Total body water (L)} = \begin{cases} \text{Adult males: weight (kg)} \times 0.6 \\ \text{Adult females: weight (kg)} \times 0.4 \end{cases} \qquad (10.1)$$

- The percentage of body weight composed of water, declines as we age. Newborns typically have around 75% to 85% body weight as water, whereas adult males have 60% and females about 40% (variable; these estimations are not valid for obese patients or patients with larger than average muscle mass).[1]
- Most body water is housed within cells. Since adult males generally have a higher muscle cell mass than adult females, they will have a higher volume of body water (accounted for in the equation by applying a higher multiplication factor).
- TBW is used to help select an appropriate IV fluid as well as to provide information for fluid and electrolyte dosing.

BOX 10.1 General Approach to IV Fluid/Electrolyte Therapy

1. Determine clinical goals based on the specific patient.
2. Identify which IV fluids and/or electrolytes will assist with achieving clinical goals and make appropriate selection. Consider the following:
   - IV access (central or peripheral IV line)
   - Oral intake capability of patient
   - All sources of fluids and/or electrolytes
   - IV fluid and electrolyte distribution characteristics
3. For fluids: determine volume needs and the associated fluid rate.
   - Consider maintenance fluid needs as well as replacement of excessive losses and requisite electrolyte content
4. For electrolytes: determine the dose and administration method (oral, IV, other).
   - Consider any electrolyte corrections necessary before assessing "true" electrolyte levels for dosing
5. Monitor the patient and reassess needs as clinical status changes.

Fluid Compartments and Determinants of Volume

- Figure 10.1 depicts the estimated typical distribution of TBW in the various body compartments of an adult. This information, together with an understanding of how different IV fluids distribute into different compartments, can be applied to determine the optimal fluid choices to meet particular clinical goals.
  - For example, a hypovolemic hypotensive patient requires fluid volume that will distribute by higher proportion into the intravascular space.

Determinants of Fluid Distribution

Osmolality, Osmolarity, Tonicity, and Free Water[1]

- *Osmolarity* is measured in mOsm/*kg solvent*, whereas *osmolality* is measured in mOsm/*L solution*. The difference between these two terms is confusing and not consistently applied in the medical literature. Clinicians typically refer to the normal serum range for the pressure exerted across semipermeable membranes by particles

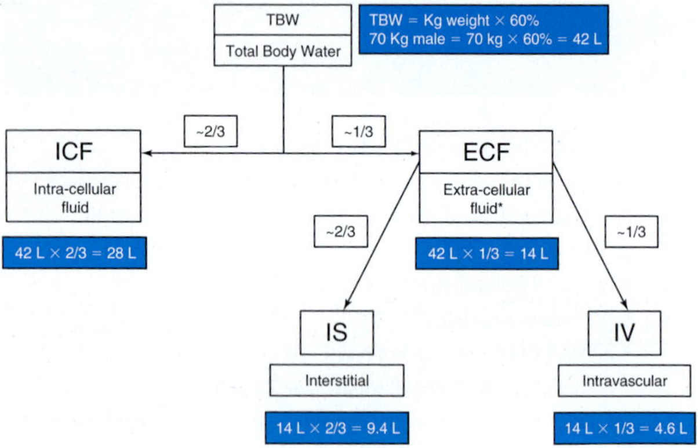

* Other extra-cellular fluid compartments not included, for diagramatic clarity, include: connective tissues, bone water, glandular secretion, and cerebrospinal fluid [1].

FIGURE 10.1 Typical distribution of body water.

in blood as 280 to 295 mOsm/L. Most commonly, this is calculated from the results of a basic metabolic panel or chem-7 using Equation 10.2, but direct lab measurement may also be obtained. Figure 10.2 describes the mathematical interconversion between the different units that may be used clinically.

$$\text{Serum osmolality}\left(\text{mOsm/L}\right) = 2 \times \text{Na} + (\text{BUN}/2.8) + (\text{Glucose}/18) \tag{10.2}$$

BUN, blood urea nitrogen; adult reference range: 280 – 295 mOsm/L

- *Tonicity* describes osmotic pressure exerted across a cell membrane by particles in plasma. Isotonicity describes equal osmotic pressure on both sides of a semipermeable membrane, so there is no net movement of the solvent across the membrane. Normal saline solution (NSS), 0.9% NaCl, is an isotonic solution, meaning that no net fluid is distributed into cells on administration.
    - Dextrose 5% in water (D5W) does distribute into cells (approximately two-thirds of the volume administered) and is therefore described as *free water*. Approximately 130 mL of a 1,000-mL infusion will remain in the intravascular compartment on administration.

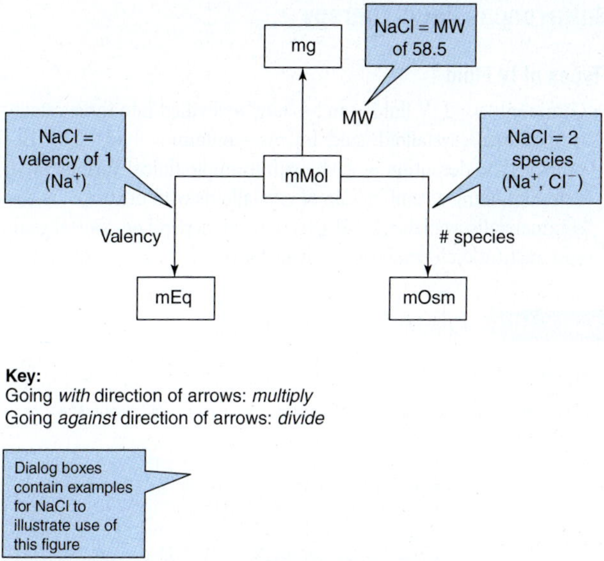

FIGURE 10.2 Unit interconversion. (MW, molecular weight.) (Adapted from Eric J. Mack, PhD, Keck Graduate Institute School of Pharmacy, with permission.)

  - NSS and lactated Ringer (LR) solution are both considered to be isotonic fluids. For each, approximately 300 to 340 mL of a 1,000-mL infusion will remain in the intravascular compartment on administration.
  - Hypotonic or hypertonic fluids may be uncomfortable or painful during the infusion and must be administered via a central IV line.
- Equation 10.2 describes the major contribution of sodium toward serum osmotic pressure. The sodium load of IV fluids will therefore be a major determinant of the volume that remains in the IV space versus distributing to other body compartments.
- Free water describes the distribution of fluids that have neither oncotic nor colloidal pressure affecting the compartment distribution. D5W is an example of a fluid that is 100% free water.

Intravenous Fluid Therapy

Types of IV Fluid

- Commonly used IV fluids can broadly be divided into three categories: colloids, crystalloids, and dextrose-containing fluids. Table 10.1 provides the definition of each, with example fluids. Various products containing a combination of crystalloids with dextrose are also commercially available. Fluid selection will depend on clinical goals, cost, institution formulary, and availability.

TABLE 10.1 Commonly Used IV Fluids

Colloid	
Definition: IV fluids containing the dispersion of large molecular weight (MW) molecules	
5% Albumin	• Iso-oncotic • Natural albumin product (possibility of sensitivity reaction) • Used for plasma volume expansion
25% Albumin	• Hyperoncotic • Natural albumin product • Used for fluid redistribution into the intravascular space
Hetastarch 6%	• Synthetic product • Used for plasma volume expansion • Can increase risk for bleeding • Less antigenic than dextran products
Dextran 6%	• Product derived from the bacterium *Leuconostoc mesenteroides* • Available as dextran 40, 70, or 75. Number refers to the average MW (×1,000 daltons) • Can increase the risk for bleeding • Incidence of antigenic reactions increased with a higher MW product
Crystalloid	
Definition: IV fluids containing sodium	
0.9% NaCl (normal saline solution, NSS)	• Isotonic • Used for plasma volume expansion • Can cause hyperchloremic metabolic acidosis if a large volume is administered
Lactated Ringer solution (LRS)	• Isotonic • Used for plasma volume expansion • Contains lactate, which is converted by a healthy liver to bicarbonate • Contains potassium. Use with caution in patients with compromised renal function

(continued)

TABLE 10.1 Commonly Used IV Fluids *(continued)*

3% NaCl	• Hypertonic • Used in patients with increased cerebral perfusion pressure due to traumatic brain injury or life-threatening hyponatremia • Extreme caution needed with this product since serum Na should not change by >10 mEq/d to avoid serious complications • Higher concentrations of NaCl solutions are available
Dextrose in Water Solutions	
Dextrose 5% in water (D5W)	• Distributes 100% as free water • Weight per volume (w/v) solution containing 5 g dextrose in 100 mL water (or 50 g in 1 L) • Since 1 g dextrose contains 3.4 kcal, each 100 mL contains 17 kcal (or 170 kcal in 1 L)
Dextrose 10% in water (D10W)	• Distributes 100% as free water • Contains 10 g dextrose in 100 mL water (or 100 g in 1 L) • Each 100 mL contains 34 kcal (or 340 kcal in 1 L) • Often used as a step-up or step-down fluid to parenteral nutrition or for patients who are consistently hypoglycemic

- Table 10.2 summarizes the fluid compartment distribution of various types of IV fluids.
- Figures 10.3 and 10.4 compare the compartment distribution of D5W and NSS, respectively (note that the D5W distribution figure matches Fig. 10.1 since D5W is 100% free water).
- Table 10.3 compares the healthy adult ranges for serum osmolality and major electrolyte concentrations with those for selected IV fluids.

TABLE 10.2 Distribution of IV Fluids

Fluid	% ICF	% ECF	Free water/L
D5W	60	40	1,000 mL
0.45% NaCl	37	73	500 mL
D5W 0.45% NaCl	37	73	500 mL
0.9% NaCl	0	100	0 mL
154 mEq/L sodium bicarbonate (compounded solution)	0	100	0 mL
3% NaCl	0	100	–2,331 mL

ICF, intracellular fluid; ECF, extracellular fluid.

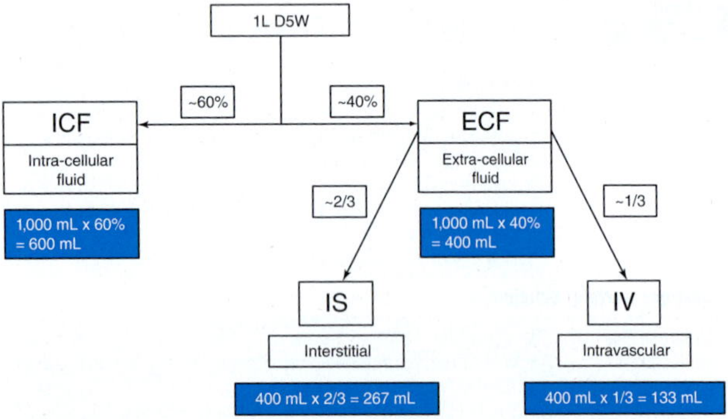

FIGURE 10.3 Typical distribution of 5% dextrose intravenous infusion.

- Since in most cases biologic fluids can shift down concentration gradients across semipermeable membranes, the expected results from administration of a fluid containing higher concentrations of a given electrolyte would include elevation of the serum electrolyte concentration. The opposite would typically occur if a relatively hypoconcentrated electrolyte-containing fluid was administered.
  - For example, administration of LR, which contains 4 mEq/L potassium, to a patient with normal renal function and a serum potassium concentration of 3 mEq/L would typically result in an increase in serum potassium concentration until an equilibrium point serum concentration of around 4 mEq/L is reached (again,

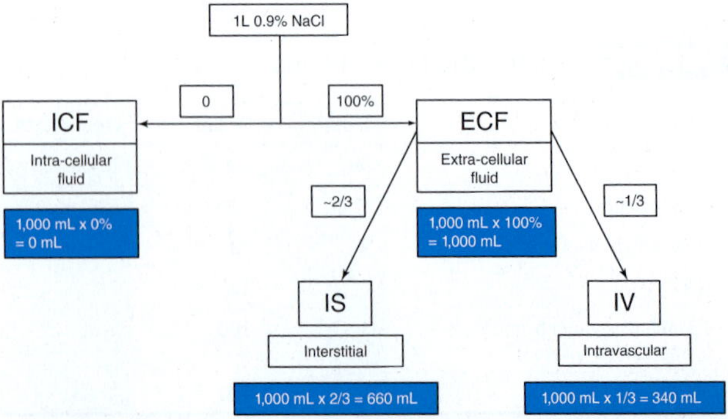

FIGURE 10.4 Typical distribution of 0.9% NaCl intravenous infusion.

TABLE 10.3 Comparison of IV Fluid Electrolyte Content with Serum

Fluid	Osm/L	Na^+, mEq/L	Cl^+, mEq/L	K^+, mEq/L	$Ca2^+$, mEq/L	Lactate,[a] mEq/L
Serum	280–295	140	100	4	9	Bicarbonate 26
0.9% NaCl	308	154	154	0	0	0
LR	274	130	109	4	1.5	28
D5W	278	0	0	0	0	0

LR, lactated Ringer.
[a]Converted by a healthy liver to bicarbonate.

depending on the rate of administration and clearance), with the rate of change depending on the rate of LR administration as well as the rate of potassium elimination. Giving LR to a patient with a serum potassium concentration of 5.4 mEq/L would typically result in a decrease in serum potassium until equilibrium is reached.

Estimated Daily Fluid Requirements

- To estimate the daily fluid requirements for a patient, the clinical situation of the patient is the primary factor governing both volume and choice of the fluid.
- General guidelines for patients without special need for fluid restriction or replacement of excessive loss are provided in Table 10.4.
- For patients with demonstrated water deficit or excess, Table 10.5 provides associated equations to help guide volume therapy decisions.
- Estimated daily urine and insensible fluid losses are provided in Table 10.6.
- Table 10.7 includes common signs and symptoms of decreased versus increased fluid within each of the major body compartments. These can be used for both assessing the patient therapy needs and monitoring. Table 10.8 provides common renal markers of fluid status.
- If a patient has a large output of body fluids, it may be necessary to replace both fluid volume and the electrolytes these fluids typically contain.
- Table 10.9 provides typical volumes per day of various biologic fluids produced, with their major electrolyte concentrations. Typically, each 1 mL of fluid loss is replaced with 0.5 to 1 mL of replacement fluid.
  - For example, if a patient is experiencing large losses of fluid through vomiting, then it may be necessary to replace sodium and

TABLE 10.4 General Guidelines for Patients Without Special Need for Fluid Restriction or Replacement of Excessive Loss

Patient Population	Estimated Daily Fluid Requirements	Example(s)
Adults and pediatrics	Holliday-Segar method[a] 100 mL/kg/d for the first 10 kg 50 mL/kg/d for the next 10 kg 20 mL/kg/d for additional weight >20 kg Add 10% for each degree of body temperature (Celsius) above normal Add extra for excessive fluid losses	8 kg child: 800 mL/d 17 kg child: 1,350 mL/d 50 kg adult: 2,100 mL/d
Adults	30–35 mL/kg/d	50 kg adult: 1,500–1,750 mL/d

[a]Holliday MA, Segar WE. The maintenance need for water in parenteral fluid therapy. *Pediatrics*. 1957;19:823–832.[2]

TABLE 10.5 Calculating Water Deficit or Excess Based on Total Body Water (TBW) and Serum Sodium Concentration

Water Deficit	Water Excess
Water deficit (L) = normal TBW – present TBW Where normal TBW = wt in kg × 40% (female) or 60% (male) $\text{Present TBW} = \frac{\text{Desired Na}^+}{\text{Current Na}^+} \times \text{normal TBW}$ Note: This equation does not account for ongoing losses such as insensible fluid loss and other sources of fluid loss.	Water excess (L) = TBW – (TBW × observed Na^+/desired Na^+)

Source: Lau A. Fluid and electrolyte disorders. In: Koda-Kimble MA, Young LY, Kradjan WA, et al., eds. *Applied Therapeutics: The Clinical Use of Drugs*. 8th ed. Philadelphia, PA: Lippincott Williams & Wilkins; 2005:12-1–12-33, with permission.

TABLE 10.6 Estimated Daily Fluid Loss

Fluid Type	Adults	Pediatrics
Urine	• 0.5–1 mL/kg/h • ~30 mL/kg/d • ~50 mL/h	1 mL/kg/h
Insensible	~1,000 mL/d	Fever adjustment = 10% × maintenance fluid for each degree C >37°C[a]

[a]Chicella MF, Hak EB. Pediatric nutrition. In: Koda-Kimble MA, Young LY, Kradjan WA, et al., eds. *Applied Therapeutics: The Clinical Use of Drugs*. 8th ed. Philadelphia, PA: Lippincott Williams & Wilkins; 2005:97-1–97-22.[3]

TABLE 10.7 Assessing and Monitoring Clinical Need for Fluid: Common Signs and Symptoms

Decreased Fluid	Increased Fluid
Total Body Water	
• Decreased body weight unrelated to changes in lean body mass • Intake and output records	• Increased body weight unrelated to changes in lean body mass • Intake and output records
Intracellular Fluid	
• Increased serum osmolality • Increased thirst sensation • Mental status changes	• Decreased serum osmolality • Decreased thirst sensation • Mental status changes
Extracellular Fluid—Interstitial	
• Dry skin and mucous membranes • Poor skin turgor • Sunken eyes • Depressed fontanelle in infants	• Peripheral or sacral edema • Pulmonary congestion (such as crackles, radiograph changes, dyspnea, hypoxia) • Ascites or other sequestered (third space) fluid
Extracellular Fluid—Intravascular	
• Decreased urine output: a sensitive indicator of intravascular volume if no organ failures are present • Oliguria • Urine chemistry (see Table 10.8) • Serum chemistry: increased values due to decreased intravascular water volume (concentration effect) • BUN:creatinine ratio >20 • Tachycardia • Signs of peripheral hypoperfusion such as increased nail bed capillary refill time • Cool temperature and color changes in extremities • Decreased level of consciousness • Orthostatic changes in pulse and blood pressure • Increased blood hematocrit and hemoglobin due to decreased intravascular water volume • Swan-Ganz catheter readings—decreased CVP, occlusion pressure, and cardiac output	• Increased urine output • Serum chemistry: decreased values due to increased intravascular water volume (dilutional effect) • S-3 heart sound • Increased CVP • Jugular venous distension • Hepatojugular reflux • Decreased blood hematocrit and hemoglobin due to increased intravascular water volume • Swan-Ganz catheter readings—increased CVP, occlusion pressure, and cardiac output

BUN, blood urea nitrogen; CVP, central venous pressure.

chloride, and potentially potassium, since these three electrolytes are the major components lost. Keeping track of vomit volume may provide valuable information on replacement needs.

TABLE 10.8 Assessing Fluid Status with Urine Markers of Decreased Renal Perfusion

Urine specific gravity	>1.022
Urine Osm	>500
Urine Na mEq/L	<20
Fractional excretion of filtered Na (FENA) $\text{FENA} = 100 \times \dfrac{(\text{Urine Na / Plasma Na})}{(\text{Urine Cr / Plasma Cr})}$	<1

Source: Trombetta DP. The kidneys. In: Lee M, ed. *Basic Skills in Interpreting Laboratory Data.* 5th ed. Bethesda, MD: American Society of Health-System Pharmacists; 2012:175–192.[4]

IV Fluids Associated with Metabolic Blood pH Alterations

- It is important to understand that IV fluid therapy can profoundly affect the blood gas status of a patient. This can be used to therapeutically treat a blood gas disorder or to prevent development or complication of an existing disorder.
- Figure 10.5 demonstrates the interrelationship between chloride and bicarbonate, as well as including the effects of an anion gap in metabolic blood gas disorders.

TABLE 10.9 Typical Electrolyte Composition of Selected Body Fluids

Fluid	Volume (mL/d)	Na^+ (mEq/L)	K^+ (mEq/L)	Cl^- (mEq/L)	HCO_3^- (mEq/L)
Plasma	—	140	4	100	26
Gastric	1,500	60	10	130	0
Bile	800	145	5	100	35
Pancreatic	1,000	140	5	75	115
Small bowel	300–1,500	140	5	80	50
Sweat	500	45	4.5	60	0
Ileal	Variable; ~3,000	140	5	105	30
Cecal	Variable	60	30	40	20

Adapted from Chicella MF, Hak EB. Pediatric nutrition. In: Koda-Kimble MA, Young LY, Kradjan WA, et al., eds. *Applied Therapeutics: The Clinical Use of Drugs.* 8th ed. Philadelphia, PA: Lippincott Williams & Wilkins; 2005:97-1–97-22, with permission.

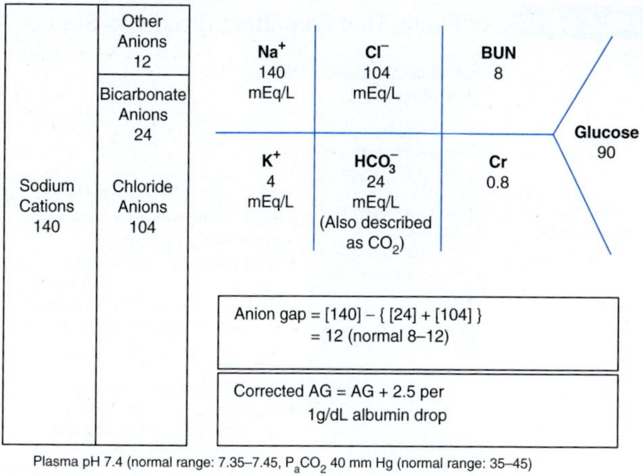

FIGURE 10.5 Diagrammatic relationship between serum chloride, bicarbonate, and anion gap. (BUN, blood urea nitrogen; AG, anion gap.)

- For example, an increase in chloride (e.g., from administration of a large volume of NSS) will typically be reflected in a decreased bicarbonate concentration, described as a hyperchloremic metabolic acidosis).

- Table 10.10 includes the IV fluids that directly affect blood gas status. These fluids may be used therapeutically for this purpose, but they have the potential to cause or complicate an existing disorder.

Clinical Goals of IV Fluid Therapy

- The therapeutic plan relating to fluids for a patient will ultimately depend on the clinical goals.
- Table 10.11 identifies a goal-based approach to patient fluid therapy.

Electrolytes

Electrolyte Reference Ranges

- Figure 10.6 provides reference ranges for adult serum electrolytes in the commonly used medical format. Table 10.12 provides pediatric reference ranges for serum electrolytes.

TABLE 10.10 IV Fluids That Can Affect Blood Gas Status

	Affect on Metabolic Acid–Base Status	Notes
Sodium chloride	• Can cause hyperchloremic metabolic acidosis	
Sodium bicarbonate	• Can cause metabolic alkalosis • Can be used to increase alkalinity of blood	• HCO_3^- deficit (mEq) = (24 – measured HCO_3^-) × TBW • Typically provide ~50% of the calculated deficit in first 24 hours. Caution not to cause rapid changes in CNS pH and/or sodium concentration (not >12 mEq/L Na change in 24 hours • Careful monitoring required • May induce intracellular acidosis. Not recommended for use when arterial pH is >7.15
Hydrochloric acid	• Can cause metabolic acidosis • Can be used to increase acidity of blood	• HCl (mmol) = (103 – measured Cl^- in mmol/L) × body weight in kg × 0.2 • Typically administer 50% over 12–24 hours to lower pH by 0.2 • Alternative dosing: 0.1–0.2 mmol/kg/h, with frequent monitoring of ABG and electrolytes • Must administer via central line • Use 0.1 N solution (10 mmol HCl/L) in D5W
THAM (tromethamine; trihydroxymethylaminomethane)	• Can be used to buffer acidity of blood as an alternative to sodium bicarbonate • Does not increase serum sodium, bicarbonate, or PCO_2	THAM mL = body weight in kg × base deficit (mEq/L) × 1.1 • Factor of 1.1 accounts for about a 10% reduction in buffering capacity due to the presence of sufficient acetic acid to lower pH of the 0.3 M solution to approximately 8.6 • Additional dosing is determined by serial measurement of base deficit

TBW, total body weight; M, molar solution; CNS, central nervous system; ABG, arterial blood gases.

Sources: Lau A. Fluid and electrolyte disorders. In: Koda-Kimble MA, Young LY, Kradjan WA, et al., eds. *Applied Therapeutics: The Clinical Use of Drugs*. 8th ed. Philadelphia, PA: Lippincott Williams & Wilkins; 2005:12-1–12-33; Dellinger RP, Carlet JM, Masur H, et al. Surviving Sepsis Campaign guidelines for management of severe sepsis and septic shock. *Crit Care Med*. 2004 Mar;32(3):858–873; Metabolic Alkalosis: Acid–base Regulation and Disorders: Merck Manual Professional Website. Available at www.merck.com/mmpe/sec12/ch157/ch157d.html. Accessed March 18, 2008; and Tham Solution [package insert]. Abbott Park, IL: Abbott Laboratories; 2000.[5–7]

TABLE 10.11 Goal-Based Approach to Patient Fluid Therapy

What is the Therapeutic Goal for Your Patient?	Possible Approach(es)
Restore circulating volume	• Provide fluid that will optimize intravascular volume (e.g., NSS, LR)
Correct electrolyte disorders	• Treat life-threatening hyperelectrolyte or hypoelectrolyte disorders as first priority • Consider need for parenteral versus enteral therapy depending on the patient status • Treat any underlying causes including adjustment of any sources of exogenous electrolytes if elevated (such as electrolyte containing IV fluids), or agents contributing to hypo conditions (such as binding agents)
Correct acid–base disorder	• Treat the underlying cause (e.g., diarrhea can cause metabolic acidosis, vomiting can cause metabolic alkalosis, blunting of respiratory drive with agents such as benzodiazepines or opiates can cause respiratory acidosis) • Consider effects of any IV fluids administered (e.g., NSS can contribute to hyperchloremic metabolic acidosis, sodium bicarbonate solutions can contribute to metabolic alkalosis) • THAM may be an option for patients with severe metabolic acidosis intolerant of the sodium bicarbonate solution (due to high sodium load, increased PCO_2, or pH outside the recommended range for use of this fluid)
Replace anticipated water and electrolyte losses	• Provide fluid and electrolyte therapy as necessary during the course of therapy • Consider options for fluid and electrolyte combination versus providing fluid separately from electrolyte therapy • Adjustments are based on repeated assessments of the patient status
Remove excessive fluid	• Consider need for diuretic therapy, depending on renal function • Adjust any fluids currently being administered

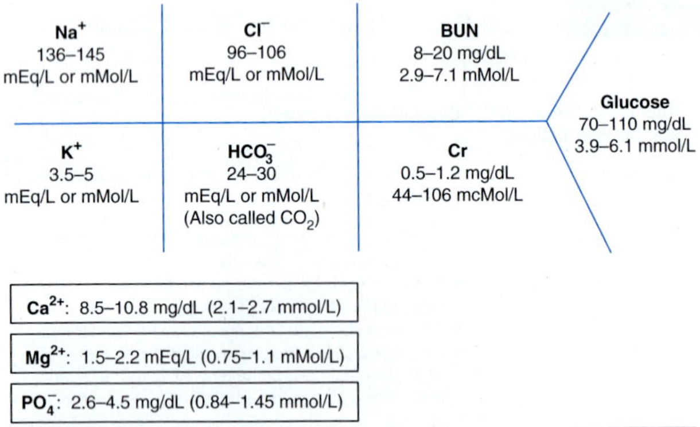

FIGURE 10.6 Adult reference ranges for serum electrolytes. (BUN, blood urea nitrogen.) (From Lau A. Fluid and electrolyte disorders. In: Koda-Kimble MA, Young LY, Kradjan WA, et al., eds. *Applied Therapeutics: The Clinical Use of Drugs*. 8th ed. Philadelphia, PA: Lippincott Williams & Wilkins; 2005:12-1–12-33, with permission.)

Electrolyte Therapies

- Table 10.13 provides any correction factors that should be accounted for prior to providing pharmacotherapy, as well homeostasis factors to consider.
- Table 10.14 provides pharmacotherapy summaries for electrolyte level reduction and replacement.
- Table 10.15 contains selected medications associated with hypoelectrolyte or hyperelectrolyte disorders.

(text continued on page 385)

TABLE 10.12 Infant and Pediatric Electrolyte Reference Ranges

	Premature Neonates	Newborns	Infants 1 Month to 1 Year	Children 1–12 Year	Adults
Na^+	48 hour life: 128–148 mEq/L or mol/L	133–146 mEq/L or mol/L	139–146 mEq/L or mol/L	138–145 mEq/L or mol/L	136–145 mEq/L or mol/L
K^+	48 hour life: 3.0–6.0 mEq/L or mol/L	3.7–5.9 mEq/L or mol/L	4.1–5.3 mEq/L or mol/L	3.4–4.7 mEq/L or mol/L	3.5–5 mEq/L or mol/L
Cr	0.3–1.0 mg/dL (27–88 µmol/L)		0.2–0.4 mg/dL (18–35 µmol/L)	0.3–0.7 mg/dL (27–62 µmol/L)	0.5–1.2 mg/dL (44–106 µmol/L)
Ca^{2+}	3–24 hour life: 9.0–10.6 mg/dL (2.3–2.65 mol/L) 24–48 hour life: 7.0–12.0 (1.75–3.0 mol/L) 4–7 days: 9.0–10.9 mg/dL (2.2–2.73 mol/L)	8.8–0.8 mg/dL (2.2–2.7 mol/L)	8.5–10.8 mg/dL (2.1–2.7 mol/L)		
Mg^{2+}	0–6 days life: 1.2–2.6 mEq/L (0.48–1.05 mmol/L)	7 days–2 years: 1.6–2.6 mEq/L (0.65–1.05 mmol/L) 2–14 years: 1.5–2.3 mEq/L (0.6–0.95 mmol/L)	1.5–2.2 mEq/L (0.75–1.1 mmol/L)		
PO_4	4.8–8.2 mg/dL (1.55–2.65 mmol/L)	1–3 years: 3.8–6.5 mg/dL (1.55–2.1 mmol/L) 4–11 years: 3.7–5.6 mg/dL (1.2–1.8 mol/L) 12–15 years: 2.9–5.4 mg/dL (0.95–1.75 mol/L)	2.6–4.5 mg/dL (0.84–1.45 mmol/L)		

Source: Kraus D. Interpreting pediatric laboratory data. In: Lee M, ed. *Basic Skills in Interpreting Laboratory Data*. 5th ed. Bethesda, MD: American Society of Health-System Pharmacists; 2012:521–544.[8]

TABLE 10.13 Select Adult Serum Electrolyte Recommended Daily Intake (RDI), Reference Ranges, Correction Factors, and Homeostasis

	Serum Concentration	Lab Value Correction Factors	Recommended Daily Intake (RDI)	Homeostasis
Sodium (Na^+)	136–145 mEq/L or mmol/L	1. Correct for hyperglycemia (falsely low sodium due to lab error) 2. For every serum glucose of 100 >100, add 1.7 to the serum sodium Na_{corr} = [(Glucose – 100)/100 × 1.7 mEq/L] + Na_{uncorr}	PO: • Variable; 50–100 mEq IV: • Per individual patient	• Antidiuretic hormone (ADH) • The renin–angiotensin–aldosterone system (RAAS)
Potassium (K^+)	3.5–5 mEq/L or mmol/L	• Correct for metabolic acidosis or alkalosis (pseudohyperkalemia as K^+ shifts from cells into the IV fluid (IVF) in exchange for hydrogen ions in acidemia; the opposite effect seen with alkalemia) • For every 0.1 pH < 7.4, deduct 0.6 from the lab reported K. For every 0.1 pH > 7.4, add 0.6 to the lab reported K (see equation below): • K_{corr} = [(7.4 – pH)/0.1 × 0.6 mEq/L] + K_{uncorr}	PO: • 50–100 mEq IV: • Per individual patient • Average 0.5–1.2 mEq/kg/d	• Renal elimination • Aldosterone • Transcellular distribution (NA^+/K^+/ATPase pump) • Metabolic plasma pH changes • Beta-adrenergic (particularly beta-2) receptor stimulation • Insulin
Magnesium (Mg^{2+})	1.5–2.2 mEq/L (0.75–1.1 mmol/L)	N/A	Based on elemental magnesium PO: • 360 mg • 30 mEq • 15 mmol IV: • 120 mg • 10 mEq • 5 mmol • (~1/3 PO RDI)	Parathyroid hormone (PTH) • 1 Alpha, 25-dihydroxy-vitamin D • Renal elimination • Mineralocorticoids • Glucagon

(continued)

TABLE 10.13 Select Adult Serum Electrolyte Recommended Daily Intake (RDI), Reference Ranges, Correction Factors, and Homeostasis *(continued)*

	Serum Concentration	Lab Value Correction Factors	Recommended Daily Intake (RDI)	Homeostasis
Calcium (Ca^{2+})	8.5–10.8 mg/dL (2.1–2.7 mmol/L)	• Correct for hypoalbuminemia: • Most accurate: obtain an ionized calcium	Based on elemental calcium • PO: • 800–1,500 mg IV: • 200 mg • 10 mEq • 5 mmol • (~1/4 of PO RDI) calcium daily	• PTH • Vitamin D • Calcitonin
Phosphate ($PO4^-$)	2.6–4.5 mg/dL (0.84–1.45 mmol/L)	N/A	PO: • 1,000 mg • 30 mmol IV: • Same as PO	• Calcium concentration • PTH • Thyroid hormone • Vitamin D • Thyrocalcitonin • Dietary intake • Renal elimination

Sources: Lau A. Fluid and electrolyte disorders. In: Koda-Kimble MA, Young LY, Kradjan WA, et al., eds. *Applied Therapeutics: The Clinical Use of Drugs.* 8th ed. Philadelphia, PA: Lippincott Williams & Wilkins; 2005:12-1–12-3; Lau A, Chan LN. Electrolytes, other minerals, and trace elements. In: Lee M, ed. *Basic Skills in Interpreting Laboratory Data.* 3rd ed. Bethesda, MD: American Society of Health-System Pharmacists; 2004:183–232; Dickerson RN. Guidelines for the intravenous management of hypophosphatemia, hypomagnesemia, hypokalemia, and hypocalcemia. *Hosp Pharm.* 2001;36:1201–1208; Baran DR, Aronin N. Disorders of mineral metabolism. In: Irwin RS, Rippe JM, eds. *Intensive Care Medicine.* 6th ed. Philadelphia, PA: Lippincott Williams & Wilkins; 2008:1287–1293; Cohen AJ. Physiologic concepts in the management of renal, fluid, and electrolyte disorders in the intensive care unit. In: Irwin RS, Rippe JM, eds. *Intensive Care Medicine.* 6th ed. Philadelphia, PA: Lippincott Williams & Wilkins; 2008:867–883; Black RM, Noroian GO. Disorders of plasma sodium and plasma potassium. In: Irwin RS, Rippe JM, eds. *Intensive Care Medicine.* 6th ed. Philadelphia, PA: Lippincott Williams & Wilkins; 2008:898–925; and Driscoll DF, Bistrian BR. Parenteral and enteral nutrition in the intensive care unit. In: Irwin RS, Rippe JM, eds. *Intensive Care Medicine.* 6th ed. Philadelphia, PA: Lippincott Williams & Wilkins; 2008:2186–2201.[9–15]

TABLE 10.14 Hyperelectrolyte and Hypoelectrolyte Therapy

Dosing weight for electrolyte therapy:

- Use current body weight (CBW) unless the patient is >130% ideal body weight (IBW), in which case, use adjusted body weight (AdjBW):
- AdjBW = [0.25 × (CBW – IBW)] + IBW

Potassium (K^+)

Hyperkalemia (assess for pseudohyperkalemia from metabolic acidosis or lab sample hemolysis)

Signs and symptoms	• Paresthesias • Weakness • Peaked T waves on the electrocardiogram (ECG)
Treatment	Shift K: 1. Ca/glucose/insulin combination a. 10 mL of 10% calcium gluconate IV over 3 minutes (to antagonize cardiac cell effects of hyperkalemia, need cardiac monitoring), 50 mL of 50% glucose IV (unless hyperglycemic), 10 units SQ/IV fast-acting insulin 2. Albuterol a. (20 mg in 4 mL NSS inhaled nasally for 10 minutes, or 0.5 mg IV) 3. Increase pH by providing bicarbonate a. 45 mEq IV over 5 minutes (variable effect on pH) Remove from body 1. Loop or thiazide diuretic a. Unpredictable response, particularly in renal insufficiency. Not recommend as primary therapy 2. Sodium polystyrene sulfonate exchange resin a. 1 g resin binds 0.5–1 mEq K^+ in exchange for Na^+ b. 20 g PO with 100 mL sorbitol solution (prevent constipation) c. 50 g PR with 50 mL 70% sorbitol and 100 mL tap water. Retained in colon for 120–180 minutes
Monitoring	• Patients require careful monitoring for hyperkalemia, including: ∘ Telemetry monitoring ∘ Serum potassium level monitoring ∘ Signs and symptoms such as weakness and paresthesias
Notes	• Do not forget to discontinue all sources of potassium while treating a patient for hyperkalemia, such as ∘ Lactated Ringer or other potassium-containing IV fluid ∘ Enteral or parenteral feedings

Hypokalemia

Signs and symptoms	• ST segment depression on ECG • QRS widening, PR prolongation • Hypotension • Decreased release of insulin • Decreased release of aldosterone • Cramps • Areflexia • Weakness • Increased risk of digoxin toxicity (for patients on digoxin)

(continued)

TABLE 10.14 Hyperelectrolyte and Hypoelectrolyte Therapy *(continued)*

Treatment • Check Mg and treat any deficiency (often difficult to correct low potassium until Mg is corrected) • BMP, basal metabolic profile	**Serum K (mEq/L)**	**KCl Dose (mEq)**	**Monitoring**
	3.5–3.9	Consider giving 40 mEq × 1	BMP and Mg next AM
	3.0–3.4	40 mEq × 2	BMP and Mg next AM Consider stat K 2 hours after the second dose
	2.0–2.9	40 mEq × 3	Stat K after second dose, reassess (may need an additional 1–2 doses. Check serum Mg

Notes	• Check Mg and treat any deficiency (often difficult to correct low potassium until Mg is corrected)
	• Reduce the dose in renal impairment (usually by ~50% depending on renal function and need)
	• Potassium acetate and potassium phosphates are alternative salt forms to chloride for patients who are hyperchloremic. Each requires sterile preparation (not commercially available as premix)
	  ∘ Acetate is converted to bicarbonate: 1 mEq acetate provides 1 mEq potassium
	  ∘ 1 mmol phosphate provides 1.47 mEq potassium
	• Maximum rate of administration and concentration:
	  ∘ Peripheral IV—10 mEq/h; 0.1 mEq/mL
	  ∘ Central IV—20 mEq/h; 0.4 Eq/mL
	  ∘ Must be administered by IV infusion (*do not use IV push*)
	• Oral potassium replacement products:
	  ∘ Potassium chloride powder for reconstitution: 20 mEq dissolved in 120 mL water
	  ∘ Potassium bicarbonate effervescent tablet: 25 mEq dissolved in 120 mL water
	  ∘ Potassium chloride liquid: 1.33 mEq/mL diluted in water or juice for palatability		

Magnesium (Mg^{2+})

Hypermagnesemia

Signs and symptoms	**Serum Magnesium Concentration**	**Possible Signs and Symptoms**
	2–5 mEq/L	• Bradycardia • Sweating • Nausea and vomiting • Decreased ability to clot
	6–9 mEq/L	• Decreased deep tendon reflexes • Drowsiness
	10–15 mEq/L	• Flaccid paralysis • Increased PR and QRS intervals
	>15 mEq/L	• Respiratory distress • Asystole

TABLE 10.14 Hyperelectrolyte and Hypoelectrolyte Therapy *(continued)*

Treatment	• 10 mL of 10% calcium gluconate in 50 mL D5W IV • Repeat as needed, serum calcium not to exceed 11 mg/dL		
Monitoring	• If the patient has received exogenous source of magnesium, note that the true serum level may not be observed until ≤48 hours after discontinuation due to tissue redistribution		
Notes	• May not see clinical signs and symptoms of hypermagnesemia until the level exceeds 5 mEq/L (2.5 mmol/L)		
Hypomagnesemia			
Signs and symptoms	• Central nervous system (CNS) excitability • Hypokalemia		
Treatment	**Serum Mg (mg/dL)**	**Magnesium IV Dose**	**Magnesium PO Dose**
	1.6–1.8	0.05 g/kg	400–800
	1–1.5	0.1 g/kg	mg magnesium oxide daily—QID as tolerated
	<1	0.15 g/kg	Use IV
Monitoring	• Successful treatment of hypomagnesemia typically takes several days since it usually takes ~48 hours for Mg to redistribute in body tissues. Checking Mg level prior to 48 hours should be undertaken with the understanding that the measured value will be falsely high until redistribution has been completed		

Notes	• Reduce dose in renal impairment (usually by ~50% depending on renal function and need)
	• Rate of administration for IV infusion: not to exceed 8 mEq/h (1 g Mg sulfate per hour); otherwise the renal threshold will be exceeded, resulting in disproportional excretion in patients with good renal function.
	• Suggested concentration: 10 mg/mL
	• Oral magnesium replacement products:
	  ◦ Magnesium oxide: 400 mg tablets contain 241 mg elemental magnesium
	  ◦ Magnesium gluconate: 1,000 mg/5 mL contains 58.5 mg elemental magnesium
	  ◦ Oral magnesium can cause diarrhea		

Calcium (Ca^{2+})			
Hypercalcemia			
Signs and symptoms	• Obtundation • Confusion • Lethargy • Decreased deep tendon reflexes • Myalgias • Decreased muscle strength • Shortened QT interval on the ECG		

(continued)

Treatment	Increase renal elimination • Hydration with NSS to stimulate diuresis (4–6 L NSS to achieve goal urine output of 3–5 L in 24 hours); can also administer furosemide, 40–80 mg IV every 1 to 2 hours, to avoid fluid overload) Shift Ca^{2+} into bone 1. Calcitonin 2. Bisphosphonates a. Etidronate disodium 7.5 mg/kg IV every 8 hours (with NSS hydration) b. Pamidronate disodium, 15 mg in 250 mL NSS once daily c. Gallium nitrate, 200 mg/m^2 continuous infusion for 5 days (with NSS hydration; avoid aminoglycosides ≥48 hours before or after administration)
Monitoring	• Serum calcium, magnesium, phosphorus, creatinine, albumin • Use of ionized calcium is preferred in acutely ill patients to corrected calcium calculations
Hypocalcemia	
Signs and symptoms	• Paresthesias • Tetany • Positive Chvostek/Trousseau (suggestive) • Increased QT interval on ECG
Treatment	**Ionized Calcium (mmol/L)** — **Dose Calcium Gluconate IV** 1–1.12 — 1–2 g 0.9–0.99 — 2 g 0.89–0.89 — 3 g Administration: Mix in 100–250 mL NSS or D5W. Rate: 1–2 g/h
Monitoring	• Check serum Mg since hypomagnesemia can induce hypocalcemia • Recheck serum Ca 2–24 hours after dose
Notes	• Serum calcium falls ~0.8 mg/dL for every 1 g/dL fall in serum albumin <4 • Use of ionized calcium is preferred in acutely ill patients to correct calcium calculations • Doses are provided as calcium gluconate. For medication safety, it is important to note the different elemental calcium content between calcium gluconate and chloride: ◦ Gluconate: 1 g (10 mL) = 93 mg (4.65 mEq) Ca^{2+} ◦ Chloride: 1 g (10 mL) = 273 mg (13.6 mEq) Ca^{2+} • Oral calcium replacement products • Calcium carbonate tablet: 1,250 mg contains 500 mg elemental calcium (40%) ◦ Calcium carbonate chewable tablet: 750 mg contains 300 mg elemental calcium (40%) ◦ Calcium carbonate suspension: 1,250 mg/5 mL contains 500 mg elemental calcium/5 mL (40%) ◦ Calcium glubionate syrup: 1,800 mg/5 mL contains 126 mg elemental calcium/5 mL (6.5%)

TABLE 10.14 Hyperelectrolyte and Hypoelectrolyte Therapy *(continued)*

Phosphate (PO_4^-)				
Hyperphosphatemia				
Signs and symptoms	Increased risk of ectopic calcification when serum calcium and phosphorus exceed 55 mg^2/dL^2			
Treatment (based on end-stage renal disease [ESRD] studies; adjust the dose to achieve the goal level)	**Per Meal**	**Phos mg/dL**		
	Initial Dose	>5.5–<7.5	≥7.5–<9	≥9
	Calcium acetate, 667 mg tab	1	2	3
	Sevelamar, 400 mg tab	2	3	4
	Sevelamar, 800 mg tab	1	2	2
Monitoring	Serum phosphorous, calcium, and creatinine			
Hypophosphatemia				
Signs and symptoms	• Decreased mentation • Weakness • Cardiomyopathy • Tachypnea • Osteomalacia • Decreased insulin sensitivity • Dysfunction of red blood cells, white blood cells, and platelets			
Treatment	**Serum Phosphorous (mg/dL)**	**Dose Sodium or Potassium Phosphate IV**		
	2.3–3	0.16 mmol/kg		
	1.6–2.2	0.32 mmol/kg		
	<1.6	0.64 mmol/kg		
	Administration: Mix in 100–250 mL NSS or D5W. Rate: maximum of 7.5 mmol/h			
Monitoring	• Serum phosphorus, calcium, creatinine, potassium • 9.15 SSRI = selective serotonin reuptake inhibitor			

(continued)

TABLE 10.14 Hyperelectrolyte and Hypoelectrolyte Therapy *(continued)*

Notes	• Use sodium phosphate if serum K^+ is >4 mEq/L • Each 3 mmol IV phosphate salt contains either 4.4 mEq K^+ or 4 mEq Na^+ • Reduce dose in renal impairment (usually by ~50% depending on renal function and need) • Oral phosphorous replacement products: ∘ Potassium and sodium phosphate powder contains 8 mmol phosphorous, 7.1 mEq K, and 7.1 mEq Na per packet; dissolve in 75 mL water ∘ Potassium phosphate powder contains 8 mmol phosphorus and 14.25 mEq K per packet; dissolve in 75 mL water ∘ Sodium phosphate oral solution contains 4.14 mmol phosphorus/mL and 4.8 mEq of Na/mL; dilute in 120 mL water ∘ Oral phosphate can cause diarrhea

Sources: Lau A. Fluid and electrolyte disorders. In: Koda-Kimble MA, Young LY, Kradjan WA, et al., eds. *Applied Therapeutics: The Clinical Use of Drugs.* 8th ed. Philadelphia, PA: Lippincott Williams & Wilkins; 2005:12-1–12-3; Lau A, Chan LN. Electrolytes, other minerals, and trace elements. In: Lee M, ed. *Basic Skills in Interpreting Laboratory Data.* 3rd ed. Bethesda, MD: American Society of Health-System Pharmacists; 2004:183–232; Dickerson RN. Guidelines for the intravenous management of hypophosphatemia, hypomagnesemia, hypokalemia, and hypocalcemia. *Hosp Pharm.* 2001;36:1201–1208; Brown KA, Dickerson RN, Morgan LM, et al. A new graduated dosing regimen for phosphorus replacement in patients receiving nutrition support. *JPEN J Parenter Enteral Nutr.* 2006;30: 209–214; Baran DR, Aronin N. Disorders of mineral metabolism. In: Irwin RS, Rippe JM, eds. *Intensive Care Medicine.* 6th ed. Philadelphia, PA: Lippincott Williams & Wilkins; 2008:1287–1293; Cohen AJ. Physiologic concepts in the management of renal, fluid, and electrolyte disorders in the intensive care unit. In: Irwin RS, Rippe JM, eds. *Care Medicine.* 6th ed. Philadelphia, PA: Lippincott Williams & Wilkins; 2008:867–883; Black RM, Noroian GO. Disorders of plasma sodium and plasma potassium. In: Irwin RS, Rippe JM, eds. *Intensive Care Medicine.* 6th ed. Philadelphia, PA: Lippincott Williams & Wilkins; 2008:898–925; Driscoll DF, Bistrian BR. Parenteral and enteral nutrition in the intensive care unit. In: Irwin RS, Rippe JM, eds. *Intensive Care Medicine.* 6th ed. Philadelphia, PA: Lippincott Williams & Wilkins; 2008:2186–2201; and Renagel [package insert]. Cambridge, MA: Genzyme Corporation; 1998.[16]

TABLE 10.15 Select Medications Associated with Electrolyte Disorders

	Drugs Associated with Hyperelectrolyte Condition	Drugs Associated with Hypoelectrolyte Condition
Sodium (Na^+)	• Sodium polystyrene sulfonate–exchange resin • Sodium (in IV fluids, parenteral and enteral nutrition) • Sodium bicarbonate	• Diuretics—loops, thiazides, SSRIs
Potassium (K^+)	• Angiotensin-converting enzyme inhibitors (ACEI) • Beta-adrenergic antagonists • Dapsone • Diuretics—K^+-sparing (amiloride, spirinolactone, triamterene) • Heparin • IV fluids containing K^+ • Nonsteroidal anti-inflammatory drugs (NSAIDs) • Penicillin (K^+ salt form) • Potassium (in IV fluids, parenteral and enteral nutrition) • Trimethoprim	• Acetazolamide • Amphotericin B • Beta-adrenergic agonists • Cisplatin • Corticosteroids • Diuretics—thiazides, loops • Insulin • Laxative abuse • Penicillins
Magnesium (Mg^{2+})	• Magnesium-containing antacids and bowel evacuant preparations	• Aminoglycosides • Cisplatin • Ethanol • Loop diuretics
Phosphate (PO_4^-)	• Phosphate-containing bowel evacuation preparations	• Antacids (containing aluminum, magnesium, and calcium) • Epinephrine • Insulin • Loop diuretics • Sevalemer • Sucralfate • Thiazide diuretics
Calcium (Ca^{2+})	• Androgenic hormones • Calcium (in antacids and supplements) • Estrogen • Lithium • Progesterone • Tamoxifen • Thiazide diuretics	• Bisphosphonates • Calcitonin • Glucocorticoids • Loop diuretics • Plicamycin

Sources: Lau A. Fluid and electrolyte disorders. In: Koda-Kimble MA, Young LY, Kradjan WA, et al., eds. *Applied Therapeutics: The Clinical Use of Drugs.* 8th ed. Philadelphia, PA: Lippincott Williams & Wilkins; 2005:12-1–12-3; Lau A, Chan LN. Electrolytes, other minerals, and trace elements. In: Lee M, ed. *Basic Skills in Interpreting Laboratory Data.* 3rd ed. Bethesda, MD: American Society of Health-System Pharmacists; 2004:183–232; Dickerson RN. Guidelines for the intravenous management of hypophosphatemia, hypomagnesemia, hypokalemia, and hypocalcemia. *Hosp Pharm.* 2001;36:1201–1208; Baran DR, Aronin N. Disorders of mineral metabolism. In: Irwin RS, Rippe JM, eds. *Intensive Care Medicine.* 6th ed. Philadelphia, PA: Lippincott Williams & Wilkins; 2008:1287–1293; and Black RM, Noroian GO. Disorders of plasma sodium and plasma potassium. In: Irwin RS, Rippe JM, eds. *Intensive Care Medicine.* 6th ed. Philadelphia, PA: Lippincott Williams & Wilkins; 2008:898–925.

References

1. Lau A. Fluid and electrolyte disorders. In: Koda-Kimble MA, Young LY, Kradjan WA, et al., eds. *Applied Therapeutics: The Clinical Use of Drugs*. 8th ed. Philadelphia, PA: Lippincott Williams & Wilkins; 2005: 12-1–12-33.
2. Segar WE, Holliday MA. The maintenance need for water in parenteral fluid therapy. *Pediatrics*. 1957;19:823–832.
3. Chicella MF, Hak EB. Pediatric nutrition. In: Koda-Kimble MA, Young LY, Kradjan WA, et al., eds. *Applied Therapeutics: The Clinical Use of Drugs*. 8th ed. Philadelphia, PA: Lippincott Williams & Wilkins; 2005:97-1–97-22.
4. Trombetta DP. The kidneys. In: Lee M, ed. *Basic Skills in Interpreting Laboratory Data*. 5th ed. Bethesda, MD: American Society of Health-System Pharmacists; 2012:175–192.
5. Dellinger RP, Carlet JM, Masur H, et al. Surviving Sepsis Campaign guidelines for management of severe sepsis and septic shock. *Crit Care Med*. 2004;32(3):858–873.
6. Metabolic Alkalosis: Acid–base Regulation and Disorders. Merck Manual Professional Web site. Available at: www.merck.com/mmpe/sec12/ch157/ch157d.html. Accessed March 18, 2008.
7. Tham Solution [package insert]. Abbott Park, IL: Abbott Laboratories; 2000.
8. Kraus D. Interpreting pediatric laboratory data. In: Lee M, ed. *Basic Skills in Interpreting Laboratory Data*. 5th ed. Bethesda, MD: American Society of Health-System Pharmacists; 2012:521–544.
9. Lau A, Chan LN. Electrolytes, other minerals, and trace elements. In: Lee M, ed. *Basic Skills in Interpreting Laboratory Data*. 3rd ed. Bethesda, MD: American Society of Health-System Pharmacists; 2004:183–232.
10. Dickerson RN. Guidelines for the intravenous management of hypophosphatemia, hypomagnesemia, hypokalemia, and hypocalcemia. *Hosp Pharm*. 2001;36:1201–1208.
11. Brown KA, Dickerson RN, Morgan LM, et al. A new graduated dosing regimen for phosphorus replacement in patients receiving nutrition support. *JPEN J Parenter Enteral Nutr*. 2006;30:209–214.
12. Baran DR, Aronin N. Disorders of mineral metabolism. In: Irwin RS, Rippe JM, eds. *Intensive Care Medicine*. 6th ed. Philadelphia, PA: Lippincott Williams & Wilkins; 2008:1287–1293.
13. Cohen AJ. Physiologic concepts in the management of renal, fluid, and electrolyte disorders in the intensive care unit. In: Irwin RS, Rippe JM, eds. *Intensive Care Medicine*. 6th ed. Philadelphia, PA: Lippincott Williams & Wilkins; 2008:867–883.
14. Black RM, Noroian GO. Disorders of plasma sodium and plasma potassium. In: Irwin RS, Rippe JM, eds. *Intensive Care Medicine*. 6th ed. Philadelphia, PA: Lippincott Williams & Wilkins; 2008:898–925.

15. Driscoll DF, Bistrian BR. Parenteral and enteral nutrition in the intensive care unit. In: Irwin RS, Rippe JM, eds. *Intensive Care Medicine*. 6th ed. Philadelphia, PA: Lippincott Williams & Wilkins; 2008:2186–2201.
16. Renagel [package insert]. Cambridge, MA: Genzyme Corporation; 1998.

11

Enteral Nutrition

Gordon Sacks and Diana Wells

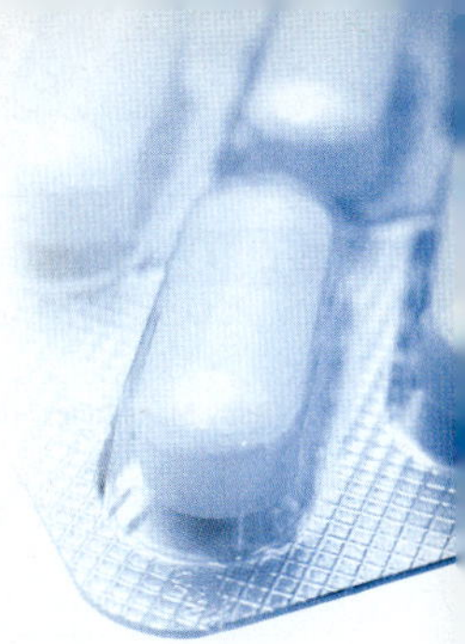

Nutritional Assessment

Nutritional assessment consists of evaluations, including patient history, physical examination, and laboratory parameters (Tables 11.1, 11.2, and 11.3). An International Consensus Guideline Committee has proposed an etiology-based approach for diagnosing adult malnutrition (Fig. 11.1). To make the diagnosis of malnutrition, identification of two or more characteristics found in Table 11.4 is recommended. Alternative methods of evaluating nutritional status include use of Subjective Global Assessment (SGA) and the Mini Nutritional Assessment (MNA®).[1–4] Physical findings of malnutrition are listed in Table 11.5. In pediatric

TABLE 11.1 Nutritional Assessment

Evaluation	Purpose
Medical and surgical history	Underlying pathology, medications, and risk factors related to nutritional status
Dietary history	Accurate food intake, weight changes, and possible food allergies
Physical examination	Lean body mass (LBM) and vitamin deficiencies
Laboratory parameters	Electrolyte abnormalities
Anthropometric measurements	Protein and fat stores
Subjective Global Assessment	Nutrition-related disease
Mini Nutritional Assessment	Nutrition-related disease

Sources: Hammond K. History and physical examination. In: Matarese LE, Gottschlich MM, eds. *Contemporary Nutrition Support Practice: A Clinical Guide*. Philadelphia, PA: WB Saunders; 1998:17–32; Mueller C, Compher C, Ellen DM, and ASPEN Board of Directors. ASPEN Clinical Guidelines: nutrition screening, assessment, and intervention in adults. *JPEN J Parenter Enteral Nutr*. 2011;35(1):16–24.

TABLE 11.2 Anthropometric Measurements: Body Mass Index

Body Mass Index[a] (kg/m^2)	Classification
<18.5	Underweight
18.5–24.9	Normal
>25.0	Overweight
25.0–29.9	Overweight
30.0–34.9	Obesity Class I
35.0–39.9	Obesity Class II
>40.0	Obesity Class III

[a]Body mass index = weight (kg)/height (m^2).
Adapted from World Health Organization Technical Report Series; 894. *Obesity: Preventing and Managing the Global Evidence: Report of a WHO Consultation.* Geneva, Switzerland: World Health Organization; 2004 (reprint). http://www.who.int/nutrition/publications/obesity/WHO_TRS_894/en, accessed October 28, 2013.

patients, height/length ratios are compared to age-related percentiles to establish malnutrition. External head dimension is an additional parameter useful in evaluating the nutritional status of infants (Table 11.6).[5,6]

Laboratory Parameters to Monitor[7]

- Serum electrolytes
- Blood glucose
- Cholesterol panel, including triglycerides
- Liver function tests
- Renal function tests

TABLE 11.3 Anthropometric Measurements: Body Composition

Body Composition[a]	Male	Female
Tricep skinfold (mm)	12.5	16.5
Midarm muscle circumference (cm)	29.3	28.5

[a]Tricep skinfold measures fat reserve. Midarm muscle circumference measures protein reserve.
Adapted from Blackburn GL, Bistrian BR, Maini BS, et al. Nutritional and metabolic assessment of the hospitalized patient. *JPEN J Parenter Enteral Nutr.* 1977;1(1):11–22.

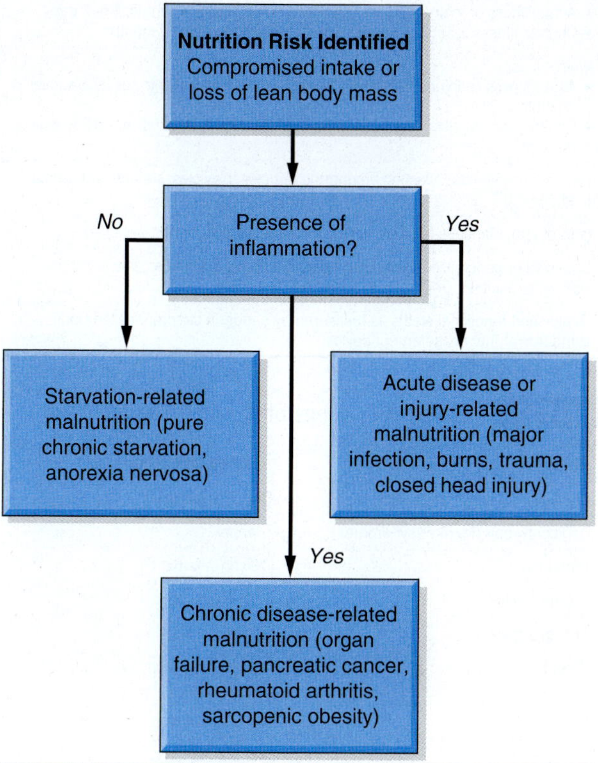

FIGURE 11.1 Nutrition care algorithm. (Adapted from White JV, Guenter P, Jensen G, et al.; the Academy Malnutrition Work Group, the ASPEN Malnutrition Task Force, the ASPEN Board of Directors. Consensus statement: Academy of Nutrition and Dietetics and the American Society for Parenteral and Enteral Nutrition: characteristics recommended for the identification and documentation of adult malnutrition (undernutrition). JPEN *J Parenter Enteral Nutr*. 2012;36:275–283. Reprinted by Permission of SAGE Publications.)

- Complete blood cell (CBC) count
- Prothrombin time (PT)
- Visceral Proteins (Table 11.7)[8]

(*Text continued on page 392*)

TABLE 11.4 Malnutrition Characteristics

Insufficient energy intake • Acute illness or injury: ≤50–75 estimated energy requirement for >5–7 days • Chronic illness: ≤75% estimated energy requirement for ≥1 month
Weight loss • Acute illness or injury: ≥2% over 1 week, ≥5% over 1 month, or ≥7.5% over 3 months • Chronic illness: ≥5% over 1 month, ≥7.5% over 3 months, or ≥10% over 6 months
Loss of muscle mass: wasting around the temples, clavicles, shoulders, scapula, thigh, or calf
Loss of subcutaneous fat: loss around the eyes, triceps, or ribs
Localized or generalized fluid accumulation: around extremities, vulvar/scrotal edema, or ascites
Diminished functional status as measured by handgrip strength: based upon standards of the measurement device

TABLE 11.5 Physical Findings of Nutrient Deficiencies

Finding	Nutrient Deficiency
Cheilosis	Niacin, riboflavin
Corkscrew hair (Menkes syndrome)	Copper
Dementia	Niacin, vitamin B_{12}
Enlarged parotids	Protein, bulimia
Enlarged thyroid	Iodine
Glossitis	Niacin, riboflavin, folic acid, iron, vitamin B_{12}
Growth retardation	Protein, calories, vitamin A
Heart failure	Thiamine
Hepatomegaly	Protein
Loss of weight, muscle mass, or fat stores	Protein, calories
Magenta tongue	Riboflavin
Nail plate and hair appear dull, lusterless	Protein
Poor wound/ulcer healing	Protein, vitamin C, zinc
Psychomotor decline/mental confusion	Protein
Rickets	Vitamin D, calcium
Swollen, painful joints	Vitamin C
Tetany	Calcium, magnesium

Adapted from Hammond K. History and physical examination. In: Matarese LE, Gottschlich MM, eds. *Contemporary Nutrition Support Practice: A Clinical Guide.* Philadelphia, PA: WB Saunders; 1998:17–32.

TABLE 11.6 Anthropometric Measurements: Pediatrics

Age	Weight (g/day)	Height (cm/month)	Head Circumference (cm/week)
0–3 months	24–35	2.8–3.4	0.5
3–6 months	15–21	1.7–2.4	0.5
6–12 months	10–13	1.3–1.6	0.5
1–3 years	5–9	0.6–1.0	—
4–6 years	5–6	0.5–0.6	—
7–10 years	7–11	0.4–0.5	—

Adapted from Chessman KH, Kumpf VJ. Assessment of nutrition status and nutrition requirements. In: DiPiro JT, Talbert RL, Yee GC, eds. *Pharmacotherapy: A Pathophysiologic Approach*. 6th ed. New York, NY: McGraw-Hill; 2005:2559–2578; Davis AM. Pediatrics. In: Matarese LE, Gottschlich MM, eds. *Contemporary Nutrition Support Practice: A Clinical Guide*. Philadelphia, PA: WB Saunders; 1998:347–364.

TABLE 11.7 Laboratory Parameters

Visceral Proteins	Normal Range	Half-Life	Severe Malnutrition
Serum Protein			
Albumin[a]	3.5–5.0 g/dL	20 days	<2.1 g/dL
Fibronectin	220–400 mg/L	15 hours	Variable
Thyroxine-binding prealbumin[b]	15.7–29.6 mg/dL	2–3	<5 mg/dL
Retinol-binding protein	3–6 mg/dL	12 hours	<2.4 mg/dL
Somatomedin C (insulin-like growth factor)	0.1–0.4 mg/L	2 hours	Variable
Transferrin[c]	200–400 mg/dL	8–10 days	<100 mg/dL

[a]Decreased in the setting of infection, inflammation, or fluid overload; increased in the setting of dehydration.
[b]Decreased in the setting of infection or inflammation; increased in the setting of renal failure or corticosteroid administration.
[c]Decreased in the setting of infection, inflammation, or iron-deficiency anemia.
Source: Russell MK, McAdams PM. Laboratory monitoring of nutritional status. In: Matarese LE, Gottschlich MM, eds. *Contemporary Nutrition Support Practice: A Clinical Guide*. Philadelphia, PA: WB Saunders; 1998:47–64.

Serum albumin is most commonly used to assess protein nutritional status, but it is of limited usefulness in determining acute nutritional changes because albumin has a long half-life. Proteins with shorter half-lives are used increasingly for monitoring improvements in protein malnutrition.[8]

- Nitrogen balance may be an indicator of the patient's catabolic state (Eq. 11.1). It is often used to assess the efficacy of nutrition support.[9]
- A 24-hour urine collection is often necessary to determine the amount of nitrogen excreted.
- Use this equation with caution because in some patient populations, nitrogen excretion may be over- or underestimated.

Calculation of Nitrogen Balance[9]

$$\begin{aligned}&\text{Nitrogen Balance} = \text{Nitrogen Intake} - \text{Nitrogen Output}\\&\text{Nitrogen Intake} = 24\text{-hour protein intake} / 6.25\\&\text{Nitrogen Output} = \left(\text{UUN}^{*}\ \text{g}/24\ \text{hour}\right) - 4^{\dagger}\end{aligned} \tag{11.1}$$

*UUN, urine urea nitrogen.
†The constant factor of 4 represents an estimated 2 g from GI and respiratory losses and 2 g derived from nonurea nitrogen losses (i.e., ammonia, uric acid, creatinine).

Enteral Nutrition

Enteral nutrition (EN) is a method of providing nutritional support to patients with normal gastrointestinal (GI) function who are unable to eat to meet metabolic demands.

- EN is preferred over parenteral nutrition because it is safe, effective, and economical for patients.[10]
- Administered by tube or mouth, enteral products can serve as the sole source of nutritional support, as a dietary supplement to oral intake, or as an adjunct during transition from parenteral to oral feedings.[10]
- EN is warranted if the GI tract is functioning and additional nutritional intake is needed.[11]
- Indications and contraindications for enteral nutrition are listed in Tables 11.8 and 11.9.
- A wide variety of dietary terms are used to describe nutrition plans for patients.
- Commonly prescribed diets are described in Table 11.10.

TABLE 11.8 Indications for Enteral Nutrition

Acquired immunodeficiency syndrome
Anorexia nervosa
Carcinoma with severe weight loss
Correction of malnutrition secondary to chronic disease
Endotracheal intubation
Esophageal stricture
Handicapping conditions
Hypermetabolic state (i.e., severe burn or trauma)
Inborn errors of metabolism
Neurologic disorders
Oral or esophageal injury
Severely impaired growth and development
Swallowing difficulties/dysphagia

Sources: Davis AM. Pediatrics. In: Matarese LE, Gottschlich MM, eds. *Contemporary Nutrition Support Practice: A Clinical Guide*. Philadelphia, PA: WB Saunders; 1998:347–364; Cresci G, Lefton J, Esper DH. Enteral formulations. In: Mueller CM, ed. *The ASPEN Adult Nutrition Support Core Curriculum*. 2nd ed. Silver Spring, MD: American Society for Parenteral and Enteral Nutrition; 2012:185–205; and Kumpf VJ, Chessman KH. Enteral nutrition. In: DiPiro JT, Talbert RL, Yee GC, et al., eds. *Pharmacotherapy: A Pathophysiologic Approach*. 6th ed. New York, NY: McGraw-Hill; 2005:2615–2634.

TABLE 11.9 Contraindications for Enteral Nutrition

GI hemorrhage
GI obstruction
High output enterocutaneous fistula (i.e., >500 mL/day)
Intestinal ischemia
Intractable diarrhea or vomiting despite medical therapy
Nutritional intervention not warranted
Paralytic ileus
Peritonitis
Severe malabsorption
Short bowel syndrome with a <100-cm small bowel remaining with malabsorption

Adapted from Brantley SL, Mills ME. Overview of Enteral Nutrition. In: Mueller CM, ed. *The A.S.P.E.N. Adult Nutrition Support Core Curriculum*. 2nd Ed. Silver Spring, MD: American Society for Parenteral and Enteral Nutrition; 2012:173 with permission from the American Society for Parenteral and Enteral Nutrition (A.S.P.E.N.).

TABLE 11.10 Types of Oral Diets

Type	Description	Indication	Example
Clear liquid	Provides fluid and calories; low in irritants and contains foods that require minimal digestion	Prior to diagnostic tests or bowel surgery; recovery phase after surgery; transition from nothing by mouth to more advanced diet	Fat-free clear broth, tea, coffee, plain flavored gelatin, carbonated beverages, hard candy, clear fruit juices, popsicles
Full liquid	Provides adequate calories and protein; requires minimal chewing and digestion	Difficulty swallowing, chewing, or digesting sold foods; transition to more advanced diet	Blenderized foods, such as soup; all liquids allowed
Pureed	Provides adequate nutrition; facilitates ingestion of food with no chewing	Very limited chewing ability; severe mouth sore; motor deficits; esophageal strictures; head and neck surgery; transition to more advanced diet	Solid foods moistened and blended to a mashed potato like consistency; all liquids allowed
Soft mechanical	Provides adequate nutrition; facilitates ingestion of solid foods with minimal chewing	Difficulty chewing and/or swallowing whole foods	Solid foods softened or moistened; all liquids allowed
General	Meets nutritional needs for maintenance, repair, growth, and development	All patients not requiring restrictions, modifications, or special additions to their dietary regimen	All foods are allowed; milk products, meat, bread and cereal products, fruits and vegetables, saturated and unsaturated fats, and added sugar

Enteral Nutrition Products

In general, EN products are selected after a thorough and complete assessment of the patient's digestive/absorptive state and fluid and electrolyte demands.

- Commonly available EN products are described in Table 11.11.[12,13]
- Starting EN within 24 to 48 hours after severe injury has positive effects, whereas postponing it for 4 to 5 days may be too late to achieve reduced infectious complications.[14]

(*Text continued on page 397*)

TABLE 11.11 Profile of Enteral Nutrition Products

Type	Description	Indication	Example
Adult			
Standard without fiber	Isotonic; 1–1.2 kcal/mL; may contain fiber; not sweetened	Most patient populations; generally for tube feeding only (not palatable for oral supplementation)	Isosource HN (No), Osmolite (MJ), Fibersource HN (No), Jevity (R)
High protein	NPC:N <125:1; may contain fiber	Critically ill (i.e., trauma, burn); pressure sores; surgical wounds; high fistula output	Isosource VHN (No), Replete (N), Promote with Fiber (R)
Concentrated	Hypertonic; 1.5–2 kcal/mL; low electrolyte content	Fluid restriction (i.e., cardiac, renal, pulmonary, or hepatic failure)	Isosource 1.5 (No), Osmolite 1.5 (N), Resource 2.0 (No), TwoCal HN (R)
Peptide-based	Protein supplied in the form of dipeptides and tripeptides; higher fat content supplied as MCT	Intolerance to standard formulations due to malabsorption; chronic pancreatitis; cystic fibrosis; celiac disease	Peptinex DT (No), Perative (R), Peptamen (N), Subdue (MJ)
Diabetic	Isotonic; 1–1.2 kcal/mL; High fat, low carbohydrate	Hyperglycemia; limited evidence	Glucerna (R), Resource Diabetic (No), Glytrol (N)
Hepatic	Hypertonic; 1.2–1.5 kcal/mL; high BCAA:AAA	Grade II or greater encephalopathy; not for use in the absence of encephalopathy	Nutri-Hep (N)
Immune modulating	Contains glutamine, arginine, nucleotides, and/or omega-3 fatty acids	Critically ill (i.e., trauma, burn, sepsis), perioperative	Impact with Glutamine (No), Perative (R), Crucial (N), AlitraQ (R)
Pulmonary	1.5 kcal/mL; contains omega-3 fatty acids, gamma-linolenic acid, and antioxidants	Acute respiratory distress syndrome	Oxepa (R)

(continued)

TABLE 11.11 Profile of Enteral Nutrition Products *(continued)*

Type	Description	Indication	Example
Renal	Hypertonic; caloric dense (2 kcal/mL); moderate protein; low electrolyte and mineral content	Renal failure with difficult to control electrolyte and mineral; not for dialyzed patients	Nepro (R), Novasource Renal (No); Renalcal (N)
Pediatric			
Standard	Isotonic; 0.8–1 kcal/mL; contains at least one source of cow milk; may contain fiber	Children 1–10 years	Enfamil Kindercal (MJ), PediaSure (R), Kindercal with Fiber (MJ), PediaSure with Fiber (R)
	0.8–1 kcal/mL	Children 1–10 years with malabsorption, cow's milk protein allergy	Neocate One + (SHS), EleCare (R), Peptamen Jr (N), Vital Jr (R), Tolerex (No)
Cow's milk-based	Isotonic; 0.67–0.8 kcal/mL; carbohydrate source is lactose (lactose-free formulations are available); high iron content	Term infants	Enfamil LIPIL (MJ), Enfamil Lactofree LIPIL (MJ), Similac Advance (R), Similac Lactose Free Advance (R)
Soy-based lactose-free	Hypotonic; 0.67 kcal/mL; cow milk protein and lactose free	Term infants who have allergies, lactose intolerance, or galactosemia	Enfamil ProSobee LIPIL (MJ), Similac Isomil Advance (R)
Preterm	Isotonic; 0.67–0.8 kcal/mL; easily digested	Preterm infants <2–3 kg	Enfamil Premature LIPIL (MJ), Similac Care Advance 20 Advance (R), Similac Care Advance 24 Advance (R)

NPC:N, nonprotein calorie:nitrogen ratio; MCT, medium-chain triglyceride; BCAA:AAA, branched-chain amino acids:aromatic amino acids; M, Mead Johnson Nutritionals; R, Ross Products; N, Nestle Clinical Nutrition; No, Novartis; SHS, SHS International Ltd.

Adapted from Kumpf VJ, Chessman KH. Enteral nutrition. In: DiPiro JT, Talbert RL, Yee GC, eds. *Pharmacotherapy: A Pathophysiologic Approach.* 6th ed. New York, NY: McGraw-Hill; 2005:2615–2634; and Carlson SJ. Enteral formulations. In: Merritt R, ed-in-chief, DeLegge MH, Holcombe B, Mueller C, et al., eds. Guenter P, managing ed., *The ASPEN Nutrition Support Practice Manual.* 2nd ed. Silver Spring, MD: American Society for Parenteral and Enteral Nutrition; 2005:63–75.

- EN may be delivered via numerous routes depending on the patient's clinical condition (see Table 11.12)[12]:
  - Nasogastric (placed from the nose into the stomach)
  - Gastrostomy (stoma created from the abdominal wall into the stomach)
  - Jejunostomy (stoma created from the abdominal wall into the jejunum)[11]
- Complications of EN are GI, metabolic, and mechanical (see Table 11.13).[2,15,16]

Administration of Enteral Nutrition

The proper administration of EN products is important to achieve and enhance patient tolerance. The following points should be considered when administering a particular product.

- Continuous drip given over a 24-hour period is the preferred method for administration of tube feedings in the hospital setting.
- Potential complications associated with tube feedings (e.g., hyperglycemia, pulmonary aspiration, and diarrhea) can be reduced by continuous feedings.
- Bolus feedings are an option if the feeding tube is in the stomach and previous feedings have been well tolerated.

Initiation of Enteral Feedings (Table 11.14)

To initiate a continuous tube feeding

1. Perform an abdominal examination. Presence of abdominal distention, nausea, bloating, and bowel sounds should be evaluated.
2. Placement of the tube should be confirmed by insufflation with air or aspiration of stomach or small bowel contents. Radiologic verification of the tube may also be used.
3. After determination of final goal rate based on energy requirements, continuous feeding may be initiated. If the patient has a gastric tube, start enteral feeding at 25 mL/h. If the tube is in the small bowel, start feeding at 25 mL/h.
4. If the tube is in the stomach, perform an abdominal examination and check gastric residuals every 4 hours. Feedings may be increased by 25 mL/h every 4 to 6 hours, if the feeding is tolerated,

(*Text continued on page 401*)

TABLE 11.12 Types of Feeding Tubes

Type	Location	Indications	Advantages	Disadvantages
Nasogastric	Stomach	Normal gastric emptying Short term (<30 days)	Easily placed at bedside Allows intermittent and bolus feeding	Aspiration risk Discomfort to the patient
Nasoduodenal/nasojejunal	Small bowel	Impaired gastric emptying Short term (<30 days)	Easily placed at bedside Reduced aspiration risk	Risk of misplacement Requires placement verification Discomfort to the patient
Percutaneous gastrostomy/ open gastrostomy	Stomach	Normal gastric emptying Long term	Allows intermittent and bolus feeding	Surgical risk Aspiration risk Requires stoma site care
Percutaneous jejunostomy/ open jejunostomy	Small bowel	Postoperative feeding Impaired gastric emptying Long term	Reduced aspiration risk	Continuous and cyclic feeding only Requires stoma site care

Source: Kumpf VJ, Chessman KH. Enteral nutrition. In: DiPiro JT, Talbert RL, Yee GC, eds. *Pharmacotherapy: A Pathophysiologic Approach*. 6th ed. New York, NY: McGraw-Hill; 2005:2615–2634.

TABLE 11.13 Tube Feeding Complications

Complication	Causes	Management
Gastrointestinal		
Diarrhea (most common)	Bacterial contamination of formula; improper administration; use of antibiotics; lactose intolerance; impaction; malnutrition; liquid drug formulations containing sorbitol; bowel infection from *C. difficile* and pseudomembranous colitis	Discard tubing after 24 hours; use only 8–12 hours of feeding; use isotonic formula at a tolerable rate by continuous delivery; avoid or recognize drugs causing diarrhea; avoid lactose containing formulas; rule out impaction before treating diarrhea; use elemental formula; add fiber to formula
Constipation	Low residue formula used in long-term, tube-fed patients, dehydration	Provide additional fluids by mouth or tube feeding; increase ambulation or use a high-fiber, high-residue formula; administer bulking agents (psyllium); administer laxatives
Bloating	Presence of a mild ileus; intolerance to lipids in formula; swallowing excessive amounts of air (e.g., head and neck surgery)	Use formulas with no fiber; increase ambulation; administer laxative; start promotility agents; check gastric residuals
Inadequate gastric emptying	Gastric atony, prepyloric ulcers, bowel ileus; drugs such as theophylline, dopamine, anticholinergics, calcium channel blockers, and narcotics that relax the lower esophageal sphincter	Verify tube placement; monitor stomach content residuals before bolus feedings or every 2–4 hours during continuous feedings
Vomiting	Psychological association with the illness; unpleasant odor of formulas containing free amino acids or the reinstilling of large amounts of aspirated gastric residuals	Reduce anxiety; use intact protein containing formulas or antiemetic when indicated; reduce the rate of delivery; feed beyond the pylorus; slowly advance the feeding rate
Nausea	Delayed gastric emptying; gastric distention; formula too hot or too cold, or given too rapidly	Stop feedings and determine cause; check gastric residual to determine the progress of gastric emptying after 1–2 hours; restart feedings at slower rate and slowly advance

(continued)

TABLE 11.13 Tube Feeding Complications *(continued)*

Complication	Causes	Management
Metabolic		
Hyperglycemia	Common in patients who are diabetic, hypermetabolic, or receiving corticosteroids	Check blood glucose and frequently with advancing enteral feedings; administer insulin as needed; hydrate the patient or change to a lower-carbohydrate content formula
Electrolyte disturbance	Fluid imbalance; medication use; renal insufficiency; feeding formulation	Monitor fluid intake and output and serum chemistries; replace electrolytes as necessary
Mechanical		
Tube obstruction	Formula with a caloric density of 1.5–2.0 kcal/mL; inadequate crushing of medications or inadequate dilution/flushing of psyllium or antacids	Use feeding pumps for dense formulas and/or larger-bore feeding tubes; give medications as elixirs; flush tube with 30 mL of water after medications; use pancreatic enzymes
Displacement	Vomiting; cough; incorrect tube placement; detached tape holding tube to nose	Check tube placement by x-ray; listen for air being injected through the tube into the stomach with a stethoscope, followed by aspiration of a small amount of gastric contents
Irritation	Esophageal reflux, peptic esophagitis; pressure necrosis of esophageal and tracheal wall at cuff inflation site	Provide nose and mouth care; change tape; increase salivation in the mouth by allowing chewing gum, hard candy, or ice chips
Aspiration	Gastric contents refluxing into bronchus secondary to delayed gastric emptying; improper placement of tube in tracheal or bronchus; incompetent lower esophageal sphincter	Place feeding tube beyond the pylorus; use small, soft feeding tube; keep maximum gastric content residuals to <250 mL; raise head of bead to 45 degrees

Sources: Mueller C, Compher C, Ellen DM, and ASPEN Board of Directors. ASPEN Clinical Guidelines: nutrition screening, assessment, and intervention in adults. *JPEN J Parenter Enteral Nutr.* 2011;35(1):16–24; Malone AM, Seres D, Lord L. Complications of enteral nutrition. In: Mueller CM, ed. *The ASPEN Adult Nutrition Support Core Curriculum.* 2nd ed. Silver Spring, MD: American Society for Parenteral and Enteral Nutrition; 2012:218–233; Haddad RY, Thomas DR. Enteral nutrition and enteral tube feeding: review of the evidence. *Clin Geriatr Med.* 2002;18(4):867–881.

TABLE 11.14 Initiation of Continuous Enteral Nutrition

Age	Initial Rate	Advance, If Tolerated	Goal Rate
0–12 months[6]	1–2 mL/kg/h	Every 2–8 hours	6 mL/kg/h
1–6 years[6]	1 mL/kg/h	Every 2–8 hours	4–5 mL/kg/h
>6 years[6]	25 mL/h	Every 2–8 hours	100–150 mL/h
Adult—gastric	25 mL/h	Every 4–6 hours	Variable
Adult—jejunal	25 mL/h	Every 24 hours	Variable

Adapted from Davis AM. Pediatrics. In: Matarese LE, Gottschlich MM, eds. *Contemporary Nutrition Support Practice: A Clinical Guide*. Philadelphia, PA: WB Saunders; 1998:347–364.

until the goal rate is achieved. If the tube is in the small bowel, feedings may be increased by 25 mL/h each day until the goal rate is achieved.

5. If diarrhea or abdominal discomfort is present after the advancement of the feeding, the previous rate may be returned to for another 24-hour period.

Monitoring Enteral Nutrition

Once tube feedings are initiated, the patient must be monitored to ascertain efficacy of the nutritional support regimen and to identify and correct intolerance problems, metabolic complications, or other adverse effects (Table 11.15).[17]

Drug–Nutrient Compatibility

Drug–nutrient interactions may occur when medications and EN are given via a tube.

- To avoid potential drug–nutrient incompatibilities, tube feedings should be discontinued and at least 30 mL of water instilled through the tube before and after drug administration.[18,19]
- The most frequent compatibility problems involve strongly acidic or buffered syrups with pH values <4 (Table 11.16).[20]

TABLE 11.15 Monitoring Parameters for Enteral Nutrition

Accurate records of input and output
Evidence of intolerance (abdominal distention/pain, nausea, emesis)
Frequency and consistency of stool output
Laboratory parameters, including serum electrolytes, complete blood count, serum glucose, inflammatory markers (i.e., CRP)
Markers for nutrition status (prealbumin, nitrogen balance)
Physical examination for hydration or nutrient deficiency or excess
Review of medications
Weight trends

Adapted from Marian M, McGinnis C. Overview of enteral nutrition. In: Gottschlich MM, ed. The A.S.P.E.N. Nutrition Support Core Curriculum: A Case-Based Approach-The Adult Patient. Silver Spring, MD: American Society for Parenteral and Enteral Nutrition; 2007:201 with permission from the American Society for Parenteral and Enteral Nutrition (A.S.P.E.N).

TABLE 11.16 Drug–Nutrient Compatibility

Product	Ensure	Osmolite	Vivonex
Acetaminophen elixir	C	C	C
Amphojel	NA	I	C
Bentyl liquid	NA	I	C
Benadryl elixir	C	C	C
Cibalith-S syrup	I	I	C
Dimetapp elixir	I	I	I
Feosol elixir	I	I	C
Guaifenesin liquid	I	I	C
Imodium	NA	C	C
KCl liquid	I	I	I
Lanoxin elixir	C	C	C
Morphine liquid	C	C	C
Phenytoin suspension	I	I	NA
Phenytoin injection	C	C	NA
Sudafed syrup	I	I	C
Thorazine concentrate	I	I	C

C, compatible; I, incompatible; NA, no data available.
Adapted from Sacks GS. Drug-nutrient considerations in patients receiving parenteral and enteral nutrition. *Pract Gastroenterol.* July 2004:39–48.

- Incompatibilities between formulas and drugs can cause immediate clumping, and the increased viscosity and particle size can clog feeding tubes.[20]
- At pH values <5, in vitro clotting has occurred with Pulmocare, Ensure Plus, Osmolite, Enrich, Ensure, and Resource.[21]

Medication Administration[18,19]

Medication dosage forms possess different characteristics that can affect how they are tolerated when administered through enteral feeding tubes.

- Immediate release tablets may be crushed and mixed with water to form a slurry and administered through a feeding tube. Similarly, capsules may be opened and the contents made into a slurry for administration.
- Sublingual, buccal, time-released, or enteric-coated tablets may have an altered therapeutic effect or increased side effects and toxicity when crushed.
- Some medications may be administered as a liquid dosage form. However, liquid dosage forms may have higher osmolality and a significant amount of sorbitol, which increase the possibility of diarrhea.
- See Table 11.17 for examples of medications that should not be given through a tube.

Pediatric Enteral Nutrition

In general, children are at an earlier risk for nutrient deficiencies than adults due to lower energy and protein stores. Therefore, earlier intervention may be required.

- Table 11.6 shows the growth targets of infants and children. Children who are unable to meet these targets may be candidates for nutrition support.[5,6]
- EN is the preferred method of nutrition support if oral access is not available. Indications for enteral nutrition in pediatrics are listed in Table 11.8.[6,12,17]

TABLE 11.17 Selected Medications That Should Not Be Given Via Feeding Tube

Medication	Dosage Form	Mechanism
Bisacodyl (Ducolax)	Tablet	Enteric coated
Bupropion (Wellbutrin XL)	Tablet	Sustained release
Carbamazepine (Tegretol XR)	Tablet	Sustained release
Carbidopa/levodopa (Sinemet CR)	Tablet	Sustained release
Clarithromycin (Biaxin-XL)	Tablet	Sustained release
Diclofenac (Voltaren)	Tablet	Delayed release
Diltiazem (Cardizem CD,[a] Cardizem SR,[a] Tiazac)	Capsule	Sustained release
Felodipine (Plendil)	Tablet	Extended release
Fluoxetine (Prozac Weekly)	Capsule	Sustained release
Lansoprazole (Prevacid[a])	Capsule	Delayed release
Mesalamine (Asacol, Pentasa)	Tablet, Capsule	Sustained release
Mycophenolate (CellCept)	Tablet, Capsule	Teratogenic
Omeprazole (Prilosec)	Capsule	Delayed release
Pancreatic enzymes (Creon 10, Creon 20, Pancrease, Ultrase, Zymase)	Capsule	Enteric coated spheres
Pantoprazole (Protonix)	Tablet	Sustained release
Verapamil (Verelan,[a] Calan SR)	Capsule, Tablet	Sustained release

[a]The capsule may be opened and contents administered by tube with fluid.
Adapted from Sacks GS. Drug-nutrient considerations in patients receiving parenteral and enteral nutrition. *Pract Gastroenterol.* 2004:39–48.

- Table 11.14 provides continuous infusion recommendations based on age and weight.[6]
- In infants, EN is intended to provide adequate replacement for human breast milk.
- For those infants allergic or intolerant to various components of human breast milk or standard infant formulas, enteral nutrition should provide adequate substitute feeding.
- Table 11.18 compares the content of cow to human milk.[6,22,23]
- Formulas may be modified to meet the protein, vitamin, and mineral requirements of the child, although this results in a concentrated formulation.[22]

TABLE 11.18 Comparison of Cow Milk to Human Milk

Nutrient	Cow Milk	Human Milk
Fat (% of total calories)	50	50–55
Triglycerides	Long-chain saturated fatty acids	Long-chain polyunsaturated and monounsaturated fatty acids
Protein (% of total calories)	22%	6%
Whey:casein[a]		55:45
Taurine and cystine[b]	Low levels	Abundant
Carbohydrate (% of total calories)	31%	42%
Carbohydrate source[c]	Lactose	Lactose
Renal solute load	228 mOsm/L	75 mOsm/L
Sodium	2.2 mmol/100 mL	0.7 mmol/100 mL
Ca/PO^4 ratio	1.3:1	2:1

[a]Whey is a soluble, noncurdling protein that remains in solution throughout the digestive process. Casein is relatively insoluble.
[b]Taurine is an essential amino acid involved with the development of the central nervous system. Cysteine is an essential amino acid in infants.
[c]Lactose enhances the absorption of calcium and magnesium.
Sources: Davis AM. Pediatrics. In: Matarese LE, Gottschlich MM, eds. *Contemporary Nutrition Support Practice: A Clinical Guide.* Philadelphia, PA: WB Saunders; 1998:347–364; Bechard LJ, Duggan C. Modifying enteral formulas. In: Corkins MR, Shulman RJ, eds. *Pediatric Nutrition in Your Pocket.* Silver Spring, MD: American Society for Parenteral and Enteral Nutrition; 2002:110–115; Magelli MA, Grinder CP. Meeting the special enteral nutrition needs of infants and children. *J Pediatr Pharm Prac.* 1996;1(2):113–129.

- Caution must be used to not exceed the kidney's ability to concentrate and excrete renal solute when concentrated EN formulations are used.[6,22]

References

1. Hammond K. History and physical examination. In: Matarese LE, Gottschlich MM, eds. *Contemporary Nutrition Support Practice: A Clinical Guide.* Philadelphia, PA: WB Saunders; 1998:17–32.
2. Mueller C, Compher C, Ellen DM, et al. ASPEN Clinical Guidelines: nutrition screening, assessment, and intervention in adults. *JPEN J Parenter Enteral Nutr.* 2011;35(1):16–24.
3. White JV, Guenter P, Jensen G, et al. Consensus statement: Academy of Nutrition and Dietetics and American Society for Parenteral and

Enteral Nutrition: characteristics recommended for the identification of adult malnutrition (undernutrition). *JPEN J Parenter Enteral Nutr.* 2012;36(3):275–283.

4. World Health Organization Technical Report Series; 894. Obesity: Preventing and Managing the Global Evidence: Report of a WHO Consultation. Geneva, Switzerland: World Health Organization; 2004 (reprint).
5. Chessman KH, Kumpf VJ. Assessment of nutrition status and nutrition requirements. In: DiPiro JT, Talbert RL, Yee GC, et al., eds. *Pharmacotherapy: A Pathophysiologic Approach.* 6th ed. New York, NY: McGraw-Hill; 2005: 2559–2578.
6. Davis AM. Pediatrics. In: Matarese LE, Gottschlich MM, eds. *Contemporary Nutrition Support Practice: A Clinical Guide.* Philadelphia, PA: WB Saunders; 1998:347–364.
7. Jensen GL, Hsiao PY, Wheeler D. Nutrition screening and assessment. In: Mueller CM, ed. *The ASPEN Adult Nutrition Support Core Curriculum.* 2nd ed. Silver Spring, MD: American Society for Parenteral and Enteral Nutrition; 2012:155–169.
8. Russell MK, McAdams PM. Laboratory monitoring of nutritional status. In: Matarese LE, Gottschlich MM, eds. *Contemporary Nutrition Support Practice: A Clinical Guide.* Philadelphia, PA: WB Saunders; 1998:47–64.
9. Dickerson RN. Using nitrogen balance in clinical practice. *Hosp Pharm.* 2005;40(12):1081–1085.
10. DeChicco RS, Matarese LE. Determining the nutrition support regimen. In: Matarese LE, Gottschlich MM, eds. *Contemporary Nutrition Support Practice: A Clinical Guide.* Philadelphia, PA: WB Saunders; 1998:185–191.
11. Kirby DF, Delegge MH, Fleming CR. American gastroenterological association technical review on tube feeding for enteral nutrition. *Gastroenterology.* 1995;108(4):1282–1301.
12. Kumpf VJ, Chessman KH. Enteral nutrition. In: DiPiro JT, Talbert RL, Yee GC, et al., eds. *Pharmacotherapy: A Pathophysiologic Approach.* 6th ed. New York, NY: McGraw-Hill; 2005:2615–2634.
13. Carlson SJ. Enteral formulations. In: Merritt R, ed-in-chief, DeLegge MH, Holcombe B, Mueller C, et al., eds. *The ASPEN Nutrition Support Practice Manual.* 2nd ed. Silver Spring, MD: American Society for Parenteral and Enteral Nutrition; 2005:63–75.
14. Minard G, Kudsk KA. Is early feeding beneficial? How early is early? *New Horiz.* 1994;2(2):156–163.
15. Malone AM, Seres D, Lord L. Complications of enteral nutrition. In: Mueller CM, ed. *The ASPEN Adult Nutrition Support Core Curriculum.* 2nd ed. Silver Spring, MD: American Society for Parenteral and Enteral Nutrition; 2012:218–233.
16. Haddad RY, Thomas DR. Enteral nutrition and enteral tube feeding: review of the evidence. *Clin Geriatr Med.* 2002;18(4):867–881.

17. Cresci G, Lefton J, Esper DH. Enteral formulations. In: Mueller CM, ed. *The ASPEN Adult Nutrition Support Core Curriculum*. 2nd ed. Silver Spring, MD: American Society for Parenteral and Enteral Nutrition; 2012:185–205.
18. Sacks GS. Drug-nutrient considerations in patients receiving parenteral and enteral nutrition. *Pract Gastroenterol*. 2004;28(7):39–48.
19. Beckwith CM, Feddema SS, Barton RG, et al. A guide to drug therapy in patients with enteral feeding tubes: dosage form selection and administration methods. *Hosp Pharm*. 2004;39(3):225–237.
20. Cutie AJ, Altman E, Lenkel L. Compatibility of enteral products with commonly employed drug additives. *JPEN J Parenter Enteral Nutr*. 1983;7(2):186–191.
21. Marcuard SP, Perkins AM. Clogging of feeding tubes. *JPEN J Parenter Enteral Nutr*. 1988;12(4):403–405.
22. Bechard LJ, Duggan C. Modifying enteral formulas. In: Corkins MR, Shulman RJ, eds. *Pediatric Nutrition in Your Pocket*. Silver Spring, MD: American Society for Parenteral and Enteral Nutrition; 2002:110–115.
23. Magelli MA, Grinder CP. Meeting the special enteral nutrition needs of infants and children. *J Pediatr Pharm Prac*. 1996;1(2):113–129.

12

Parenteral Nutrition

Gordon Sacks and Diana Wells

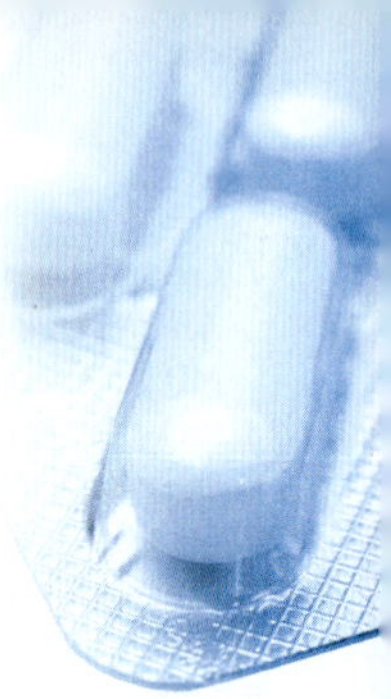

Parenteral Nutrition

Parenteral nutrition (PN) provides carbohydrate, protein, lipid, electrolytes, vitamins, and minerals intravenously to patients who are unable to assimilate nutrients via the gastrointestinal (GI) tract. It can maintain weight and metabolic integrity, replete malnourished patients with deficits in lean body mass, and restore hematologic and immune function integrity:

- PN may be started and given in a hospital, a skilled nursing facility, or a patient's home.
- PN should be used only when the gut is unavailable or dysfunctional.
- Indications and contraindications for PN are listed in Tables 12.1 and 12.2.

Central Versus Peripheral Administration

PN may be given via a peripheral or a central intravenous line:

- Central PN (CPN) refers to PN infused through central veins, including the subclavian, internal jugular, and femoral veins.
  - PN via a central vein requires a central venous access device due to its hyperosmolarity (>1,000 mOsm/L).[1]
  - Total nutrient admixture, also known as 3-in-1, refers to a solution containing dextrose, amino acids, and intravenous lipid emulsion (Table 12.3).
- Peripheral PN (PPN) is used when a patient requires intravenous nutritional support, but does not have a central access device.
- Guidelines for administering PPN are listed in Table 12.4.
- Providing nutrition through a central line is the preferred method.
- Table 12.5 lists common access devices for CPN.

(*Text continued on page 411*)

TABLE 12.1 Indications for PN

Anticipated a nonfunctioning GI tract for at least 5–7 days
Enterocutaneous fistula (high output >500 mL/day)
Short bowel syndrome
Intestinal obstruction
Radiation enteritis
Motility disorders (ileus, intestinal pseudoobstruction)
Severe malnutrition with a dysfunctional or inaccessible GI tract
Severe pancreatitis with intolerance to EN
Hyperemesis of pregnancy with intolerance to EN
Severe hypermetabolic states in which enteral feeding is contraindicated or inadequate
Inborn errors of metabolism (pediatrics)
Intractable diarrhea of infancy (pediatrics)
Extreme prematurity (pediatrics)

Sources: Mirtallo J, Canada T, Johnson D, et al. Safe practices for parenteral nutrition. *JPEN J Parenter Enteral Nutr*. 2004;28:S39–S70; Mehta NM, Compher C, ASPEN Board of Directors. A.S.P.E.N. clinical guidelines: nutrition support of the critically ill child. *JPEN J Parenter Enteral Nutr*. 2009;33(3):260–276.

TABLE 12.2 Contraindications for PN

Adequate nutrition stores and expected GI function returning within 5–7 days
GI function is not impaired.
Nutritional intervention not warranted

TABLE 12.3 Components of 2-in-1 Versus 3-in-1 Solutions

Component	2-in-1	3-in-1/Total Nutrient Admixture
Dextrose	Yes	Yes
Amino acids	Yes	Yes
Lipid	No	Yes

TABLE 12.4 Guidelines for PPN

Used for <7 days
Hypoosmolar solution (600–900 mOsm/L)
Final dextrose concentration: <10% (adults), 12.5% (children)
Final amino acid concentration: <5% (adults), 3.5% (children)
Large volume is required for compatibility; limit PPN to patients with no fluid restriction.
Monitor for vein irritation.
Consider addition of hydrocortisone 5 mg/day and heparin 100–1,000 units/day to decrease the risk of vein irritation.

Sources: Isaacs JW, Millikan WJ, Stackhouse J, et al. Parenteral nutrition of adults with 900-milliosmolar solution via peripheral vein. *Am J Clin Nutr.* 1977;30:552–559; Payne-James JJ, Khawaja HT. First choice for total parenteral nutrition: the peripheral route. *JPEN J Parenter Enteral Nutr.* 1993;17:468–478.[2,3]

TABLE 12.5 Types of Central Venous Access Devices

Type	Description	Advantages	Disadvantages
Peripheral catheter	Short-term access; may be placed at the bedside	Easily placed	Increased infection risk
Peripherally inserted central catheter (PICC)	Short- or long-term access; may be placed at the bedside; enters the antecubital vein and threaded into the subclavian vein; placement verified radiographically	Easily placed; decreased infection risk; less expensive than other long-term options	
Tunneled	Long-term access; placed surgically through the vein on the upper chest; useful for home total parenteral nutrition (TPN) patients	Decreased infection risk; increased patient comfort	Surgical risks; requires proper care
Implanted port	Long-term access; placed surgically underneath the skin near the clavicle; useful for home TPN patients	Decreased infection risk; increased patient comfort; aesthetically pleasing	Surgical risks; requires proper care; requires needle changes to gain access to port

Reprinted with permission from Krzywda EA, Andris DA, Edmiston CE, et al. Parenteral access devices. In: Mueller CM, ed. *The A.S.P.E.N. Adult Nutrition Support Core Curriculum.* 2nd ed. Silver Spring, MD: A.S.P.E.N.; 2012:265–283.[4] Reprinted by permission of SAGE Publications.

TABLE 12.6 Common Prescribing Errors

Prescribing practices
Formulation compatibilities
Prescribing nomenclature
Calculation of dosages

Source: Mirtallo J, Canada T, Johnson D, et al. Safe practices for parenteral nutrition. *JPEN J Parenter Enteral Nutr.* 2004;28:S39–S70.

Safe Prescribing Practices

Guidelines published by the American Society of Parenteral and Enteral Nutrition (ASPEN) are considered the gold standard for PN[1]:

- PN orders commonly contain abbreviated guidelines and information enabling physicians to devise patient-specific PN.
- Each institution should create guidelines for the uniform prescribing of PN in order to decrease the risk for errors (Table 12.6).
- Components that should be considered for inclusion on the PN order form are listed in Table 12.7.

Fluid Requirements

Fluid requirements should be considered in PN in order to prevent overhydration or dehydration:

- In healthy adult individuals, a fluid intake of 30 to 40 mL/kg maintains normal fluid balance.[1]

TABLE 12.7 Components of Order Form

Organized and clearly written for prescribers and anyone else who may use the form
Ingredients listed in the same format and order as the PN label
Components ordered in units per day (i.e., mg/day, mcg/day) or kg per day
Specify central or peripheral access device
Infusion rate guidelines
Dosing guidelines
Recommended laboratory tests

Reprinted with permission from Mirtallo J, Canada T, Johnson D, et al. Task force for the Revision of Safe Practices for Parenteral Nutrition. Safe practices for parenteral nutrition. *JPEN J Parenter Enter Nutr.* 2004;28:S39-S70. Reprinted with permission of SAGE Publications.

TABLE 12.8 Calculation of Fluid Requirements

	Daily Baseline Fluid Requirements
Adult	35 mL/kg
Children	
0–10 kg	100 mL/kg
11–20 kg	1,000 mL + 50 mL/kg for each kg >10 kg
>20 kg	1,500 mL + 20 mL/kg for each kg >20 kg

Reprinted with permission from Mirtallo J, Canada T, Johnson D, et al. Task force for the Revision of Safe Practices for Parenteral Nutrition. Safe practices for parenteral nutrition. JPEN *J Parenter Enter Nutr.* 2004;28:S39-S70. Reprinted with permission of SAGE Publications.

- Fluid requirements can be increased by fever, losses from vomiting, diarrhea, nasogastric suction, fistula drainage, and underlying disease.
- Most adults require 35 mL/kg actual body weight (ABW) to maintain fluid balance.
- A method for calculating fluid requirements in children is displayed in Table 12.8.
    - In infants, use of radiant warmers and treatment with phototherapy increases fluid requirements by 10% to 20%.

Minimizing Fluid in PN

Under certain clinical conditions when a patient is fluid overloaded (e.g., congestive heart failure, chronic renal failure, hypoproteinemia, pulmonary edema), the fluid in PN must be minimized:

- Commercial amino acids are available as diluted (8.5%, 10%) and concentrated (15%, 20%) solutions.
- Because of the low concentrations, amino acid stock solutions add considerable fluid to PN.
- In patients who require less fluid, a more concentrated amino acid solution (15%, 20%) and lipid emulsion (30%) should be used.

Nutritional Requirements

Energy Requirements

The kilocalories a patient needs daily are determined by the basal metabolic rate, level of activity, and increased metabolism caused by the stress of trauma or disease. The basal metabolic rate varies with age, weight, height, gender, and disease state:

- True basal energy expenditure (BEE) can only be measured in a contained metabolic chamber.

- Resting energy expenditure (REE) can be determined by using formulas based on population studies or at a patient's bedside using indirect calorimetry with a metabolic measurement cart.[5]
- Indirect calorimetry is a useful tool, but is expensive and reproducible results require a skilled and experienced technician.
- Underlying disease and trauma influence indirect calorimetry results.
- Indirect calorimetry cannot be used in patients on continuous airway pressure with chest tubes or when the fraction of inspired air is ≥50%.
- Indirect calorimetry has limited validity in infants and small children in whom a large amount of physiologic "dead space" is present.

Calculating Energy Requirements

It has been estimated that almost 200 different published formulas derived from population studies are available to calculate REE. Because these formulas are derived from population studies, they are approximations, and the clinical response of the patient should be monitored to determine if the correct kilocalories are being supplied. When energy requirements are calculated, the patient's ABW is customarily used.

Method 1

Harris-Benedict Equation[5]

$$\text{Male: } 66.5 + (13.75 \times \text{Wt}) + (5 \times \text{Ht}) - (6.8 \times \text{Age})^{*}$$
$$\text{Female: } 655 + (9.6 \times \text{Wt}) + (1.7 \times \text{Ht}) - (4.7 \times \text{Age})^{*}$$
$$^{*}\text{Wt (kg), Ht (cm), Age (yr)}$$

Multiplying REE by activity and stress factors in Table 12.9 gives the approximate kilocalories needed. In practice, multiplying REE by 1.2 to 1.4 should supply sufficient kilocalories to account for activity and the stress of trauma and/or disease for most patients.

Method 2

kcal/kg/day

The kcal/kg/day method is often used because most patients will require 25 to 35 kcal/kg/day[7,8]:

- Current practice advocates estimating 25 total kcal/kg/day in most adult patients.
- Table 12.10 lists estimated energy requirements for different stress situations.

TABLE 12.9 Activity and Stress Factors for the Harris-Benedict Equation

Activity Factors	Use	Stress Factors	Use
Confined to bed	1.2	Minor operation	1.2
Ambulatory	1.3	Skeletal trauma	1.3
Sepsis	1.6	Major burn	1.5–2.1

Reprinted with permission from Long C. Metabolic response to injury and illness: estimation of energy and protein needs from indirect calorimetry and nitrogen balance. *JPEN J Parenter Enteral Nutr.* 1979;3:452. Reprinted with permission of SAGE Publishing.

Method 3

Hypocaloric Feeding for Obese Patients

Patients with excess body stores of fat (BMI > 30 kg/m^2) may be hypocalorically fed:

- Table 12.11 summarizes energy requirements.
- Clinical outcomes to support this strategy include improved wound healing, decreased insulin requirements, and decreased number intensive care unit days.[9,10]

Dextrose Requirement

Adults

- Maximum glucose oxidation rate of 5 mg/kg/min
- Provides 70% to 85% of nonprotein calories (NPC)
- Available as stock concentrations 2.5%, 20%, 30%, 40%, 50%, and 70% for compounding

TABLE 12.10 Energy Requirements Using the kcal/kg/day Method

Stress	Energy (kcal/kg/day)
Maintenance/routine surgery	25–30
Moderate stress/minor infection	30
Major surgery/sepsis/severe stress/trauma/head injury	30–35
Thermal	40

Source: Mirtallo J, Canada T, Johnson D, et al. Safe practices for parenteral nutrition. *JPEN J Parenter Enteral Nutr.* 2004;28:S39–S70.

TABLE 12.11 Hypocaloric Regimen Strategies

22–25 kcal/kg IBW/day
11–14 kcal/kg ABW/day

IBW, ideal body weight; ABW, actual body weight.
Sources: Choban PS, Dickerson RN. Morbid obesity and nutrition support: is bigger different? *Nutr Clin Pract.* 2005;20:480–487; Dickerson RN. Hypocaloric feeding of obese patients in the intensive care unit. *Curr Opin Clin Nutr Metab Care.* 2005;8: 189–196.

Pediatrics

- Maximum glucose oxidation rate of 14 mg/kg/min in neonates
- Provides 50% of caloric intake
- Available as 50% and 70% concentrations for compounding

Protein Requirement

Protein requirement is closely related to the patient's clinical situation:

- Protein requirements vary with degree of metabolic stress (Table 12.12).
- For healthy adults, 0.8 g/kg/d has proven enough to maintain positive nitrogen balance.[11]

TABLE 12.12 Protein Requirements

Clinical Situation	Protein (g/kg/day)
Maintenance	0.8–1.0
Moderately stressed	1.1–2
Severely stressed	2.0–2.5
Chronic renal failure, no dialysis	0.8–1.2
• Peritoneal dialysis	1.2–1.3
• Hemodialysis	1.2–1.5
Acute kidney injury	
• Hemodialysis	1.5–1.8
• Continuous renal replacement therapy (CRRT)	1.5–2.5
Obese, hypocaloric feeding	
• BMI 30–40	2
• BMI >40	2.5

Adapted from Mirtallo J, Canada T, Johnson D, et al. Safe practices for parenteral nutrition. *JPEN J Parenter Enteral Nutr.* 2004;28:S39–S70.Reprinted with permission of SAGE Publications.

- Critically ill or hypermetabolic patients generally require 1.5 to 2 g/kg/d.[1]
- Patients with chronic renal failure may require slightly less protein, while patients with acute renal failure probably do not need protein restriction.
- Daily protein requirements are based on the ABW.
- If a patient is obese (BMI > 30 kg/m^2), IBW should be used.
- If a patient is edematous, estimated dry weight should be used.

Lipid Emulsion

Lipid emulsion is used to deliver calories and to prevent and treat essential fatty acid deficiency (EFAD)[7]:

- To prevent EFAD, at least 8% of the total kcal/day must be given as lipid emulsions.
- The usual proportion of fat kilocalories is 15% to 30% of total kcal/day.
- In adults who tolerate lipid emulsion (i.e., those whose serum triglycerides do not rise above 500 mg/dL), a greater proportion of fat calories (up to 40%) may provide a balanced nutrient solution.
- The percentage of total kcal/day contributed by lipid should not exceed 60% or an infusion rate >0.11 g/kg/h).[1]

Electrolytes[1]

Standard concentrations of electrolytes in PN solutions vary with institutional guidelines:

- The concentrations shown in Table 12.13 are derived from healthy populations and are general guidelines.
- The electrolyte concentration of a PN solution should be based on the patient's chemistries and clinical condition. Patients may have significant deficits or excesses of serum electrolytes.
- Baseline laboratories and the patient's clinical situation should be considered when determining electrolyte requirements.
- In the institutionalized setting, PN formulations are infused over 24 hours, and electrolyte imbalances should be taken care of immediately.
- Oral or intravenous supplementation of electrolytes may be used in addition to the PN.
- Early after nutrition support is instituted in the malnourished patient, potassium, magnesium, and phosphate shift intracellularly because of increased synthesis of cells.

TABLE 12.13 Guidelines for Amount of Electrolytes to be Added to PN Solutions

Electrolyte	Adults	Children
Sodium	1–2 mEq/kg	2–4 mEq/kg (max, 100–120 mEq/day)
Potassium	1–2 mEq/kg (max, 100 mEq/L)	2–3 mEq/kg (max, 100–120 mEq/day)
Chloride	As needed to maintain acid–base balance	3–5 mEq/kg
Phosphate	20–40 mmol/day	0.3–1 mmol/kg
Calcium	10–15 mEq/day	0.5–1.0 mEq/kg
Magnesium	8–24 mEq/day	0.2–1 mEq/kg
Acetate	As needed to maintain acid–base balance	As needed to maintain acid–base balance

Sources: Mirtallo J, Canada T, Johnson D, et al. Safe practices for parenteral nutrition. *JPEN J Parenter Enteral Nutr.* 2004;28:S39–S70; Mehta NM, Compher C; ASPEN Board of Directors. A.S.P.E.N. clinical guidelines: nutrition support of the critically ill child. *JPEN J Parenter Enteral Nutr.* 2009;33(3):260–276.

- As a result, serum concentrations of potassium, magnesium, and phosphate fall. This is known as the refeeding syndrome. It should be anticipated in malnourished patients and serum electrolytes monitored carefully during this period.[12]
- Commercially available stock solutions of the salts used to provide electrolytes in PN solutions are listed in Table 12.14.
- Under conditions of metabolic acidosis, it is common to increase or maximize the concentration of acetate salts because acetate is

TABLE 12.14 Electrolyte Salts of Commercially Available Solutions

Sodium chloride
Sodium acetate
Sodium phosphate
Potassium chloride
Potassium acetate
Potassium phosphate
Calcium gluconate
Magnesium sulfate

converted metabolically to bicarbonate by the liver, which raises pH. The concentration of chloride salts, which lower pH, is minimized.[13]

- It is not always possible to entirely remove chloride because amino acid solutions contain intrinsic amounts of chloride counterions.
- Under conditions of metabolic alkalosis, acetate is minimized to avoid raising pH and chloride maximized to lower pH. Eliminating acetate completely is not possible because there are acetate salts intrinsically in amino acid solutions.[13]
- Severe cases of metabolic acidosis or alkalosis should be resolved by fluids and electrolyte solutions and not by PN.

Vitamins[1]

Vitamin requirements for adults and children are based on the recommended daily allowances. The compositions of the most used adult and pediatric preparations are shown in Table 12.15.

TABLE 12.15 Composition of Adult and Pediatric Multivitamin Solutions

Vitamins	Adult Multivitamins/10 mL	Pediatric Multivitamins
A	3,300 IU	2,300 IU
D	200 IU	400 IU
C	200 mg	80 mg
Thiamine (B_1)	6 mg	1.2 mg
Pyridoxine (B_6)	6 mg	1.0 mg
Riboflavin (B_2)	3.6 mg	1.4 mg
Niacin (B_3)	40 mg	17 mg
Pantothenic acid	15 mg	5 mg
E	10 IU	7 IU
Folic acid	600 mcg	140 mcg
Cyanocobalamin (B_{12})	5 mcg	1.0 mcg
K	150 mcg	200 mcg
Biotin	60 mcg	20 mcg

Reprinted with permission from Mirtallo J, Canada T, Johnson D, et al. Task force for the Revision of Safe Practices for Parenteral Nutrition. Safe practices for parenteral nutrition. *JPEN J Parenter Enter Nutr.* 2004;28:S39-S70. Reprinted with permission of SAGE Publications.

TABLE 12.16 Composition of Adult and Pediatric Trace Element Solutions

Trace Elements	Adult Solution	Pediatric Solution
Zinc	5 mg	100 mcg
Manganese	0.5 mg	6 mcg
Copper	2 mg	20 mcg
Chromium	20 mcg	0.2 mcg
Selenium	100 mcg	—

Reprinted with permission from Mirtallo J, Canada T, Johnson D, et al. Task force for the Revision of Safe Practices for Parenteral Nutrition. Safe practices for parenteral nutrition. *JPEN J Parenter Enter Nutr.* 2004;28:S39-S70. Reprinted with permission of SAGE Publications.

Trace Elements[1]

Concentrations of trace elements in commonly used commercial preparations are listed in Table 12.16:

- Copper and manganese are eliminated primarily via the bile. For adult patients with cholestasis, copper and manganese are withheld, and appropriate amounts of zinc, selenium, and copper are added to the PN separately.
- Patients receiving PN for long periods may develop deficiencies in trace elements due to inadequate intake or underlying diseases.[14]

Additions to PN Formulations

Many compounds can be added safely to PN and total nutrient admixtures (TNAs) although it is usually best to keep the formulation as simple as possible:

- Additions to TNAs should be very limited because of the risk of "cracking" the emulsion. To determine whether a compound is compatible, major references of intravenous stability and compatibility should be consulted such as Trissel's Compatibility for PN.[15]
- If no data can be found, any requested addition should be considered incompatible.
- Table 12.17 lists commonly added components to PN formulations.

Characteristics of PN Components

These major components of PN (dextrose, amino acids, lipid emulsions) are typically prescribed in terms of grams. Therefore, the amount of

TABLE 12.17 Common Additions to PN Solutions

Component	Usual Dose	Indication
Regular insulin	0.1 units/g of dextrose; adjust for blood glucose.	Hyperglycemia
H2 antagonists	Ranitidine: 150 mg; adjust for renal dysfunction.	Stress ulcer prophylaxis if has risk factors; gastroesophageal reflux disease

calories must be considered when determining energy requirements. Table 12.18 lists common components of PN and the amount of energy provided per gram. Certain clinical situations may exclude the use of lipid emulsions. Contraindications to the use of lipid emulsions are listed in Table 12.19.

Compatibility Issues with PN

Although TNAs must be compounded carefully because precipitates cannot be seen by the unaided eye, any PN formulation can form precipitates either during compounding, storage, or administration. See Table 12.20 for ways to prevent incompatibility when compounding a PN formulation.

Administration of PN

PN should be initiated slowly in order to prevent intolerance. Because of the risk of hyperglycemia with large doses of dextrose, the initial day of nutrition support should not contain >200 g/d.

To initiate continuous PN

1. Calculate final goal fluid, energy, and protein requirements. Protein and a maximum of dextrose 200 g may be initiated on the first

TABLE 12.18 Typical Components of PN Solutions

Component	kcal/g	Comments
Dextrose 70%	3.4	Maximum infusion rate: 5 mg/kg/min (adult), 20 mg/kg/min (pediatric)
Amino acid 10%	4.0	
Amino acid 15%	4.0	Concentrated form of amino acid
Lipid, intravenous 10%	10	Should not be used for nutrition support
Lipid, intravenous 20%, 30%	10	

TABLE 12.19 Lipid Emulsion Contraindications

Triglyceride levels >400–500 mg/dL
Acute pancreatitis with hyperlipidemia
Lipoid nephrosis when accompanied by hyperlipidemia
Neonates with hyperbilirubinemia since lipids displace bilirubin from albumin. If bilirubin is <10 mg/dL (direct <2 mg/dL) and the free fatty acid-to-albumin ratio is 4, lipids may be given because displacement is unlikely
Egg allergy because egg yolk phospholipids are used as emulsifiers
The dose of lipid emulsion should be adjusted to account for kilocalories during propofol administration

day. If lipid emulsion is included in the PN formulation, it should be withheld until it is verified that the triglyceride concentration is <400 mg/dL.

2. Start at a rate of 25 mL/h.
3. Check blood glucose via fingersticks every 6 hours. If blood glucose remains <180 mg/dL, the rate may be increased by 25 mL/h, until the goal rate is reached.
4. On day 2, if the patient has tolerated, PN may be adjusted to include the goal amount of dextrose, protein, and lipid. If the lipid emulsion is to be hung separately, it may be ordered on this day.
5. If the patient does not tolerate the dextrose load, do not advance to goal calories on day 2. Adjust insulin and reassess the next day.
6. If PN must be discontinued, the rate of administration is gradually tapered to prevent rebound hypoglycemia. A typical approach is to reduce the hourly rate by 50% per hour until the final rate is

TABLE 12.20 Prevention of Precipitation

Use calcium gluconate for compounding, rather than calcium chloride.
Phosphate should be added near the beginning and calcium near the end of compounding.
Do not add ascorbic acid to solution due to its degradation of calcium.
The sum of calcium and magnesium should be <20 mEq/L.
Add iron with caution secondary to higher cation valence and increased destabilizing potential.
Keep the solution away from high temperatures.

Source: Trissel LA. *Calcium and Phosphate Compatibility in Parenteral Nutrition.* 1st ed. Houston, TX: TriPharma Communications; 2001.

TABLE 12.21 Monitoring Parameters for PN

Weight trends
Accurate records of input and output
Evidence of intolerance
Laboratory parameters, including serum electrolytes, complete blood count, glucose, inflammatory markers
Markers for nutrition status (prealbumin, nitrogen balance)
Physical examination for hydration or nutrient deficiency or excess
Review of medications

≤25 mL/h. If the solution is discontinued abruptly, infuse 10% dextrose until nutrition is able to be restarted.

Monitoring PN

PN is an invasive therapy, and patients should be monitored carefully for metabolic abnormalities throughout the course of the therapy. The suggested regimen in Table 12.21 provides some guidelines for monitoring patients who require PN. Monitoring of patients receiving PN should be individualized according to clinical status, chemical abnormalities, and severity of illness.

Complications of PN

Complications of PN can be categorized as mechanical, metabolic, hepatobiliary, and infectious. The complications associated with PN, as well as possible causes and suggested management, are given in Table 12.22. Health care professionals caring for patients receiving PN should be experienced in the detection and resolution of these complications.

Pediatric Considerations

Enteral nutrition (EN) is the preferred method of nutrition support. However, when this route is contraindicated or inaccessible, PN may be instituted.[7] Typical indications for PN in pediatrics are shown in Table 12.23.

Nutrient requirements for infants and children vary with gender, age, growth rate, and disease state:

- Numerous equations and methods exist to estimate nutrient needs.
- Premature infants may require greater amount of calories for the "catch-up" growth period.

(*Text continued on page 425*)

TABLE 12.22 PN Complications

Complication	Causes	Management
Mechanical		
Pneumothorax	Placement by inexperienced personnel	Possible chest tube placement; minimize the number of catheter insertions; placement by experienced personnel
Air embolism	Air inspiration during line placement	Placement by experienced personnel
Catheter occlusion	Formation of the fibrin sheath outside of the catheter	Anticoagulation locally with tissue plasminogen activator (tPA); routine line flushing
Venous thrombosis	Trauma to the vein, hypercoagulopathy, sepsis	Anticoagulation; catheter removal
Metabolic		
Hyperglycemia	Common in patients who are diabetic, hypermetabolic, or receiving corticosteroids	Slowly initiate PN; check blood glucose and frequently prior to advancing nutrition; administer insulin if needed
Hypoglycemia	Overuse of insulin in PN; abrupt discontinuation of PN	Decrease amount of insulin administered; avoid abrupt discontinuation of PN by tapering the rate of infusion; administer 10% dextrose if PN is abruptly discontinued
Hypertriglyceridemia	Inadequate clearing of lipids from bloodstream; pathologic hyperlipidemia	Decrease lipid volume administered; increase length of infusion time; avoid lipid administration >60% of total calories; assess risk factors for hypertriglyceridemia.
Electrolyte disturbance	Fluid imbalance; refeeding syndrome; medication use; renal insufficiency	Monitor fluid intake and output, and serum chemistries; replace electrolytes as necessary

TABLE 12.22 PN Complications *(continued)*

Complication	Causes	Management
Essential fatty acid deficiency	Inadequate lipid intake	Provide 8%–10% of total calories as lipid
Prerenal azotemia	Excessive protein administration; dehydration; insufficient NPC	Increase fluid intake; decrease protein administered; increase NPC; analyze nitrogen balance
Gastrointestinal		
Cholestasis	Exact cause unknown; possible excess glucose, protein, amino acid; impaired bile flow; absence of intraluminal nutrients needed to stimulate hepatic bile secretion	Avoid overfeeding; use the GI tract as soon as clinically able
GI atrophy	Atrophy of villi; colonic hypoplasia	Use the GI tract as soon as clinically able
Infectious		
Catheter-related sepsis	Inappropriate line placement technique; inadequate catheter care; type, location, and duration of the catheter	Remove the catheter and place at an alternate site; adequately care for the catheter site; possible treatment with intravenous antibiotics

Sources: Btaiche IF, Khalidi N. Metabolic complications of parenteral nutrition in adults, part 1. *Am J Health Syst Pharm.* 2004;61:1938–1949; Btaiche IF, Khalidi N. Metabolic complications of parenteral nutrition in adults, part 2. *Am J Health Syst Pharm.* 2004;61:2050–2059.[16,17]

TABLE 12.23 Indications for PN—Pediatrics

Omphalocele
Short bowel syndrome
Congenital malformation
Gastroschisis
Malrotation/volvulus
Intestinal pseudoobstruction
Hirschsprung disease

Source: Mehta NM, Compher C, ASPEN Board of Directors. A.S.P.E.N. clinical guidelines: nutrition support of the critically ill child. *JPEN J Parenter Enteral Nutr.* 2009;33(3):260–276.

- Table 12.24 summarizes estimated energy and protein requirements dependent on age.
- Electrolyte requirements are similar to that of adults.
- Table 12.25 gives dose ranges for electrolyte goals according to age and weight.
- Children are at risk for EFAD; therefore, most regimens should include lipid emulsion.
- Stability of 3-in-1 formulations has not been verified in this population. Intravenous lipid emulsions should be infused separately from the dextrose/amino acid formulation.

TABLE 12.24 Energy and Protein Requirements—Pediatrics

Age	Calories (kcal/kg/day)	Protein (g/kg/day)
Preterm	120–150	2.5–3
<6 months	90–120	2.5–3
6–12 months	80–100	2–2.5
Toddler	80–12	1.5–2
Child	60–90	1.5–2
Adolescent	30–75	0.8–2

Sources: Mirtallo J, Canada T, Johnson D, et al. Safe practices for parenteral nutrition. *JPEN J Parenter Enteral Nutr.* 2004;28:S39–S70; Mehta NM, Compher C; ASPEN Board of Directors. A.S.P.E.N. clinical guidelines: nutrition support of the critically ill child. *JPEN J Parenter Enteral Nutr.* 2009;33(3):260–276.

TABLE 12.25 Intravenous Electrolyte Requirements—Pediatrics

Electrolyte	Neonates	Infants/Children	Adolescents
Sodium	2–5 mEq/kg/d	2–6 mEq/kg/d	60–150 mEq/d
Potassium	1–4 mEq/kg/d	2–3 mEq/kg/d	70–180 mEq/d
Chloride	1–5 mEq/kg/d	2–5 mEq/kg/d	60–150 mEq/d
Magnesium	0.3–0.5 mEq/kg/d	0.3–0.5 mEq/kg/d	10–30 mEq/d
Calcium	3–4 mEq/kg/d	1–2.5 mEq/kg/d	10–20 mEq/d
Phosphorus	1–2 mmol/kg/d	0.5–1 mmol/kg/d	10–40 mmol/d

Sources: Mirtallo J, Canada T, Johnson D, et al. Safe practices for parenteral nutrition. *JPEN J Parenter Enteral Nutr.* 2004;28:S39–S70; Mehta NM, Compher C; ASPEN Board of Directors. A.S.P.E.N. clinical guidelines: nutrition support of the critically ill child. *JPEN J Parenter Enteral Nutr.* 2009;33(3):260–276.

- Pediatric PN formulations contain significant amounts of cysteine, histidine, and tyrosine, amino acids that are considered semiessential for infants. In addition, taurine is included because it has been reported to prevent cholestasis associated with PN in children.

References

1. Mirtallo J, Canada T, Johnson D, et al. Safe practices for parenteral nutrition. *JPEN J Parenter Enteral Nutr.* 2004;28:S39–S70.
2. Isaacs JW, Millikan WJ, Stackhouse J, et al. Parenteral nutrition of adults with 900-milliosmolar solution via peripheral vein. *Am J Clin Nutr.* 1977;30: 552–559.
3. Payne-James JJ, Khawaja HT. First choice for total parenteral nutrition: the peripheral route. *JPEN J Parenter Enteral Nutr.* 1993;17:468–478.
4. Krzywda EA, Andris DA, Edmiston CE, et al. Parenteral access devices. In: Mueller CM, ed. *The A.S.P.E.N. Adult Nutrition Support Core Curriculum.* 2nd ed. Silver Spring, MD: A.S.P.E.N.; 2012:265–283.
5. Harris JA, Benedict FG. *A Biometric Study of Basal Metabolism in Man. Publication No. 279.* Washington, DC: Carnegie Institute; 1919.
6. Long C. Metabolic response to injury and illness: estimation of energy and protein needs from indirect calorimetry and nitrogen balance. *JPEN J Parenter Enteral Nutr.* 1979;3:452.
7. Mehta NM, Compher C; ASPEN Board of Directors. A.S.P.E.N. clinical guidelines: nutrition support of the critically ill child. *JPEN J Parenter Enteral Nutr.* 2009;33(3):260–276.

8. Cerra FB, Benitez MR, Blackburn GL, et al. Applied nutrition in ICU patients. A consensus statement of the American College of Chest Physicians. *Chest.* 1997;111:769–778.
9. Choban PS, Dickerson RN. Morbid obesity and nutrition support: is bigger different? *Nutr Clin Pract.* 2005;20:480–487.
10. Dickerson RN. Hypocaloric feeding of obese patients in the intensive care unit. *Curr Opin Clin Nutr Metab Care.* 2005;8:189–196.
11. Miles JM. Yes, protein should be included in calorie calculations for a TPN prescription. *Nutr Clin Pract.* 1996;11:204–205.
12. Kraft MD, Btaiche IF, Sacks GS. Review of refeeding syndrome. *Nutr Clin Pract.* 2005;20:625–633.
13. Sacks GS. The ABC's of acid–base balance. *J Pediatr Pharmacol Ther.* 2004;9:235–242.
14. Triplett WC. Clinical aspects of zinc, copper, manganese, chromium and selenium metabolism. *Nutr Int.* 1985;1(2):60.
15. Trissel LA. *Calcium and Phosphate Compatibility in Parenteral Nutrition.* 1st ed. Houston, TX: TriPharma Communications; 2001.
16. Btaiche IF, Khalidi N. Metabolic complications of parenteral nutrition in adults, part 1. *Am J Health Syst Pharm.* 2004;61:1938–1949.
17. Btaiche IF, Khalidi N. Metabolic complications of parenteral nutrition in adults, part 2. *Am J Health Syst Pharm.* 2004;61:2050–2059.

13

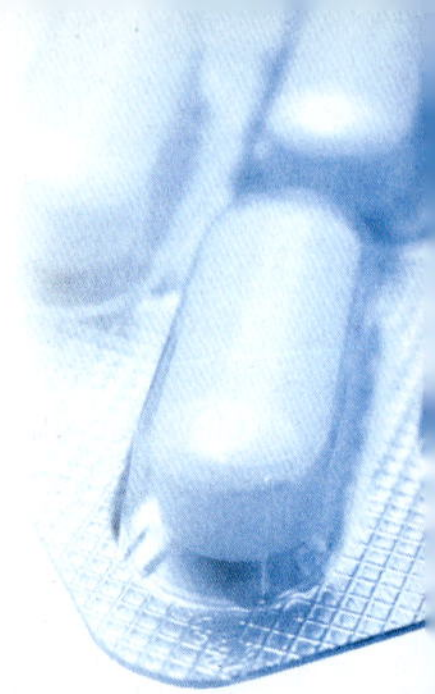

Pharmacy Calculations

Shelley L. Chambers-Fox
and Teresa A. O'Sullivan

The practice of pharmacy requires proficiency in calculations, so during both early and advanced practice experiences, students should take every opportunity to practice and perfect their ability to accurately perform calculations. This chapter is a collection of both common and rare (but complex) calculations encountered in pharmacy practice.

General Principles for Solving Pharmacy Calculations

- Calculation accuracy is greatly improved by independent double checks (i.e., two trained practitioners independently calculate and then compare answers). The calculation error rate for a single individual is around 10% (based on results from comprehensive exams). Independent double checks catch 95% of errors,[1] so double checks will catch all but 5% of an individual's errors, reducing the likelihood that a calculation error will reach the patient from 10% to 0.5% $(0.1 \times 0.05 \times 100 = 0.5\%)$.
- Published[2] strategies for increasing accuracy in pharmacy calculations include the following:
  - Using references to identify unknown definitions or equations
  - Writing equations on a paper or screen rather than trying to solve mentally
  - Identifying related terms that can be used to construct proportions or dimension analysis strings (e.g., 1 kg/2.2 lb, 250 mg/5 mL, 1 g/100 mL)
  - Labeling substance and units for each number in the related term
  - Using proportional/ratio analysis for calculations involving two different but related expressions of drug amounts

  - Using dimensional analysis for calculations involving more than two different expressions of drug amounts
  - Consciously double-checking the accuracy by ensuring that all numbers, units, and substances are correctly transcribed/identified and that all substances and their units on either side of an equation's equal sign (after crossing out matching numerator–denominator substances and their units on either side of the equal sign) are the same
- Medications are manufactured in forms allowing most recipients to receive small but measurable drug amounts. In general, doses of oral solid medications will be one or two tablets or capsules; doses of liquid medications will be anywhere from 1 mL to 2 teaspoonfuls. If a calculation results in a drug amount that is unreasonably high (e.g., 75 tablets of a manufactured dosage form) or low (e.g., 0.0005 mL of a manufactured liquid dosage form), then the calculation is probably incorrect.
- Many medication dosing recommendations are expressed as a range. Dose calculations for individual patients must identify a single dose, not a dosing range.
- Tablets can be cut in half, but cutting exact half tablets is difficult even when tablets are scored. Avoid recommending doses that require a patient to cut tablets in half unless there is a clear benefit to the patient. *Capsules cannot be cut in half.*
- Calculated doses should be rounded to a measurable number, requiring familiarity with the precision of the measurement device used for medication dosing. For example, if a medication is being administered orally using a teaspoon as the measuring device, it is difficult to give even a half teaspoon with any degree of precision.
- Many widely used methods of communicating information about medications have been identified as potentially dangerous.[3] Health care professionals need to avoid using abbreviations in general See Table 13.1 for a list of abbreviations to avoid.

Calculation Basics

Conversion Factors and Definitions

A list of conversion factors between the systems commonly used in the United States and the metric system is presented in Table 13.2. Three approaches for converting between the Celsius and Fahrenheit systems

TABLE 13.1 Abbreviations to Avoid

Do Not Use	To Mean	Because	Instead
Trailing zero[a]	For example, "2.0 mg"	Decimal point is missed: interpreted number higher than actual number by factor of 10	Use 2 mg rather than 2.0 mg
Lack of leading zero	For example, "0.2 mg"	Decimal point is missed: interpreted number higher than actual number by factor of 10	Use a leading zero, for example, 0.2 mg
U	Unit	Mistaken for "0," the number "4," or "cc"	Write out "unit"
IU	International unit	Mistaken for "IV" or the number "10"	Write out "international unit"
μ	Micro	Mistaken for either u (unit) or m (milli)	Write "micro" or use mc (e.g., mcg = microgram)
QD, qd	Every day	Mistaken for QOD or qod	Write "daily"
QOD, qod	Every other day	Mistaken for QD or qd	Write "every other day"
DC	"Discharged" or "discontinue"	Confused for one another	Write out full word
Abbreviations for drug names, for example, NTG, HCTZ	Full drug names, for example, nitroglycerin, hydrochlorothiazide	Abbreviations can be misunderstood and misinterpreted	Write out full name of drug
Chemical-like abbreviations MS, MSO_4, and $MgSO_4$	Morphine sulfate or magnesium sulfate	Confused for one another	Write "morphine sulfate" and "magnesium sulfate"

[a]A trailing 0 can be used when needed to identify the level of measurement precision, such as for compounding and reporting of laboratory values and imaging studies. A trailing zero should never be used on a medication order.

TABLE 13.2 Conversion Factors

Unit of Measure	Exact Equivalent	Approximate Equivalent
1 meter (m)	39.4 in.	—
1 inch (in.)	2.54 cm	—
1 kilogram (kg)	2.2 pounds (lb avoir)	—
1 gram (g)	15.4 grain (gr)	—
1 grain (gr avoir)	64.8 mg	60 or 65 mg
1 ounce (oz avoir)	28.35 g	30 g
1 pound (lb avoir)	454 g	—
1 teaspoon (tsp)	5 mL	—
1 tablespoon (tbs or Tbsp)	15 mL	—
1 fluid dram (fʒ)	3.69 mL	5 mL (1 tsp)
1 fluid ounce (f℥)	29.57 mL	30 mL
1 pint (pt; 16 f℥)	473 mL	480 mL
1 quart (32 f℥; 2 pt)	946 mL	1 liter (1 L)
1 gallon (gal; 4 qt)	3,785 mL	—

are shown in Table 13.3, and the equations and definitions commonly used in pharmacy calculations are presented in Table 13.4.

Dosing Calculations

As delineation of drug pharmacokinetic properties has increased, so have the variety of ways used to determine drug doses. These include dosing by weight, by body surface area (BSA), by kidney function, and by titration to a therapeutic concentration and by using pharmacokinetic parameters. Drug doses should be individualized whenever

TABLE 13.3 Thermometry Conversions

$°F = \frac{(°C)(9)}{5} + 32$	or	$°F = (°C \times 1.8) + 32$	or	$(5)(°F) = (9)(°C) + 160$
$°C = \left(\frac{°F - 32}{9}\right)(5)$	or	$°C = (°F - 32) \times 0.556$	or	$(9)(°C) = (5)(°F) - 160$

(*Text continued on page 434*)

TABLE 13.4 Formulas and Definitions Used in Pharmacy Practice

Term	Definition	Formula
Actual body weight (ABW) or total body weight (TBW) in kg	An individual's actual weight, measured in kg	(ABW in lb)(1 kg/2.2 lb) = ABW in kg
Adjusted body weight in kg	An adjustment made to ideal body weight (IBW) to account for drug distribution	AdjBW = 0.4 (TBW – LBW) + IBW
Body surface area (BSA) in meters squared	Size of body surface provides a dose adjustment with better relationship to drug clearance than weight	$BSA = \sqrt{\frac{\text{Height (in cm)} \times \text{Weight (in kg)}}{3{,}600}}$
Creatinine clearance (CrCl) in mL/min	The rate at which creatinine is cleared by the kidneys; approximates how well kidneys are functioning	(Cockcroft-Gault equation) $\frac{(140 - \text{age}) \times (\text{actual BW in kg})}{(GF)(S_{cr})}$ GF (gender factor) = 72 for males, 85 for females S_{cr}, serum creatinine
Ideal body weight (IBW) in males in kg	Fat-free weight in males	50 kg + (2.3 × inches over 5 ft)
Ideal body weight (IBW) in females in kg	Fat-free weight in females	45.5 kg + (2.3 × inches over 5 ft)
Milliequivalent (mEq)	1 mEq = weight of a substance that can replace or combine with 1 millimole (1 mg) of H^+	$1\ mEq = \frac{\text{mg FW weight}}{(\text{ions} \times \text{valence})}$ where MW is molecular weight
Milliosmole (mOsm)	A millimole (6.022×10^{20}) of dissolved particles	$= \frac{\text{weight in g} \times \text{no. species} \times 1{,}000}{\text{MW in g}}$ where MW is molecular weight

(continued)

TABLE 13.4 Formulas and Definitions Used in Pharmacy Practice *(continued)*

Term	Definition	Formula
Minimum weighable quantity (MWQ)	The smallest weight of the substance that can be measured with ≤5% error	$= \frac{\text{Balance sensitivity requirement}}{\text{Acceptable error rate (5\%)}}$
Osmolarity (mOsm/L)	Number of milliosmoles in a liter of solution	$= \frac{\text{concentration in g / L} \times \text{no.species} \times 1{,}000}{\text{MW in g}}$
Parts per million; ppm (weight/volume)	g per 1,000,000 mL solution	g/mL × 1,000,000
Parts per million; ppm (weight/weight)	g per 1,000,000 g mixture	g/g × 1,000,000
Parts per billion; ppb (volume/volume)	mL per 1,000,000,000 mL solution	mL/mL × 1,000,000,000
Percent (% weight/volume)	g per 100 or in 100 mL	g/mL × 100
Percent (% volume/volume)	mL per 100 or in 100 mL	mL/mL × 100
Percent (% weight/weight)	g per 100 or in 100 g	g/g × 100
Ratio strength (1:1,000 weight/volume)	g in 1,000 mL solution	g/mL × 1,000
Ratio strength (1:2,500 volume/volume)	mL in 2,500 mL solution	mL/mL × 2,500
Ratio strength (1:500 weight/weight)	g in 500 g mixture	g/g × 500
Sodium chloride equivalent (E value)	Weight of sodium chloride equivalent to 1 g of drug	E g NaCl = 1 g drug
Specific gravity	The ratio of the weight of a substance to the weight of an equal volume of water	$S_pG = \frac{\text{g / mL substance}}{\text{g / mL water}}$
USP volume	The volume of an isotonic solution that can be made from 1 g of drug and water	USP mL isotonic solution = 1 g drug

possible to elicit the desired therapeutic response with minimal side effects. The preferred method for determining a drug's dose depends on its margin of safety as well as the drug's pharmacokinetic profile.

Dosing Based on Body Weight

Actual Body Weight (ABW): Some doses are calculated based on body weight. As long as the individual is not overweight, the dose in mg/kg should be multiplied by the patient's actual body weight in kilograms; for example, a 3-year-old, 36-lb patient with otitis media is to receive cephalexin. The recommended dose is 75 to 100 mg/kg per day in four divided doses. If 90 mg/kg is used, what volume in teaspoons of Keflex suspension, 250 mg/5 mL, should the child receive in each dose?

$$(36\text{ lb})\frac{(1\text{ kg})}{(2.2\text{ lb})}\frac{(90\text{ mg})}{(\text{kg / day})}\frac{(\text{day})(1\text{ tsp})}{(4\text{ doses})(250\text{ mg})}=1.47\text{ tsp}=1.5\text{ tsp / dose}$$

Ideal Body Weight and Lean Body Weight: Some drugs partition mainly into lean tissues such that fat-free mass will be a better predictor of drug concentration than total body weight. This means an overweight or obese patient could receive more drug than needed to produce therapeutic concentrations in the lean tissues, if the dose were based on actual body weight. Overweight is defined as a body mass index (BMI) over 25 kg/m^2, and obesity is defined as a BMI > 30 kg/m^2 in non-Asian ethnic groups. *Ideal body weight (IBW)* is usually estimated from an equation[4]:

$$\text{IBW (males)}=50\text{ kg}+(2.3\times\#\text{inches over 5 ft})$$

$$\text{IBW (females)}=45.5\text{ kg}+(2.3\times\#\text{inches over 5 ft})$$

Example: The digitalizing or loading dose of digoxin tablets is 10 to 15 mcg/kg. What is the appropriate dose for a 62-year-old woman who is 5 ft. 1 inch and weighs 188 pounds (85.5 kg)?

First calculate IBW body weight:

$$\text{IBW (females)}=45.5\text{ kg}+(2.3\times 1)=47.8\text{ kg}$$

Then, calculate the digitalizing dose:

$$(47.8\text{ kg})\frac{(12.5\text{ mcg})}{(1\text{ kg})}=597.5\text{ mcg}$$

The patient should receive one 250-mcg tablet immediately and a second 250-mcg tablet in 6 to 8 hours.

Several formulas designed to calculate fat-free weight in various groups of adults have been proposed and validated. One formula[5] for calculating *lean body weight*, often referred to as LBW_{2005}, has been used in a number of drug dosing and other studies conducted with overweight and obese individuals; LBW_{2005} is available on several online calculators.

Adjusted Body Weight (AdjBW): Some dosing calculations for patients over 130% of ideal body weight use a value for body weight that is between ideal body weight and actual body weight. For example, the traditional recommendation[6] for dosing aminoglycosides in obese individuals add to IBW 40% of the difference between IBW and ABW. This method has been referred to as $AdjBW_{40}$: IBW + (0.4)(ABW − IBW).

Dosing Based on Body Surface Area

Dosing for many chemotherapeutic agents is based on a patient's BSA, where desired units are BSA in square meter (m^2). The most common equation used for determining BSA for adults is the Mosteller equation.[7] The form of the equation using metric measurements is slightly more accurate than the variation using pounds and inches.

$$\text{BSA in m}^2 = \sqrt{\frac{(\text{ht})(\text{wt})}{3{,}600}} \quad \text{where height is in cm and weight in kg}$$

$$\text{BSA in m}^2 = \sqrt{\frac{(\text{ht})(\text{wt})}{3{,}131}} \quad \text{where height is in inches and weight in pounds}$$

One equation for BSA validated in both adults and children is the Haycock equation:[8]

$$\text{BSA in m}^2 = (\text{H}^{0.3964})(\text{W}^{0.5378})(0.024265) \text{ where height is in cm and weight in kg}$$

Dosing Based on Kidney Function

Drugs that are primarily cleared from the body by the kidneys may accumulate to toxic concentrations in patients with kidney dysfunction, so either the dose or the frequency of administration must be modified. The most widely used estimates of renal function are based on serum creatinine, an endogenous substance that is filtered by the kidneys and not significantly reabsorbed, but is secreted to a small extent. Thus, the clearance of creatinine will slightly exceed the glomerular filtration rate (ClCr normal range, 100 to 140 mL/min, GFR ~ 125 mL/min). The estimate of kidney function most widely used for drug dosing is the Cockcroft-Gault equation.

Cockcroft-Gault (C-G) Equation[9]

$$\text{eCrCl in mL / min} = \frac{(140 - \text{age})(\text{ABW})}{(72)(\text{SCr})} \text{ multiply this result by 0.85 for females}$$

where age is in years, ABW is weight in kg, and SCr is serum creatinine in mg/dL.

This equation was developed from a study of 249 males. Problems[10] include

- The adjustment factor of 0.85 for females was added by the authors without validation.
- The largest of the subjects in the study was only 130% of his IBW, so this equation has not been validated in people who are over 130% of ideal body weight. Various "fixes" have been proposed for patients who are overweight or obese, including use of IBW, LBW, $\text{AdjBW}_{0.3}$, $\text{AdjBW}_{0.4}$, and no body weight.
- The equation was developed before the standardization of laboratory methods for the measurement of SCr (labs now use isotope dilution mass spectrometry).
- All patients had stable kidney function so the C-G equation is not accurate in patients with acute kidney function changes.

Despite its limitations, in 1998, the FDA listed the original (actual body weight) C-G equation as a recommended method of estimating creatinine clearance (CrCl) based on serum creatinine in its *Guidance for the Industry: Pharmacokinetics in Patients with Impaired Renal Function.* As a result, much of the drug literature available uses the C-G equation to estimate renal function or does not specify the method used to estimate renal function, increasing the uncertainty in dosing decisions based on renal function. The literature on a number of drugs has been summarized in dosing tables[11] for adjusting drug regimens based on the extent of renal dysfunction.

One note with regard to serum creatinine used in Cockcroft-Gault. Historically, some clinicians have advocated correcting low serum creatinine concentrations in the elderly to 1.0 mg/dL, due to decreased kidney function that occurs as part of the aging process. Not only is there no literature to support this practice, but there is good evidence that using the real serum creatinine will produce a value closer to the measured creatinine clearance.[12]

Chronic Kidney Disease Epidemiology Collaboration (CKD-EPI) Equation

The most accurate estimate of the glomerular filtration rate (eGFR) is the CKD-EPI equation developed by a group of clinician scientists based on data from 8,254 patients and published in 2009.[13] This approach is actually a series of equations developed to estimate GFR in various subpopulations. The CKD-EPI equation provides the eGFR in the units of mL/min/1.73 m^2. Most laboratories will calculate this value for clinicians; there are also several online calculators available that can be used for calculation.

Kidney-Adjusted Drug Dosing in Children

The Schwartz equation developed in 2009[14] for the estimation of the GFR in children is the most widely used equation:

$$\text{eGFR in mL/min/1.73m}^2 = (0.413)(\text{ht in cm/SCr in mg/dL})$$

This equation is even more accurate, if blood urea nitrogen (BUN) and serum cystatin C concentrations are available:

$$\begin{aligned}\text{eGFR} = {} & (39.1)(\text{ht/SCr})^{0.516}(1.8/\text{SCysC})^{0.294}(30/\text{BUN})^{0.169} \\ & (1.099 \text{ if male})(\text{ht}/1.4)^{0.188}\end{aligned}$$

where ht is in m, SCr is in mg/dL, SCysC is in mg/L, and BUN is in mg/dL.

Using Normalized GFR Equations for Drug Dosing

Note that the estimate of GFR calculated by all of the above-referenced equations (except for the Cockcroft-Gault equation, which calculates unnormalized eCrCl) is normalized over the surface area of the 5'9", 70-kilogram average person (1.73 m^2). These equations should NOT be used in this normalized form for the dosing of drugs. The normalized equation must be corrected for the specific patient by multiplying the eGFR by the patient's estimated BSA.[10] For example, a 5'6", 103-lb patient with eGFR of 47 mL/min/1.73 m² can be individualized as follows:

$$\text{GFR in mL / min} = (\text{eGFR in mL / min/1.73 m}^2)(\text{eBSA})$$

$$(103\text{ lb})(1\text{ kg / 2.2 lb}) = 46.8\text{ kg}\quad (66\text{ inches})(2.54\text{ cm / inch}) = 167.6\text{ cm}$$

$$\text{BSA} = 1.48\text{ m}^2\sqrt{\frac{(167.6\text{ cm})\times(46.8\text{ kg})}{3{,}600}} = 1.14\text{ m}^2$$

$$\text{iGFR} = (47\text{ mL / min/1.73 m}^2)(1.48\text{ m}^2) = 40\text{ mL / min}$$

Example: A 79-year-old male patient has a urinary tract infection. He is 69 inches tall and 155 lb, and his S_{cr} = 1.7 mg/dL. Calculate this patient's estimated CrCl:

$$\text{LBW} = 50 + (2.3\times 9) = 70.7\text{ kg}\quad 155\text{ lb / 2.2 lb / kg} = 70.5\text{ kg}$$

$$\text{CrCl} = \frac{(140-79)\times 70.5}{72\times 1.7} = \frac{4300.5}{122.4} = 35.1\text{ mL / min}$$

The labeling of cefixime makes the following recommendations for patients with kidney dysfunction:

CrCl >60 mL/min:	No dosage adjustment needed
CrCl 20 to 60 mL/min:	300 mg daily
CrCl <20 mL/min:	200 mg daily

How many 100-mL bottles of cefixime suspension, 100 mg/5 mL, should be dispensed to provide the patient above with 14 days' therapy?

$$\frac{300\text{ mg}}{\text{day}}\ \frac{5\text{ mL}}{100\text{ mg}}\ \frac{1\text{ bottle}}{100\text{ mL}}(14\text{ d}) = 2.1\text{ bottle}(3\text{ bottle})$$

Parenteral Calculations

Calculation of Injectable Volumes

The pharmacy has an order for a 120-lb patient for amikacin sulfate, 7.5 mg/kg loading dose, in 100 mL D5W. Amikacin is available in vials containing 100 mg/2 mL, 500 mg/2 mL, and 1 g/4 mL:

$$120\ \text{lb}\frac{(1\ \text{kg})}{(2.2\ \text{lb})}\frac{(7.5\ \text{mg})}{(\text{kg})} = 409\ \text{mg amikacin}$$

$$\text{Use the 500 mg vial}: \frac{500\ \text{mg}}{2\ \text{mL}} = \frac{409\ \text{mg}}{\text{y mL}} \quad \text{y} = 1.64\ \text{mL}$$

- Note: this volume, 1.64 mL, would be added to a 100-mL bag of D5W, which means that the resulting volume would be 101.64 mL.
- This is typically how IV additives are made *rather* than first withdrawing 1.64 mL of D5W and then adding the drug solution so that the final volume is 100 mL.
- Although small volumes of overfill are sometimes ignored in subsequent calculations, this example will include them.
- This practice will vary from hospital to hospital.

Administration Rate Calculations

Large-volume parenterals and small-volume parenterals can be administered using a drip set or via infusion pump, a programmable device that allows the nurse/pharmacist to set the number of *milliliters per hour or milligrams per hour* that it will deliver through the tubing to the patient. In general, an infusion pump will be used when it is important to control the rate of fluid entry into the patient, and drip sets will be used when tight control of the infusion rate is not necessary.

In addition to the overfill created by additives, most parenteral products contain some planned overfill. Manufacturers provide a slight excess volume since it is impossible to transfer 100% of the volume from a container into a syringe. Some pharmacies ignore overfill in their calculations of volume and flow rate and others do not.

Administration Rate Using Infusion Pumps

A patient is to receive dopamine at 2 μg/kg/min. The patient weighs 70 kg. The concentration of drug in the bag is 80 mg/100 mL. At what flow rate in milliliter per hour should the dopamine solution be infused?

$$(70)\text{kg}\ \frac{2\ \mu\text{g}}{\text{kg/min}}\ \frac{1\ \text{mg}}{1{,}000\ \mu\text{g}}\ \frac{100\ \text{mL}}{80\ \text{mg}}\ \frac{60\ \text{min}}{1\ \text{h}} = \frac{10.5\ \text{mL}}{\text{h}}$$

The 2004 Joint Commission on Accreditation of Healthcare Organizations (JCAHO) medication error reduction program recommended programming pumps in milligram per hour instead of milliliter per hour. What is the infusion rate in milligram per hour?

$$(70)\text{kg}\frac{2\ \mu\text{g}}{\text{kg/min}}\frac{1\ \text{mg}}{1{,}000\ \mu\text{g}}\frac{60\ \text{min}}{1\ \text{h}}=\frac{8.4\ \text{mL}}{\text{h}}$$

Calculating Osmolarity

In clinical practice, the pharmacist may need to know the concentration of particles exerting osmotic pressure in a parenteral product in order to know whether the product can be infused through a peripheral line or whether it will need to be administered through a central line. The osmolarity or moles of solute particles per liter of most body fluids is between 275 and 295 mOsm/L.

Osmolality and Osmolarity

- The United States Pharmacopeia (USP) designates the units for expressing the osmotic pressure exerted by a real solution across a semipermeable membrane as osmoles per kilogram or milliosmoles per kilogram of water.
- One osmole equals 1 mole of dissolved particles, meaning, for a nonelectrolyte, 1 mole equals 1 osmole and, by definition, would lower the freezing point of water by 1.86°C.
- The osmolality of blood and other body fluids is between 285 and 310 mOsm/kg, and drug solutions typically have osmotic concentrations in the milliosmolal range.
- Osmolarity, the number of osmoles or milliosmoles per liter of the solution, is calculated and cannot be directly measured.
- The USP provides the following equation for calculation of the theoretical osmolar concentration of multicomponent drug solutions:

$$\text{Osmolarity}=\sum i_i C_i$$

where i_i is the van't Hoff factor of each component and C_i is the molar concentration. Table 13.5 includes the van't Hoff factors for various types of solutes encountered in drug products.

We can calculate the osmolarity of a 0.9% sodium chloride solution using this equation:

$$\frac{(9\ \text{g})}{(\text{L})}\frac{(1\ \text{mole})}{(58.5\ \text{g})}=0.1538\ \text{M NaCl}$$

$$\begin{aligned}\text{Osmolarity}&=(1.823)(0.1538\ \text{M})\\&=0.280\ \text{Osmoles/L or }280\ \text{mOsm/L}\end{aligned}$$

TABLE 13.5 van't Hoff Factors for Different Solute Classes

Class	Examples	$L_{iso} = K_f\, i$	*i* Factor
Nonelectrolyte	Dextrose	1.86	1.0
Weak electrolyte	Weak acids or bases, boric acid, citric acid, acetic acid	2.0	1.053
Divalent–divalent salts, 2 ions	$ZnSO_4$, $MgSO_4$	2.0	1.053
Univalent–univalent salts, 2 ions	KCl, dipivefrin hydrochloride, cephalothin sodium	3.4	1.79
Univalent–divalent salts, 3 ions, anion polyvalent	Atropine sulfate, ticarcillin disodium, dibasic sodium phosphate, morphine sulfate	4.3	2.26
Divalent–univalent salt, 3 ions, anion univalent	$CaCl_2$, magnesium gluconate, hydroxyzine dihydrochloride	4.8	2.53
Univalent–trivalent salts, 4 ions, anion polyvalent	Sodium citrate, sodium phosphate	5.2	2.74
Trivalent–univalent salts, 4 ions, anion univalent	Aluminum chloride, ferric chloride	6.0	3.16
Tetraborates	Sodium borate	7.6	4.0

Source: Goyan FM, Enright JM, Wells JM. Rapid method for calculating isotonic solutions. *J Am Pharm Assoc Pract Ed.* 1944;5:99.[16]

You can see that this equation ignores the difference between osmolality and osmolarity. In practice, calculated values for osmolality and osmolarity are very close, and the terms are used interchangeably. To illustrate the calculation for a multicomponent solution, osmolarity of 1 g of ampicillin sodium (FW 371.4, van't Hoff factor for a univalent salt from Table 13.5 is 1.79) in 10 mL of normal saline would be

Molarity of ampicillin 1 g/10 mL:

$$\frac{(1\text{ g})}{(10\text{ mL})}\frac{(1{,}000\text{ mL})}{(\text{L})}\frac{(1\text{ mole})}{(371.4\text{ g})} = 0.269\text{ M ampicillin}$$

Calculating its osmolarity:

$$\begin{aligned}\text{Osmolarity} &= (1.79)(0.269\text{M})\\ &= 0.482\text{ Osmoles / L or }482\text{ mOsmol / L}\end{aligned}$$

The osmolarities are additive:

$$280 \text{ mOsm} / \text{L} + 482 \text{ mOsmol} / \text{L} = 762 \text{ mOsmol} / \text{L}$$

Bulky Powders for Reconstitution

Many drugs are not stable in solution:

- Manufactured as powders for reconstitution, the pharmacy adds a diluent before they can be administered.
- Some of these powders represent a very large volume; they may include buffers or with oral products, flavors, sweeteners, and dyes, which increase the volume of the powders to be dissolved.
- It cannot be assumed that the volume of the powder to be reconstituted is negligible; that is, dissolving 1 g of ampicillin in 10 mL water produces a concentration of 100 mg per milliliter.
- The manufacturer will give specific instructions on how much diluent to use to produce a specified concentration.

A pharmacist needs to make cefazolin injection for ophthalmic use at a concentration of 25 mg/0.1 mL. He has cefazolin powder for reconstitution: to 1 g, add 2.5 mL of diluent, for a resulting concentration of 333.3 mg/mL. How many milliliters of normal saline should be added to make the 25 mg/0.1 mL for ophthalmic use?

$$\frac{1 \text{ g}}{x \text{ mL}} = \frac{0.3333 \text{ g}}{1 \text{ mL}} \quad x = 3 \text{ mL} \quad 3 - 2.5 \text{ mL} = 0.5 \text{ mL}$$

represented by the powder

$$\frac{1{,}000 \text{mg}}{x \text{ mL}} = \frac{25 \text{ mg}}{0.1 \text{ mL}} \quad x = 4 \text{ mL} \quad 4 - 0.5 \text{ mL} = 3.5 \text{mL}$$

saline to add

Milliequivalents

One milliequivalent is the weight of a substance that can replace or combine with 1 millimole (1 mg) of H^+.

Example: How many milliequivalents of Ca are there per milliliter of a 10% calcium gluconate injection?

Formula:	$C_{12}H_{22}CaO_{14}$
FW:	430
Valence:	2×1 Ca ion

There is one calcium in calcium gluconate, and it has a valence of 2+, thus a related term that can be used in the calculation:

$$\frac{2\text{ mEq Ca ion}}{430\text{ mg Ca gluc}}$$

$$10\%\text{ Ca gluc} = \frac{10\text{ g Ca gluc}}{100\text{ mL}}\frac{(2\text{ mEq Ca})}{(0.43\text{ g Ca gluc})} = 0.465\text{ mEq Ca / mL}$$

Compounding Calculations

Percent Volume/Volume (v/v) Concentration Example

A pharmacist needs 38% alcohol in a vehicle to dissolve a drug at the required concentration. The prescription requires 120 mL of an oral liquid solution (soln). How much alcohol is needed to make 120 mL 38% (v/v) alcohol?

$$38\% = \frac{38\text{ mL alcohol}}{100\text{ mL soln}} = \frac{x\text{ mL alcohol}}{120\text{ mL soln}} \quad x = 45.6\text{ mL alcohol}$$

The alcohol the pharmacist will use to make this is alcohol USP, which is 95% ethanol:

$$95\% = \frac{95\text{ mL ethanol}}{100\text{ mL alcohol USP}} = \frac{45.6\text{ mL ethanol}}{y\text{ mL alcohol USP}}$$

$$y = 48\text{ mL alcohol USP}$$

Percent of Concentrated and Dilute Acids

Remember that chemists use the convention of % weight/weight (w/w) for concentrated acids and % weight/volume (w/v) for dilute acids. If a pharmacist uses 50 mL concentrated phosphoric acid (85%, sp gr 1.71) to make 500 mL of diluted phosphoric acid, what is the percent concentration of the dilution (w/v)?

What weight of phosphoric acid does 50 mL of the concentrated acid contain?

$$\frac{85\text{ g PA}(1.71\text{ g soln})}{100\text{ g solution}(1\text{ mL soln})} = \frac{145\text{ g PA}}{100\text{ mL soln}}$$

$$\frac{145\text{ g PA}}{100\text{ mL soln}} = \frac{x\text{ g PA}}{50\text{ mL soln}} \quad x = 72.7\text{ g PA}$$

What is the new concentration w/v?

$$\frac{72.7\ \text{g}}{500\ \text{mL}} = \frac{x\ \text{g}}{100\ \text{mL}} \quad x = 14.5\ \text{g and as a percent } 14.5\%$$

Ratio Strength Calculations

The dose of epinephrine required for a child is 0.022 mg. Can this volume be more conveniently drawn from epinephrine 1:1,000 or 1:10,000?

$$\frac{1\ \text{g epi}}{1{,}000\ \text{mL}} = \frac{1{,}000\ \text{mg epi}}{1{,}000\ \text{mL}} = 1\ \text{mg epi / mL} \quad 0.022\ \text{mg}\frac{1\ \text{mL}}{1\ \text{mg}} = 0.022\ \text{mL}$$

$$\frac{1\ \text{g epi}}{10{,}000\ \text{mL}} = \frac{1{,}000\ \text{mg epi}}{10{,}000\ \text{mL}} = 0.1\ \text{mg / mL} \quad 0.022\ \text{mg}\frac{(1\ \text{mL})}{0.1\ \text{mg}} = 0.22\ \text{mL}$$

The 0.22-mL amount can be more accurately measured than the 0.022-mL amount, so the epinephrine 1:10,000 strength would be the more convenient strength of epinephrine to select for this dose.

Parts per Million Calculation

A patient reads that the fluoride concentration of her drinking water is 0.8 ppm. How much fluoride does she consume from drinking three 8-oz glasses of water per day?

$$\frac{8\ \text{oz}}{\text{glass}}\ \frac{(3\ \text{glasses})}{(\text{day})}\ \frac{(30\ \text{mL})}{(\text{oz})}\ \frac{(0.8\ \text{g})}{10^6\ \text{mL}}\ \frac{(1{,}000\ \text{mg})}{(1\ \text{g})}$$

$$= \text{weight / day} = \frac{0.576\ \text{mg fluoride}}{\text{day}}$$

Simple Dilutions

What volume of adult strength acetazolamide injection, 100 mg/mL, should be used to make 10 mL of the neonatal concentration, 5 mg/mL?

$$\frac{\text{Original concentration}}{\text{Diluted concentration}} = \frac{\text{Diluted volume}}{\text{Original volume}}$$

$$\frac{100\ \text{mg / mL}}{5\ \text{mg / mL}} = \frac{10\ \text{mL}}{y\ \text{mL}}$$

Rearranging for y,

$$(100\ \text{mg / mL})(y\ \text{mL}) = (5\ \text{mg / mL})(10\ \text{mL})$$
$$C_1V_1 = C_2V_2$$

$$V_1 = \frac{(5\ \text{mg / mL})(10\ \text{mL})}{(100\ \text{mg / mL})} = 0.5\ \text{mL adult strength acetazolamide}$$

Blending Two Concentrations

Rx: Tobramycin 1% eye drops
Disp 10 mL
Sig: 1 gtt od tid

The pharmacist will make these drops from the commercially available eye drops, which have a strength of 0.3%, and the injectable tobramycin, 40 mg/mL. What volume of each strength should be used to make the 10-mL eye drops?

$$40\ \text{mg / mL} \times 100 = 4{,}000\ \text{mg / 100 mL} = 4\ \text{g / 100 mL} = 4\%$$

Set

$$x = \text{fraction of tobramycin injection}$$
$$1 - x = \text{fraction of tobramycin eye drops}$$

The equation is

$$1\% = 4\%\,x + (1 - x)0.3\%$$

Multiplying by 0.3,

$$1 = 4x + 0.3 - 0.3x$$

Combine the like terms:

$$1 - 0.3 = 4x + 0.3 - 0.3 - 0.3x$$
$$0.7 = 3.7x$$

Solving for x:

$$\frac{0.7}{3.7} = \frac{3.7x}{3.7} \qquad x = 0.19 = \text{fraction of injectable tobramycin}$$
$$1 - x = 0.81 = \text{fraction of tobramycin eyedrops}$$

To make 10 mL:

$$0.19 \times 10 \text{ mL} = 1.9 \text{ mL injectable tobramycin}$$
$$0.81 \times 10 \text{ mL} = 8.1 \text{ mL tobramycin eye drops}$$

Aliquot Dilutions

If the available balance or volumetric equipment cannot accurately measure the quantity required, the pharmacist can weigh out a multiple of the quantity and dilute it such that the desired amount is contained in a measurable quantity. This is called an aliquot dilution and can be done as follows:

Example: The pharmacist needs 30 mg Klonopin (clonazepam) to compound capsules for a child with seizures. She has a typical torsion balance with a sensitivity of 5 mg and

$$\text{Minimum weighable quantity (MWQ)} = \frac{\text{sensitivity or linear accuracy}}{\text{fraction error}}$$

$$\text{Minimum weighable quantity} = \frac{5 \text{ mg}}{0.05} = 100 \text{ mg}$$

1. Select a multiple of the amount that will equal or exceed the minimum weighable quantity (MWQ) for the balance

$$30 \text{ mg} \times 4 = 120 \text{ mg clonazepam to weigh out}$$

2. Select the weight of the dilution that will contain the amount of active ingredient that is needed (the aliquot weight). This number must also equal or exceed the MWQ.

   The pharmacist decides that 1/4 of the dilution will weigh 200 mg. Multiply it by the same factor:

$$200 \times 4 = 800 \text{ mg total dilution} - \frac{120 \text{ mg drug}}{680 \text{ mg lactose}}$$

   Mix these two well.

3. Take 1/4 or 200 mg of the dilution, and it will contain 30 mg clonazepam.

Tonicity Calculations

- *E* value calculates the weight of sodium chloride equivalent to 1 g of drug or other solute.

- In some cases, the *E* value of the drug has been tabulated,[11] and the amounts of water and isotonic vehicle to be added to prepare an isotonic product can be calculated using proportions.

E Value Calculation

Rx: Cromolyn sodium 40 mg/mL
Benzalkonium chloride 0.01%
Dispense 10 mL

How much sodium chloride is required to make the solution isotonic if the *E* for cromolyn sodium = 0.11?

1. Amount of NaCl equivalent to drug: For cromolyn,

$$40\ \text{mg}/\text{mL} \times 10\ \text{mL} = 400\ \text{mg} = 0.4\ \text{g cromolyn} \quad E\ \text{value} = 0.11$$

$$\frac{0.4\ \text{g drug}}{1\ \text{g drug}} = \frac{x\ \text{g NaCl}}{0.11\ \text{g NaCl}} \quad x = 0.044\ \text{g NaCl}$$

For benzalkonium chloride,

$$0.01/100 \times 10\ \text{mL} = 0.001\ \text{g benzalkonium chloride} \quad E\ \text{value} = 0.16$$

$$\frac{0.001\ \text{g drug}}{1\ \text{g drug}} = \frac{x\ \text{g NaCl}}{0.16\ \text{g NaCl}} \quad x = 0.00016\ \text{g NaCl}$$

2. How much NaCl is needed to make the solution isotonic?

$$\frac{0.9\ \text{g NaCl}}{100\ \text{mL}} = \frac{y\ \text{g NaCl}}{10\ \text{mL}} \quad y = 0.09\ \text{g NaCl}$$

3. How much NaCl is needed to be added?

0.09 g	NaCl
−0.044 g	Contributed by the cromolyn
−0.00016 g	Contributed by the benzalkonium chloride
0.04584 =	0.046 g NaCl to add

Oral Suspensions for Reconstitution

Rx: Zithromax 250 mg/5 mL
Sig: 2 tsp today and 1 tsp qd × 4 additional days

The patient is an 87-year-old man with pneumonia. The pharmacist has a 30-mL size bottle of azithromycin (Zithromax) powder for reconstitution that if reconstituted with 18 mL water will have a concentration of 200 mg/5 mL. How many milliliters of water should be added to prepare it in the prescribed concentration?

What volume is the powder?

$$30 - 18 \text{ mL} = 12 \text{ mL represented by the powder}$$

How much total drug is in the bottle?

$$\frac{200 \text{ mg}}{5 \text{ mL}} \times 30 \text{ mL} = 1{,}200 \text{ mg drug total}$$

What total volume should be used to make the concentration equal 250 mg/5 mL?

$$\frac{5 \text{ mL}}{250 \text{ mg}} \times 1{,}200 \text{ mg} = 24 \text{ mL total volume}$$

How much water should be added?

24-mL total volume
−12 mL represented by the powder
12 mL water to add

Proportionate Parts

A convenient method for recording formulas that are made in widely varying amounts is proportionate parts. For example, the formula of a popular suppository base consists of

PEG 1000	3 parts
PEG 4000	1 part

A prescription requires 22 g of the suppository base. How much of each component does the pharmacist need?

PEG 1000	3 parts
PEG 4000	1 part
Total	4 parts

$$\frac{3 \text{ parts PEG 1000}}{4 \text{ parts total}} = \frac{x \text{ g PEG 1000}}{22 \text{ g total}} \qquad x = 16.5 \text{ g PEG 1000}$$

$$\frac{1 \text{ parts PEG 4000}}{4 \text{ parts total}} = \frac{x \text{ g PEG 4000}}{22 \text{ g total}} \qquad x = 5.5 \text{ g PEG 4000}$$

Compounding with Commercially Available Dosage Forms

- Pharmacists will often use commercially available dosage forms in compounding rather than drug powders.
- For example, an ointment may be prepared from so many milliliters of an injection and an ointment base that absorbs solutions, or a suspension may be compounded by crushing tablets or opening capsules.
- When using an injectable product, the volume of the solution that contains a specified amount of drug can be easily calculated *because the weight per unit volume is on the label.*
- With solid dosage forms, the concentration of drug in solid mixture is specified per tablet or per capsule rather than per gram or milligram.
- Tablets and capsules will always have ingredients other than drug in the dosage form.
  - One hydralazine tablet contains 50-mg drug; 10 tablets are required to provide 500 mg.
  - But what if a prescription requires 480 mg?
- It will be necessary to know the weight of the tablet or in the case of capsules *of the capsule contents*, to determine what weight of hydralazine tablets contains 480 mg.

Rx: Lamotrigine 4-mg capsules
Make capsules
Dispense 28
Sig: Open 1 capsule on soft food twice daily

Lamotrigine is an anticonvulsant drug available as 25-, 100-, 150-, and 200-mg tablets.

How much drug is required to make the 28 capsules?

$$4\text{ mg / cap} \times 28\text{ caps} = 112\text{ mg is needed}$$

If the pharmacist uses 25-mg tablets and they weigh 80 mg each, how much crushed tablet powder is required to make the 28 capsules?

$$(112\text{ mg drug})\frac{(80\text{ mg tab powder})}{25\text{ mg drug}} = 358.4\text{ mg tab powder}$$

And what weight of tablet powder will contain the dose?

$$\frac{358.4\text{ mg tablet powder}}{28\text{ doses}} = 12.8\text{ mg tab powder / dose}$$

Test Capsules, Test Suppositories

- When making capsules or suppositories, the pharmacist is faced with determining what weight of the drug mixture will fit in the volume dictated by a capsule shell or suppository mold.
- This is done by preparing a test capsule or suppository using diluent and drug.
- The weight of the test capsule or suppository can be used to determine how much diluent or suppository base to use for a given batch.

Consider the lamotrigine capsules above. The pharmacist plans to pack them into a no. 4 capsule. If the test capsule weighs 135 mg, how much lactose should be used to make the 28 lamotrigine capsules?

$$\begin{aligned} 135\text{ mg / capsule} \times 28\text{ capsules} = {} & 3{,}780\text{ mg total mixture} \\ & \underline{-358.4\text{ mg tablet powder}} \\ & \text{containing our drug} \\ & 3{,}421.6\text{ mg lactose to add} \end{aligned}$$

Rx: Avandia 8-mg suppositories
Dispense 7
Sig: 1 rectally q AM.

These suppositories can be made from Avandia tablets. A batch of five Avandia 8-mg tablets weighs 1,570 mg. If the test suppository weighs 2.4 g, how many grams PEG 1000 and PEG 4000 should be used to make the seven suppositories?

$$\begin{aligned} & 1{,}570\text{ mg / 5 tab} = 314\text{ mg / tab} = 0.314\text{ g} \\ & 2.4\text{ g} \times 7 = 16.8\text{ g suppository mixture} \\ & \text{tablets weigh } 0.314\text{ g} \times 7 = 2.198 \\ & 16.8 - 2.198 = 14.602\text{ g base needed} \end{aligned}$$

$$\frac{3\text{ parts PEG1000}}{4\text{ parts total}} = \frac{x\text{ g PEG1000}}{14.602\text{g total}} \quad x = 10.95\text{ g PEG1000}$$

$$\frac{1\text{ parts PEG 4000}}{4\text{ parts total}} = \frac{x\text{ g PEG 4000}}{14.602\text{ g total}} \quad x = 3.65\text{ g PEG 4000}$$

References

1. The virtues of independent double checks—they really are worth your time? In: *Institute for Safe Medication Practices Medication Safety Alert [Internet]*. Horsham, PA: Institute for Safe Medication Practices; 2003 March 6. Available at: www.ismp.org/newsletters/acutecare/articles/20030306.asp. Accessed April 19, 2013.
2. Brown MC. Introduction to pharmaceutical calculations. *Am J Pharm Educ.* 2003;67(2): Article 67.
3. Anonymous. ISMP's List of Error-Prone Abbreviations, Symbols and Dose Designations [Internet]. Horsham, PA: Institute for Safe Medication Practices; ©2013. Available at www.ismp.org. Accessed April 19, 2013.
4. Shargel L, Wu-Pong S, Yu ABC. *Applied Biopharmaceutics and Pharmacokinetics*. 6th ed. New York, NY: McGraw Hill; 2012.
5. Janmahasatian S, Duffull SB, Ash S, et al. Quantification of lean bodyweight. *Clin Pharmacokinet.* 2005; 44:1051–1065.
6. Bauer LA, Edwards WA, Dellinger EP, et al. Influence of weight on aminoglycoside pharmacokinetics in normal weight and morbidly obese patients. *Eur J Clin Pharmacol.* 1983;24:643–647.
7. Mosteller RD. Simplified calculation of body-surface area. *N Engl J Med.* 1987;317:1098.
8. Haycock GB, Schwartz GJ, Wisotsky DH. Geometric method for measuring body surface area: a height-weight formula validated in infants, children, and adults. *J Pediatr.* 1987;93:62–66.
9. Cockcroft DW, Gault MH. Prediction of creatinine clearance from serum creatinine. *Nephron.* 1976;16:31–41.
10. Richardson M. Trade offs in assessing kidney function and drug dosing. *Pharmacotherapy.* 2010;30:(8):758–761.
11. Aronoff GR, Bennett WM, Berns JS, et al. *Drug Prescribing in Renal Failure.* 5th ed. Philadelphia, PA: American College of Physicians; 2007.
12. Winter MA, Guhr KN, Berg GM. Impact of various body weights and serum creatinine concentrations on the bias and accuracy of the Cockcroft-Gault equation. *Pharmacotherapy.* 2012;32:604–612.
13. Levey AS, Stevens LA, Schmid CH, et al. A new equation to estimate glomerular filtration rate. *Ann Intern Med.* 2009;150(9):604–612.
14. Schwartz GJ, Munoz A, Schneider MF, et al. New equations to estimate GFR in children with CKD. *J Am Soc Nephrol.* 2009;20:629–637.
15. Thompson, JE, Davidow, LE. *A Practical Guide to Contemporary Pharmacy Practice.* 3rd ed. Philadelphia, PA: Lippincott Williams & Wilkins; 2009.
16. Goyan FM, Enright JM, Wells JM. Rapid method for calculating isotonic solutions. *J Am Pharm Assoc Pract Ed.* 1944;5:99.

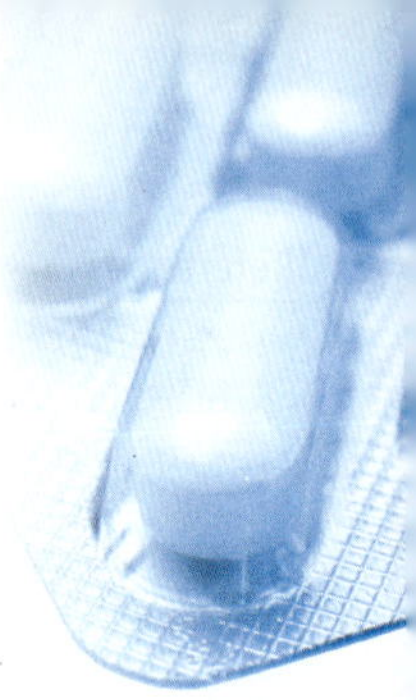

14

Clinical Pharmacokinetics

Sandra B. Earle and Molly E. Bruvold

Use of Pharmacokinetic Principles to Enhance Drug Therapy

Pharmacists are uniquely qualified in their understanding and application of pharmacokinetic (PK) principles as tools to optimize the use of drugs in patients. Using PK principles, the pharmacist can properly evaluate measured drug concentrations and design dosage regimens. In addition, by understanding what determines PK parameters, drug and disease interactions can be predicted. This chapter provides a table of equations, a glossary, and some general concepts of clinical therapeutic drug monitoring (TDM) and dosage regimen design. This is not an all-encompassing review of clinical PKs, but can serve as a refresher of basic ideas and important caveats. Please see more detailed texts and literature references for further details.

Evaluation of Measured Drug Concentrations: Therapeutic Drug Monitoring

Indications for Therapeutic Drug Monitoring

Most drugs do not require determination of drug concentrations for optimization of drug therapy. If you can give a standard dosage regimen and get the wanted effect in all/most patients, there is no reason to measure drug concentrations. TDM may be useful only if the following criteria are in place:

- Absence of a well-defined dose–response relationship
- A well-defined concentration–response relationship (pharmacodyamics)
- A relatively narrow therapeutic range
- Interpatient variability in the dose regimen–concentration relationship (pharmacokinetics)
- Accurate drug assays available

In addition to serving as a guide for dosage adjustment, drug concentrations may be used to assess patient adherence.

For appropriate interpretation of the measured drug concentrations, the following information should be either known or obtained:

- What condition is being treated?
- Is the patient suffering from any dose-related toxicities and/or signs of lack of efficacy?
- Is the patient at steady state (SS)?
- Were all doses given at the appropriate time and if not, when were they given?
- When was(were) the sample(s) drawn in relation to the dose given?
- Are there any patient-specific factors that can influence PK parameters? (i.e., volume status, albumin concentrations, renal function, obesity, genomics, other drugs)

Unbound "Free" Versus Total Concentrations

Total concentrations of drugs are made up of the sum of both drugs bound to plasma proteins as well as the drug that is free from the binding proteins. Only "free" or unbound drug molecules can interact at the pharmacologic sites. Therefore, free concentrations correlate more closely with the drug effect. It is much easier (and therefore less expensive) for the lab to measure the total drug rather than just the free drug concentration. Thus, most drug concentrations are reported as total concentrations and most therapeutic ranges are in terms of total drug concentrations. As long as the free fraction of drug in the plasma (fraction unbound in plasma [fup]) remains constant, the total concentration will be proportional to the free concentration. As soon as the fup changes, this will no longer be true. It is almost always acceptable to look at total concentrations and feel confident that they are proportional to the free concentration, except when fup is thought to be altered by drugs or disease or is changing with concentration.

Sampling Times

As a general rule, the trough concentration (C_{min}) is usually monitored. If the C_{min} (trough) is within the therapeutic range (TR), the patient is likely not suffering from lack of efficacy due to inadequate serum concentrations. This does not ensure, however, that the patient's average concentration at steady state ($C_{ss,avg}$) and maximum concentration at steady state ($C_{ss,max}$) are appropriate. Since the time to C_{max} can vary significantly for orally administered drugs, it is hard to determine when to draw a concentration to capture the C_{max}. If any two concentrations are drawn during the elimination phase, an elimination rate constant (k), half-life (t½), volume of distribution (V), and drug out (CL) can be determined along with C_{max}, C_{min}, and any other concentration. There are drugs for which both the trough and the peak concentrations may be monitored (e.g., aminoglycosides). If trying to determine k when giving a short infusion, be sure to allow sufficient time after giving a drug for initial distribution. A good rule of thumb is to wait 1 hour after giving a ½ hour infusion and wait ½ hour if giving an infusion over an hour.

It is important to be sure that the blood sample drawn will have a concentration that will be above the minimum detection limit of your lab. The pharmacist should predict what the concentration will be before it is drawn, to ensure it is within the detectable range. A C_{min} measurement may be too low. If a concentration-related toxicity is suspected, a serum concentration sample should be drawn as soon as possible to determine the toxicity range for that patient.

Dosage Regimen Design

Initial Dosing

Depending upon the therapeutic concentration goals, a loading dose (LD) may or may not be needed. An LD is needed when it will take too long to achieve therapeutic concentrations when using a maintenance dosing regimen. Since it takes about five half-lives to attain steady state, this usually includes drugs with a long t½. An LD is based upon the target concentration and the V_c. Giving an LD does not change the time to steady state (SS), only t½ determines when SS will be achieved.

$$LD = V_c \times C_{target}$$

Initial maintenance dosage regimens are determined by choosing a target $C_{ss,avg}$ and target peak-to-trough ratio (P:T). The dosage regimen is made up of the dose rate (DR) and the dose interval (τ). The DR is a determinant of the $C_{ss,avg}$ achieved, and the τ determines what the P:T will be seen, or the variance around the average concentration. When a drug is given to a patient for the first time, population averages are employed as the patient's PK parameters. Target $C_{ss,avg}$ along with population CL and F estimates determine the initial DR:

$$C_{ss,avg} = \frac{F \times DR}{CL}$$

Dosing once every t½ is a good rule of thumb, but the P:T can be targeted using a population k, until an individual k can be determined.

$$P:T = \frac{1}{e^{-k\tau}}$$

Modification of a Dosing Regimen

After starting a patient on a dosage regimen based upon population information, optimization of the individual patient's drug therapy must be verified. This includes evaluating the patient clinically. The drug concentrations are only one tool in evaluating therapy. Evaluating the patient's clinical status in light of their drug concentrations will help to determine if a change in the dosing regimen is necessary. To evaluate $C_{ss,avg}$, you must be at SS. It is often appropriate to measure concentrations before reaching SS to avoid toxicity or lack of efficacy.

If the patient is at SS, the pharmacist should determine if the $C_{ss,avg}$ is appropriate for the patient. If the $C_{ss,avg}$ is too high, the patient's drug exposure may be too high, putting them at risk for concentration-related toxicity; therefore, the DR should be decreased. If the $C_{ss,avg}$ is too low, the opposite would be true and the DR should be increased. What would cause a change in $C_{ss,avg}$? The determinants of $C_{ss,avg}$ are drug in (F × DR) and drug out (CL).

$$C_{ss,avg} = \frac{F \times DR}{CL} = \frac{\text{Drug In}}{\text{Drug Out}}$$

If CL or F are altered, there will be a resulting change in $C_{ss,avg}$, possibly necessitating a change in DR. If there is a possible change in plasma protein binding, it will be important to consider the $C_{ss,avg}$, free rather than just the $C_{ss,avg}$. If a change in DR is deemed necessary and the patient is at SS, as long as there is no reason to think there might be a change in CL or F, $C_{ss,avg}$ becomes proportional to DR. Therefore, the adjustment in DR can be made using a simple proportion:

$$\frac{DR_1}{C_{ss,avg_1}} = \frac{DR_2}{C_{ss,avg_2}}$$

It is often important to consider the variability in the C_{max} and C_{min} concentrations (P:T). If the C_{max} is too high and the C_{min} is too low (large P:T), the dosing interval may be too long, so the dosing interval should be shortened, giving the drug more often during the day. It is rare (with the exception of aminoglycosides) that a C_{max} would be too low and the C_{min} too high (too small P:T). In this case, the τ should be increased. This would allow for greater change between the C_{max} and C_{min}. What would cause a change in this variability (P:T)? Changes in V or CL will cause a change in t½, therefore changing the P:T.

Determination of Concentrations Other Than Those Measured

If a drug follows a first-order, one-compartment elimination model, concentrations at any time during the dosing interval can be determined if one concentration and a k is known. Therefore, $C_{ss,max}$, $C_{ss,min}$, and any other concentration can be quantified using the one-compartment decay equation. k can be determined if two concentration–time points are known. $C_{ss,avg}$ can be determined by calculating the area under the concentration–time curve ($AUC_{0-\tau}$) at SS.

$$C_t = C_0 e^{-kt}$$

$$k = \frac{\ln C_2 - \ln C_1}{t_2 - t_1}$$

$$C_{ss,avg} = \frac{AUC_{ss,0-\tau}}{\tau}$$

Predicting Drug and Disease Interactions

Drugs administered concurrently and diseases that patients have can alter PK parameters. This may result in changes in $C_{ss,avg}$ or P:T ratios that could cause concentration-related toxicity or lack of efficacy. To predict these changes, the determinants of $C_{ss,avg}$ and P:T must be understood.

Altered $C_{ss,avg}$ can come about from a change in F and/or a change in CL. A change in F can occur due to a change in the fraction absorbed (fa), the fraction escaping the gut wall (fg), and/or the fraction escaping the first-pass effect (ffp). A change in formulation or addition of drug that adsorbs the first drug, for example, could decrease fa causing a decrease in F and therefore a decrease in $C_{ss,avg}$. The DR should be increased to maintain a given $C_{ss,avg}$. Inhibiting enzymes in the gut wall by grapefruit juice has become a well-known interaction. This results in an increase in fg, increasing the F and the $C_{ss,avg}$. This could cause dose-related toxicity symptoms. In this case, the DR may need to be decreased. The determinants of CL are complex as many organs may be involved. To simplify, consider a drug cleared only by the liver. Hepatic clearance is also complex depending upon blood flow to an organ (Q), enzyme activity (CL_{int}), and free fraction (fup) for clearance. To make predictions possible, it is helpful to consider two extremes: drugs with high extraction efficiencies (and therefore significant first-pass effects) and drugs with low extraction efficiencies (no or little first-pass effect). Low first-pass drugs are dependent upon enzyme activity and fup to determine CL_H. If the object (first) drug was a CYP P450 2D6 substrate and a new drug is added, that is, a CYP P450 2D6 inhibitor, a decrease in the CL of the object drug would be expected. This would cause an increase in $C_{ss,avg}$ possibly resulting in concentration-dependent toxicity. The DR should be decreased before the patient would possibly suffer from a toxicity. A good resource for updated CYP P450 data is http://medicine.iupui.edu/flockhart/table.htm. There are many variations of drug and disease interactions that can alter $C_{ss,avg}$.

$$C_{ss,avg} = \frac{F \times DR}{CL} = \frac{\text{Drug In}}{\text{Drug Out}}$$

Changes in the P:T are rarely as clinically significant as changes in $C_{ss,avg}$, but still should not be ignored. For example, if there is a decrease in V, the t½ would decrease and k would increase. This results in more variation between the $C_{ss,max}$ and $C_{ss,min}$ (increase P:T). This may result in C_{max} causing toxicity and/or C_{min} causing lack of efficacy. Decreasing the τ (giving the drug more often) should allieviate the problem. A change in CL or V resulting in a smaller P:T (less variance between $C_{ss,max}$ and $C_{ss,min}$) probably does not require a change in τ, but τ could be extended allowing the patient to take a drug less often.

Glossary

Bioavailability (F): units—none (fraction). The fraction of the administered dose that is available to the systemic circulation. Determined by fa, fg, and ffp. It is important in determining the DR needed to achieve a certain targeted $C_{ss,avg}$ if given other than by intravenous route.

Fraction absorbed (fa): fraction of drug given that is able to be absorbed into the circulation.

Fraction that escapes gut metabolism (fg): fraction of drug absorbed that is able to escape metabolism in the gut and escape efflux pumps that are in the gut wall (like P-glycoprotein).

Fraction that escapes first-pass effect (ffp): fraction of drug that escapes metabolism in the liver as the blood passes through the liver before reaching the systemic circulation. ffp is related to the hepatic extraction ratio of a drug (E): ffp = 1 − E.

Clearance (CL): units—vol/time. The volume of serum, plasma, or blood that has all of the drug removed per unit of time by the eliminating organ. Total body clearance is the sum of the clearances of all the eliminating organs. It is also the rate of elimination with respect to the given plasma concentration $(CL = k/c)$. Clearance of any organ is determined by the blood flow to that organ (Q) and the extraction efficiency of that organ (E): $CL = Q \times E$.

First order or linear elimination: the rate of elimination is directly proportional to the conentration of drug in the serum. It is independent of concentration.

Michaelis-Menten or nonlinear elimination: the rate of elimination does not change in proportion to the concentration of drug in the serum. As serum drug concentrations rise, the rate of elimination increases less than proportionally. This occurs when there is a capacity-limited elimination process. Examples are the hepatic enzymes and the transport sites for renal tubular secretion. When all available or nearly all available receptors are in use, the process reaches a saturation point, which results in the rate of elimination becoming fixed.

$$CL = \frac{V_{max}}{K_m + c}$$

Hepatic extraction ratio (E): units—none fraction of the absorbed dose metabolized during each pass through the liver. It is determined by Q_H, $CLint_H$, and fup and is an important determinant of CL_H.

Dose regimen (DR): units—amt/time. The amount of drug administered per time. May be thought of as daily dose. Important in determining the $C_{ss,avg}$. One of the factors that pharmacists can control.

Dose interval (τ): units—time. The frequency of intermittent drug administration. Important in determining the variance between the $C_{ss,max}$ and $C_{min,ss}$ or P:T. One of the factors that pharmacists can control. As a rule of thumb, drugs can be given once every half-life.

Peak-to-trough ratio (P:T): comparison of C_{max} to C_{min}. Important for understanding how much variation there is between the C_{max} and C_{min} concentrations within a dosing interval.

Half-life (t½): units—time. Time it takes for one-half of the drug to be removed from the body if eliminated by first-order elimination. Important for determining how often to dose a drug and how long it will take to get to SS. Determined by total body clearance (CL) and volume of distribution (V). Inversely related to elimination rate constant (k).

Elimination rate constant (k): units—time. The fraction of drug removed in a given time. Determined by measuring the slope of the terminal portion of the slope of the line formed by log serum concentrations versus time. Important for determining how often to dose a drug and how long it will take to get to steady state. Determined by total body clearance (CL) and volume of distribution (V). Inversely realted to half-life (t½).

Area under the concentration–time curve (AUC): units—$\frac{amt \times time}{vol}$. The area measured under the concentration–time curve that reults after administration of the drug. It relates patient exposure to a drug better than just a concentration at a point in time. In some cases, it may be helpful in determining efficacy and/or toxicity of a given drug. It is determined by the dose given, F if given other than IV and CL.

Steady state (SS): the point in therapy when the amount of drug administered exactly replaces the amount of drug removed. SS is never technically achieved, but for clinical purposes, 5 t½s (97% of SS) is considered to be at SS.

Maximum concentration at steady state ($C_{max,ss}$): units—amt/vol. The highest concentration achieved after intermittent dosage administration at SS. $C_{max,ss}$ will remain constant from dose to dose. May correlate to possible dose-related toxicity problems.

Minimum concentration at steady state ($C_{min,ss}$): units—amt/vol. The lowest concentration within an SS dosing interval. $C_{min,ss}$ will remain constant from dose to dose. May correlate to possible dose-related lack of efficacy.

Average concentration at steady state ($C_{ss,avg}$): units—amt/vol. The drug concentration representing the average concentration achieved during an SS dosing interval. It is similar but not determined by the average of the $C_{ss,max}$ and $C_{ss,min}$. It is often the target concentration when determining what dose rate to administer.

Therapeutic range (TR): a statistical range of desirable drug concentrations, for which the *majority* of patients show effective therapeutic response with minimal drug-related side effects. Is *not* an absolute for every patient. Individual patients can have good therapeutic response with "subtherapeutic" drug concentrations or can experience toxicity with "therapeutic" drug concentrations. Therapeutic ranges are indication specific.

Volume of distribution (V): units—volume. Where the drug distributes in the body. Important for determining how long the drug stays in the body (determinant of t½) and whether a drug will be removed by hemodialysis (larger volumes will not be removed significantly). Is primarily determined by binding of the drug to plasma and tissue binding sites as well as lipophilicity.

Central volume of distribution (V_c): hypothetical volume into which a drug initially distributes. It includes blood and highly perfused tissues. It is important for determining loading doses.

Apparent volume of distribution (V_d): calculated volume that would be necessary to account for all the drugs or the concentration of drug in the body. It is calculated by $V_d = \frac{Dose}{C}$ or by relating clearance and $KV_d = \frac{CL}{k}$.

Volume of distribution at steady state (V_{ss}): actual blood and tissue volumes into which the drug distributes. Can estimate the amount of drug in the body. Amount of drug in body = $V_{ss} \times C_{ss,avg}$.

Drugs Commonly Using TDM

Aminoglycosides (Gentamicin and Tobramycin)

Use: parenteral antibiotics, gram-negative infections

TR: extended interval dosing: peak 20 mg/L, trough too low to measure

Traditional dosing: peak 5 to 10 mg/L, trough <2 mg/L

CL: renal

Approximated by glomerular filtration rate (GFR)

V_d: 0.25 L/kg

Adjust for obesity and/or alterations in the extracellular fluid status

t½: 2 to 3 hours

Concentration-related side effects: nephrotoxicity and ototoxicity[1–4]

Aminoglycoside dose regimens are determined in an unusual way because it targets peak and trough levels rather than targeting a $C_{ss,avg}$. The dosing goals go on to be unconventional because a high peak concentration is the best predictor of efficacy, and low troughs are necessary to avoid toxicity. Because of these goals, a relatively new dosing method has been used called extended interval or "once-daily" dosing.[5] To improve the chance for a high peak and low trough, a longer dose interval is desirable. So, rather than a conventional q8- or q12-hour dosing schedule, longer schedules of q24 hours have been used, targeting higher peaks and lower troughs during a dosing interval. This method has been tested in many patient groups with good success.

Clinical Insights

1. Serum concentrations should be monitored if aminoglycoside therapy is expected to be continued for more than a few days. Determination of two serum concentrations would enable the patient's PK parameters to be determined and the dosage regimen to be optimized for the treatment, but nomograms for extended interval dosing allows for only one midpoint concentration to be drawn.[5]
2. Athough the disposition of aminoglycosides is better described by a two- or three-compartment model, no clinically significant difference is seen in predicted trough concentration using a

one-compartment model versus a two-compartment model.[6] Be sure to wait for ½ to 1 hour after the end of infusion to ensure the distribution phase has ended before drawing a "peak."

3. Serum creatinine lags change in renal function by at least 24 hours. Therefore, urine output, if available, should be used in conjunction with the serum creatinine to monitor aminoglycoside therapy.
4. Nephrotoxicity induced by aminoglycosides is usually reversible on discontinuance of the drug. Although high trough concentrations have been associated with renal toxicity, the high trough concentrations may also be the result, and not the cause, of renal dysfunction. In fact, elevated trough concentrations are an early indicator of renal damage.[2,7]

Carbamazepine

Use: antiepileptic, generalized seizures
TR: 4 to 12 mg/L
CL: Hepatic3A4
  Epoxide active metabolite
  Autoinduction
V_d: 1.4 L/kg
t½: initial 15 hours; after induction of 10 hours
Concentration-related side effects: central nervous system (CNS) (nystagmus, ataxia, blurred vision, and drowsiness). *Not* concentration-related dermatologic and hemalotologic, the most serious of which is the rare, but potentially fatal aplastic anemia[8–10]

Carbamazepine undergoes autoinduction. It induces the enzymes responsible for its own clearance and the clearance of other drugs. Clearance increases with time of exposure. It takes 3 to 4 weeks for full induction. Therfore, as clearance increases, concentrations and t½ decrease. Therefore, dose rate should increase and τ decrease over the first month of administration. Also carbamazepine can induce the metabolism of other drugs, specifically other antiepileptics.

Clinical Insights

1. A baseline complete blood cell count (CBC) with differential, platelet count, serum sodium, and liver function tests should be obtained before the initiation of therapy. If possible, a baseline evaluation of gait and nystagmus should be obtained for future comparisons.

2. Rare but potentially fatal blood dyscrasias (aplastic anemia, agranulocytosis, thrombocytopenia, and leukopenia) have been reported. Signs of bone marrow toxicity (e.g., fever, sore throat, easy bruising) should be monitored. On the other hand, frequent monitoring of the CBC after the patient's condition is stabilized with carbamazepine is unnecessary and unlikely to detect toxicity.
3. Most of the CNS side effects can be minimized by a slow titration of dose increases.

Cyclosporine

Use: immunosuppression
TR: depends upon assay
CL: Hepatic
  P-gp substrate
  3A4 substrate
V_d: 4 to 5 L/kg
t½: 6 to 12 hours
fu: <0.1 bound to lipoproteins
Concentration-related side effects: renal vasoconstriction (renal impairment), neurotoxicity (headache, tremor, paresthesias, seizures), and hypertension

Cyclosporine is at risk for many interactions. Being a CYP 3A4 and P-glycoprotein substrate, there are many drugs and diseases that can alter these causing changes in CL and F. Also, cyclosporine is highly plasma protein bound making binding displacement situations significant. The result of subtherapeutic concentrations is very serious. There are many cases of organ rejection resulting from drug–drug or drug–disease interactions that alter CL, F, or V of cyclosporine.

Digoxin

Use: congestive heart failure (CHF) and atrial fibrillation (a fib)
TR: CHF 0.5 to 1 μg/L
  a fib 1.5 to 2.5 μg/L
CL: renal (primarily) + hepatic
  P-gp substrate
  CHF decreases CL_H
  CL_R approximated by GFR

V_d: 3.8 (weight kg) + (3.1 × creatinine clearance [CrCl])
Dosed on ideal body weight (IBW)
Decreased in renal failure
t½: 36 to 48 hours
Dose-related side effects: decreased heart rate, arrhythmias, and vision changes

Digoxin has a relatively large volume of distribution and long half-life. Volume and clearance are affected by many diseases and drugs.

Clinical Insights[11–13]

1. Interpretation of serum digoxin concentrations for optimal dosing design should ideally be made after a steady state is attained.
2. Blood sampling for determination of any digoxin serum concentrations must take into account its prolonged distribution phase. The clinician should wait at least 6 hours after an intravenous dose and 8 hours after an oral dose to obtain the blood sample. Therefore, a standard collection time (preferably as a trough concentration before administration of the patient's daily dose) should be instituted.
3. For rapid control of ventricular rate in the acute management of atrial fibrillation, digoxin loading doses generally are divided into 3 or 4 doses (e.g., one-half, one-quarter, one-quarter given every 6 hours) to assess the clinical effect of each dose before administration of the next. In this clinical setting, determination of digoxin concentration in between dosing is likely of minimal benefit and is not cost-effective.
4. Determination of digoxin concentrations is appropriate for patients with significant renal impairment, for patients with clinical deterioration after initial good response, when toxicity or drug interaction (e.g., with quinidine) is suspected, and for evaluating noncompliance and/or the need for continued therapy.
5. Some medical conditions (e.g., hypokalemia, hyperthyroidism, and hypothyroidism) can change the sensitivity of the patient to pharmacologic effects of digoxin independent of any change in concentration. Therefore, in addition to renal function and concurrent therapy, electrolytes (especially potassium) and thyroid status should be assessed.

Ethosuximide

Use: antiepileptic; absence
TR: 40 to 100 mg/L[14–17]
CL: hepatic
3A4 (subject to induction and inhibition)
V_d: 0.7 L/kg
t½: 50 hours

Clinical Insights

1. The incidence of adverse effects associated with ethosuximide therapy is relatively low and does not correlate well with drug concentrations. Many patients with concentrations in excess of 100 mg/L experience no side effects.[18] Drug concentrations are, therefore, primarily used to evaluate a patient's potential for clinical response and compliance.
2. Ethosuximide may exhibit nonlinear kinetics in the higher concentrations.[19,20] Therefore, caution needs to be exercised with dosage increments at the upper end of the therapeutic range.

Lidocaine

Use: local anesthetic, antiarrhythmic
TR: 2 to 5 mg/L[21–25]
CL: hepatic
High E; therefore, a high first-pass drug
CHF, cirrhosis (↓Q) decrease CL
Active metabolites: MEGX and GX
V_1: 0.5 L/kg
V_2: 1.3 L/kg
t½: 100 minutes
fu: 0.3 (α_1-acid glycoprotein [AAG])
Concentration-related side effects: CNS side effects (e.g., dizziness, mental confusion, and blurred vision). Seizures are usually associated with concentrations exceeding 9 mg/L.[21–25]

Lidocaine is highly extracted by the liver, which results in a very low oral bioavailability. Its pharmacokinetic profile follows a two-compartment model. To maintain lidocaine concentration within the therapeutic range, it is necessary to administer "mini" bolus doses (one-half of original loading dose) every 8 to 10 minutes.

Clinical Insights

1. Concurrent medical conditions such as congestive heart failure and liver disease can decrease the clearance of lidocaine and the expected therapeutic responses with the usual doses. Therefore, a reduction of dose by as much as 40% may be necessary for these patients.
2. MEGX is primarily eliminated by the liver, and GX is eliminated by both the liver and the kidney. Therefore, in patients with liver and/or renal disease, accumulation of the metabolites may contribute to CNS toxicity.
3. AAG is an acute phase reactant; as such, its concentration can increase with stress or pathophysiologic conditions such as acute myocardial infarction (especially during the first week after infarction). An increase in the serum concentration of AAG decreases the free fraction of lidocaine temporarily due to enhanced protein binding. The increase and subsequent decrease in AAG concentration can further complicate interpretation of lidocaine kinetics and effects in patients. Careful concentration and clinical monitoring are required.
4. Because lidocaine is rapidly distributed to the brain and the heart, intravenous bolus doses should be administered at a rate not faster than 50 mg/min, so that the patient is not exposed to transient but toxic concentrations of lidocaine, especially in the brain. Seizures and arrhythmias may occur and may not always be preceded by other toxic signs (e.g., confusion, dizziness).
5. The clearance of lidocaine decreases with continuous dosing.[25,26]
6. Therefore, infusions lasting longer than 24 hours require diligent monitoring of concentrations and of clinical responses. If necessary, doses should be reduced.

Lithium

Use: treat bipolar disease
TR: 0.6 to 0.8 mEq/L
CL: renal
  Treated like Na
  Actively reabsorbed
  0.25 × CrCl
V: 0.7 L/kg
t½: 20 hours

Concentration-related side effects: gastrointestinal (i.e., nausea, vomiting, anorexia, epigastric bloating, abdominal pain) and CNS (i.e., lethargy, fatigue, muscle weakness, and tremor)[27–29]

Clinical Insights

1. Administering lithium preparations with meals will decrease both the rate of absorption and the achievable peak concentration. Meals, therefore, may help minimize the incidence of some of the adverse effects (e.g., tremor and polyuria). Side effects may also be minimized in some patients by use of the slow-release lithium dosage formulations.
2. The daily dose of lithium should be divided into two or more doses, and trough concentrations should be obtained 12 hours after the last dose.
3. Lithium reabsorption follows sodium reabsorption in the proximal tubule. Therefore, patients with precipitous changes in fluid balance or electrolytes due to drug therapy (e.g., thiazide diuretics) that result in increased sodium (and lithium) reabsorption are at increased risk of toxicity.

Phenobarbital

Use: antiepileptic
TR: 15 to 40 mg/L[30,31]
CL: hepatic (primary) + renal
  Low E
  Enzyme inducer
V: 0.7 L/kg
t½: 5 days
fu: 0.5
Concentration-related side effects: depression and ataxia[31]

Clinical Insights

1. For the treatment of status epilepticus, an LD of 15 mg/kg can be administered intravenously, usually in 3 divided doses of 5 mg/kg.
2. Because phenobarbital distributes to fatty tissue, loading doses for morbidly obese patients should be based on total body weight.[32]

Phenytoin

Use: antiepileptic
TR: 10 to 20 mg/L
Free: 1 to 2 mg/L
CL: hepatic
nonlinear
enzyme inducer 3A4
subject to induction and inhibition
V: 0.65 L/kg
t½: nonlinear since nonlinear CL
fu: 0.1 (albumin)
Concentration-related side effects: nystagmus, ataxia, and diminished mental capacity.[33] Gingival hyperplasia, folate deficiency, and peripheral neuropathy are not related to concentration.

Phenytoin has nonlinear clearance in the TR and high plasma protein binding makes dosing very difficult. The metabolism of phenytoin is saturable. Therefore, modest changes in DR can result in disproportionate changes in steady-state plasma concentrations. The high binding provides a challenge in the interpretation of phenytoin concentration in patients with altered protein binding (e.g., patients with renal failure or hypoalbuminemia and patients with concurrent drugs that displace phenytoin from the binding sites).

Clinical Insights

1. Oral bioavailability of phenytoin can be reduced significantly by concomitant oral nutrition supplements (e.g., Osmolite) administered as nasogastric feedings. The most practical way of circumventing this problem is to administer phenytoin intravenously. If that is not possible, then stop NG feeding 2 hours before dose administration, flush the NG tube with 60 mL of water after dose administration, and then wait 2 hours before resuming NG feeding.
2. Only Dilantin capsules should be dosed once daily. As with other sustained-release formulations, the capsules should not be crushed.
3. Hypotension can occur with intravenous administration due to the propylene glycol diluent.[34] Therefore, the rate of phenytoin infusion should not be >50 mg/min. Fosphenytoin, a prodrug of phenytoin, is available for parenteral use. The addition of a phosphate group to the chemical structure of phenytoin results in a more soluble

chemical entity; therefore, there is no need for the propylene glycol as a diluent for fosphenytoin.

4. Fosphenytoin dosing should be based on phenytoin equivalent (the molecular weight of fosphenytoin is 1.5 times that of phenytoin).
5. Protein binding displacement make interpretation of a total concentration difficult.[35–37] In this case, the total concentration of phenytoin would be lower once a new steady-state condition is established. However, the unbound (pharmacologically active) concentration remains the same. Dose regimen adjustment is again not necessary in patients with an altered degree of binding only.
6. Equations to "equate" the measured total phenytoin concentration to that which would be observed under normal binding conditions should be used so that inappropriate dosage adjustments can be avoided.[38,39]

Procainamide[40–45]

Use: antiarrhythmic
TR: 4 to 8 mg/L
  May need much higher concentrations in some patients
CL: hepatic and renal
  CLH by acetylation (acetylation phenotype: slow and fast acetylators)
  Active metabolite: n-acetylprocainamide (NAPA) (renal clearance)
V: 2 L/kg
t½: 3 hours
Concentration-related side effects: gastrointestinal disturbances, weakness, mild hypotension, and electrocardiogram (ECG) changes (10% to 30% prolongation of the PR, QT, or QRS intervals)

Clinical Insights

1. Hypotension may occur if intravenous procainamide is administered too quickly. The rate of infusion should not be faster than 25 mg/min.
2. The short plasma half-life of procainamide requires the use of 3- to 4-hour dosing intervals for the rapid-release products and every 6-hour intervals for the sustained-release formulations. This is in contrast to the usual longer dosing intervals with sustained-release formulations of other drugs.
3. Wax matrix carcasses or "skeletons" of the sustained-release tablets may come through intact in the stool. This is not a concern

because the drug is absorbed despite the recovery of the wax matrix.

4. Most clinical laboratories report the concentrations of both procainamide and NAPA. The electrophysiologic activity of NAPA is different from that of procainamide, and monitoring of NAPA concentration is not necessary to evaluate efficacy. However, assessment of NAPA concentrations may be appropriate in some patients[46] (e.g., those with diminished renal function), because NAPA is primarily eliminated by the kidneys and accumulates to a much greater extent than procainamide.
5. In addition to concentration monitoring, a baseline QT interval should be obtained, if possible, before initiation of therapy or before dosage increases. Prolongation of QT interval >25% to 50% of the baseline value necessitates at least the consideration of dosage reduction.

Valproic Acid[47–52]

Use: antiepileptic

TR: 50 to 100 mg/L

Nonlinear protein binding at upper ranges

CL: hepatic

Nonlinear clearance due to nonlinear protein binding

3A4 substrate

Can induce and inhibit CL_{int} of other drugs

V: 0.14 L/kg

fu = 0.005 to 0.2 (albumin). Nonlinear in upper end of therapeutic range

t½: 10 to 12 hours

Concentration-related side effects: gastrointestinal disturbances, sedation, drowsiness, and hepatotoxicity. NOT concentration-related alopecia, a benign essential tremor, and thrombocytopenia

Clinical Insights

1. Although the rate of absorption from the use of enteric-coated tablets may be slower, this formulation can be used to minimize gastrointestinal side effects.
2. Diurnal variation in valproic acid clearance has been reported, and the concentrations of valproic acid in the afternoon or evening are

lower than in the morning. Therefore, it is important to standardize consistent blood sampling times (e.g., morning trough concentration) for TDM.

3. Valproic acid can inhibit the metabolism of a number of other drugs such as phenobarbital. In addition, valproic acid can displace highly protein-bound drugs such as phenytoin from their albumin-binding sites. Therefore, similar to other antiepileptic drugs, the potential of drug–drug interactions should be considered when adding or deleting drugs to a patient's regimen.
4. Although valproic acid–induced hepatotoxicity is rare, it is a serious complication of therapy and should be considered in any patient with elevated liver enzymes. Unfortunately, the predictive value of laboratory monitoring for occurrence of hepatotoxicity induced by valproic acid is low.

Vancomycin[46,53–63]

Use: antibiotic used for gram-positive infections

TR: peak <40 to 50 mg/L, trough 15 to 20 mg/L (depending upon resistance)

CL: renal

Approximated by CrCl

V: 0.7 L/kg OR $0.17 \times (\text{age}) + (0.22 \times \text{TBW in kg}) + 15$

$fu = 0.5$

t½: 6 to 7 hours

Concentration-related side effects: nephrotoxicity when combined with other nephrotoxins or other assaults to the kidney rarely ototoxicity.

Clinical Insights

1. Red man syndrome (characterized by flushing, tachycardia, and hypotension) is associated with histamine release. Its incidence is higher with rapid infusion rates. To minimize its occurrence, vancomycin should be infused slowly (e.g., 1 g over at least 60 minutes). Even at this rate of infusion, some patients will experience flushing and tachycardia. The syndrome may also be managed by premedication with an antihistamine and slowing the infusion rate even more.
2. Efficacy is tied to having adequate concentrations of drugs available. Therefore, keeping a "therapeutic trough" is very important.

(Text continued on page 480)

Pharmacokinetic Equations

	Equations	When to Use	When Not to Use
Area under the Concentration–time curve (AUC) Units: (amt/vol) × time	$AUC_{0-\infty} = \left[\frac{C_1 + C_2}{2} \times (t_2 - t_1)\right]\left[\frac{C_2 + C_3}{2} \times (t_3 - t_2)\right] + \cdots + \frac{C_{last}}{k}$ 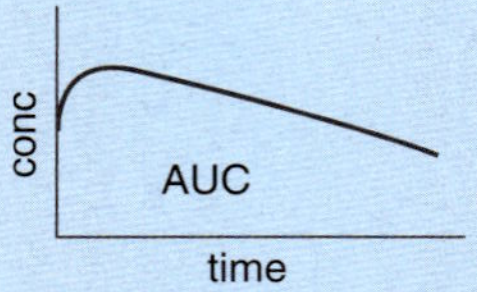 	To determine $AUC_{0-\infty}$, given concentration–time data after administration of the drug	If only want to measure to end of τ
	$AUC_{0-\infty} = \left[\frac{C_1 + C_2}{2} \times (t_2 - t_1)\right]\left[\frac{C_2 + C_3}{2} \times (t_3 - t_2)\right] + \cdots + \left[\frac{C_{next\,to\,last} + C_{last}}{2} \times (t_{next\,to\,last} - t_{last})\right]$	To determine $AUC_{0-\tau}$, given concentration–time data after administration of the drug	If want to measure to ∞
	$AUC_{0-\infty} = \frac{Dose_{IV}}{CL}$	Determine AUC or CL from AUC if the dose given IV	If given by other than IV

	$AUC_{0-\infty} = \frac{F \times Dose_{PO}}{CL}$	Determine AUC or CL from AUC if dose given other than IV	
Bioavailability (F) Units: no units (fraction)	$F = fa \times fg \times ffp$	Determine F, fa, fg, or ffp, given the others	
	$ffp = \frac{Q_H}{Q_H + (CL_{int} \times fup)}$ Low hepatic extraction drugs: $ffp \sim 1$ High hepatic extraction drug: $ffp \sim \frac{Q}{CL_{int} \times fup}$	Determine ffp Assume the well-stirred jar model	Assume the parallel tube model
	$F = \frac{AUC_{nonIV}}{AUC_{IV}}$	Used to determine F when same dose is given by IV and nonintravenous routes	If different doses given
	$F = \frac{AUC_{nonIV}}{AUC_{IV}} \times \frac{Dose_{IV}}{Dose_{nonIV}}$	To determine F when comparing differing doses	
Total body clearance (CL) Units: vol/time	$CL = CL_H + CL_R + \cdots$	To determine total body clearance, all organ clearances must be summed	

(continued)

Pharmacokinetic Equations *(continued)*

	Equations	When to Use	When Not to Use
Hepatic CL (CL_H) Units: vol/time	$CL_H = Q_H \times E_H$ Low extraction: $CL_H \cong CLint \times fup$ High extraction: $CL_H \cong Q_H$	• To determine what will alter hepatic clearance. • Low extraction drugs, the rate limitation to clearance is the enzyme activity (CL_{int}) and fraction unbound in plasma (fup). • High extraction drugs: the rate limitation to clearance is liver blood flow (Q)	
Hepatic extraction efficiency (E_H) Units: none	$E_H = \dfrac{CL_{int} \times fup}{Q_H + (CL_{int} \times fup)}$	According to the well-stirred jar model	
Hepatic intrinsic clearance = enzyme activity (CL_{int}) Units: vol/time	$CL_{int} = \dfrac{V_{max}}{K_m + C}$	Michealis-Menten V_{max}: maximum rate of metabolism, capacity of the system, or number of enzymes available K_m: concentration at which ½ V_{max} is reached, measure of affinity	
Renal clearance (CLR) Units: vol/time	$CL_R = (CL_{gf} + CL_{TS})(1 - E_{TR})$	CL_{gf} = filtration clearance CL_{ts} = tubular secretion clearance ETR = efficiency of tubular reabsorption	

Elimination rate constant (k) Units: vol/time	$k = \frac{\ln C_2 - \ln C_1}{t_2 - t_1}$ 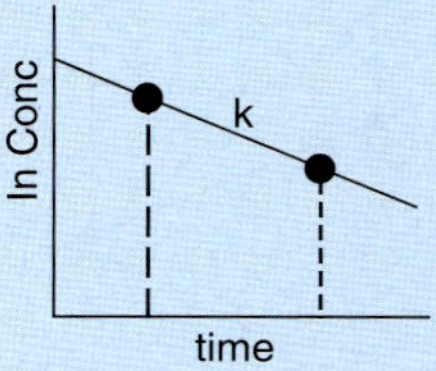 	To determine k when given two concentration–time points during the decay phase of a drug considered to be linear and gathered during a time that is considered to be reflecting only one compartment	If the concentrations given are not gathered during the decay phase of a drug that is considered to be linear and within one compartment
	$k = \frac{CL}{V}$	• To determine how changes in V and/or CL might alter k • To determine k if given CL and V • To determine CL if given k and V • To determine V if given K and CL	
Half-life (t½) Units: time	$t_{1/2} = \frac{0.693}{k}$	To determine t½ from k or vice versa	
	$t_{1/2} = \frac{0.693 \times V}{CL}$	To determine how changes in V and/or CL might alter t½	
Central volume of distribution (Vc) Units: vol	$V_C = \frac{\text{Dose (injected instanteneously)}}{C_0}$	Used to determine V_c or dose to achieve a target C_0	

(continued)

Pharmacokinetic Equations *(continued)*

	Equations	When to Use	When Not to Use
Apparent volume of distribution (V_d) Units: vol	$V_d = \frac{Dose}{C}$ $k = \frac{CL}{V_d}$		
Volume of distribution at steady state (V_{ss}) Units: vol	$V_{ss} = V_p + \left[V_T \times \frac{fup}{fut}\right]$ Given: Vp = 0.07 L/kg V_T = 0.53 L/kg	Determine V_{ss}, fut, or fup; given the other parameters	
Dosing Equations			
A model of decay of one compartment, first-order elimination	$C_t = C_0e^{-kt}$ 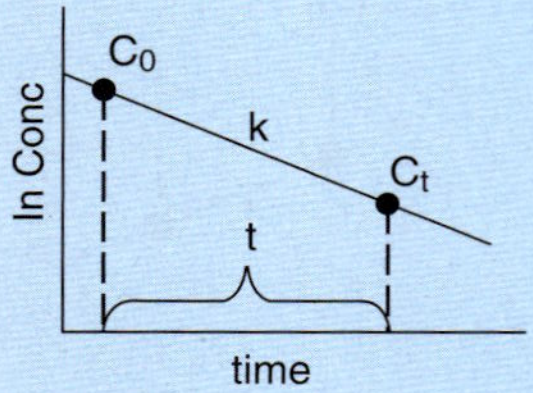	• To determine the concentration at any time (C_t) during the decay of a drug following one compartment, linear kinetics when given k, an earlier concentration (C_0), and the time between C_0 and C_t (t) • To determine the concentration of an earlier concentration (C_0) when all the above conditions are met • To determine the time (t) between two given concentrations (C_0 and C_t) when all the above conditions are met • To determine elimination rate constant (k) when all the above conditions are met	• Multiple compartments • Nonlinear clearance

Model of decay, two compartments, linear	$C_t = C_1 e^{-k_1 t} + C_2 e^{-k_2 t}$	To determine the concentration at any time t during the decay of the drug if a two-compartment model	Nonlinear
Loading dose (LD) Units: amt	$LD = V_c \times (C_{target} - C_{observed})$	Determine LD when V_c, target concentration, and any drug already in the body are known	
Concentration at steady state Units: amt/vol	$C_{ss} = \frac{DR}{CL}$	• To determine the plasma concentration at steady state (C_{ss}) when a constant infusion is given at a certain dose rate (DR) and CL • To determine a DR if given a target C_{ss} and CL • To determine CL if given a DR and resulting C_{ss}	If not at steady state If nonlinear CL
	$C_{ss,avg} = \frac{S \times F \times DR}{CL}$	• To determine the average concentration during a dosing interval at steady state • To determine how changes in DR, CL, and F will affect $C_{ss,avg}$	
	$C_{ss,avg} = \frac{AUC_{ss,0-\tau}}{\tau}$	• To determine the $C_{ss,avg}$ given AUCss and τ	
Concentration before steady state, constant infusion Units: amt/vol	$C_t = \frac{DR}{CL}\left(1 - e^{-kt}\right)$	To determine the plasma concentration at time t prior to reaching steady state if given a constant infusion and the DR, CL, and k are known	

(continued)

Pharmacokinetic Equations *(continued)*

	Equations	When to Use	When Not to Use
Multiple dosing function (MDF) Units: none	$MDF = \frac{1 - e^{-nkt}}{1 - e^{-kt}}$ Ct at dose *n* = Ct at first dose × MDF	Use to multiply times any known concentration after first dose to any concentration at that same time on subsequent doses (n)	
Accumulation factor (Rac) Units: none	$Rac = \frac{1}{1 - e^{-kt}}$ CtSS = Ct at first dose × Rac	Use to multiply times any known concentration after first dose to any concentration at that same time at SS	
Calculating new DR if known $C_{ss,avg}$ at DR known	$DR_{new} = \frac{DR_{given} \times C_{ss,target}}{C_{ss,observed}}$	Determine new DR when measured concentration at SS and assumes CL and F remain constant	Nonlinear CL or Nonlinear F C observed not at SS
Calculating a new dose regimen based upon $C_{ss,avg}$	Determine DR $DR = \frac{C_{target} \times CL}{F}$	Determine DR if CL and F are known at SS	Must be linear clearance and bioavailability
	Determine τ, dose q t½ $t_{1/2} = \frac{0.693 \times V}{CL}$ OR based upon known target peak and trough as below	Determine τ if can dose every t½	

Calculating a new dose regimen based upon target C_{max} and C_{min} (i.e., aminoglycosides)	Determine optimal τ $\tau = \left\|-\frac{1}{k}\right\| \left[\ln \frac{C_{min,target}}{C_{max,target}}\right] + t_i$ t_i = time of infusion	Determine optimal dosing interval given target peak and troughs K must have been determined at SS	Multicompartmental Not at SS
	Determine optimal dose (using optimal τ from above) $DR = V \times k \times C_{max,target} \left(\frac{1 - e^{-kt}}{1 - e^{-kti}}\right)$ DR is in terms of amt/time NOT dose	Determine optimal dose using optimal τ and target C_{max} V and k must have been determined at SS	
	Determine what $C_{ss,max}$ would be expected using a given dosing regimen $C_{max} = \frac{DR}{V \times k} \left(\frac{1 - e^{-kti}}{1 - e^{-kt}}\right)$	Determine $C_{ss,max}$ when giving a defined dosing regimen	
	Determine what $C_{ss,min}$ would be expected using a given dosing regimen $C_{min} = C_{max} e^{-k(\tau - ti)}$	Determine $C_{ss,min}$ when giving a defined dosing regimen	
Adjustment of total phenytoin concentrations when protein binding displacement	In hypoalbuminemia: $C_{normal} = \frac{C_{observed}}{[(0.2)(Alb) + (0.1)]}$	Determine what would have been the observed concentration if normal-binding Alb in g/dL	
	In renal failure: $C_{normal} = \frac{C_{observed}}{[(0.1)(Alb) + (0.1)]}$	Determine what would have been the observed concentration if normal-binding Alb in g/dL	

References

1. Jackson GG, Arcieri G. Ototoxicity of gentamicin in man: a survey and controlled analysis of clinical experience in the United States. *J Infect Dis.* 1971;124(Suppl):130.
2. Schentag JJ, et al. Clinical and pharmacokinetic characteristics of aminoglycoside nephrotoxicity in 201 critically ill patients. *Antimicrob Agents Chemother.* 1982;5:721.
3. Wilfret JN, et al. Renal insufficiency associated with gentamicin therapy. *J Infect Dis.* 1971;124(Suppl):148.
4. Federspil P, et al. Pharmacokinetics and ototoxicity of gentamicin, tobramycin, and amikacin. *J Infect Dis.* 1976;134(Suppl):200.
5. Nicolau D, et al. Experience with a once-daily aminoglycoside dosing program administered to 2,184 adult patients. *Antimicrob Agents Chemother.* 1995;39:650–655.
6. Hatton RC, Massey KL, Russell WL. Comparison of the predictions of one- and two-compartment microcomputer programs for long-term tobramycin therapy. *Ther Drug Monit.* 1984;6:432–437.
7. Goodman EL, et al. Prospective comparative study of variable dosage and variable frequency regimens for administrations of gentamicin. *Antimicrob Agents Chemother.* 1975;8:434.
8. So EL, et al. Seizure exacerbation and status epilepticus related to carbamazepine-10,11 epoxide. *Ann Neurol.* 1994;35:743–746.
9. Rane A, Hojer B, Wilson JT. Kinetics of carbamazepine and its 10.11-epoxide metabolite in children. *Clin Pharmacol Ther.* 1976;19:276–283.
10. Bertilsson L. Clinical pharmacokinetics of carbamazepine. *Clin Pharmacokinet.* 1978;3:128.
11. Smith TW. Digitalis toxicity: epidemiology and clinical use of serum concentration measurements. *Am J Med.* 1975;58:470.
12. Smith TW, Harber E. Digoxin intoxication: the relationship of clinical presentation to serum digoxin concentration. *J Clin Invest.* 1970;49:2377.
13. Aronson JK, Hardman M. ABC of monitoring drug therapy: digoxin. *Br J Med.* 1992;305:1149–1152.
14. Browne TR, et al. Ethosuximide in the treatment of absence seizures. *Neurology.* 1975;25:515.
15. Sherwin AL, et al. Improved control of epilepsy by monitoring plasma ethosuximide. *Arch Neurol.* 1973;27:178.
16. Penry JK, et al. Ethosuximide: relation of plasma levels to clinical control. In: Woodbury DM, Penry JK, Schmidt RP, eds. *Anti-epileptic Drugs.* New York, NY: Raven Press; 1972:431–441.
17. Sherwin AL, Robb JP. Ethosuximide: relation of plasma levels to clinical control. In: Woodbury DM, Penry JK, Schmidt RP, eds. *Anti-epileptic Drugs.* New York, NY: Raven Press; 1972:443–448.

18. Sherwin AL, et al. Plasma ethosuximide levels: a new aid in the management of epilepsy. *Ann Royal Coll Surg Can.* 1971;14:48.
19. Bauer LA, et al. Ethosuximide kinetics: possible interactions with valproic acid. *Clin Pharmacol Ther.* 1982;31:741–745.
20. Smith GA, et al. Factors influencing plasma concentrations of ethosuximide. *Clin Pharmacokinet.* 1979;4:38–52.
21. Gianelly R, et al. Effect of lidocaine on ventricular arrhythmias in patients with coronary heart disease. *N Engl J Med.* 1967;277:1215.
22. Jewett DE, et al. Lidocaine in the management of arrhythmias after acute myocardial infarction. *Lancet.* 1968;1:266.
23. Seldon R, Sasahara AA. Central nervous system toxicity induced by lidocaine. *JAMA.* 1967;202:908.
24. Thompson PD. Lidocaine pharmacokinetics in advanced heart failure, liver disease, and renal failure in humans. *Ann Intern Med.* 1973;78:499.
25. LeLorier J, et al. Pharmacokinetics of lidocaine after prolonged intravenous administrations in uncomplicated myocardial infarction. *Ann Intern Med.* 1977;87:700–702.
26. Davidson R, Parker M, Atkinson A. Excessive serum lidocaine levels during maintenance infusions: mechanisms and prevention. *Am Heart J.* 1982;104:203–208.
27. Elizur A, et al. Intra:extracellular lithium ratios and clinical course in affective states. *Clin Pharm Ther.* 1972;13:947.
28. Salem RB. A pharmacist's guide to monitoring lithium drug–drug interactions. *Drug Intell Clin Pharm.* 1982;16:745.
29. Amdisen A. Lithium. In: Evans WE, Schentag JJ, Jusko WJ, eds. *Applied Pharmacokinetics: Principles of Therapeutic Drug Monitoring.* 2nd ed. Vancouver, WA: Applied Therapeutics; 1986:978–1002.
30. Buchthal F, et al. Relation of EEG and seizures to phenobarbital in serum. *Arch Neurol.* 1968;19:567.
31. Plass GL, Hine CH. Hydantoin and barbiturate blood levels observed in epileptics. *Arch Int Pharmacodyn Ther.* 1960;128:375.
32. Wilkes L, Danziger LH, Rodvold KA. Phenobarbital pharmacokinetics in obesity: a case report. *Clin Pharmacokinet.* 1992;22:481–484.
33. Kutt H, et al. Diphenylhydantoin metabolism, blood levels and toxicity. *Arch Neurol.* 1964;11:642–648.
34. Louis S, et al. The cardiocirculatory changes caused by intravenous dilantin and its solvent. *Am Heart J.* 1967;74:523.
35. Lund L. Effects of phenytoin in patients with epilepsy in relation to its concentration in plasma. In: David DS, Prichard NBC, eds. *Biological Effects of Drugs in Relation to Their Concentration in Plasma.* Baltimore, MD: University Park Press; 1972:227.
36. Lascelles PT, et al. The distribution of plasma phenytoin levels in epileptic patients. *J Neurol Neurosurg Psychiatry.* 1970;33:501.

37. Reidenberg MM. The binding of drugs to plasma proteins and the interpretation of measurements of plasma concentrations of drugs in patients with poor renal function. *Am J Med.* 1977;62:466.
38. Winter M. *Basic Clinical Pharmacokinetics.* 3rd ed. Vancouver, WA: Applied Therapeutics; 1994:312–316.
39. Liponi DL, et al. Renal function and therapeutic concentrations of phenytoin. *Neurology.* 1984;34:395.
40. Koch-Weser J. Pharmacokinetics of procainamide in man. *Ann N Y Acad Sci.* 1971;169:370.
41. Koch-Weser J, Klein SW. Procainamide dosage schedules, plasma concentrations and clinical effects. *JAMA.* 1971;215:1454.
42. Engel TR, et al. Modification of ventricular tachycardia by procainamide in patients with coronary artery disease. *Am J Cardiol.* 1980;46:1033.
43. Giardina EV, et al. Efficacy, plasma concentrations and adverse effects of a new sustained release procainamide preparation. *Am J Cardiol.* 1980;46:855.
44. Greenspan AM, et al. Large dose procainamide therapy for ventricular tachyarrhythmia. *Am J Cardiol.* 1980;46:453.
45. Vlasses PH, et al. Lethal accumulations of procainamide metabolite in renal insufficiency [abstract]. *Drug Intell Clin Pharm.* 1984;18:493.
46. Newfield P, Roizen MF. Hazards of rapid administration of vancomycin. *Ann Intern Med.* 1979;91:581.
47. Kodama Y, et al. Binding parameters of valproic acid to serum protein in healthy adults at steady-state. *Ther Drug Monit.* 1992;14:55–60.
48. Pinder RM, et al. Sodium valproate: a review of its pharmacological properties in therapeutic efficacy in epilepsy. *Drugs.* 1977;13:81.
49. Graham L, et al. Sodium valproate, serum level, and critical effect in epilepsy: a controlled study. *Epilepsia.* 1979;20:303.
50. Sherard ES, et al. Treatment of childhood epilepsy with valproic acid: result of the first 100 patients in a 6-month trial. *Neurology.* 1980;30:31.
51. Suchy FJ, et al. Acute hepatic failure associated with the use of sodium valproate. *N Engl J Med.* 1979;300:962.
52. Donalt JT, et al. Valproic acid and fatal hepatitis. *Neurology.* 1979;29:273.
53. Alexander MB. A review of vancomycin. *Drug Intell Clin Pharm.* 1974;8:520.
54. Kirby WMM, et al. Treatment of staphylococcal septicemia with vancomycin. *N Engl J Med.* 1960;262:49.
55. Banner WN Jr, Ray CG. Vancomycin in perspective. *Am J Dis Child.* 1984; 183:14.
56. Cunha BA, Ristuccia AM. Clinical usefulness of vancomycin. *Clin Pharm.* 1982;2:417.
57. Rotschafer JC, et al. Pharmacokinetics of vancomycin: observations in 28 patients and dosage recommendations. *Antimicrob Agents Chemother.* 1982;22:391.

58. Blouin RA, et al. Vancomycin pharmacokinetics in normal and morbidly obese subjects. *Antimicrob Agents Chemother.* 1982;21:575.
59. Mollering RC, et al. Vancomycin therapy in patients with impaired renal function; a nomogram for dosage. *Ann Intern Med.* 1981;94:343.
60. Farber BF, Mollering RC Jr. Retrospective study of the toxicity of preparations of vancomycin from 1974 to 1981. *Antimicrob Agents Chemother.* 1983;23:138.
61. Ryback MJ, et al. Nephrotoxicity of vancomycin, alone and with an aminoglycoside. *J Antimicrob Chemother.* 1990;25:679–687.
62. Cook FV, Farrar WE. Vancomycin revisited. *Ann Intern Med.* 1978;88:813.
63. Lanese DM, et al. Markedly increased clearance of vancomycin during hemodialysis using polysulfone dialyzers. *Kidney Int.* 1989;35:1409.

15

Clinical Drug Monitoring

Teresa A. O'Sullivan and Ann K. Wittkowsky

Clinical drug monitoring is the most basic element of pharmaceutical care.[1] All the therapeutic knowledge the pharmacy student possesses is useless unless it can be applied in a structured and consistent manner to detect and solve the patient's problems. This structured process is considered clinical drug monitoring. It includes each of the following activities[2]:

- Gathering objective and subjective patient information
- Analyzing that information to determine medical and drug-related problems (DRPs)
- Setting therapeutic goals for each medical and DRP
- Developing and enacting a treatment plan to reach the therapeutic goals
- Developing and enacting a monitoring plan to see if the treatment works or causes any harm
- Documenting all of the above (subjective and objective information, analysis, and plan) in a coherent and systematic manner so that the next care provider can continue the process

Each of these activities is a necessary component of clinical drug monitoring. No single activity can be skipped, or good patient care will be sacrificed. The following steps provide a linear and methodic approach to these activities for the pharmacy student to follow when providing patient care.

Step 1. Gather Information: Prepare for the Interview

To effectively provide care, a pharmacist *must* talk to the patient. The discussion will be more comfortable and productive if the clinician first scans the patient's chart or profile to determine some discussion issues. The following should be considered:

- The current medication list (patient profile or most recent medication administration record [MAR])
  - What medications has the patient been prescribed?
  - What likely disease states are present?
- Patient compliance/adherence (patient profile or most recent MAR)
  - How often does the patient get his or her medications for chronic conditions refilled? In an institutional setting, the pharmacist will want to check the MAR to see if the patient has been receiving or refusing medications.
- Disease state control (recent progress notes)
  - Monitoring notes written by other health care providers will be useful in an institutional or clinic ambulatory setting. Some community pharmacy practitioners are starting to document previous disease state control in their electronic profiles.
  - The pharmacist should look for disease state monitoring data obtained through interview, physical examination, and laboratory values. Well-written progress notes will include this information. In the absence of well-written progress notes, information from previous visits or admissions, an admission or discharge summary (for hospitals or long-term care settings), or current laboratory data can be reviewed to gain an idea of the patient's medical problems. In this situation, an interview with the patient or caregiver will provide invaluable information to determine disease state control.
- Cost (patient profile will contain costs; most recent MAR will not)
  - Are any chronic medications relatively expensive?
  - Is there any indication that lower-cost agents have not worked? Physicians distributing drug samples can facilitate the initiation of high-cost, brand name products without initial trials of low-cost agents.
  - Which agents are covered by the health insurance provider?
- Adverse drug effects (recent progress notes), including drug allergy information
  - Are there any medications that may have been prescribed to treat side effects from other medications? When thinking about adverse drug reactions, the "as needed" or "prn" portion of the MAR is useful because prn medications are often given to combat

side effects from routinely scheduled medications. For instance, if the patient begins asking for a laxative shortly after beginning opiate therapy for pain, opiate-induced constipation should be suspected.

The goal of this first step is to identify discussion questions quickly, *not* to read the patient's chart from beginning to end. The most important sources of information regarding patient problems are the patients themselves, not their charts. Only after the patient interview can the chart information be used efficiently.

To summarize, before interviewing the patient, the pharmacy student should look at the patient's medication list in the chart or profile in any setting, the MAR in an institutional setting, and any previous care notes that would indicate how well the patient's disease states are controlled.

Step 2. Gather Information: Interview the Patient

Obtaining subjective information from the patient is the most important step in the database-building process. The pharmacist must make it a priority to interview every patient to whom he or she provides care. If an interview with the patient is not possible (e.g., the patient is intubated) or unlikely to be informative (e.g., a patient has moderate to severe dementia), then the pharmacy student should interview the patient's caregiver:

- Before beginning the interview, the pharmacist should
  - Introduce himself or herself and explain the role of the pharmacist on the health care team (which is to optimize the patient's drug therapy).
  - Ask if this is a good time to ask some questions about medication use. If it is not a good time for the interview (e.g., the patient is in a hurry, has visitors, or is going for a diagnostic test), another time should be scheduled.
- Many experienced clinicians use the standard organization for patient history and physical database (the "patient H&P database," Box 15.1) as a mental nudge for directing an interview. This helps to ensure that the proper information is gathered completely and consistently. The H&P database is also a standard format to use when presenting patient information at a formal case presentation.

BOX 15.1 Standard Organization of Patient History and Physical Data

ID (identifying information): patient age, sex, race

CC (chief complaint): a one-phrase description of the patient's reason(s) for seeking medical and/or pharmaceutical care. Identification of the probable diagnosis is sometimes given as a chief complaint but is not strictly correct.

HPI (history of the present illness): a summary of the events leading to the chief complaint. Organize chronologically if possible.

PMH (past medical history): a brief summary of current diagnosed medical problems

- Organized by problem in order of most important (top) to the least important (bottom). Numbering or bulleting each medical problem will enhance organization. A pharmacist's PMH list should prioritize conditions based on the need for drug therapy monitoring.
- Information about past health events can also be listed if they affect or explain current conditions.
- Where possible, indicate time period since onset or duration of each problem.

DH (drug history): some data may be obtained from the chart, but most will be obtained by interviewing the patient and, where possible, the patient's pharmacy. The drug history includes the following:

- Name, dose, frequency, reason for use, duration of use, efficacy, toxicity, and indication of all prescription, over-the-counter (OTC), and herbal medications that the patient has taken during the past month
  - All drug indications should be reflected in the past medical history.
  - Note name and telephone number of pharmacy(ies) where the patient obtains medications and medication-related information.
- Medications previously (but not currently) used for a current medical condition; note why they were discontinued.
- Recreational drug use, including current or past use of tobacco, ethanol, or illicit drugs
- Allergies or contraindications for drug use. The allergy history should include a detailed description of the allergic reaction, where possible.
- Compliance/adherence. Assess the patient's comprehension of drug therapy, knowledge of side effects/toxicity, compliance to the drug

BOX 15.1 Standard Organization of Patient History and Physical Data *(continued)*

regimen (including reliability), compliance aids, and needs for further intervention. Note any language or other barriers to compliance.

FH (family history): genetic predisposition or occurrence of relevant diseases in other family members. Only include if pertinent.

SH (social history): includes pertinent information regarding living situation, support systems, lifestyle, employment, and work environment (risks/chemical exposure) that may affect drug therapy

ROS (review of systems): a subjective review of bodily systems as voiced by the patient during the interview

PE (physical examination): an objective review of bodily systems obtained during the examination of the patient. At the very least, this should include vital signs (heart rate, blood pressure [BP], respiratory rate, temperature), weight, and height:

- Both the ROS and the PE begin with general statements about the patient (subjective for ROS and objective for PE) and then move on to specific findings starting at the patient's head and moving down the body to the feet ("head to toe").

Labs (laboratory data): obtain all laboratory data pertinent to the problem list. At a minimum, report the baseline seven laboratory values (Na, K, Cl, CO_2, glucose, BUN [blood urea nitrogen], and Cr), CBC (complete blood count) (WBC [white blood cell]/diff, Hct [hematocrit], and platelets), and liver function tests (AST, ALT, alkaline phosphatase, and total bilirubin; albumin and PT/INR are reasonable indicators of metabolic capacity). If the patient is febrile and/or an infection is suspected, report Gram stain and C&S findings.

Dx (diagnosis): any diagnosis made by the physician regarding the chief complaint, particularly if the patient will require pharmacotherapy for the condition

Gathering Information about Prescription Medications

All prescription medications that the patient is currently taking should be reviewed. For each drug, the following should be noted:

- Drug, dose, route, frequency, indication (this is the *patient's* version of the indication)
- Efficacy ("Tell me how you know that this medication is working for you")
- Toxicity ("What problems do you think may be caused by this medication?"). If the patient says "none," the pharmacist can probe with a few of the most common side effects.
- Height and weight (if not otherwise available)
- Compliance ("How often do you actually take this medication?" or "Tell me what interferes with your ability to take the medication regularly." "What do you do if you miss a dose?"). The pharmacist should try to verify if cost, dosing frequency, adverse effects, or personal beliefs may be an obstacle to compliance.
- Medication management issues including the following:
  - How/where the patient stores medications
  - Ease of administration for each dosage form
  - The number and names of physicians the patient sees
  - The name and telephone number of each pharmacy the patient uses
  - How the patient remembers to order/pick up refills and transportation limitations (to the physician or pharmacy)
  - Technique and maintenance of devices used to facilitate drug delivery or monitor drug therapy

Gathering Information About Nonprescription Medications

These include OTC medications, herbal and other natural remedies, vitamins and minerals, and nondrug therapy. The following "head to toe" review of systems approach should be used to inquire about nonprescription agents used by the patient. In addition to gaining valuable information about nonprescription agents the patient uses routinely or infrequently, it will also often identify disease states that may not have been identified through the prescription medication portion of the interview:

- Head, eyes, ears, nose, and throat (HEENT): nose, ear, or eye drops; nasal inhalers; analgesics used for headache or sinus pain; and dental products
- Respiratory tract: antihistamines, decongestants, and OTC inhalers
- Gastrointestinal: antacids, antiflatulents, antidiarrheals, laxatives, and hemorrhoidal preparations

- Genitourinary: urinary antibacterials, vaginal anti-infectives; usual amount of fluid consumed daily; and what kind of fluid (e.g., soda versus water versus light beer)
- Musculoskeletal: aspirin, anti-inflammatory agents, acetaminophen, or combination pain medications
- Hematologic: iron, B_{12}, and folate
- Dermatologic: psoriatic, seborrheic, anti-infective, or analgesic topical preparations; corn/callus pads or other foot care
- Neurologic: medications for insomnia, motion sickness, anxiety, and lethargy
- Overall/system-wide: vitamins; naturopathic, homeopathic, or other alternative health care products. Tobacco and alcohol use, noting favored product, quantity, frequency, and duration of use. Nonprescribed (illicit) drugs for recreational purposes (patients are more likely to be honest if asked questions about illicit drug use in a matter-of-fact manner)

If the patient uses nonprescription products for a particular medical problem, the pharmacy student should establish how often the medical problem occurs, if the nonprescription therapy works, and if the therapy causes any side effects. Patients should be asked where they usually buy nonprescription products and how they obtain answers to questions about the products (i.e., if there is a pharmacist or other health care professional available to answer their questions).

Review of Disease States, Conditions, and Medications

These lists should be reviewed with the patient for confirmation. The pharmacy student should ask if there are other conditions that are not included on the list. Patients should be asked to describe their disease (e.g., "Just to give me an idea of your understanding of congestive heart failure [CHF], please describe what is happening"). The pharmacy student should probe for understanding of the effects of overtreatment, undertreatment, or sporadic treatment of the disease (e.g., "Tell me what long-term complications you may avoid if your blood pressure is lowered.") and any cultural and personal beliefs that might affect current or future drug therapy ("Tell me how you feel about medication use, in general." or "How do you feel your medications affect your quality of life?"). Information about therapies used *previously* for each disease state may also be valuable.

Drug Allergies and Other Conditions

If a patient states that he or she is allergic to a certain drug or has had an adverse reaction to a certain drug, as much of the following information as possible should be obtained. This information should be obtained for every drug that the patient notes:

- Name of the drug to which the reaction occurred and information about similar reactions
  - Occurrence of similar reaction when drugs in same class previously taken
  - Number of times the drug was used previously without adverse sequelae
- Reason the patient took the drug (and likelihood of viral infection within 2 weeks preceding drug use, if the reaction was a rash)
- Complete description of physical symptoms of the reaction. A physical assessment should be conducted if the adverse drug reaction is currently in progress.
- Timing of reaction versus administration of the drug ("How soon after you took the drug did this reaction happen?" "How many days or doses into therapy were you when this reaction occurred?"). Any information about other medications administered around the same time that the reaction occurred may also be useful.
- Other allergies or intolerances (e.g., food, nickel, latex). Drug vehicles or inert ingredients may contain something to which the patient will react.

If it is determined that a patient is incorrectly labeled as allergic to a drug or other substance, the primary care provider should be consulted about the possibility of removing the allergy label and flag from the patient's chart or profile.

Medication Reconciliation

Medication reconciliation is the process of comparing a patient's new medication list with a patient's previous medication list when that patient transitions from one care setting to another.[3,4] The tricky part of medication reconciliation is identifying an accurate list of the patient's previous medications. One of the obvious ways to obtain information about prior medication use is to interview the patient and/or their caregiver. Thus, it is vital for students to learn how to successfully interview patients. Other steps in the medication reconciliation process include contacting a previous care site (e.g., a patient came to hospital from a skilled nursing facility or vice versa), contacting the patient's pharmacy, having a patient caregiver bring in all prescription and nonprescription medication bottles for inspection, and calling the office(s) of the patient's health care providers to obtain chart information about what has been prescribed.

Step 3. Gather Information: Examine the Patient

Immediately after or during the interview, any physical examination necessary to test a hypothesis about DRPs should be conducted. Current and past laboratory data and diagnostic tests should be checked to determine changes that might indicate drug efficacy or toxicity. The patient's pharmacy should be contacted to confirm current prescription drugs and regimens. Questions about refill patterns will confirm compliance. A patient's family members, caregivers, or physician can be contacted if they can provide valuable information regarding the patient's response to therapy.

If a pharmacy student wishes to obtain information about an objective parameter that has not been previously measured, he or she must justify to the preceptor why the information would be helpful and cost justified. The student should also identify tests or procedures that must be done immediately versus those that can be delayed until the most emergent problem(s) is/are addressed.

Step 4. Determine and Prioritize Medical and Drug-Related Problems

A list of all the patient's current medical problems—conditions that the patient is experiencing or being treated for—should be identified. These medical problems should be numbered and placed in order of importance, starting with the medical problems needing the most immediate attention and ending with problems that can be addressed later. In a hospital setting, many of the patient's medical conditions will be identified by the physician in the patient chart. In the community pharmacy, medical problems may need to be inferred from the patient's drug therapy list and confirmed through the patient interview.

Alongside each medical condition should be a corresponding list of DRPs. DRPs are issues pertaining specifically to drug therapy. Although eight DRPs were identified in the seminal publication[2] distinguishing the role of the pharmacist in the patient care team, these DRPs can be further consolidated into five easily remembered issues:

- Drug needed (i.e., drug indicated but not prescribed, correct drug prescribed but not taken)
- Wrong drug (i.e., inappropriate drug prescribed—no apparent current medical problem justifying use of drug, unneeded duplication of therapy, less expensive alternative available or drug not covered by formulary, drug not available; failure to account for pregnancy status, age of the patient, or other contraindications; incorrect nonprescription agent self-prescribed by the patient; harmful recreational drug use)
- Wrong dose (i.e., prescribed dose too high, needs adjustments for kidney, liver function, age, or body size; correct prescribed dose but overuse by the patient; prescribed dose too low, needs adjustment for age or body size; correct prescribed dose but underuse by the patient; incorrect, inconvenient, or less than optimal dosing interval)
- Adverse drug reaction (i.e., unwanted side effect, allergy, drug-induced medical problem, or laboratory change)
- Drug interaction (i.e., unwanted drug–drug, drug–disease, drug–nutrient, or drug–laboratory interaction)

Questions that a pharmacist should consider while examining a patient's list of medications to determine whether any of these issues are occurring are as follows:

- Are there any medical problems (diagnoses) identified by the prescriber or pharmacist for which no drug therapy has been prescribed? If so, does the condition probably need drug therapy?
- Are there any drugs prescribed for the patient with no apparent indication?
- Is the patient taking the medications as prescribed? If not, why not?
- Is the treatment working? If not, why not?
- Is the treatment causing intolerable side effects?

- Are the doses correct/optimal?
- Are any abnormal laboratory values drug induced?
- Could lower-cost medications produce a similar effect?

Step 5. Determine the Therapeutic Goal for Each Medical Problem

The four primary goals for any drug therapy are to accomplish the following as needed:

- Cure a disease (e.g., infection)
- Eliminate or reduce a patient's symptoms (e.g., pain, CHF)
- Arrest or slow a disease process (e.g., kidney dysfunction, atherosclerosis)
- Prevent an unwanted condition (e.g., stroke, infection, pregnancy)

There are also general secondary goals that, if achieved, can aid in attaining the patient's primary goals. Secondary goals include the following:

- Avoiding unwanted adverse effects
- Attaining medication regimen convenience
- Achieving cost-effectiveness
- Enhancing patient education

Proxy or intermediate end points are most often monitored to determine the therapeutic efficacy of a medication regimen:

- The best intermediate end points are predictive of the primary goals (which are essentially avoidance of adverse health-related events); for example, there is a reasonable correlation between a systolic blood pressure (SBP) <130 mm Hg (an intermediate end point) and a lower risk of stroke (an unwanted condition).
- Many intermediate end points, however, are not strongly correlated with lower risk of adverse health events. For example, although it is true that the risk of stage 5 chronic kidney disease increases as BP increases, it has not been shown definitively that lowering BP lowers risk of progression to stage 5 chronic kidney disease.

Pharmacy students need to identify which intermediate end points most strongly predict achievement of the overall health goal.

Step 6. Identify Reasonable Therapeutic Alternatives for Each DRP

All reasonable therapeutic options (drug classes and nondrug therapies) used for a medical problem should be considered in the process of solving a DRP. For each therapeutic option, the following should be determined:

- The evidence for efficacy
- The likelihood and severity of adverse medication effects
- The number of daily doses
- The effects (either positive or negative) of the option on the patient's other diseases
- The cost relative to the other agents

The pharmacy student should review this information during the practice experience for each treatment received by or considered for each assigned patient. The ability to clearly summarize the most recent evidence supporting (or disputing) each treatment option will facilitate providing the best possible care. The preceptor will query students extensively about therapeutic alternatives, so this important step should not be neglected.

Step 7. Choose and Individualize the Best Therapeutic Option

If a thorough job has been done collecting and evaluating the benefits and limitations of each therapeutic option, choosing the most reasonable therapeutic option should be easy. The option must then be individualized to fit the characteristics of the patient. This is where knowledge about height and weight (for pharmacokinetic dose considerations), concomitant diseases and medications (for drug–disease and drug–drug interactions), and adherence history (to determine frequency of doses) will be vital. If the plan includes drug therapy, then drug, dose, route, frequency, and duration of therapy need to be specified. All drug and nondrug plans should include some degree of patient education.

Step 8. Design a Monitoring Plan for Efficacy and Toxicity

After choosing a therapeutic regimen, a monitoring plan needs to be designed. The monitoring plan should include the following:

- Exactly what will be measured
- Who will do the measuring
- How often it will be done
- When it may be time to change or discontinue the therapy
- Why the backup plan is the next best option

The student must be able to defend all of the above measures. This will be easy if the monitoring parameters are cheap, quick, and noninvasive but more difficult if they are expensive, lengthy, or invasive.

Step 9. Discuss the Care Plan with a Preceptor

Students are expected to have all decision making reviewed by a preceptor prior to plan implementation, until the preceptor is satisfied that the student can be trusted to make independent recommendations. One tool useful for presenting patient information verbally to a preceptor is SBAR: situation, background, assessment, and recommendation. An example of an SBAR is included in the sample workup at the end of this chapter.

Step 10. Document the Decision-Making Process

It is professionally unacceptable and legally dangerous to provide care for a patient and not record both care decisions and the reasoning behind those decisions.[5–7] Practice-based experiences are valuable because they allow students the necessary practice to eventually produce a brief yet informative note in a short amount of time.

All documentation notes should begin with the date and time that the information is recorded. Good notes will also include before the start of the note a brief one-phrase overview of the reason for the note. This one-phrase overview should identify the pharmacy origin of the note (making it easier for other health care providers to locate) and some indication of the problem (e.g., "Pharmacy note suboptimally controlled blood pressure," "Pharmacy note regarding probable adverse drug reaction").

Format

There are several formats for documentation of medication regimen decision making, but all follow the same general flow of ideas:

- Pertinent patient data are listed.
- Data analysis identifies an actual or potential DRP.
- A plan or recommendation is identified to address or prevent the identified DRP. The plan or recommendation includes monitoring parameters to determine success of the proposed treatment plan.

The most widely used format for documentation is the SOAP format, which is outlined in Box 15.2. Other written formats for communicating information include FARM (findings, assessment, recommendations, monitoring), DAP (data, assessment, plan), and preprinted checkoff forms, such as care pathways or protocols. Because patient care activities such as unexpected DRPs cannot be recorded completely using a preprinted form, these activities should be documented by adding a written addendum to the progress notes.

BOX 15.2 Components of a SOAP Note

S—**Subjective** information is obtained verbally from the patient or caregiver and therefore is not directly observed or measured by the SOAP writer.

O—**Objective** information is presented next and details data directly measured or observed by the SOAP writer. One example of objective information is a diagnosis that has been made by a qualified health care practitioner.

Information in the subjective and objective sections of a SOAP note do not use the subheadings of ID, CC, HPI, DH, SH, ROS, and PE used in the patient H&P database (see Box 15.1 for definitions of abbreviations). The subjective and objective information in a SOAP note should be limited to information that pertains directly to the assessment or plan/recommendation.

BOX 15.2 Components of a SOAP Note *(continued)*

A—The **assessment** section of a SOAP note communicates the critical thinking of the writer. The assessment section should

- Identify a DRP and explain why the identified DRP needs correcting.
- Contain a short list of reasonable therapeutic alternatives with a brief explanation of benefits and potential problems associated with each option and treatment goals.
- Reference evidence from the medical literature where appropriate. It is conventional to use a brief reference format of acceptable journal name/abbreviation, year of publication, volume, and first page number.
- *When written optimally, by the time the reader reaches the end of the assessment section, that reader will know exactly what is going to be recommended by the writer and why.*

P—The **plan** section, which is the final step, identifies the actions proposed by the writer. A pharmacist's recommendation or plan should include the following:

- Drug, dose, route, frequency, and duration (when applicable)
- What will be measured to determine if the therapy is working (i.e., effective), who will measure it, and how frequently this will be done
- What will be measured to determine if the recommended drug is causing a problem (i.e., toxicity), who will measure it, and what will be done if toxicity occurs. Toxicity monitoring will usually involve different monitoring parameters than the efficacy measures.
- Specific counseling points about administration, dose, frequency of use, side effects, or precautions if the writer's purpose is to document patient counseling
- When follow-up will occur (e.g., follow-up in 3 months for repeat BP check)
- The alternatives to treatment if efficacy is not achieved or if toxicity occurs

Written notes in the ambulatory care setting are often used to document patient interactions for billing purposes. In such cases, it is important to include in the note the number of minutes spent on the interaction/workup. This number is usually placed at the end of the note.

Pharmacy students who present oral or written information about patients to people outside the care team (e.g., a care note submitted to their school as part of a professional portfolio) need to remember that certain health-related information cannot be included in their reports. The Health Insurance Portability and Accountability Act (HIPAA) identifies specific information that cannot be shared outside of the care team. This information is summarized in Box 15.3; some recommendations (e.g., dates) have been broadened for simplicity.

Tips for Writing Patient Care Notes

- **Length.** As a general rule, care notes should not exceed one page. This can be most easily accomplished through careful use of phrases, rather than sentences, and by including *only* the information needed to support the assessment and plan and nothing more.
- **Number of problems.** Practitioners working in the inpatient setting often only have time to address one problem in each patient each day, so inpatient notes tend to be brief. An exception is notes written after medication reconciliation has been performed. In these cases, all medications will need to be listed and assessed. Practitioners working in the non–specialty clinic setting and pharmacists completing medication therapy management (MTM) in the community pharmacy setting will usually address the effectiveness and concerns associated with each medication that the patient is taking and so will assess each control of each medical condition by the therapy taken for that condition.
- **Abbreviations.** It is reasonably safe to abbreviate common laboratory values (e.g., white blood cells [WBCs], hemoglobin [Hgb]),

BOX 15.3 Information That Cannot Leave the Care Site

- Calendar dates of any kind (instead, organize by time around a single event, e.g., day 4 after admission, 4 months prior to this appointment)
- Names or initials of any patient, caregiver, health care provider, or any other individual
- Names or locations of any business, institution, care facility, or residence (the HIPAA specifies no geographical area smaller than a state)
- Patient or medical identification numbers or codes of any kind, including phone numbers and email addresses

the four main vital signs, and common diagnostic tests (e.g., chest x-ray study [CXR], radiograph [x-ray], computed tomography [CT], magnetic resonance imaging [MRI], forced expiratory volume [FEV_1], forced vital capacity [FVC]), but abbreviation of anything else may result in miscommunication among health care providers, increasing the risk of medication errors. Drug names should never be abbreviated. Many institutions have an approved abbreviations list; the pharmacy student should obtain a copy of this list on the first day at a new site. Pharmacy students should be well acquainted with potentially dangerous abbreviations and avoid their use.

- **Common problems** seen in care notes written by new or untrained writers include the following:
  - Inclusion of extraneous information (e.g., identification of all medications a patient is receiving in the subjective or objective section when the assessment addresses only one or two of those medications)
  - Exclusion of important information (e.g., identification of uncontrolled hypertension in the assessment with no or only one BP reading in the objective section)
  - Information in the wrong place (e.g., assessment information in the plan)
  - Vague or unclear information. Avoid use of nonspecific words such as "decreased," "increased," "recent," "symptoms," "problems," "changes," "monitor," "review," and "follow"
  - Lack of clear reasoning to support problem existence or choice of recommendation

Step 11. Meet with the Patient After Plan Implementation

It is important to meet with the patient after plan implementation to determine the success of the plan and the need for modification.

Example

The following example of a complete patient workup will illustrate the patient care process:

It is the first day of the clinical clerkship at a community pharmacy. Mr. Smith, a 68-year-old man who has been a patient at this pharmacy for several years, presents a prescription for "Coumadin 2 mg #30, 1 PO daily" to the pharmacy student. The information sources available to the student are Mr. Smith, his pharmacy profile, and a log of his laboratory values, which the pharmacist has asked him to bring every time he comes to the pharmacy. The following information is the patient history and physical data, the student's assessment of Mr. Smith's therapy, the review of the student's findings with the preceptor, and the care note.

Patient History and Physical Database

ID: A 68-year-old man

CC: Needs an increase in warfarin dose due to decreased efficacy of past dose

HPI: The patient takes warfarin daily for deep venous thrombosis (DVT) prevention. The INR (international normalized ratio) today was 1.5, and the physician has decided to increase the warfarin dose from 5 mg by mouth daily to 7 mg by mouth daily. The patient has been instructed to take one 5-mg tablet and one 2-mg tablet daily and to return for reassessment in 2 weeks.

PMH:

- DVT, 2 months ago
- Hip replacement surgery, 3 months ago
- Atrial fibrillation, single episode 4 years ago; no symptoms are currently reported.
- Congestive heart failure (CHF), diagnosed 7 years ago
- Chronic obstructive pulmonary disease (COPD), diagnosed 5 years ago
- Anterior myocardial infarction (MI) 14 years ago indicating coronary artery disease (CAD); no current chest pain

DH:

Prescription medications:

- Warfarin, 5 mg by mouth every day for 2 months (DVT; same dose since discharge from hospital 2 months ago)
- Digoxin, 0.25 mg by mouth every day for 7 years (CHF)
- Ipratropium, two puffs four times a day for 5 years (COPD)
- Albuterol, two puffs four times a day for 5 years (COPD)

Nonprescription medications:

- Multivitamin with iron and minerals, one by mouth daily for 7 months

- Psyllium, one scoop in a glass of water for constipation daily for 4 years
- Bismuth salicylate, four tablespoonfuls as needed for diarrhea (took one dose twice in the past year for stomach flu)
- Alfalfa tablet two to three every day for health; a friend recommended this to him about 1 month ago.

Adherence information:

- Medication refill records indicate that the patient obtains refills on time.
- The patient obtains all prescription and OTC medications from this pharmacy.
- The patient bought alfalfa tablets at a health food store.

Recreational drug use:

- 40-pack/year smoking history: quit 2 years ago
- Occasional alcohol use: 1 to 2 drinks/week; no recent change in this amount

Allergies: denies history of medication or environmental allergies

FH: Father died of acute MI at age 54

SH: Retired; lives with spouse who assists with medication management at home; denies any changes in ingestion of vitamin K–containing foods

ROS: No current complaints

- Lungs: clear sputum, no spells of coughing recently; denies shortness of breath (SOB), dyspnea on exertion (DOE), and paroxysmal nocturnal dyspnea (PND); sleeps with one pillow; is comfortable walking short distances (no change from 3 months ago)
- CV (cardiovascular): denies chest pain
- Skin: denies bleeding or bruising
- GI (gastrointestinal): stools are dark brown.
- GU (genitourinary): urine is clear, yellow, no blood.

PE: 5'10", 80 kg today (usual weight); HR (heart rate): 85, regular rhythm; BP: 135/82; RR (respiratory rate): 20; temp: 37.2°C; no bruising found on arms, legs, or face

Pertinent Labs:

Today	2 Weeks Ago	4 Weeks Ago	6 Weeks Ago	8 Weeks Ago (at Discharge)	8 Weeks Ago
INR: 1.5	INR: 1.9	INR: 2.4	INR: 2.6	INR: 2.3	Alb: 4.5

Current Medical Problems	Goal of Therapy	Measurable End Point
1. Recent DVT	Prevent recurrent thromboembolism	Therapeutic INR
2. CAD	Prevent angina and MI	No anginal episodes
3. CHF	Symptom control	No episodes SOB, edema, PND
4. COPD	Symptom control	No DOE, SOB, PND

Current Drug-Related Problems	Justification	Therapeutic Alternatives
1a. Under anticoagulation (wrong dose? drug interaction?)	Subtherapeutic INR Possible causes: • Diet (no recent change) • EtOH (the patient denies) • Underlying disease state change (no evidence to support) • Drug interaction (recent addition of natural product that contains varying amounts of vitamin K) • Compliance (no evidence of noncompliance)	• Increase warfarin dose (problematic, considering the inconsistent amount of vitamin K in alfalfa tablets). • Discontinue (D/C) alfalfa. • Heparin (prolonged heparin use would be more expensive than warfarin; short-term LMW heparin use might save cost of ultrasound to check for clot formation.)
2a. Inadequate MI prophylaxis (needs drug?)	Current AHCPR guidelines recommend aspirin and beta-blocker for all patients post-MI unless contraindicated.	• ASA, 81 mg PO daily (lower dose will minimize the risk of bleeding) • ASA, 325 mg PO daily • Beta-blocker (contraindicated secondary to CHF + COPD)
3a. Inadequate CHF and post-MI mortality benefit (needs drug?)	Current ACC/AHA guidelines recommend ACEI for all patients with CHF; SAVE, AIRE, and TRACE trials support use post-MI to reduce mortality.	• ACE inhibitor • Angiotensin receptor antagonist

(continued)

4a. COPD overmedicated (wrong drug?)	1995 study conducted in the Netherlands showed increased costs and no additional benefit of two bronchodilators over one alone	• D/C albuterol (preferred due to CHF) • D/C ipratropium

EtOH, ethyl alcohol; LMW, low molecular weight; AHCPR, Agency for Health Care Policy Research; ACC/AHA, American College of Cardiology/American Heart Association.

Recommendation	**Monitoring Plan**
1. Anticoagulation • D/C alfalfa tablets • Start enoxaparin, 80 mg (1 mg/kg) SQ q12h. D/C when INR ≥ 2.0. • Continue warfarin at current dose. Instruct the patient to self-administer SQ medication.	• Return for INR check in 5 days • The patient to self-monitor for signs/symptoms (S/S) of DVT: calf warmth, tenderness, or pain. The patient to call provider immediately if experiences chest pain or SOB • The patient to self-monitor for S/S minor, moderate, and major bleed: visual check for gum, urine, stool, skin bruising, epistaxis
2. MI prophylaxis • ASA, 81 mg PO daily	• The patient to self-check for bleeding as noted above. Stool guaiac in 3 months
3. CHF/post-MI mortality benefit • Lisinopril, 5 mg PO daily; first dose at bedtime; titrate dose upward weekly to maximal doses (20 mg PO q12hr) as tolerated per BP and serum creatinine (SCr).	• Check BP in 1 week (goal SBP 100–120). • Check SCr now for baseline and again in 1 week. • The patient to self-monitor for and report dizziness/light-headedness and any increase in coughing frequency
4. COPD • D/C albuterol	• The patient to self-monitor for and report any increased incidence of SOB, DOE, PND

Example SBAR Presentation by Student to Preceptor

Situation: This is a 68-year-old white male presenting with an increase in warfarin dose due to recently elevated INR.

Background: This patient is 2 months out from hospitalization for DVT. His INR was therapeutic at discharge and 1 month ago. Two weeks ago, his INR started trending downward, and today, it was 1.5. Other medical conditions he is being treated for is CHF and COPD. Apparently, a friend recommended he take alfalfa tablets about a month ago so he has been taking 2 to 3 tablets daily since then.

Assessment: His INR started decreasing after he started taking the alfalfa tablets. Since they are a known source of vitamin K, it would be prudent to have him discontinue the alfalfa. He will likely return to a stable INR in the normal range within a few days of resuming his warfarin 5-mg dose, but it would be a good idea to provide extra support with a low molecular weight heparin until he is again at therapeutic INR. Goal INR is 2.0 to 3.0. Given that he has taken two alfalfa tablets already today, I expect that it will take 3 to 4 days before the effect of the alfalfa on the clotting cascade disappears.

Plan: Call physician and explain situation. Recommend no increase in warfarin dose at this time. Recommend enoxaparin 1 mg/kg (80 mg) SC q12h until INR >2.0. Have the patient return for INR check in 5 days.

Example SOAP Note

Today's Date and Time

Pharmacy note regarding anticoagulation and other drug therapy for a 68-year-old white male is as follows:

S: DVT, 2 months ago; CHF for 7 years; COPD for 5 years; anterior MI, 14 years ago. Denies coughing, SOB, DOE, PND, chest pain, bleeding or bruising, blood in stool or urine. Occasional alcohol use: 1 to 2 drinks/week; no recent change in that amount. Denies any changes in ingestion of vitamin K–containing foods; has taken alfalfa tabs 2 or 3 daily for approximately 1 month per friend's advice (for general health)

O:

- 5'10", 80 kg today (usual weight); HR: 85, regular rhythm; BP: 135/82; RR: 20
- No bruising found on arms, legs, or face
- INR: 1.5 today; 1.9, 2 weeks ago; 2.4, 4 weeks ago; 2.6, 6 weeks ago; 2.3 at discharge 8 weeks ago
- Pertinent prescription medications: warfarin, 5 mg PO daily (same dose for last 2 months); ipratropium, 2 puffs QID; albuterol, 2 puffs QID

A:

1. INR ≤ 2.0 associated with ↑ risk of recurrent DVT. Addition of alfalfa coincides with ↓ INR control. Discontinuing alfalfa preferable to increasing warfarin dose since varying vitamin K tablet amount confounds dose titration. Since the patient shows no

signs/symptoms of acute DVT, addition of outpatient enoxaparin for a few days until INR in therapeutic range would be more cost-effective than admission to hospital to watch for recurrent DVT.

2. Suboptimal CHF and post-MI mortality benefit. Addition of aspirin for CAD and ACE inhibitor for CHF and post-MI associated with ↓ mortality. Beta-blocker use also associated with ↓ risk of subsequent MI but is relatively contraindicated in this patient because of CHF and COPD.
3. Dual-bronchodilator therapy not superior to single-bronchodilator therapy for COPD.[8] Ipratropium preferred over albuterol in this patient due to CHF

P:

1. D/C alfalfa tabs. Start enoxaparin, 80 mg SQ (subcutaneous) q12h. D/C when INR ≥ 2.0. Continue warfarin at current dose. Teach the patient how to self-administer SQ medication. Return for INR check in 5 days. Instruct the patient to self-monitor and report calf warmth, tenderness, or pain; chest pain or SOB; and excessive blood in gums, urine, stool, nose, and dermis.
2. Start ASA (acetylsalicylic acid; aspirin), 81 mg PO daily; lisinopril 5 mg PO daily; first dose at bedtime; titrate dose up by 5 mg every week to maximum 20 mg PO daily as tolerated per BP (✓ in 1 week; goal: SBP [systolic BP] 100 to 120) and SCr (✓ today and in 1 week). The patient to report any dizziness or ↑ coughing
3. D/C albuterol. The patient to report any ↑ in SOB, DOE, PND

Summary

In summary, whether with a patient in the hospital, in the clinic, or at the pharmacy counter, the student should perform the following steps:

- Quickly scan the chart or profile to identify issues that need to be discussed with the patient.
- Obtain subjective data by interviewing the patient.
- Gather objective data by physical examination and review of pertinent laboratory parameters, MAR or patient fill records, and diagnostic tests and consultations.

- Summarize the patient's medical problems and DRPs, and set goals for the therapy of those problems that need to be addressed immediately.
- Consider the potential benefits and hazards of all reasonable therapeutic alternatives. Select the alternative that has the highest likelihood of efficacy and a minimum of toxicity and that seems the most cost-effective.
- Determine the optimal dose, route, frequency, and duration for the patient's pharmacokinetic, concomitant drug and disease state, economic, and compliance needs.
- Design and implement a monitoring plan to determine if the recommendation works or causes unreasonable toxicity.
- Document the decision-making process.

At first, this process will seem long and cumbersome, but with practice, it will become quick and effortless. By taking the responsibility for clinical drug monitoring, the student will become a practitioner whom patients and health care colleagues will respect and trust.

References

1. Hepler CD, Strand LM. Opportunities and responsibilities in pharmaceutical care. *Am J Hosp Pharm.* 1990;47:533–543.
2. Strand LM, Cipolle RJ, Morley PC. Documenting the clinical pharmacist's activities: back to basics. *Drug Intell Clin Pharm.* 1988;22:63–66.
3. ASHP Council on Pharmacy Practice. ASHP statement on the pharmacist's role in medication reconciliation. *Am J Health Syst Pharm.* 2013; 70:453–456.
4. Kwan JL, Lo L, Sampson M, et al. Medication reconciliation during transitions of care as a patient safety strategy. *Ann Intern Med.* 2013;158:397–403.
5. Canaday BR, Yarborough PC. Documenting pharmaceutical care: creating a standard. *Ann Pharmacother.* 1994;28(11):1292–1296.
6. Zierler-Brown S, Brown TR, Chen D, et al. Clinical documentation for patient care: models, concepts, and liability considerations for pharmacists. *Am J Health Syst Pharm.* 2007;64:1851–1858.
7. Kennie N, Farrell B, Dolovich L. Demonstrating value, documenting care: lessons learned about writing comprehensive patient medication assessments in the IMPACT project. *Can Pharm J.* 2008;141:114–119.
8. Rutten-van Molken MP, Van Doorslaer EK, Jansen MC, et al. Costs and effects of inhaled corticosteroids and bronchodilators in asthma and chronic obstructive pulmonary disease. *Am J Resp Crit Care Med.* 1995; 151(4):975–982.

16

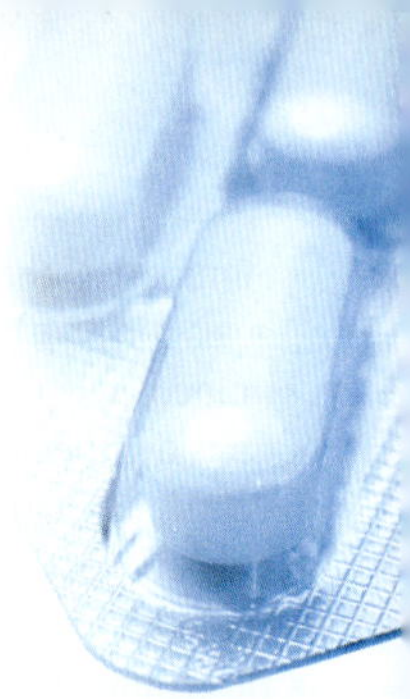

Antibiotics, Antivirals, and Infection

Jennifer M. Jordan, Devon Flynn, and David T. Bearden

Signs and Symptoms of Infection

Fever and an elevation in peripheral white blood cell (WBC) count are the classic nonspecific signs of infection. Fever is inexactly defined, but most clinicians consider temperatures >100.4°F (38°C) to be abnormal.[1] An increase in neutrophils, termed a "left shift" in WBCs, is also frequently noted. It is important to note that some individuals may display neither sign of infection, due to a diminished host response. Reasons to lack a fever include advanced age, use of antipyretics, or sepsis. A low temperature in sepsis of <96.8°F (36°C) is actually a worse prognostic sign than a high temperature. Similarly, neutropenic oncology patients may not have an infection-related WBC increase. Other signs and symptoms depend on the specific site of infection.

Cultures and Sensitivities Time Line

The treatment of infectious diseases is predicated on identifying and obtaining the pathogen causing the disease. This frequently occurs in several steps that may require several days (see Table 16.1) for completion. Each step reveals more data to aid in clinical decision making but also requires careful interpretation. It is important to note that the approximate times listed in Table 16.1 apply to most common bacterial cultures. Some more-difficult-to-grow organisms (fastidious organisms) can take several days to several weeks (*Mycobacterium tuberculosis*) to become positive.

Early Gram stain distinction of the organism shape and grouping provides important clues to the pathogen likely to be isolated (Table 16.2).

TABLE 16.1 The Typical Bacterial Culture Time Line

Step	Time Frame	Antibiotic Choices	Example	Notes
1. Obtaining a specimen for culture	—	Broad empiric coverage for the likely pathogens at the suspected site of infection	Blood culture obtained; initially started empirically on vancomycin	—
2. Gram stain	Minutes	Add or alter therapy if empiric selection does not cover this group of organisms	No Gram stains are done on blood; no change in therapy	The presence of organisms does not always mean infection. Some sites are not sterile, and colonization cannot always be differentiated
3. Initial positive culture	12–48 hours	Add or alter therapy if empiric selection does not cover this group of organisms; stop unnecessary additional coverage	Gram strain of growing organism reveals gram-negative bacilli; stop vancomycin, start ceftazidime	The lack of a positive culture does not rule out infection. For most infections, a positive culture may never be isolated due to technical issues, a difficult-to-grow organisms, or transient bacterial appearance
4. Identification of species	24–48 hours	Add or alter therapy if empiric selection does not typically cover this organism	Organism identified as *Klebsiella pneumoniae*; continue ceftazidime	Using local susceptibility patterns at this step can give a better indication of the likelihood that initial therapy will be adequate
5. Anti-infective susceptibilities	48–72 hours	Narrow therapy to the specific organism's data	Susceptibilities reveal organism is resistant to ceftazidime but sensitive to ciprofloxacin; stop ceftazidime, start ciprofloxacin	Final antibiotic recommendations can now be made

TABLE 16.2 Bacterial Shapes and Gram Stains

Gram Stain and Shape	Likely Pathogen
Gram Positive	
Cocci in clusters	*Staphylococcus* species
Cocci in chains	*Streptococcus* species (not *S. pneumoniae*)
Cocci in pairs and chains	*Enterococcus* species
Diplococci	*S. pneumoniae*
Gram Negative	
Bacilli (rods)	Many species
Diplococci	*Neisseria* species

Source: Koneman EW, Allen SD, Janda WM, et al. *Color Atlas and Textbook of Diagnostic Microbiology*. 5th ed. Philadelphia, PA: Lippincott-Raven; 1997:2.[2]

In instances where only a single pathogen from a normally sterile site is likely, this information can be very helpful early in the treatment course.

Not all positive cultures are clinically relevant. Attention to the type of organism isolated is also revealing. Normal flora is present at nonsterile sites and may contaminate samples (e.g., skin flora in blood samples or oral flora in sputum samples). Positive cultures of this sort that lack clinical symptoms (e.g., coagulase-negative staphylococci in a blood culture) are often considered contaminants. Similarly, not all negative cultures confirm a lack of infection. Even with documented infections, it is often difficult to isolate a specific bacterial cause. Finally, some types of organisms are notoriously difficult to culture. For example, anaerobes are often missed by typical cultures and need to be assumed present in some infections (e.g., diabetic foot, intra-abdominal infections).

Newer, rapid technology tests are currently being more widely used for the identification of important pathogens. For instance, polymerase chain reaction (PCR) testing can detect the gene responsible for methicillin-resistant *Staphylococcus aureus* (*mec*A) within hours, cutting substantial time off selecting appropriate therapy. Mass spectrometry is also being utilized for rapid identification of a variety of bacterial isolates.

Susceptibility Testing

The minimum inhibitory concentration (MIC) of an antibiotic against an organism is the concentration that inhibits growth in the laboratory. This concentration is determined and then compared to established guidelines that categorize the value into one of the three groups—sensitive, intermediate, or resistant. Many laboratories will report only one of these three categories and not the exact concentration of the MIC. Clinically, the categories should generally guide antibiotic selection. An "intermediate" determination generally weighs against the use of that anti-infective.

There are times when a specific MIC may be important in decision making, and the laboratory can be asked to provide the actual concentration. Knowledge of the specific MIC is imperative for use in maximizing pharmacodynamic parameters in dosing regimens (see Pharmacokinetic- Pharmacodynamics of Antimicrobial Therapy: Optimizing Dosing). It is important to note that comparing a list of MIC values for various anti-infectives without knowing the concentrations required for a determination of sensitive, intermediate, or resistant is of little value. Lower does not always mean better. The typical concentration of the anti-infective in the blood and at the site of infection plays an important role in setting the break-point values for determining susceptibility. An antibacterial with an MIC of 4 μg/mL can be preferable to one with an MIC of 2 μg/mL in the context of the tissue concentrations typically achieved.

Choosing the Appropriate Antimicrobial Agent

The delay of appropriate antimicrobial therapy is often related to higher rates of morbidity and mortality. This relationship creates a difficult challenge for clinicians who want to treat all the major pathogens until microbiologic laboratory data are available, while minimizing a patient's drug exposure to avoid toxicities, excessive costs, and the development of superinfections and resistance. The principles of treating infection can be simplified into the following steps:

1. Diagnosis of the infectious disease state (e.g., cellulitis)
2. Consideration of likely pathogens consistent with the patient history, clinical presentation, and epidemiologic data (e.g., streptococcus or staphylococcus)

3. Choosing an antimicrobial regimen that has activity against the most likely pathogens and achieves adequate drug concentrations at the site of infection, and the patient is likely to tolerate (e.g., dicloxacillin)
4. Monitoring the patient for improvement and adjusting therapy based on clinical and microbiology data

Pharmacists can play a key role in assisting prescribers with antimicrobial selection, dose optimization, and monitoring therapy for efficacy as well as toxicity.

Table 16.3 consists of the more common infectious diseases seen in clinical practice, likely pathogens, and possible empiric antibiotic regimens. A detailed patient history, including history of present illness, allergy data, previous antibiotic therapy, health care exposure, presence of comorbidities, and laboratory data should be considered before recommending or starting any antimicrobial regimen. Complicated cases should be referred to an infectious disease specialist.

Unfortunately, the regimens as listed in Table 16.3 do not fit all patients. One must consider allergies, severity of disease, and local resistance patterns. Also, there are many drugs that would be effective, but listing every regimen is beyond the scope of this chapter. To assist in choosing alternative regimens, Table 16.4 lists most antimicrobials with their general spectrum of activity.

Special Bugs

Multidrug-resistant pathogens are becoming relatively common. The armamentarium to treat *Acinetobacter*, *Pseudomonas*, and *Enterobacter* species is becoming small with the increasing development of resistance.

Special Considerations

- *Acinetobacter*: There have been several outbreaks of multidrug-resistant *Acinetobacter* in the United States. Many of these strains are susceptible only to colistin and tigecycline.
- *Enterobacter*: Inducible β-lactamases not seen with routine susceptibility tests may be present. Do not use third-generation cephalosporins. Drugs of choice for serious infections include carbapenems or cefepime.
- *Pseudomonas*: Fluoroquinolones or aminoglycosides should not be used as monotherapy for serious infections outside the urinary tract.

(Text continued on page 520)

TABLE 16.3 Common Infectious Diseases and Recommended Treatment

Disease State	Typical Pathogens	Oral/IV Options	Comments
Cellulitis (uncomplicated, community acquired)	*S. pyogenes, S. aureus*	Dicloxacillin, clindamycin, nafcillin, oxacillin, or vancomycin	Emergence of CA-MRSA Bactrim, doxycycline, vancomycin, linezolid
Bacterial meningitis (age ≥1 month, without head trauma or recent neurosurgery)	*S. pneumoniae* *N. meningitidis*	Vancomycin *plus* ceftriaxone *or* cefotaxime	Age >50 years, add ampicillin for *Listeria* species
Acute otitis media	*S. pneumoniae* Viral *H. influenzae* *M. catarrhalis*	Amoxicillin	High-dose amoxicillin recommended; delay in therapy may be appropriate
Acute rhinosinusitis	*S. pneumoniae* *H. influenzae* *M. catarrhalis* Viral	Amoxicillin/clavulanate	Observation with analgesics recommended in some cases
Acute pharyngitis	Viral streptococci	Penicillin	Document group A *Streptococcus* before treatment
Community-acquired pneumonia (previously healthy individual with no risk factors for drug resistant streptococcus pneumoniae)	*S. pneumoniae* *M. pneumoniae* *H. influenzae* *C. pneumoniae* Viral newline	Macrolide Doxycycline	Hospitalized patients should receive a respiratory fluoroquinolone or a β-lactam plus macrolide

(continued)

TABLE 16.3 Common Infectious Diseases and Recommended Treatment *(continued)*

Disease State	Typical Pathogens	Oral/IV Options	Comments
Community-acquired pneumonia (comorbidities or antibiotics in previous 3 months or high prevalence of macrolide resistance)	*S. pneumoniae* *M. pneumoniae* *H. influenzae* *C. pneumoniae* Viral	Respiratory FQ Macrolide *plus* amoxicillin or cefpodoxime or ceftriaxone or cefuroxime	If admitted to the ICU, an IV β-lactam *plus* a macrolide or fluoroquinolone is recommended
Health care–associated pneumonia (hospitalized <5 days, low risk for a multidrug-resistant pathogen)	*S. pneumoniae* *H. influenzae* MSSA GNB	Ceftriaxone Quinolone Ampicillin/sulbactam Ertapenem	Empiric regimens should cover >90% of the local pathogens
Health care–associated pneumonia (hospitalized ≥5 days and risk for a multidrug-resistant pathogen)	Above pathogens *Pseudomonas* *Klebsiella* *Acinetobacter* MRSA	Anti–pseudomonal β-lactam *plus* ciprofloxacin or levofloxacin *plus* vancomycin or linezolid	Empiric regimens should cover >90% of the local pathogens
Urinary tract infections (UTIs) (acute, female, uncomplicated)	*E. coli* Enteric GNB *S. saprophyticus*	TMP/SMX Nitrofurantoin Fosfomycin Fluoroquinolone	Moxifloxacin and gemifloxacin are not FDA approved for UTIs

Intra-abdominal infections (mild to moderate, community acquired)	*E. coli* Enteric GNB *B. fragilis* Streptococci Enterococci	β-Lactam/β-lactamase inhibitor Third-generation cephalosporin *plus* metronidazole Fluoroquinolone *plus* metronidazole	Initial regimen should be based on local resistance patterns and severity of illness
Clostridium difficile diarrhea	*C. difficile*	Metronidazole Vancomycin oral Fidaxomicin	Vancomycin preferred for moderate to severe infections

CA-MRSA, community-acquired methicillin-resistant *Staphylococcus aureus*; GNB, gram-negative bacilli; TMP/SMX, trimethoprim/sulfamethoxazole; ICU, intensive care unit; MSSA, methicillin-susceptible *Staphylococcus aureus*.

Sources: Lieberthal AS, et al. The diagnosis and management of acute otitis media. *Pediatrics*. 2013;131(3):e964–e999; Shulman ST, et al. Clinical practice guideline for the diagnosis and management of group A streptococcal pharyngitis: 2012 update by the Infectious Diseases Society of America. *Clin Infect Dis*. 2012;55(10):1279–1282; American Thoracic Society Infectious Diseases Society of America. Guidelines for the management of adults with hospital-acquired, ventilator-associated, and healthcare-associated pneumonia. *Am J Respir Crit Care Med*. 2005;171:388–416; Mandell LA, et al. Infectious Diseases Society of America/American Thoracic Society consensus guidelines on the management of community-acquired pneumonia in adults. *Clin Infect Dis*. 2007;44:S27–S72; Chow AW, et al. IDSA clinical practice guideline for acute bacterial rhinosinusitis in children and adults. *Clin Infect Dis*. 2012;54(8):e72–e112; Solomkin JS, et al. Diagnosis and management of complicated intra-abdominal infection in adults and children: guidelines by the Surgical Infection Society and the Infectious Diseases Society of America. *Clin Infect Dis*. 2010;50(2):133–164; Stevens DL, Bisno AL, Chambers HF, et al. Practice guidelines for the diagnosis and management of skin and soft-tissue infections. *Clin Infect Dis*. 2005;41:1373–1406; Tunkel AR, Hartman BJ, Kaplan SL, et al. Practice guidelines for the management of bacterial meningitis. *Clin Infect Dis*. 2004;39:1267–1284; and Gupta K, et al. International clinical practice guidelines for the treatment of acute uncomplicated cystitis and pyelonephritis in women: a 2010 update by the Infectious Diseases Society of America and the European Society for Microbiology and Infectious Diseases. *Clin Infect Dis*. 2010;52(5):e103–e120.[3-11]

TABLE 16.4 Spectrum of Antimicrobial Activity to Common Pathogens

	Gram Positive				Gram Negative				Anaerobes		
	Streptococci	**MSSA**	**MRSA**	***Enterococcus***	***E. coli***	***Klebsiella***	***H. influenzae***	***Pseudomonas***	**Oral Anaerobes**	***B. fragilis***	**Comments**
Penicillins											
Penicillin	+	–	–	–	–	–	–	–	+	–	Drug of choice for susceptible streptococci
Ampicillin Amoxicillin	+	–	–	+	+/–	–	+/–	–	+	–	Drug of choice for susceptible enterococci
Ampicillin/ sulbactam	+	+	–	+	+	+	+	–	+	+	
Amoxicillin/ clavulanate	+	+	–	+	+	+	+	–	+	+	
Dicloxacillin	+	+	–	–	–	–	–	–	+	–	Drug of choice for MSSA
Nafcillin Oxacillin	+	+	–	–	–	–	–	–	+	–	Drug of choice for MSSA
Piperacillin/ tazobactam	+	+	–	+	+	+	+	+	+	+	

Cephalosporins											
Cefazolin	+	+	–	–	+	+	–	–	+	–	First generation
Cephalexin	+	+	–	–	+	+	–	–	+	–	First generation
Cefuroxime	+	+	–	–	+	+	+	–	+	–	Second generation
Cefoxitin	+	+	–	–	+	+	+	–	+	+	Second generation
Ceftriaxone and cefotaxime	+	+	–	–	+	+	+	–	+	–	Third generation
Ceftazidime	+/–	+/–	–	–	+	+	+	+	+/–	–	Third generation
Cefepime	+	+	–	–	+	+	+	+	+	–	Fourth generation
Ceftaroline	+	+	+	–	+	+	+	–	+	–	Fifth Generation
Aminoglycosides											
Gentamicin Tobramycin Amikacin	Syn	Syn	Not tested in vivo	Syn	+	+	+	+	–	–	Gentamicin is drug of choice for gram-positive synergy Tobramycin and amikacin more potent against *Pseudomonas*

(continued)

TABLE 16.4 Spectrum of Antimicrobial Activity to Common Pathogens *(continued)*

	Gram Positive				Gram Negative				Anaerobes		
	Streptococci	**MSSA**	**MRSA**	***Enterococcus***	***E. coli***	***Klebsiella***	***H. influenzae***	***Pseudomonas***	**Oral Anaerobes**	***B. fragilis***	**Comments**
Fluoroquinolones											
Ciprofloxacin	–	+/–	–	–	+	+	+	+	–	–	Atypicals, poor gram positive
Levofloxacin	+	+	–	+/–	+	+	+	+	+/–	–	Atypicals
Moxifloxacin	+	+	–	+/–	+	+	+	–	+	+	Atypicals, most potent gram positive
Others											
Trimethoprim/ sulfamethoxazole	+/–	+	+	–	+	+	+	–	+	–	
Clindamycin	+	+	–	–	–	–	–	–	+	+	
Metronidazole	–	–	–	–	–	–	–	–	+	+	
Aztreonam	–	–	–	–	+	+	+	+	–	–	OK for β-lactam allergy
Ertapenem	+	+	–	–	+	+	+	–	+	+	
Imipenem Meropenem	+	+	–	+/–	+	+	+	+	+	+	

Azithromycin Clarithromycin	+	+/–	–	–	–	–	+	–	+	–	Atypicals
Daptomycin	+	+	+	+	–	–	–	–	–	–	Activity against VRE
Linezolid	+	+	+	+	–	–	+/–	–	–	–	Activity against VRE
Telavancin	+	+	+	+	–	–	–	–	–	–	
Tigecycline	+	+	+	+	+	+	+	–	+	+	Activity against VRE
Vancomycin	+	+	+	+	–	–	–	–	+	–	

Note: Susceptibilities in this table are from national trends and should serve as a guide for selection of empiric antibiotics. Choice of initial antimicrobials should depend on local susceptibilities, presence of drug-resistance risk factors, previous susceptibilities and antimicrobial use, and severity of illness.

MSSA, methicillin-susceptible *Staphylococcus aureus*; MRSA, methicillin-resistant *Staphylococcus aureus*; Syn, synergy only, not likely to yield clinical cure as monotherapy; VRE, vancomycin-resistant *Enterococcus*; +, typically susceptible; –, typically resistant or no clinical activity.

Sources: Gales AC, Jones RN, Sader HS. Global assessment of the antimicrobial activity of polymyxin B against 54,731 clinical isolates of Gram-negative bacilli: report from the SENTRY Antimicrobial Surveillance Programme (2001–2004). *Clin Microbiol Infect.* 2006;12:315–321; Jones RN, et al. Ceftaroline activity against pathogens associated with complicated skin and skin structure infections: results from an international surveillance study. *J Antimicrob Chemother.* 2010;65(Suppl 4):iv17–iv31; and Hope R, et al. In vitro activity of telavancin and comparators against selected groups of Gram-positive cocci. *Int J Antimicrob Agents.* 2013;41(3):213–217.[12–14]

- Methicillin-resistant *Staphylococcus aureus* (MRSA) is a particular problem in the inpatient and outpatient setting. MRSA isolates with a vancomycin MIC >2 mg/L should be treated with an alternative anti-MRSA agent.[15] Community-acquired *methicillin*-resistant *Staphylococcus aureus* (CA-MRSA) may cause necrosis and rapidly progressing life-threatening infections. This staphylococcus can usually be treated with several antibiotics, including trimethoprim/sulfamethoxazole (TMP/SMX) or doxycycline for mild infections, but daptomycin, linezolid, ceftaroline, or vancomycin is preferred for severe infections.
- Fungus and mold: See Table 16.5 for susceptibilities.

Pharmacokinetics–Pharmacodynamics of Antimicrobial Therapy: Optimizing Dosing

To optimize antimicrobial dosing, one must first understand pharmacokinetic/pharmacodynamic (PK/PD) principles that relate to the antimicrobial agent being used and take into account pharmacokinetics for the individual patient. Pharmacodynamics is the correlation of drug concentration and response, whereas pharmacokinetics describes absorption, distribution, metabolism, and elimination of the drug from the body. PK/PD parameters may be used to optimize clinical outcomes and avoid the development of antimicrobial resistance.[18,19] Overly simplified, an antimicrobial's effectiveness can be categorized as a concentration-dependent or time-dependent activity.

- Time-dependent killers: Frequent administration, prolonged infusion times, or continuous infusion is optimal. In cases of renal insufficiency, a dose reduction while maintaining a normal dosing interval is typically preferred.
- Concentration-dependent killers: Killing activity is related to peak:MIC or area under the curve (AUC):MIC ratios.[18,19] These antimicrobials may be dosed less frequently but in high doses. Once-daily aminoglycoside administration is an example of maximizing killing and postantibiotic effects. In patients with renal insufficiency, doses of concentration-dependent antimicrobials should generally be maintained while extending the dosing interval.

See Table 16.6 for PK/PD properties of antimicrobial drug classes.

TABLE 16.5 Antifungal Spectrum of Activity and Concentrations in the Urine

Drug	Activity Against *Candida* Species				*Aspergillus* Activity	Urine Concentrations	Comments
	Candida albicans	*Candida glabrata*	*Candida parapsilosis*	*Candida krusei*			
Azoles							
Fluconazole	+++	+	+++	–	–	Excellent	*C. glabrata* may need high doses
Itraconazole	+++	+	+++	+/–	+	Poor	Needs acidic environment for PO absorption, unless suspension is used
Posaconazole	+++	++	+++	++	+++	Poor	Activity against some zygomycetes
Voriconazole	+++	++	+++	+	+++	Poor	IV and PO
Echinocandins							
Anidulafungin	+++	+++	++	+++	+++	Poor	Not metabolized
Caspofungin	+++	+++	++	+++	+++	Poor	
Micafungin	+++	+++	++	+++	+++	Poor	
Polyenes							
Amphotericin	+++	++	+++	++	+++	Poor	Nephrotoxicity, electrolyte disturbances

Sources: Pappas PG, et al. Clinical practice guidelines for the management of candidiasis: 2009 update by the Infectious Diseases Society of America. *Clin Infect Dis.* 2009;48(5):503–535; and Walsh TJ, et al. Treatment of aspergillosis: clinical practice guidelines of the Infectious Diseases Society of America. *Clin Infect Dis.* 2008;46(3):327–360.[16,17]

TABLE 16.6 Pharmacodynamic Properties of Individual Antimicrobials

Drug	PD Property	Notes
Aminoglycoside	Concentration dependent	Peak:MIC, 10–12× MIC
Fluoroquinolones	Concentration dependent	AUC:MIC >100–125 for GNB, AUC:MIC >30 for *S. pneumoniae*
Metronidazole	Concentration dependent	AUC:MIC, C_{max}:MIC
Daptomycin	Concentration dependent	AUC:MIC, C_{max}:MIC
Cephalosporins	Time dependent	50%–60% of T > MIC
Penicillins	Time dependent	40%–50% of T > MIC
Carbapenems	Time dependent	40%–50% of T > MIC
Macrolides	Time dependent	T > MIC, AUC:MIC
Clindamycin	Time dependent	T > MIC
Linezolid	Time dependent	T > MIC
Vancomycin	Time dependent	AUC:MIC
Tetracyclines	Time dependent	AUC:MIC

PD, pharmacodynamic; MIC, minimum inhibitory concentration; GNB, gram-negative bacilli; AUC, area under the curve; C_{max}, maximum concentration.
Sources: Ambrose PG, Bhavnani SM, Rubino CM, et al. Pharmacokinetics-pharmacodynamics of antimicrobial therapy: it's not just for mice anymore. *Clin Infect Dis.* 2007;44:79–86; and Craig WA. Does the dose matter? *Clin Infect Dis.* 2001;33(Suppl 3):S233–S237.

Synergy and Double Coverage

Synergy occurs when the effects of two drugs combined are greater than the addition of the individual drug's effects acting separately. Although the term is used frequently in the infectious disease realm, it is clinically relevant in only a few circumstances. Some of the most popular drug combinations for synergy are β-lactams and aminoglycosides or rifampin combinations.

- Aminoglycosides: Addition of gentamicin or streptomycin is essential when treating enterococcal endocarditis. Bactericidal effects of the penicillin or ampicillin are not seen in the absence of the aminoglycoside. Note: The dose of gentamicin is only 1 mg/kg every 8 hours in a patient with normal renal function, as gentamicin peaks of 3 to 5 mg/L have been studied for gram-positive synergy. This is in contrast to once-daily administration mentioned previously in this chapter.

- Rifampin: Rifampin is frequently used in combination with other antibiotics for infections involving bone and prosthetic material. The dose and timing of rifampin in therapy is somewhat questionable since large, randomized, placebo-controlled trials are lacking.

In the era of multidrug-resistant gram-negative pathogens, it may be acceptable to use combination therapy empirically to provide appropriate antibiotic therapy to moderately to severely ill patients. In this circumstance, the clinician may choose drugs that may be additive or synergistic initially and adjust therapy when cultures and susceptibilities are available.

IV or PO Therapy?

After choosing the correct antimicrobial spectrum and coverage, the next question is usually related to the appropriate route of administration.

While it is appealing to maximize the oral route to minimize the cost and risks of complications associated with intravenous (IV) access, in many clinical instances, the IV route is preferred.

Oral medications are preferred for mild to moderate infections when adequate drug levels reach the site of infection. Oral formulations are acceptable in more severe infections if they have a high bioavailability (Table 16.7), the patient has a functioning gastrointestinal (GI) tract in which drug absorption can occur, and there is an absence of drug or food interactions that would interfere with drug absorption. Most oral antimicrobials, even with high bioavailability, have not been well studied and should not be used for endocarditis, meningitis, sepsis, or other life-threatening infections. Oral antimicrobials may serve a role in step-down therapy or initial therapy when no IV formulations are available.

Antimicrobial Stewardship

Many health systems are incorporating antimicrobial stewardship programs to improve patient care, decrease health care costs, and decrease the development of antibiotic resistance. The antimicrobial stewardship team is typically composed of an infectious disease physician, an infectious

TABLE 16.7 Oral Antimicrobials with High Bioavailability

Antifungals	**Notes**
Fluconazole	—
Voriconazole	Take 1 hour before or after a meal
Antibiotics	
Clindamycin	Large oral doses may cause GI distress
Doxycycline and minocycline	Absorption may be hindered by divalent and trivalent cations (calcium, iron, magnesium) in food or medication
Linezolid	—
Metronidazole	—
Fluoroquinolones	Absorption may be hindered by divalent and trivalent cations (e.g., aluminum, calcium, iron, magnesium) in food or medication
Trimethoprim/sulfamethoxazole	—

disease–trained pharmacist, a microbiologist, an epidemiologist, and several other specialists who contribute to patient care and quality initiatives. Antibiotic resistance is becoming prevalent, with few new antibiotics in development. Every pharmacist plays role in preventing further resistance and preserving our current antibiotic armamentarium by reviewing each antimicrobial order for the appropriate drug choice, dose, route, and duration. Many hospitals have pharmacy protocols for IV to oral conversion, dosing of antimicrobials, and prospective antibiotic reviews. Other pharmacist involvement may include the development of infectious disease order sets, drug use evaluation, and formulary decisions.[20]

Human Immunodeficiency Virus/Acquired Immunodeficiency Syndrome

Treatment of the human immunodeficiency virus (HIV) has come a long way since the first antiretroviral (Retrovir or zidovudine or AZT) was approved by the U.S. Food and Drug Administration (FDA) in 1987. Early antiretroviral (ARV) regimens presented many administration issues due to high pill burden and dosing frequencies greater than twice daily. Current ARV regimens require fewer tablets/capsules per day and once- or twice-daily dosing frequencies.

However, the regimens remain complex due to the potential for adverse drug reactions, drug–drug interactions, and development of resistance.

In the United States, there are approximately 1.2 million people living with HIV[21] and another approximately 50,000 new diagnoses per year.[22] Terminology used in the area of HIV can be confusing and is not always intuitive. The following section includes explanations of terminology as well as basic medication and treatment information of which you should be aware.

Basic Terminology and Information

HIV Testing[23,24]

- HIV testing generally begins with an antibody test, which if positive is followed by a confirmatory test (in the United States, this is usually a Western blot). However, new diagnostic testing algorithms are currently being reviewed.
- HIV antibody tests may be negative if testing is <3 months after the exposure.
- If suspicion for acute retroviral syndrome is high, it may be appropriate to check an HIV RNA viral load (VL). HIV RNA is detectable at approximately 9 to 11 days following initial infection.

Viral Load

- The VL is a measure of the number of HIV viral RNA copies per milliliter of plasma and is used as a surrogate marker for measuring response to ARV treatment.
- One goal of ARV treatment is to achieve an undetectable VL. This means that the number of HIV RNA copies per milliliter of plasma is less than the lower limit of detection of the process being used. "Undetectable" is reported as <20 to <75 copies/mL depending on the assay used.

CD4 Cell Count[23]

- The CD4 cell count is an absolute measurement of CD4 cells (also known as T cells or helper T cells).
- The CD4 cell count is used as a measure of the immune system's competency.
- CD4 cell count cutoffs may be used to determine the urgency of when to begin ARV treatment as well as when patients should receive prophylaxis for specific opportunistic infections (OIs).

Highly Active Antiretroviral Therapy

- Highly active antiretroviral therapy (HAART) refers to combination antiretroviral therapy (i.e., using at least three ARVs from at least two different classes of ARV medications in the regimen). It is now the standard of treatment.
- When people refer to "antiretroviral therapy" or ART, combination treatment is implied.

Boosting

- A boosted ARV regimen refers to a regimen including a pharmacokinetic booster. Ritonavir (Norvir) is generally the "booster" of choice for protease inhibitor (PI)-based regimens (although cobicistat is also being studied for use with some PIs). Cobicistat is generally used as the boosting agent for the integrase inhibitor, elvitegravir.
- When ritonavir is used as a boosting agent, the ritonavir is being used for its strong CYP P450 3A4 inhibitory properties to increase trough levels of the active ARV. Ritonavir is *not* being used for its ARV effects. Cobicistat does not have any ARV activity and only serves as a pharmacokinetic booster.
- Boosted PI regimens with ritonavir are preferred to unboosted (i.e., a PI-based regimen that does not include ritonavir) regimens.[25]
- Nelfinavir is the only PI that is never boosted.

Opportunistic Infections

- An OI is an infection that causes symptoms in people who have a dysfunctional immune system.
- OIs may be due to a new exposure to the pathogen (such as with *Mycobacterium avium* complex) or may be due to reactivation of latent infection (such as with cytomegalovirus).[26]
- Common OIs affecting patients with HIV/AIDS include the following: *Pneumocystis jirovecii* pneumonia (PJP; formerly *Pneumocystis carinii* pneumonia or PCP), *Mycobacterium avium* complex (MAC), oral candidiasis, *Toxoplasmosis gondii.*

HIV Versus AIDS Diagnosis

- HIV is the virus that causes the acquired immunodeficiency syndrome (AIDS).
- HIV diagnosis is based on HIV antibody and confirmatory follow-up testing.

- AIDS is a syndrome of immunodeficiency. Diagnosis of AIDS is based on the following:
  1. Having tested positive for HIV.
  2. Signs of severe immunodeficiency are present.[27]
- Signs of AIDS immunodeficiency may be based on laboratory data (i.e., a CD4 cell count <200 cells/mm^3 or CD4 percent <14%, and/or clinical consequences due to immunodeficiency (such as infection with an OI or development of Kaposi sarcoma or other types of malignancies).[27]

Genotype and Phenotype Testing

- The genotype reports the genetic sequence of the HIV viral genome to detect any genetic mutations that may result in decreased or increased ARV susceptibilities.
- See the International AIDS Society-USA (IAS-USA) and the Stanford Resistance Database references listed in the recommended Web sites list at the end of this chapter to help interpret the significance of specific HIV mutations.
- Phenotypic testing is similar to a bacterial culture susceptibility test. Results are reported based on how well the patient's virus survives and replicates in the presence of each ARV medication. The phenotype may be the preferred method of evaluating treatment options in highly treatment-experienced patients.
- Note: Both tests require that the HIV plasma VL be ≥500 to 1,000 copies/mL at the time the sample is collected for testing.

Antiretroviral Information

- See Table 16.8 for a list of currently available ARV medication brand names, generic names, three-letter abbreviations, and the ARV class designated for each ARV.

Common Drug–Drug Interactions to Watch for (*Note*: See the Department of Human Health Services [DHHS] guidelines in the recommended Web sites list at the end of this chapter for more detailed information regarding these and other ARV drug–drug interactions):

In General:

- PIs (except tipranavir + ritonavir): *inhibit* and are *substrates* of CYP 3A4 metabolism.

TABLE 16.8 Antiretroviral Names, Classes, and Dosing Frequencies

Brand Name	Generic Name	Three-Letter Abbreviation	ARV Class	Dosing
Aptivus	Tipranavir	TPV	PI	bid
Atripla	Emtricitabine/ tenofovir/efavirenz	FTC/TDF/ EFV	NRTI + NNRTI	qday
Combivir	Lamivudine/ zidovudine	3TC/AZT	NRTI	bid
Complera	Emtricitabine/ tenofovir/rilpivirine	FTC/TDF/ RPV	NRTI + NNRTI	qday
Crixivan	Indinavir	IDV	PI	bid or tid
Edurant	Rilpivirine	RPV	NNRTI	qday
Emtriva	Emtricitabine	FTC	NRTI	qday
Epivir	Lamivudine	3TC	NRTI	qday or bid
Epzicom	Lamivudine/abacavir	3TC/ABC	NRTI	qday
Fuzeon	Enfuvirtide	T20	EI	bid
Intelence	Etravirine	ETR	NNRTI	bid
Invirase	Saquinavir	SQV	PI	bid
Isentress	Raltegravir	RAL	InSTi	bid
Kaletra	Lopinavir/Ritonavir	LPV/r	PI	qday or bid
Lexiva	Fosamprenavir	FPV	PI	qday or bid
Norvir	Ritonavir	RTV	PI	See note[a]
Prezista	Darunavir	DRV	PI	qday or bid
Rescriptor	Delavirdine	DLV	NNRTI	tid
Retrovir	Zidovudine	AZT (or ZDV)	NRTI	bid
Reyataz	Atazanavir	ATV	PI	qday
Selzentry	Maraviroc	MVC	EI	bid
Stribild	Emtricitabine/ Tenofovir/Elvitegravir/ Cobicistat	FTC/TDF/ EVG/COBI	NRTI + InSTi + PK booster	qday
Sustiva	Efavirenz	EFV	NNRTI	qday
Trizivir	Lamivudine/ Zidovudine/Abacavir	3TC/AZT/ ABC	NRTI	bid
Truvada	Emtricitabine/ Tenofovir	FTC/TDF	NRTI	qday

TABLE 16.8 Antiretroviral Names, Classes, and Dosing Frequencies *(continued)*

Brand Name	Generic Name	Three-Letter Abbreviation	ARV Class	Dosing
Videx EC	Didanosine EC	ddI (or ddI-EC)	NRTI	qday
Viracept	Nelfinavir	NFV	PI	bid
Viramune	Nevirapine	NVP	NNRTI	qday XR or bid
Viread	Tenofovir	TDF	NtRTI	qday
Zerit	Stavudine	d4T	NRTI	bid
Ziagen	Abacavir	ABC	NRTI	qday or bid

[a]Bid dosing if used for treatment (very rare); qday to bid dosing as booster with another PI.
PI, protease inhibitor; NRTI, nucleoside reverse transcriptase inhibitor; NNRTI, nonnucleoside reverse transcriptase inhibitor; EI, entry inhibitor; InSTi, integrase inhibitor; NtRTI, nucleotide reverse transcriptase inhibitor.
Source: Panel on Antiretroviral Guidelines for Adult and Adolescents. Guidelines for the use of antiretroviral agents in HIV-infected adults and adolescents. Department of Health and Human Services. February 12, 2013:1–267.[25]

- Nonnucleoside reverse transcriptase inhibitors (NNRTIs) (plus tipranavir + ritonavir): *induce* and are *substrates* of CYP 3A4 metabolism.

Atazanavir (Reyataz)[28]

- Dose times must be spaced with dose times of H2 blockers and antacids.
- Proton pump inhibitors (PPIs) should be avoided altogether in highly treatment-experienced patients taking atazanavir but may be used in treatment-naive patients taking boosted atazanavir (up to a maximum dose equivalent of omeprazole 20 mg).
- Patients taking antacids, H2 blockers, or a PPI with atazanavir should be taking the atazanavir with ritonavir (Norvir) (i.e., the atazanavir should be boosted).
- Be aware of patients admitted to the hospital and administered an H2 blocker or PPI for stress ulcer prophylaxis.
- Be aware of patients taking over-the-counter acid-reducing products.

HMG-Coenzyme Inhibitor (Statin) Interactions with PIs (Especially with Regimens Containing Ritonavir)

- Simvastatin and lovastatin are contraindicated for use with regimens containing ritonavir.[25]
- Atorvastatin may be used but initiated at lower doses.[25]

- Pravastatin is another option (used with caution with darunavir).[25]
- Rosuvastatin may be used with the PIs, but caution is advised; start with a low dose and do not exceed 10 mg/d.[25]

Oral Contraceptives

- Many NNRTIs and PIs reduce the levels of ethinyl estradiol in oral contraceptives.[25]
- Medroxyprogesterone injection may be an option.
- Women of childbearing age should be counseled regarding the risk of pregnancy and additional contraception techniques discussed when taking oral contraceptives for birth control. Other contraception options should be considered.

Tuberculosis

Tuberculosis (TB) and other mycobacterial treatment regimens should be carefully selected in patients also taking ARV medications.

- Rifampin is contraindicated for use with many ARVs. Rifabutin is often used in its place.
- The dosing of rifabutin and ARVs (NNRTIs, PIs, and maraviroc) are often different from standard doses when used concomitantly. Double-check doses of both the TB regimen and the ARV regimen to ensure that the patient receives optimal treatment for both TB and HIV.

Methadone

- Some ARVs (especially efavirenz, nevirapine, and some PIs) may decrease levels of methadone and cause signs/symptoms of opiate withdrawal.[25]

Laboratory Interference

- Efavirenz (Sustiva) may cause a false-positive result on some cannabinoid urine drug assays.[29] Be aware of this counseling point for patients who may be involved in addiction recovery programs or have employment that requires periodic urine drug tests.

Renal Dosing[25]

- Renal dosing is required for all of the nucleoside reverse transcriptase inhibitors (NRTIs) (zidovudine, stavudine, didanosine, tenofovir, lamivudine, and emtricitabine) *except* abacavir.
- Combination tablets should be avoided when renal dosing is required.

Antiretroviral Regimens[25]

- In general, a first option ARV treatment regimen should include one NNRTI *or* one PI *or* one InSTi in addition to two NRTIs for a total of three different medications from at least two different classes of ARVs.
  - Two NRTIs + one NNRTI
  - Two NRTIs + one PI. Note: "One PI" includes boosted PI regimens (see "boosting" explanation above)
  - Two NRTIs + one InSTi
- More highly treatment-experienced patients may take ARV regimens that do not look like the above formulas.

Dosing Matters!

- Pay attention to ARV dosing, especially during medication reconciliation and when ARVs are ordered in the hospital setting.
- Pay close attention to timing of doses and food requirements, as they may differ from the hospital's standard meal and dose times and are important to achieve and maintain adequate ARV blood levels.
- ARV doses may be different when used with other specific ARVs. For example, the recommended dose for lopinavir/ritonavir (Kaletra) when given with efavirenz (Sustiva) is three tablets twice a day instead of just two tablets twice a day when efavirenz is not a component of the regimen. See the DHHS guidelines in the recommended Web sites list at the end of this chapter for more information.

Patients Coinfected with Hepatitis B

- Lamivudine, tenofovir, and emtricitabine are also active against hepatitis B.
- If a patient with HIV is treated only for the hepatitis B with one of these medications, there is a risk of HIV resistance developing during hepatitis B treatment. Adefovir continues to have a theoretical risk for promoting HIV resistance (especially to tenofovir) due to its anti-HIV activity at high doses.
- Case reports of HIV resistance developing with entecavir (previously thought to have no activity against HIV) have been reported.
- If a patient requires treatment for hepatitis B, he or she must be treated with a fully suppressive HIV regimen that (preferably) includes either lamivudine or emtricitabine and tenofovir.[25]

- Keep in mind that patients with hepatitis B who are taking an HIV regimen that includes lamivudine, emtricitabine (a close relative of lamivudine), or tenofovir may experience an acute flare, or worsening, of hepatitis B if the HIV regimen is discontinued.

Discontinuation of ARVs

- If one drug of the ARV regimen needs to be stopped, it must be replaced with another ARV medication or *all* of the ARV medications need to be stopped together.
- Note that the half-life of efavirenz (Sustiva) is 40 to 55 hours, making it take longer to clear efavirenz from the blood after stopping the medication. Therefore, the other ARVs in the regimen may be continued for 7 to 10 days after stopping efavirenz to avoid exposing the patient to monotherapy that may promote resistance. This is referred to as providing an ARV "tail."
- Nevirapine (Viramune) may also require an ARV tail of 3 to 7 days when the ARV regimen is discontinued.

ARV Treatment During Pregnancy[30]

- *All* pregnant women with HIV should be treated for HIV regardless of CD4 cell count and VL.
- A three-medication regimen should be used, as discussed above. It is preferable to include zidovudine as one of the medications in the ARV regimen.
- If the mother is on an ARV regimen at the time she becomes pregnant, assess the regimen for safety in pregnancy and determine whether to change or continue the regimen.
- If the mother is not on ARV treatment at the time of pregnancy, treatment initiations may be delayed until 14 to 16 weeks' gestation to begin an ARV regimen compatible with pregnancy. However, earlier initiation may be more effective to prevent mother-to-child transmission.
- PIs in pregnancy: Levels of lopinavir/ritonavir (Kaletra) and atazanavir (Reyataz) may be decreased during the third trimester and require increased dosing.
- NNRTIs in pregnancy: Nevirapine (Viramune) may be used, although there is an increased risk of hepatotoxicity in pregnant women. Efavirenz (Sustiva) is FDA pregnancy category D and should not be used in pregnant women or women planning to become pregnant.

- Zidovudine should be administered intravenously during labor and delivery. In some instances, single-dose nevirapine may be used during the intrapartum period; however, the risk of nevirapine resistance is high. The mother should receive a tail of ARVs for 3 to 7 days postpartum if she received single-dose nevirapine. The infant should receive oral zidovudine treatment for 6 weeks postpartum. In some high risk of transmission cases, the infant may also receive three doses of nevirapine.

Opportunistic Infections Prophylaxis

- Preventive medications for OIs are indicated based on CD4 cell count. See Table 16.9 for CD4 cell count cutoffs for specific OI prophylaxis and the preferred regimens for prophylaxis.

Helpful Infectious Diseases Web Sites

Table 16.10 includes several electronic links to important infectious diseases–related Web sites commonly visited by practicing infectious diseases pharmacists.

TABLE 16.9 CD4 Cell Count and Preferred Primary Prophylactic Regimens for Prevention of Opportunistic Infections

CD4 Cell Count	OI Risk	Preferred Prophylaxis
<200 cells/mm^3	*Pneumocystis jirovecii* pneumonia (PCP)	TMP/SMX DS 1 daily or SS 1 daily
<100 cells/mm^3	*Toxoplasmosis gondii*	TMP/SMX DS 1 daily
<50 cells/mm^3	*Mycobacterium avium* complex	Azithromycin, 1,200 mg weekly (once weekly or 600 mg twice weekly) *or* clarithromycin, 500 mg twice daily

Note: This table is *not* all inclusive. OIs listed above are those that require primary prophylaxis only. Patients are at risk for other acquired or reactivated OIs at the CD4 cell counts listed above; however, primary prophylaxis is not routinely recommended for these other OIs. See the references listed at the end of this chapter for further information regarding OIs and risk.
OI, opportunistic infection; TMP/SMX, trimethoprim/sulfamethoxazole.
Adapted from Guidelines for Prophylaxis and Treatment of Opportunistic Infections in HIV-infected Adults and Adolescents. May 7, 2013. Available at www.aidsinfo.nih.gov

TABLE 16.10 Helpful Infectious Diseases Web Sites

Web Site	Contents
Centers for Disease Control and Prevention—Sexually Transmitted Diseases (www.cdc.gov/std/)	Sexually transmitted diseases guidelines and updates
Centers for Disease Control and Prevention—Travel (www.cdc.gov/travel)	Travel-related immunizations and travel medicine
Centers for Disease Control and Prevention—Vaccine Schedules (www.cdc.gov/vaccines/recs)	Adult and pediatric vaccination schedules and resources
Infectious Diseases Society of America (www.idsociety.org)	Primary site for clinical guidelines for numerous infections and pathogens
Society of Infectious Diseases Pharmacists (www.sidp.org)	Pharmacist training, research, antibiotic stewardship
Department of Health and Human Services: AIDS info Web site (www.aidsinfo.nih.gov)	Adult, adolescent, pediatric, and perinatal HIV/AIDS treatment guidelines as well as OIs prophylaxis and treatment guidelines
International AIDS Society—USA (www.iasusa.org)	HIV/AIDS treatment guidelines and great HIV mutation database with ARV resistance information
University of California, San Francisco—National HIV/AIDS Clinician's Consultation Center (www.ucsf.edu/hivcntr)	General HIV/AIDS information, hotline information, great resource for ARV tablet crushing/capsule opening information
UCSF HIV InSite Web site (www.hivinsite.ucsf.edu/insite)	General HIV/AIDS information and extensive links to other resources
Stanford University HIV Resistance Database (hivdb.stanford.edu)	Great resource to help in evaluating genotype results
The HIV Book (hivbook.com)	General information about HIV, ARVs, and OIs. Overview of medical care for persons living with HIV

HIV/AIDS, human immunodeficiency virus/acquired immunodeficiency syndrome; ARV, antiretroviral; OIs, opportunistic infections.

References

1. Mackowiak PA, Bartlett JG, Borden EC, et al. Concepts of fever: recent advances and lingering dogma. *Clin Infect Dis*. 1997;25:119–138.
2. Koneman EW, Allen SD, Janda WM, et al. *Color Atlas and Textbook of Diagnostic Microbiology*. 5th ed. Philadelphia, PA: Lippincott-Raven; 1997:2.

3. Lieberthal AS, et al. The diagnosis and management of acute otitis media. *Pediatrics.* 2013;131(3):e964–e999.
4. Shulman ST, et al. Clinical practice guideline for the diagnosis and management of group A streptococcal pharyngitis: 2012 update by the Infectious Diseases Society of America. *Clin Infect Dis.* 2012;55(10):1279–1282.
5. American Thoracic Society; Infectious Diseases Society of America. Guidelines for the management of adults with hospital-acquired, ventilator-associated, and healthcare-associated pneumonia. *Am J Respir Crit Care Med.* 2005;171:388–416.
6. Mandell LA, Wunderink RG, Anzueto A, et al. Infectious Diseases Society of America/American Thoracic Society consensus guidelines on the management of community-acquired pneumonia in adults. *Clin Infect Dis.* 2007;44:S27–S72.
7. Chow AW, et al. IDSA clinical practice guideline for acute bacterial rhinosinusitis in children and adults. *Clin Infect Dis.* 2012;54(8):e72–e112.
8. Solomkin JS, et al. Diagnosis and management of complicated intra-abdominal infection in adults and children: guidelines by the Surgical Infection Society and the Infectious Diseases Society of America. *Clin Infect Dis.* 2010;50(2):133–164.
9. Stevens DL, Bisno AL, Chambers HF, et al. Practice guidelines for the diagnosis and management of skin and soft-tissue infections. *Clin Infect Dis.* 2005;41:1373–1406.
10. Tunkel AR, Hartman BJ, Kaplan SL, et al. Practice guidelines for the management of bacterial meningitis. *Clin Infect Dis.* 2004;39:1267–1284.
11. Gupta K, et al. International clinical practice guidelines for the treatment of acute uncomplicated cystitis and pyelonephritis in women: a 2010 update by the Infectious Diseases Society of America and the European Society for Microbiology and Infectious Diseases. *Clin Infect Dis.* 2010;52(5): e103–e120.
12. Gales AC, Jones RN, Sader HS. Global assessment of the antimicrobial activity of polymyxin B against 54,731 clinical isolates of Gram-negative bacilli: report from the SENTRY Antimicrobial Surveillance Programme (2001–2004). *Clin Microbiol Infect.* 2006;12:315–321.
13. Jones RN, et al. Ceftaroline activity against pathogens associated with complicated skin and skin structure infections: results from an international surveillance study. *J Antimicrob Chemother.* 2010;65(Suppl 4):iv17–iv31.
14. Hope R, et al. In vitro activity of telavancin and comparators against selected groups of Gram-positive cocci. *Int J Antimicrob Agents.* 2013;41(3): 213–217.
15. Liu C, Bayer A, Cosgrove SE, et al. Clinical Practice Guidelines by the Infectious Diseases Society of America for the treatment of methicillin-resistant *Staphylococcus aureus* infections in adults and children. *Clin Infect Dis.* 2011;52:1–38.

16. Pappas PG, et al. Clinical practice guidelines for the management of candidiasis: 2009 update by the Infectious Diseases Society of America. *Clin Infect Dis.* 2009;48(5):503–535.
17. Walsh TJ, et al. Treatment of aspergillosis: clinical practice guidelines of the Infectious Diseases Society of America. *Clin Infect Dis.* 2008;46(3): 327–360.
18. Ambrose PG, Bhavnani SM, Rubino CM, et al. Pharmacokinetics-pharmacodynamics of antimicrobial therapy: it's not just for mice any-more. *Clin Infect Dis.* 2007;44:79–86.
19. Craig WA. Does the dose matter? *Clin Infect Dis.* 2001;33(Suppl 3): S233–S237.
20. Dellit TH, Owens RC, McGowan JE, et al. Infectious Diseases Society of America and the Society for Healthcare Epidemiology of America guide-lines for developing an institutional program to enhance antimicrobial stewardship. *Clin Infect Dis.* 2007;44:159–177.
21. Centers for Disease Control and Prevention. Monitoring Selected National HIV Prevention and Care Objectives by using HIV Surveillance Data—United States and 6 U.S. Dependent Areas—2010. *HIV Surveillance Supplemental Report* 2012;17(No. 3, part A). http://www.cdc.gov/hiv/topics/surveillance/resources/reports/. Published June 2012. Accessed May 11, 2013.
22. Centers for Disease Control and Prevention. *HIV Surveillance Report, 2010.* Vol. 22. http://www.cdc.gov/hiv/topics/surveillance/resources/reports/. Published March 2012. Accessed May 11, 2013.
23. *AAHIVM Fundamentals of HIV Medicine.* 2012 ed. Washington, DC: American Academy of HIV Medicine; 2012.
24. Cheever, Laura W (Acting Associate Administrator and Chief Medical Officer HIV/AIDS, Bureau Health Resources and Services Administration) and Mermin Jonathan H (Director, Division of HIV/AIDS Prevention). Letter to: Dear Colleagues. February 8, 2013.
25. Panel on Antiretroviral Guidelines for Adult and Adolescents. Guidelines for the use of antiretroviral agents in HIV-infected adults and adolescents. Department of Health and Human Services. February 12, 2013:1–267.
26. Panel on Opportunistic Infections in HIV-Infected Adults and Adolescents. Guidelines for the prevention and treatment of opportunistic infections in HIV-infected adults and adolescents: recommendations from the Centers for Disease Control and Prevention, the National Institutes of Health, and the HIV Medical Association of the Infectious Diseases Society of America. http://aidsinfo.nih.gov/contentfiles/lvguidelines/adult_oi.pdf. Accessed May 1, 2013.
27. Centers for Disease Control and Prevention, National Center for Infectious Diseases Division of HIV/AIDS. 1993 Revised classification system for HIV infection and expanded surveillance case definition for AIDS among ado-lescents and adults. *MMWR Recomm Rep.* 1992;41(RR-17):1–19.

28. Atazanavir [package insert]. Princeton, NJ: Bristol-Myers Squibb Company; 2013.
29. Sustiva [package insert]. Princeton, NJ: Bristol-Myers Squibb Company; 2013.
30. Panel on Treatment of HIV-Infected Pregnant Women and Prevention of Perinatal Transmission. Recommendations for Use of Antiretroviral Drugs in Pregnant HIV-1-Infected Women for Maternal Health *and* Interventions to Reduce Perinatal HIV Transmission in the United States. http://aidsinfo.nih.gov/contentfiles/lvguidelines/PerinatalGL.pdf

17

Home Test Kits and Monitoring Devices

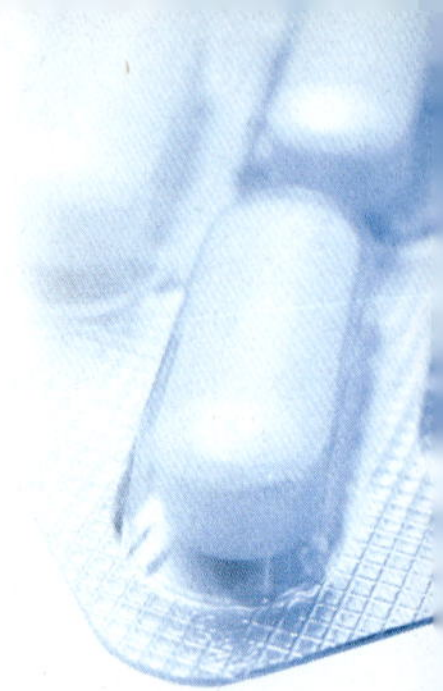

Ty Vo, Melanie Petilla Foeppel,

and Devon Flynn

Home self-test kits and monitoring devices are valuable tools and have become increasingly easier to use. The kits and devices provide patients with an opportunity to participate actively in early disease detection and monitoring. Pharmacists play an essential role in helping patients select the appropriate product, counseling them on appropriate use, interpreting results, and identifying limitations. Pharmacists should help patients make educated choices regarding product selection for home testing and monitoring. Product selection should be guided by accuracy, reliability, specificity, and sensitivity, as well as professional judgment.

To achieve an appropriate rate of accuracy and to ensure safety and efficacy, the pharmacist should assess and counsel the patient on the following points:

1. General questions to consider in patient assessment include the following[1]:
   a. What is the purpose of using this product?
   b. What chronic medical conditions does the patient have?
   c. What prescription or nonprescription medications or herbal products is the patient taking?
   d. What limitations does the patient have, including visual (i.e., poor vision, difficulty with color vision) or physical (i.e., limited dexterity, arthritis, peripheral neuropathies) that may affect the use of the product?
   e. What other health care practitioners have been consulted?
2. These products are for self-testing, not self-diagnosing. As a general principle, the patient should be advised to report positive results to the primary care clinician immediately, and negative results should be questioned if the patient is experiencing symptoms of a suspected condition. Some test results need to be reported

whether they are positive or negative because they convey useful information.

3. A family member, friend, or caregiver may need to assist if it is determined that the patient is unable to perform and interpret the test results.

The following factors should be considered when selecting a product:

- Complexity of the test procedure
- Ease of reading the results
- Presence of a control to determine if the test is functioning appropriately
- Cost

The patient should be instructed on the following guidelines[2]:

- Check the test kit expiration date, and follow the manufacturer's instructions for storage.
- Read the instructions entirely before attempting to perform a test. Note the time of day the test is to be conducted, necessary equipment, and length of time required.
- Use an accurate timing device that measures seconds if needed.
- Follow directions exactly and in sequence. A toll-free number is often available for assistance.

This chapter focuses on those products most commonly available: pregnancy tests, ovulation tests, thermometers, fecal occult blood tests (FOBTs), blood pressure monitors, blood glucose (diabetes) monitoring including ketones, cholesterol tests, human immunodeficiency virus (HIV) tests, illicit drug tests, and urinary tract infection (UTI) tests. The products listed in this chapter are representative but not exhaustive of those currently available.

Pregnancy Tests[3,4]

Additional Questions to Ask the Patient

1. How late is your menstrual period?
2. Have you used a pregnancy test before?
    a. If so, which one did you use?
    b. Did you have difficulty with it?

Home pregnancy tests are designed to detect the presence of human chorionic gonadotropic (hCG) hormone in the urine. This is detectable in the urine within 1 to 2 weeks after fertilization. The tests are indicated for use as early as the first day of a missed menstrual period but are most accurate by waiting ≥1 week after the first day of the missed period. The most current products available use monoclonal or polyclonal antibodies specific for detecting hCG hormone. Blood tests can detect a pregnancy earlier, usually 6 to 8 days after ovulation. They are useful for the health care provider in tracking certain problems of early pregnancy. However, urine pregnancy tests are the most common type and claim to have 99% accuracy when used appropriately. Most tests have hCG sensitivity limits of 25 to 100 mIU/mL; however, First Response Early Result has been shown to detect hCG levels as low as 6.3 mIU/mL. Though First Response Early Result may be the most sensitive test at detecting pregnancy before the 4th week of gestation, most tests have equivalent reliability after the 4th week. Table 17.1 lists selected home pregnancy tests.

Considerations

- OTC pregnancy tests differ in reaction times and hCG sensitivity.
- Most pregnancy tests are one-step procedures.
- Some tests have clear test sticks that allow the woman to see the reaction occurring as a check that sufficient urine was collected. Other tests include two devices, which can be helpful if a negative test is obtained first.
- The newest tests are digital and display the results as "pregnant" or "not pregnant" instead of colored lines. These eliminate the need to interpret the results, which may be especially difficult for patients who have color-defective vision or other visual impairments.

TABLE 17.1 Selected Pregnancy Tests

Product Name	Sensitivity (mIU/mL)	Comments
First Response Early Result	<6.3	Uses test sticks
Clearblue Easy +/– Results	25	Uses test sticks; Clearblue Easy Digital displays "pregnant" or "not pregnant"
E.P.T	100	Uses test sticks; E.P.T. Certainty has digital display
Accu-Clear	>100	Uses test sticks or cassettes
Fact Plus Select	>100	Uses test sticks or cassettes

- False-positive results can occur if
  - The patient has had a birth or miscarriage within the previous 8 weeks. This is due to residual levels of hCG hormone present in the body.
  - The patient is taking medications such as menotropins (Pergonal) injection and chorionic gonadotropin (Profasi) injection.
  - The patient has ovarian cysts or an ectopic pregnancy.
- False-negative results may occur if tests are performed on or before the 1st day of a missed period. This is a concern because a false-positive result may lead to a delay in prenatal care and appropriate behavior modification.

Patient Education

- The most accurate results will be obtained by waiting ≥1 week after the first day of a missed period.
- Unless the package instructions state otherwise, use the first morning urine because hCG hormone is most concentrated then.
- If testing at other times of the day, avoid fluid intake for 4 to 6 hours before urine collection to avoid dilution of the urine sample.
- Use the urine collection device provided in the kit.
- Apply urine to the testing device using one of the following methods provided in the package instructions:
  - Hold the test stick in the urine stream for the designated time.
  - Urinate into the testing well of the test cassette.
  - Collect urine in a collection cup and dip the strip into the sample or use a dropper to apply the urine.
- After the urine is applied, lay the testing device on a flat surface. Wait for the recommended time of 1 to 5 minutes before reading results. Waiting for the maximum allowed time may improve the sensitivity of the test.
- If the test result is negative, verify that the test was performed correctly and test again in 1 week if menstruation has not started. If the second test is negative and menstruation has not begun, a health care provider should be contacted.

Ovulation Prediction Tests[3]

Additional Questions to Ask the Patient

1. Are your menstrual cycles regular?
2. Have you consulted your primary care provider or a fertility specialist?

3. Have you used an ovulation prediction test?
   a. If so, which one did you use?
   b. Did you have difficulty with it?

Ovulation prediction tests (Table 17.2) measure levels of luteinizing hormone (LH) in the urine. Current products available on the market include basal thermometers, urine tests, and saliva tests. Each detection method has a different mechanism of action and method of use.

TABLE 17.2 Selected Ovulation Prediction Tests and Devices

Product Name	Reaction Time	Product Features
Clearblue Easy Ovulation Test Pack	3 minutes	7-day kit; uses urine test sticks; predicts ovulation within 24–36 hours; most sensitive product in the Consumer Reports test; easy to read
Clearblue Easy Digital Ovulation Test	3 minutes	7-day kit; uses urine test sticks; clear and easy to read with no lines to interpret; digital smiley face technology
Clearblue Easy Fertility Monitor	5 minutes	Reusable monitor; uses urine test sticks; predicts 1- to 5-day window of peak fertility; stores daily fertility information; easy to read; test for LH and E3g, an estrogen metabolite
Answer 1-Step Ovulation	5 minutes	7-day kit; uses urine test sticks; predicts ovulation within 24–36 hours
First Response 1-Step Ovulation Predictor Test	5 minutes	7-day kit; uses urine test sticks; predicts ovulation within 24–36 hours
Accu-Clear Early Ovulation Predictor Test	3 minutes	5-day kit; uses urine test sticks; predicts ovulation within 24–48 hours
BD Basal Thermometer	1 minute	Digital thermometer; auto memory for last reading; continuous beep to indicate it is working; signals when done; large lighted display
OV-Watch	Measures chloride ions every 30 minutes up to 12 readings	Lightweight; worn during sleep; detects up to 4 days prior to ovulation; easy to use and read

Reprinted with permission from the American Pharmacists Association. Briggs CB, Hurley H, Home Testing and Monitoring Devices. In: Krinsky DL, Berardi RR, et al., eds. Handbook of Nonprescription Drugs: An Interactive Approach to Self-Care. 17 ed. Washington, DC: American Pharmacists Association; 2012:915.

Urinary Hormone Tests

Urinary hormone tests use monoclonal antibodies specific to the detection of the LH surge. The LH surge is noted by changes in the color or color intensity directly proportional to the LH concentration in the urine sample.

Considerations

- Fertility medications, polycystic ovary syndrome, menopause, and pregnancy can cause false-positive results for ovulation.
- Patients receiving clomiphene should not test until the 2nd day after drug therapy ends when the true LH surge can be detected.
- Recent pregnancy, discontinuation of oral contraceptives, or breast-feeding will delay ovulation for one or two cycles. Patients should wait to start testing until after two natural menstrual cycles have occurred.

Patient Education

Ovulation Prediction Tests (Excluding Clearblue Easy Fertility Monitor)

- Test 2 to 3 days before ovulation is expected.
- Unless otherwise instructed by the manufacturer, early morning urine collection is recommended since the LH surge occurs early in the day and the urine concentration is relatively consistent at this time.
- If using a kit designed to be passed through the urine stream, either hold a test stick in the urine stream for the specified time or collect urine in a collection cup and dip the stick in the urine.
- If using a kit designed to test collected urine, collect the urine in the provided cup, and then dip the testing stick in the urine:
  - If immediate testing is not feasible, refrigerate the urine sample for the length of time specified in the directions for each product. Allow the sample to stand at room temperature for 20 to 30 minutes before beginning the test.
- Wait for the time recommended by the manufacturer before reading the test results.
- The test's first significant increase in color intensity indicates that the LH surge has occurred and ovulation will occur within a day or two.
- Once the surge is detected, verify that the test was performed correctly:
  - If the testing procedure was accurate, discontinue testing.
  - Discard the test stick after use.
  - Remaining tests can be used later, if necessary.

- If the LH surge is not detected and the test procedure was correct, ovulation may not have occurred, or testing may have occurred too late in the cycle. Consider testing for a longer duration next cycle to increase the chances of detecting the LH surge.

Clearblue Easy Fertility Monitor Test

- For the first month, test on the 6th day after beginning menstruation. The monitor will then dictate how many total days the user should test.
- For subsequent months, test the number of days indicated by the monitor.
- Remove the test stick from its packaging before use and hold in the urine stream.
- Insert the stick in the monitor.
- Discard the test stick after use.

Basal Thermometry[3]

Basal body temperature (BBT) is the temperature of the body at rest. A "normal" oral BBT is 98.6°F or 37°C. For years, women have measured BBT to predict the time of ovulation. Usually, resting BBT is below normal during the first part of the female reproductive cycle and rises to normal temperature 24 to 48 hours after ovulation.

Considerations

- Fertility specialists require a woman to chart her BBT for at least 3 consecutive months or menstrual cycles to identify cyclic patterns.
- Basal digital thermometers do not require the patient to interpret the reading, they track multiple temperature readings, and they are more expensive.
- Eating, drinking, talking, and smoking should be postponed until after taking each temperature reading as they can influence the basal metabolic temperature.

Patient Education

- Before using the basal thermometer, read the instructions thoroughly.
- Choose one method of taking temperatures—orally, vaginally, or rectally—and use the same method consistently.
- If using a nondigital basal thermometer, it should be shaken down to ≤96°F or 35.6°C.

- Place the thermometer on the nightstand or within reach before going to bed.
- Take the temperature readings at approximately the same time each morning before rising after ≥5 hours of sleep.
- Plot the temperatures on a graph.
- A rise in BBT by approximately 0.4°F (0.2°C) to 1°F (0.5°C) indicates that ovulation has occurred. To maximize the chances of becoming pregnant, women should have intercourse as soon as the increase in BBT occurs.

Thermometers[5]

A normal temperature is between 97.5°F and 98.9°F (36.4°C to 37.2°C; Box 17.1). Each person has his or her own normal temperature, which may be slightly higher or lower than average (Table 17.3). Rectal temperature is not affected by environmental factors. It is accurate, reproducible, and considered the gold standard. Rectal temperatures are approximately 1° higher than oral temperatures and 2° higher than axillary temperatures.

Temperatures can be measured in different ways with different types of thermometers. Product selection considerations include ease of use, safety, accuracy, reliability, and cost. Types of thermometers include mercury-free glass thermometers, digital thermometers, infrared thermometers, and color-change thermometers.

Mercury-Free Glass Thermometers

- Alternative to mercury-in-glass thermometer to measure body temperature
- Prevents environmental mercury contamination and exposures

BOX 17.1 Conversion of Temperatures (°F to °C)

Celsius	Fahrenheit
37°	98.6°
38°	100.4°
39°	102.2°
40°	104°

Celsius = 5/9 (°F – 32); Fahrenheit = (9/5 × °C) + 32

TABLE 17.3 Body Temperature Range Depending on the Site of Measurement

Route	Normal	Fever
Rectal	97.9°F–100.4°F (36.6°C–38°C)	>100.4°F (38.0°C)
Oral	95.9°F–99.5°F (35.5°C–37.5°C)	>99.5°F (37.5°C)
Axillary	94.5°F–99.3°F (34.7°C–37.4°C)	>99.3°F (37.4°C)
Tympanic	96.3°F–100°F (35.7°C–37.8°C)	>100°F (38°C)
Temporal	97.9°F–100.1°F (36.6°C–37.8°C)	>100.7°F (38.1°C) for 0–2 months old >100.3°F (37.9°C) for 3–47 months old >100.1°F (37.8°C) for >4 years old

Reprinted with permission from the American Pharmacists Association. Feret BM. Fever: Patient assessment and Consultation. In: Krinsky DL, Berardi RR, et al., eds. *Handbook of Nonprescription Drugs: An Interactive Approach to Self-Care.* 17ed. Washington, DC: American Pharmacists Assosciation; 2012:89.

- Are available for oral and rectal use
- Are low cost, light weight, and of compact size
- Are difficult to read and take ≤5 minutes for an accurate reading
- Are subject to breakage and may cause injuries

Digital Thermometers

- Are easier and quicker to use than glass thermometers
- Are available for oral, rectal, and axillary use
- Provide a temperature reading in about 30 to 60 seconds
- Eliminate the risk of glass breakage, mercury toxicity, and cuts
- Are easier to read with digital temperature displays
- Require batteries and need to be calibrated periodically

Infrared Thermometers

- Are very accurate, if used appropriately
- Are available for tympanic and temporal temperature measurements
- Measure the emitted infrared energy from the surface of the tympanic membrane and temporal artery
- Measure body temperature in <5 seconds
- Are relatively expensive
- Require batteries and routine calibration

Color-Change Thermometers

- Are less accurate or reliable than other available devices
- Have a heat-sensitive adhesive strip that changes color in response to different temperature gradients
- May be placed anywhere on the skin but show less variation in temperature on the forehead

Fecal Occult Blood Tests[3]

Additional Questions to Ask the Patient

1. What is your purpose for using this product?
2. Have you ever used a product like this? If so, which product have you used?
3. What type of diet do you follow?

The FOBT detects blood in the stool with a colorimetric assay for hemoglobin. It is noninvasive and easy to use in the privacy of the patient's home. Detection of blood in the stool may signify several conditions that include, but are not limited to, Crohn disease, colitis, anal fissures, diverticulitis, hemorrhoids, or colon or rectal cancer. The blue-green color indicates a positive test. The presence of blood from the lower GI tract is more likely to be detected. Currently, three categories of FOBTs are available—the toilet test, manual stool application device, and collection kit that is sent to a laboratory.

Considerations

- EZ-Detect Stool Blood Test does not require a diet or medication change.
- ColonTest-Sensitive has a card for recording results to give to the primary care clinician.
- Avoid nonsteroidal anti-inflammatory drugs, aspirin, antiplatelet drugs, steroids, vitamin C 250 mg or more per day, and red meat for 2 to 3 days before and during testing period because they can interfere with test results.
- Increase dietary fiber intake for several days before testing to stimulate bleeding from lesions that might not otherwise bleed and to increase the frequency of bowel movements.
- The patient should consult his or her health care provider before discontinuing any prescribed medication.

Patient Education

EZ-Detect[3,6]

- Before testing, remove toilet tank cleansers and deodorizers and flush toilet twice.
- Use one test pad to perform a water quality test. If any trace of blue appears in the cross-shaped area, use another toilet to test and perform a water quality test on the second toilet.
- After a bowel movement, place a pad printed side up in the toilet bowl. Check after 2 minutes for the appearance of a blue cross on the test pad (positive result).
- Repeat the test on the next two bowel movements.
- Report any positive results to the primary care clinician.

ColonTest-Sensitive[3,7]

- Open the test lid device and apply stool sample to wells A and B.
- Close the lid and press on the label "press last" to break the test ampule.
- Turn the test device over and hold vertical for 15 seconds.
- The test is positive if wells are partially or completely blue.
- The test is negative if wells are beige or brown.
- Repeat the test on the next two bowel movements.
- Report any positive results to the primary care clinician.

Blood Pressure Monitors[3,8,9]

Hypertension is a risk factor for many serious conditions including coronary heart disease, congestive heart failure, stroke, kidney disease, and eye problems. It is asymptomatic and often called a "silent killer." Monitoring blood pressure is indicated for patients with or who are at risk of developing hypertension. Refer to Table 17.4 for the classification of blood pressure by the Joint National Committee on Prevention, Detection, Evaluation, and Treatment of High Blood Pressure (JNC 7). Patients should know their treatment goals for hypertension (Box 17.2). The JNC 7 guideline is available online at www.nhlbi.nih.gov/guidelines/index.htm. At the time this chapter was written, the JNC 8 guideline had completed the expert review process. Next steps include advisory council review, public comment, and the U.S. Department of Health and Human Services' approval prior to its release.[10]

TABLE 17.4 Classification of Blood Pressure for Adults

Category	Systolic (mm Hg)		Diastolic (mm Hg)
Normal	<120	and	<80
Prehypertension	<120–139	or	80–89
Hypertension, stage 1	140–159	or	90–99
Hypertension, stage 2	≥160	or	≥100

There are three types of blood pressure measuring devices: mercury, aneroid, and automatic. Mercury column devices are expensive and not recommended for home use because they pose a potential risk of mercury toxicity should the glass tubing break. Aneroid devices are light, portable, affordable, reliable, and most accurate. Many come with a stethoscope attached to the cuff, which frees the patient from having to hold the bell of the stethoscope in place. Good eyesight and hearing are necessary for accurate readings. Digital blood pressure monitors have become more accurate, reliable, and easy to use but are most expensive. They require less manual dexterity. Digital displays are easy to read for patients with visual impairments. In addition to the standard monitors, finger and wrist monitors are available. Wrist monitors are accurate as long as the cuff size is appropriate and the wrist is at the heart level during measurement. They may be considered as another option for obese patients. Finger monitors are considered inaccurate and are not recommended.

It is important to choose an appropriate cuff size for accurate blood pressure measurement. To determine the proper cuff size, measure the circumference of the arm. Arm cuff sizes are available in child/small adult (7 to 10.25 in.), standard (9 to 13 in.), and large (13 to 17 in.). Refer to the product package for specifications to help determine the appropriate size for the patient. Table 17.5 lists selected blood pressure monitors.

BOX 17.2 Hypertension Treatment Goals

Essential hypertension	<140/90 mm Hg
Diabetes	<140/90 mm Hg
Renal disease	<130/80 mm Hg
Renal disease with >1 g/24 h proteinuria	<125/75 mm Hg

TABLE 17.5 Selected Blood Pressure Monitors

Manufacturer	Model	Automatic/Manual	Arm/Wrist
Welch Allyn www.welchallyn.com	7052-33 7052-34 7052-40	Manual Automatic Automatic	Arm Arm Wrist
Lumiscope www.grahamfield.com	1133 1137 1147	Automatic (a two-user mode) Automatic (a four-user mode) Automatic (a four-user mode)	Arm Arm Wrist
Omron www.omronhealthcare.com	BP710 BP742 BP760 BP785 BP791IT BP620 BP760	Automatic Automatic (a two-user mode) Automatic Automatic Automatic Automatic Automatic (a two-user mode)	Arm Wrist
LifeSource http://www.andonline.com/medical	UA-704V UA-705V UA631 UA-767 UA-787 UA-851 UB-512 UB-521	Manual Automatic Automatic 	Arm Arm Wrist

General guiding principles for patients when measuring blood pressure include the following:

- Sit comfortably with the back supported.
- Keep arms free of constrictive clothing.
- Position upper arm at the heart level. If using a wrist blood pressure monitor, use pillow(s) to elevate the wrist to the heart level.
- Keep legs uncrossed and feet flat on floor.
- Sit for a minimum of 5 minutes before the first reading.
- Avoid talking while taking blood pressure.
- Avoid physical activity, alcohol, caffeine, or nicotine consumption for 30 minutes before taking blood pressure.

Diabetes (Blood Glucose) Monitoring

A home glucose monitoring system, in conjunction with pharmacotherapy, is essential in assisting patients with managing and achieving glycemic goals. Routine monitoring of blood glucose is an integral

BOX 17.3 ADA Glycemic Recommendations for Adults

Hemoglobin A1c	<7%
Fasting plasma glucose	70–130 mg/dL
Postprandial plasma glucose	<180 mg/dL

component of diabetes self-care. The knowledge of current glycemic status provides patients with immediate feedback on their disease control status. Patient can use this information to determine their glycemic control, prevent and detect hypoglycemia, or assess their care in response to changes in lifestyle or medications.[11–13] Patients are encouraged to keep a daily record of all monitoring results. The American Diabetes Association (ADA) glycemic recommendations for adults with diabetes are summarized in Box 17.3. The Standards of Medical Care in Diabetes, 2013, is available online at www.diabetes.org. Most glucometers report the concentrations of plasma glucose, which is about 10% to 15% higher than whole blood. Refer to Table 17.6 for a selected list of blood glucometers.[11,14,15]

Considerations

- Determine the best glucometer for patients based on (but not limited to) size and shape, visual display, blood sample size, time to results, alternate testing site capabilities, calibration, memory capacity, and cost.
- Testing requires a single fingerstick to obtain a blood sample.
- Blood sample size varies with each meter from 0.3 to 1 μL.
- Glucose detection range varies with each monitor from 0 to 500 or 600 mg/dL.
- Some insurance plans cover all or part of the cost of monitors and/or strips under prescription or durable medical supply deductibles.

Patient Education

- Supplies needed include strips, a lancet, and a lancing device as well as a glucometer.
- Calibrate the glucose meter if required.
- Perform quality control as recommended by the meter manufacturer.

TABLE 17.6 Selected Glucose Monitors

Product	Test Strips	Blood Sample Size (μL)	Time to Result	Requires Coding	Alternate Site Testing
Accu-Chek Aviva	Accu-Chek Aviva	0.6	5	Yes	Yes
Accu-Chek Compact Plus	Accu-Chek Compact	1.5	5	No	Yes
Accu-Chek Nano	Accu-Chek SmartView	0.6	5	No	Yes
Breeze 2	Breeze 2	1	7	No	Yes
Contour	Contour	0.6	5	No	Yes
Contour USB	Contour	0.6	5	No	Yes
Freestyle Freedom Lite	Freestyle	0.3	5	No	Yes
Freestyle Lite	Freestyle Lite	0.3	5	No	Yes
One Touch Ultra 2	One Touch Ultra	1	5	Yes	Yes
One Touch UltraMini	One Touch Ultra	1	5	Yes	Yes
ReliOn Confirm	ReliOn Confirm/ micro Test Strips	0.3	7	No	Yes
ReliOn Micro	ReliOn Confirm/ micro Test Strips	0.3	7	No	Yes
ReliOn Prime	ReliOn Prime Strips	0.5	7	No	Yes
Relion Ultima	ReliOn Ultima Strips	0.6	5	No	Yes

- Wash the hand properly and dry thoroughly before obtaining a blood sample.
- Lance the side of the fingertip to obtain the blood sample, and rotate the sites. (Avoid the pad of the finger because there are more nerves in this area, which may cause pain.)
- Place the blood sample on the strip as recommended by the manufacturer.
- Dispose of lancets and strips properly in a sharps disposal container.
- Store glucometer at room temperature.

Urine Ketone Testing[3,16]

Home blood ketone monitoring is used to detect or predict ketoacidosis. When the body is lacking insulin, the uptake of glucose into the cells for energy and storage is inhibited. During these times, the liver breaks down fat as an alternative source of energy and produces ketone bodies and acetone as by-products. An accumulation of ketones in the blood can result in diabetic ketoacidosis, a potentially fatal condition if not treated. The excess ketones in the blood that spill into the urine can be detected. Table 17.7 lists selected urine ketone testing products.

Patient Education

- Patients with type I diabetes should test for ketones when plasma glucose is ≥240 mg/dL.
- All patients should test for ketones when experiencing any of the following: extreme stress, illness, pregnancy, and symptoms such as diarrhea, vomiting, loss of appetite, increased urine production, fruity-smelling breath, high fever, or when ketoacidosis is suspected.
- If ketones are present on two or more consecutive times, the patient should report to the primary care clinician.

Hemoglobin A1c Testing

Hemoglobin A1c testing provides useful information about a patient's glycemic control over the past 3 months. The American Diabetes Association recommends testing every 3 months for patients not at goal and every 6 months for patients who are stable and meeting glycemic goals. The goal for most patients with diabetes is <7%, and

TABLE 17.7 Selected Urine Ketone-Testing Products

Product	Measures Glucose/Ketones
Acetest tablets	Ketones
Chemstrip uGK	Glucose and ketones
Chemstrip K	Ketones
DiaScreen 1K	Ketones
DiaScreen 2GK	Glucose and ketones
Ketostix Reagent Strips	Ketones
Ketocare Ketone Test Strips	Ketones
Keto-Diastix Reagent Strips	Glucose and ketones

TABLE 17.8 Selected Home Hemoglobin A1c Tests

AccuBase A1c Test Kit (www.diabetestechnologies.com)
Bayer A1cNow® SelfCheck (www.a1cnow.com)
Biosafe Diabetes (A1c) Test Kit (www.safehomeproducts.com)
ReliOn® A1c Test (www.relion.com)

the normal range is 4% to 6%.[13] Many A1c kits allow patients to perform the test at home and mail the sample to the clinical laboratory for analysis. The test results are typically available via mail, email, or online within 7 days. Patients who prefer immediate feedback may consider Bayer A1cNow SelfCheck. Test results are available in approximately 5 minutes. It is currently the only product that does not require patients to mail the blood sample to the clinical laboratory for analysis. Table 17.8 lists selected hemoglobin A1c kits.[17–20]

Patient Education

- Read the instructions thoroughly before performing the test.
- Proper sample collection and handling techniques are important for accurate results.
- Testing hemoglobin A1c should not replace daily glucose testing.
- Discuss the use and results with the primary care clinician.
- Perform quality control and procedures as recommended by the manufacturer.

Additional Patient Information

Patients with diabetes should wear an identification bracelet, necklace, or tag. Additional information may be found for MedicAlert at www.medicalert.com or by calling 888-633-4298. Patients should carry an identification card including their name, address, phone number, medications, and name of the primary care clinician and phone number.

Cholesterol Tests[3]

Additional Questions to Ask the Patient

1. What is the purpose of your using this product?
2. Which product have you used?

3. Have you consulted the primary care clinician?
4. What are your current medications?

Many current home cholesterol tests measure only total cholesterol. However, a few tests also measure low-density lipoprotein cholesterol (LDL-C), high-density lipoprotein cholesterol (HDL-C), triglycerides, and/or glucose. With the exception of CheckUp America Cholesterol Panel, the patient may perform the test at home and is required to mail the blood sample to the clinical laboratory.[21] The test results may be obtained from home, via fax, or online. Patients should be informed that home cholesterol tests should not replace a complete lipid panel and the results should be shared with the primary care clinician. Refer to Table 17.9 for a list of selected home cholesterol tests.[3]

Patient Education

- Read the instructions thoroughly before performing the test.
- Proper sample collection and handling techniques are important for accurate results.
- Wash hands thoroughly with soap and warm water and dry them.
- Sit for 5 minutes before testing.
- Lance the side of one finger.
- Wipe the first drop of blood with the gauze pad.
- Apply adequate hanging/free-flowing drops of blood required by the specific test.
- Avoid excessive squeezing or milking of the finger.
- Use a different finger if there is an insufficient blood sample from the first fingerstick.
- Dispose the lancet in a sharps disposal container or puncture-resistant container.

TABLE 17.9 Selected Home Cholesterol Tests

Product	Measures
Accutrend Cholesterol	Total cholesterol
CholesTrak Total Cholesterol Kit	Total cholesterol
CholesTrak HDL and Total Cholesterol Kit	Total cholesterol, HDL-C
First Check Home Cholesterol Test	Total cholesterol
CardioChek	Total cholesterol, HDL-C, triglycerides. Can also measure glucose and ketone
CheckUp America Cholesterol Panel	Total cholesterol, triglycerides, HDL-C, LDL-C. Mail sample to clinical laboratory.

- Patients who have coagulation disorders or take anticoagulants should not self-test.
- Home cholesterol testing should not replace a complete lipid panel.
- Report test results to the primary care clinician.

HIV Testing[3,22–24]

The U.S. Centers for Disease Control and Prevention (CDC) estimates that 20% of persons living with HIV are not aware of their diagnosis. In an effort to decrease the number of people living with HIV who are undiagnosed, the CDC has worked to increase HIV testing. There are also now three U.S. Food and Drug Administration (FDA)-approved home HIV-1 testing kits.

The first two, approved in 1996, are the Home Access HIV-1 Test System and the Home Access Express HIV-1 Test System (both manufactured by Home Access Health Corporation). Both of these testing kits have been shown to have >99.9% sensitivity and specificity. They do not test for HIV-2 (a much less common subtype of HIV).

The third home HIV testing kit, the OraQuick In-Home HIV Test (manufactured by OraSure Technologies, Inc.), was approved in July 2012. It is based on the OraQuick ADVANCE Rapid HIV-1/2 Antibody Test that was approved for professional use in 2004. The OraQuick HIV test uses oral fluids to test for HIV-1 and HIV-2. Results are available after 20 minutes without the need to mail the sample for clinical laboratory analysis. The OraQuick has a sensitivity of 91.7% and a specificity of 99.9%. See Table 17.10 for a comparison of the three home HIV testing options.

Considerations for Home HIV Testing

- Is the patient physically able to perform a fingerstick and collect his or her own blood sample on a small piece of paper? Is the patient physically able to use the oral swab device and place it in the developer pouch?
- Was the patient's potential exposure to HIV ≥3 months before he or she will use the test? (See Chapter 16 section on HIV/AIDS for explanation of the window period of false-negative HIV test results.)
- The Home Access test systems are not recommended for use by patients with hemophilia.

Table 17.11 summarizes some of the potential advantages and disadvantages of at-home HIV testing.

TABLE 17.10 Comparison of Currently Available HIV Home Tests

	OraQuick In-Home HIV Test	Home Access HIV-1	Home Access Express HIV-1
Antibodies tested	HIV-1 and HIV-2	HIV-1 only	HIV-1 only
Bodily fluid tested	Oral fluids via oral swab	Blood via fingerstick	Blood via fingerstick
Time to receive test result	20 minutes (result must be read after 20 minutes, but before 40 minutes have elapsed)	Within 7 days after shipment of the collected sample	Within 3 days after shipment of the collected sample
Cost	$39.99 (as of May 2013)	~$30–$44	~$48–$60

Illicit Drug Use Tests

Home drug tests are marketed as an aid to alleviate concerns from parents who suspect illicit drug use in their children and those seeking employment. It is not meant to be substituted for open communication between the parents and their children regarding drug use. Samples of urine, hair, or saliva may be used to test. Hair and some urine tests are required to be mailed to a clinical laboratory for analysis. Results are obtained by telephone or internet using the code accompanying the test kit. Other urine and saliva tests can be performed at home. Currently, saliva tests are marketed only to drug testing programs and employers.[3] Table 17.12 lists selected home drug abuse tests available.[25–28]

TABLE 17.11 Potential Advantages and Disadvantages of At-Home HIV-1 Testing

Advantages	Disadvantages
Anonymous	Requires relatively high level of health literacy to navigate the large amount of written materials
Widely available and easily accessible	The patient does not receive behavior risk assessment and counseling.
Results within 20 minutes to 7 business days depending on the test used	Expensive ($30–$60 usually)

TABLE 17.12 Selected Home Drug Abuse Tests

Product	Time to Result	Specimen	Detection
Teensavers	4–5 minutes for initial screen at home; 7–10 days for send away laboratory confirmation (if positive screen)	Urine	Marijuana—all products Cocaine—3, 5, 7, and 12 panel Methamphetamine—3, 5, 7, and 12 panel Opiates—5, 7, and 12 panel Oxycodone—5, 7, and 12 panel MDMA—7 and 12 panel Benzodiazepine—7 and 12 panel Barbiturate—12 panel only Amphetamine—12 panel only PCP—12 panel only Methadone—12 panel only Tricyclic antidepressants—12 panel only
First Check Home Drug Test	5 to <10 minutes for initial screen at home; 5–7 days for send away laboratory confirmation	Urine	A: marijuana B: marijuana and cocaine C: marijuana and methamphetamine D (4 drugs): marijuana, cocaine, opiates, methamphetamine E (7 drugs): marijuana, cocaine, opiates, methamphetamine, amphetamine, MDMA, PCP F (12 drugs): five prescription drugs (tricyclic antidepressants, barbiturates, methadone, benzodiazepines, oxycodone), seven illicit drugs (marijuana, cocaine, opiates, MDMA, methamphetamine, PCP, amphetamine)

(continued)

TABLE 17.12 Selected Home Drug Abuse Tests *(continued)*

Product	Time to Result	Specimen	Detection
Drug confirm	4–7 minutes for initial screen at home; 3–10 days for send away laboratory confirmation	Urine	Marijuana—all panels Cocaine—4, 6, and 12 panel Opiates—4, 6, and 12 panel Amphetamine—4 and 6 panel Methamphetamine—6 and 12 panel PCP—6 and 12 panel MDMA—12 panel only Barbiturates—12 panel only Benzodiazepines—12 panel only Methadone—12 panel only Tricyclic antidepressants—12 panel only Oxycodone—12 panel only
At Home Drug Test	~10 minutes (has “result ready” panel)	Urine	Marijuana, cocaine, methamphetamine, opiates, amphetamine
Hair Confirm	1–2 business days after receipt in laboratory; express product comes with overnight mail packaging.	Hair	Marijuana, cocaine, opiates, methamphetamine, amphetamine, PCP, MDMA; prescription product label also includes oxycodone, hydrocodone, and hydromorphone testing.

Considerations

- Each kit varies by drug(s) suspected.
- The urine test detects drug use within hours to several days.
- The hair test detects drug use within 5 to 90 days.

Patient Education

- Read directions carefully before collecting samples.
- Urine samples report positive or negative results (they are qualitative tests).
- Collect the urine sample using the collection devices included.
- The temperature of the urine sample should be between 90°F (32°C) and 100°F (38°C).
- Hair samples report a low, medium, or high level of drug use.
- Obtain a ½-inch hair sample and one strand deep from the crown of the head and place in the collection package included.
- Hair from a hairbrush, comb, or clothing is not recommended.
- Medications such as codeine, decongestants, antidiarrheals, and possibly poppy seeds may cause false-positive test results.
- Open communication and discussion of test results are best conducted in a nonthreatening manner.

Additional Information

Information on FDA approval of a test for illicit drugs for home use is available at http://www.accessdata.fda.gov/scripts/cdrh/devicesatfda/

Urinary Tract Infection Tests[3]

Home UTI tests are used for detection of UTI infection and confirmation of infection resolution after treatment. Symptoms of UTI include frequency, urgency, and burning with urination. Two types of UTI tests are available (Table 17.13), and the primary difference is mechanism of

TABLE 17.13 Selected Urinary Tract Infection Test

Product	Reaction Time	Positive Indicator
AZO Test Strips	30–60 seconds	Color change to pink/dark/purple
UTI Home Screening Test	30–60 seconds	Color change to pink

action. UTI Home Screening Test detects nitrites in the urine reduced from nitrate by gram-negative bacteria. AZO Test Strips detect both nitrite and leukocyte esterase.

Patient Education

- Testing the first urine of the morning is preferred. If tested later, urine must dwell in the bladder for at least 4 hours.
- Pass the test pad or stick through the urine stream.
- Wait for 30 to 60 seconds and compare the color on the sensor pad with the color chart provided:
  - Pink indicates a positive result for the UTI Home Screening Test.
  - Pink, dark tan, and/or purple indicates a positive result for the AZO Test.
- If the test result is positive, contact the primary care provider immediately.
- If symptoms of UTI are present, contact the primary care provider immediately.
- If the test result is negative but UTI symptoms persist, contact the primary care provider immediately.

References

1. Limon L, Cimmino A, Lakamp J, eds. *APhA Nonprescription Products: Patient Assessment Handbook*. Washington, DC: American Pharmaceutical Association; 1997:25, 201.
2. Munroe WP. Home diagnostic kits. *Am Pharm*. 1994;34:50–59.
3. Briggs GC, Hurley H. Home testing and monitoring devices. In: Krinsky DL, Berardi RR, Ferreri SP, et al., eds. *Handbook of Nonprescription Drugs: An Interactive Approach to Self-Care*. 17th ed. Washington, DC: American Pharmacists Association; 2012.
4. Cole LA, Khanlian SA, Sutton JM, et al. Accuracy of home pregnancy tests at the time of missed menses. *Am J Obstet Gynecol*. 2004;190:100–105.
5. Feret BM. Fever. In: Krinsky DL, Berardi RR, Ferreri SP, et al., eds. *Handbook of Nonprescription Drugs: An Interactive Approach to Self-Care*. 17th ed. Washington, DC: American Pharmacists Association; 2012.
6. EZ-Detect [product information]. Available at www.ezdetect.com. Accessed May 6, 2013.
7. ColonTest-Sensitive [product information]. Available at www.colontest.com. Accessed May 6, 2013.
8. National Heart Lung and Blood Institute. Clinical Practice Guidelines on Hypertension. Available at www.nhlbi.nih.gov/guidelines/hypertension/jnc7full.pdf. Accessed May 22, 2013.

9. National Kidney Foundation. K/DOQI Clinical Practice Guidelines on Hypertension and Hypertensive Agents in Chronic Kidney Disease. Available at www.kidney.org/professionals/kdoqi/guidelines_bp. Accessed May 22, 2013.
10. National Heart Lung and Blood Institute. Blood Pressure in Adults: Report from the Joint National Committee (JNC). Available at http://www.nhlbi.nih.gov/guidelines/hypertension/jnc8. Accessed May 22, 2013.
11. Ulbrich TR, Krinsky DL. Self-care components of selected chronic disorder. In: Krinsky DL, Berardi RR, Ferreri SP, et al., eds. *Handbook of Nonprescription Drugs: An Interactive Approach to Self-Care*. 17th ed. Washington, DC: American Pharmacists Association; 2012.
12. Vo T, Foeppel MP, Flynn D. Point-of-sale: a review of home blood glucose meters. *J Pharm Technol*. 2011;27:76–83.
13. American Diabetes Association. Standard of medical care in diabetes—2013. *Diabetes Care*. 2013;36:S1–S66.
14. Chmielewski SA. Advances and strategies for glucose monitoring. *Am J Clin Pathol*. 1994;104(Suppl 1):S59–S71.
15. Clark WL, Cox D, Gonder-Frederick LA, et al. Evaluating clinical accuracy of systems for self-monitoring of blood glucose. *Diabetes Care*. 1987;10:622–628.
16. American Diabetes Association Diabetes Forecast 2009 Resource Guide. Ketone Testing. Available at www.forecast.diabetes.org/magazine/resource-guide/ketone-testing. Accessed May 13, 2013.
17. AccuBase A1c Test Kit [product information]. Available at www.diabetestechnologies.com. Accessed May 15, 2013.
18. A1c Now SelfCheck [product information]. Available at www.a1cnow.com. Accessed May 15, 2013.
19. Biosafe Diabetes (A1c) Test Kit [product information]. Available at www.safehomeproducts.com. Accessed May 15, 2013.
20. ReliOn A1c Test [product information]. Available at www.relion.com. Accessed May 15, 2013.
21. CheckUp America Cholesterol Panel [product information]. Available at www.homeaccess.com/checkupamericacholesterolpanel.asp. Accessed May 15, 2013.
22. Chen M, Rhodes PA, Hall HI, et al. Prevalence of undiagnosed HIV infection among persons aged ≥13 years—National HIV Surveillance System, United States, 2005–2008. *MMWR Morb Mortal Wkly Rep*. 2012;61(2):57–64.
23. Home Access HIV-1 Test System. [Label]. Home Access Health Corporation, Hoffman Estates, IL. July 1996.
24. FDA Center for Biologics Evaluation and Research (CBER). Summary of Safety and Effectiveness: OraQuick In-Home HIV Test. 15 May 2012. Available at www.fda.gov/BiologicsBloodVaccines/BloodBloodProducts/ApprovedProducts/PremarketApprovalsPMAs/ucm310436.htm. Accessed May 12, 2013.

25. Teensavers [product information]. Available at www.myteensavers.com. Accessed May 14, 2013.
26. Drug Confirm [product information]. Available at www.drugconfirm.com. Accessed May 14, 2013.
27. At Home Drug Test [product information]. Available at www.pharmatech.com. Accessed May 14, 2013.
28. Hair Confirm [product information]. Available at www.hairconfirm.com. Accessed May 14, 2013.

18

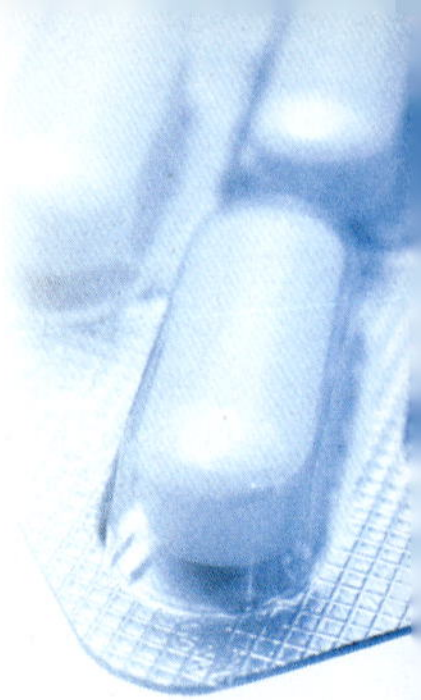

Pain Management

Daniel R. Neal

and Kenneth C. Jackson II

Pain Epidemic

From headaches to stubbing your toe, just about everybody experiences pain. Approximately 100 million US adults—more than the number affected by heart disease, diabetes, and cancer combined—suffer from common chronic pain conditions.[1] Pain is one of the most frequent reasons for physician visits, among the most common reasons for taking medications (including herbal medication), and a major cause of work disability. The annual economic cost of chronic pain in adults, including health care expenses and lost productivity, is $560 to $630 billion.[2]

Pain Defined

Pain is defined by the International Association for the Study of Pain (IASP) as an unpleasant sensory and emotional experience associated with actual or potential tissue damage, or described in terms of such damage.[3]

Consequences of Pain

Poorly treated or untreated pain has many negative consequences as described in Table 18.1.[4,5] These consequences range from the more obvious physiologic issues to more overt issues that affect not only the patient but our larger society. Pharmacists should be vigilant in assessing these issues, both in the setting of prevention and aggressive treatment to reverse these sequelae.

TABLE 18.1 Potential Clinical Consequences Related to Pain

Physical	Psychological	Immunologic	Sociologic
Increased catabolic demands: • Poor wound healing • Asthenia, fatigue	Mood disorders: • Anxiety • Depression	Decreased host defenses: • Decreased natural killer cell function • Increased risk of infection • Poor response to chemotherapy	Increased health care use: • Increased ED visits • Increased use of pharmaco-therapy
Respiratory effects: • Shallow breathing • Tachypnea (acutely) • Atelectasis • Pneumonia	Sleep disorders		Decreased productivity: • Decreased performance • Lost work days
Gastrointestinal: • Decreased GI motility • Constipation • Nausea • Vomiting	Existential suffering		Societal interaction: • Lack of family involvement • Decreased ability to inter-act in society
Cardiorenal: • Tachycardia • Hypertension • Increased sodium and water retention			

ED, emergency department; GI, gastrointestinal.

Barriers to Pain Management

Table 18.2 provides an overview of the common issues that serve to preclude effective and necessary pain management. These issues span the entire health care spectrum. Patients, clinicians, health care systems, health care educational units, and the various regulatory bodies all play a part in the poor delivery of pain management.[6] It is incumbent on the practicing pharmacist to understand good analgesic pharmacotherapy and the potential impact of each of these areas of potential conflict in providing analgesia to patients.

TABLE 18.2 Barriers to Pain Management

Patient-related Barriers:	• Reluctance to report pain
	• Reluctance to take certain medications
	  ∘ Fear of adverse effects
	  ∘ Fear of social stigma
	• Poor adherence

Clinician-related Barriers:	• Lack of training • Lack of pain assessment skills • Insufficient attention to patients • Difficulty in assessing pain • Rigidity or timidity in prescribing practices • Regulatory oversight
System-related Barriers:	• Low institutional priority • Medication availability • Issues related to cost • Poor access to pain specialists • Regulatory inconsistency

Medication History

An accurate and organized medication history is an area where the pharmacist can provide great utility to the health care team.[7] This is especially salient for patients with multiple chronic conditions and pharmacotherapies, which is often the case for patients with chronic pain. Drug–disease and drug–drug interactions are common in this patient population. Another confounder is that many patients may seek health care from multiple sources, including multiple prescribers and pharmacies. Most states now offer a Prescription Drug Monitoring Program that can be used to identify controlled substances patients may be getting from different prescribers and pharmacies. Obtaining a medication history has been further compounded by the increased use of over-the-counter medications and complementary medicinal agents. A thorough medication history will allow the pharmacist to identify both actual and potential drug-related problems. When interviewing the patient, a number of facets related to the patient's pharmacotherapy must be evaluated. For each drug assessed, the length of therapy, dose, duration, indication, and reason for discontinuation should be documented. Any pertinent information related to the effects of pain pharmacotherapy, both analgesic and adverse, should be noted as well. The components of pain medication history are presented in Table 18.3.

TABLE 18.3 Components of a Pain Medication History

- *All* current medication use
- *All* medications used in the past 6 months
- *All* current analgesic use
- *All* pertinent past analgesic use
- *All* drug-related problems related to the current regimen
- Social substance use (current and historical)
  - Caffeine, alcohol, tobacco, recreational drugs
- Nutritional dietary supplements

Pain Assessment

Patient self-report should be the primary source of pain assessment whenever feasible or possible.[8,9] Clinician observations and physiologic parameters or measurements may provide additional information but should be avoided as the primary pain assessment. Two exceptions may include preverbal children and nonverbal, cognitively impaired individuals. In these cases, behavioral observations may be required to function as the primary source of pain assessment.

The most common and easiest method for assessing pain intensity in adults is the numeric rating scale (NRS). On the NRS, the patient is asked to select a number (e.g., from 0 = no pain to 10 = pain as bad as it can be) that best describes the intensity of the pain. To obtain an accurate assessment of variations in pain, it is often useful to have patients rate the intensity of current pain, as well as the worst pain, least pain, and average pain the person has experienced in a given time frame. This time frame may be over the past 24 hours in the setting of acute pain to several weeks for patients with chronic pain. Pain intensity measures such as the NRS are easy to use and can be used repeatedly over the course of treatment to monitor progress.

The NRS is based on an older scale known as the visual analog scale (VAS). The NRS and VAS correlate well with one another and can be used at the discretion of a clinician for an individual patient. The VAS requires the patient to make a mark representing his or her pain intensity on a 10-cm line with the same anchors used on the NRS. The VAS may be useful for patients who are more visually oriented. The VAS can prove challenging, if not inappropriate, for patients with poor vision or manual dexterity.

The Wong-Baker FACES scale (Fig. 18.1) is another commonly used assessment tool that has been validated for use with children and cognitively impaired adults.[10] The basic premise is similar to that discussed above with the NRS and VAS.

0
no hurt
1
hurts little bit
2
hurts little more
3
hurts even more
4
hurts whole lot
5
hurts worst

FIGURE 18.1 The Wong-Baker FACES pain rating scale. (Reprinted from Hockenberry MJ, Wilson D. *Wong's Essentials of Pediatric Nursing*. 8th ed. St. Louis, MO: Mosby; 2009, with permission. Copyright, Mosby.)

Good analgesic pharmacotherapy requires thorough patient assessment. The best approach to accomplishing this goal is the use of the interdisciplinary team, where physicians, nurses, social workers, psychologists, therapists, and pharmacists each contribute their expertise to understanding the multidimensional nature of a patient's pain experience. The interdisciplinary approach affords each member of the team to have access to a comprehensive assessment that includes the medical history, physical and psychological pain assessments, and access to appropriate laboratory and imaging studies.[7] The pain-specific components of the assessment include those components in Table 18.4.

Pain Differentiation

Pain, like most conditions, is often categorized into acute and chronic presentations. Table 18.5 provides common differences between acute, chronic nonmalignant, and chronic cancer pain. A consensus panel

TABLE 18.4 Components of Pain Assessment

- Pain type (nociceptive versus neuropathic)
- Pain intensity (the numeric rating scale)
- Pain source (if known—e.g., tumor, arthritis)
- Pain location (can use body map)
- Pain duration (hours, days, weeks, months, years)
- Time course (persistent, intermittent, fluctuating)
- Alleviating factors (specific medications, positioning, heat, cold, etc.)
- Aggravating factors (walking, sitting, lying on back, etc.)
- Pain affect (depression, anxiety, etc.)
- Effects on activities of daily life (e.g., unable to bathe)
- Effects on quality of life
- Effects on functional capacity (e.g., unable to perform certain tasks)
- Presence of common barriers
- The patient's goal

TABLE 18.5 Types of Pain

	Acute Pain	Chronic Noncancer Pain	Chronic Malignant Pain
Cause	Usually related to an injury	Chronic condition, may or may not have started from an injury	Cancer, neoplasm
Duration	Pain resolved when injury is healed	Pain continues after healing has occurred	Until cancer resolved
Activity recommendations	Rest is good until injury resolves	Stay active	As tolerated
Medications	Short-acting medications used PRN	Short-acting or long-acting pain medications used on scheduled basis and/or PRN	Short- and long-acting pain medications used on scheduled and PRN basis
Goal	Pain relief	Increasing function	Comfort

commissioned by the National Institute of Health used this as the basis for categorizing pain, providing for three discreet types of pain[11]:

- Acute—primarily the consequence of physical injury, often related to traumatic situations such as accidents or surgical procedures. Acute pain is time limited and often lasts only hours to days. In some situations, the pain may last several weeks as a consequence of the clinical paradigm that has initiated the pain experience.
- Chronic cancer or malignant pain—persistent pain (e.g., >3 months) that is the consequence of an underlying neoplasm or the result of cancer treatment
- Chronic nonmalignant pain—a diverse group of pain conditions that are unrelated but share the common thread that the pain is ongoing (e.g., >3 months) and typically does not have any useful biologic value to patients or clinicians

All chronic pain is pain that lasts longer than would be normally anticipated or is associated with a chronic condition that produces persistent ongoing pain. The length of time for chronic pain is difficult to ascertain, but many would consider persistent pain that lasts >3 months to be chronic in nature. In the setting of chronic pain, it should be noted that the intensity of pain can wax and wane over time.

This is an especially useful construct to understand as many patients can have various pain experiences that can be affected by several factors that may include daily activity, pain treatments (e.g., pharmacologic, physical, and psychological), and/or diurnal variation. Moreover, patients may have additional pain experiences in addition to their underlying persistent pain. This additional pain experience is often defined as breakthrough pain. This additional pain experience is often severe and can become debilitating.[12,13]

Pathologic Differentiation

Pain is often described clinically in relation to the underlying pathologic properties, where in essence, the pain signaling process is initiated. It should be noted that regardless of the initiating mechanism, pain as a construct does not occur until a patient's somatosensory cortex receives and recognizes the pain signal. Although nociceptive and neuropathic pains are described below as separate entities, it should be remembered that patients can manifest both pain types concurrently. Table 18.6 provides a comparison of nociceptive and neuropathic pain.

TABLE 18.6 Comparison of Nociceptive and Neuropathic Pain

	Somatic	Visceral	Neuropathic
Causes	Osteoarthritis, postsurgical, bone fractures, sprains	Surgery, appendicitis, gall bladder disease, etc.	Diabetic neuropathy, radiculopathy, postherpetic neuralgia
Usual descriptions	Dull, achy, stabbing, sharp	Dull, achy, stabbing	Burning, tingling, numb, pins and needles
Location	Usually localized in joints	Diffuse over the abdomen	Spread over an area of the body, often travels along a dermatome
Medications used to treat	Acetaminophen NSAIDS Muscle relaxants Opioids	Antidepressants (SNRI, TCA) NSAIDs Antispasmodics Opioids	Antidepressants (SNRI, TCA) Anticonvulsants Opioids

Nociceptive Pain

Nociceptive pain is pain signaling emanating from activation of peripheral receptors that propagate pain along undamaged neuronal tissue:

- Somatic pain (also known as [AKA] musculoskeletal pain) involves tissues such as skin, soft tissues, muscle, and bone structures. Pain results from stimulation of "normal" peripheral nociceptors within the somatic nervous system. Pain may be described as sharp, aching, and/or throbbing. Often, this type of pain is easily localized by patient report.
- Visceral pain (AKA organ pain) involves organ systems such as the heart, lungs, and gastrointestinal and genitourinary tracts. This type of pain emanates from stimulation of the autonomic nervous system. Pain may be described as sharp, aching, and/or throbbing but is often difficult to describe in relation to a specific location.

Neuropathic Pain

Neuropathic pain is pain that results from damage to nerve tissue in the peripheral nervous system, the central nervous system (CNS), or sometimes both concurrently. Pain descriptors for neuropathic pain include burning, tingling, numbness, shooting, stabbing, and electrical:

- Peripheral neuropathic pain includes malignant plexopathies, painful polyneuropathy, postherpetic neuropathy, and diabetic peripheral neuropathy.
- Central neuropathic pain includes phantom pain and poststroke/thalamic pain.
- Mixed neuropathic pain includes CRPS (complex regional pain syndromes AKA causalgia or reflex sympathetic dystrophies).

Analgesic Classes

Acetaminophen

Acetaminophen is an effective analgesic for mild to moderate pain that is often useful as a coanalgesic but does not have any significant anti-inflammatory effect. Caution is needed to not exceed 4 g/24 h as this may lead to hepatotoxicity. This appears to be more problematic for patients with prior hepatic disease, with poor nutritional status, or with heavy alcohol use. Acetaminophen does maintain an analgesic ceiling, such that doses >4 g/24 h do not provide additional analgesia.

Nonsteroidal Anti-Inflammatory Drugs

Nonsteroidal anti-inflammatory drugs (NSAIDs, including aspirin) are effective analgesics for mild to moderate pain and, like acetaminophen, are often useful as coanalgesics. They differ from acetaminophen in that they do maintain anti-inflammatory properties. Several classes of NSAIDs exist (Table 18.7), and some patients may respond better to one class than another. There is no a priori test to determine which NSAID a patient may benefit from, and as such, serial trials may be necessary to determine efficacy with this drug class. NSAIDs can have significant adverse effects, especially from a gastrointestinal standpoint. All NSAIDs maintain an analgesic ceiling, so exceeding the maximum listed doses only promotes adverse effects.

Opioids

Opioids are effective analgesics for moderate to severe pain. Indeed, opioids are useful for most nociceptive pain and can sometimes be useful for some patients with neuropathic pain.[14] Opioid analgesics (Table 18.8) have traditionally been classified into three pharmacologic classes: the full agonists, partial agonists, and mixed agonist–antagonists. A more detailed description of opioid pharmacotherapy follows later in this chapter.

Adjuvant Analgesics

Adjuvant analgesics constitute a diverse group of medications that are effective for pain that is neuropathic in origin. These substances provide analgesia in addition to or improves pain treated with acetaminophen, NSAIDs, or opioids. Common adjuvant medications include tricyclic antidepressants (TCAs) (e.g., nortriptyline, desipramine), serotonin/norepinephrine reuptake inhibitors (SNRIs) (e.g., duloxetine, venlafaxine), and anticonvulsants (e.g., gabapentin, pregabalin). Other medications may include bisphosphonates (e.g., alendronate, pamidronate), calcitonin, radiopharmaceuticals, steroids, and psychostimulants (e.g., methylphenidate).

Pain Pharmacotherapy

Selection of the appropriate pharmacotherapy is predicated on two primary issues: pain intensity and presentation. Using the NRS, a clinician can choose the appropriate set of medication classes to evaluate.

(Text continued on page 580)

TABLE 18.7 Oral Nonsteroidal Anti-Inflammatory Drugs

Drug	Class	Average Analgesic Dose (mg)	Dose Interval (Hours)	Maximal Daily Dose (mg)	Comments
Aspirin	Acetylated salicylate	500–1,000	4–6	4,000	Due to risk of Reye syndrome, should not be used in children <12 years of age with possible viral illness
Diflunisal	Nonacetylated salicylate	1,000 initial, 500	8–12	1,500	Dose in elderly 500–1,000 mg/d does not yield salicylate.
Choline magnesium trisalicylate	Nonacetylated salicylate	1,000–1,500	12	2,000–3,000	Unlike aspirin and NSAIDs, does not increase bleeding time
Ibuprofen	Propionic acid	200–800	4–8	2,400	Available OTC
Naproxen	Propionic acid	250–500	6–8	1,500	—
Naproxen sodium	Propionic acid	275–550	6–8	1,650	Available OTC
Fenoprofen	Propionic acid	200	4–6	3,200	—
Ketoprofen	Propionic acid	25–50	6–8	300	Available OTC
Oxaprozin	Propionic acid	600	12–24	1,200	—
Indomethacin	Acetic acid	25	8–12	200	Rectal, IV, and sustained-release forms available for adults
Sulindac	Acetic acid	150	12	400	—

(continued)

TABLE 18.7 Oral Nonsteroidal Anti-Inflammatory Drugs *(continued)*

Drug	Class	Average Analgesic Dose (mg)	Dose Interval (Hours)	Maximal Daily Dose (mg)	Comments
Etodolac	Acetic acid	300–400	8–12	1,000	—
Ketorolac	Acetic acid	10	6	40	Also available in the parenteral dosage form Limit treatment to 5 days. Caution: may precipitate renal failure in dehydrated patients
Tolmetin	Acetic acid	200–600	8	1,800	—
Diclofenac potassium	Acetic acid	25–75	8–12	150	—
Mefenamic acid	Fenamate	500 initial, 250 subsequent	6	1,500	—
Meloxicam	Oxicam	7.5–15	24	15	—
Piroxicam	Oxicam	20–40	24	40	—
Nabumetone	Naphthylalkanone	500–750	8–12	2,000	—
Celecoxib	COX-2	100–200	12–24	400	—

OTC, over the counter; IV, intravenous.

TABLE 18.8 Common Opioid Analgesics

Generic Name	Opioid Chemical Class	Common Available Dosage Forms and Strengths	Comments
		Full Agonists	
Codeine	Phenanthrene	*Injectable*: 50 μg/mL *Tablets*: 15, 30, and 60 mg	Available as a combination product with either APAP (Tylenol with codeine #1–4) or ASA
Hydrocodone	Phenanthrene	*Tablets with APAP*: 2.5 mg + 500 mg APAP (Lortab®) 5 mg + 325 mg APAP (Norco®) 5 mg + 300 mg APAP (Vicodin®) 5 mg + 500 mg APAP (Lortab®, Lorcet-HD®) 7.5 mg + 325 mg APAP (Norco®) 7.5 mg + 500 mg APAP (Lortab®) 7.5 mg + 650 mg APAP (Lorcet Plus®) 7.5 mg + 300 mg APAP (Vicodin ES®) 10 mg + 325 mg APAP (Norco®) 10 mg + 500 mg (Lortab®) 10 mg + 650 mg APAP (Lorcet®) 10 mg + 300 mg APAP (Vicodin HP®) *Oral elixir with APAP*: 7.5 mg + 500 mg APAP per 15 mL (Lortab®) *Tablets with ibuprofen*: 7.5 mg + 200 mg (Vicoprofen®)	Lacks the 6-OH group of morphine, possibly decreasing cross-sensitivity within the phenanthrene group

(continued)

TABLE 18.8 Common Opioid Analgesics *(continued)*

Generic Name	Opioid Chemical Class	Common Available Dosage Forms and Strengths	Comments
Hydromorphone	Phenanthrene	*Injectable*: 1, 2, 3, 4, 10 mg/mL *Tablets*: 1, 2, 3, 4, 8 mg *Oral liquid*: 5 mg/5 mL *Suppositories*: 3 mg	Lacks the 6-OH group of morphine, possibly decreasing cross-sensitivity within the phenanthrene group
Levorphanol	Phenanthrene	*Tablets*: 2 mg	Lacks the 6-OH group of morphine, possibly decreasing cross-sensitivity within the phenanthrene group
Morphine	Phenanthrene	*Injectable*: 0.5, 1, 2, 3, 4, 5, 8, 10, 15, 25, 50 mg/mL *Immediate release tablets*: 15, 30 mg *Controlled release tablets (MS Contin®)*: 15, 30, 60, 100, 200 mg *Controlled release tablets (Kadian®)*: 15, 30, 60, 100, 200 mg *Controlled release tablets (Avinza®)*: 15, 30, 60, 100, 200 mg *Oral liquid*: 10 mg/5 mL, 10 mg/2.5 mL, 20 mg/5 mL, 20 mg/mL, 100 mg/5 mL *Suppositories*: 5, 10, 20, and 30 mg	Avinza® dosing interval every 24 hours; Kadian® dosing intervals every 12–24 hours; MS Contin® dosing intervals every 8–12 hours

Generic Name	Opioid Chemical Class	Common Available Dosage Forms and Strengths	Comments
Oxycodone	Phenanthrene	*Immediate release tablets:* 5 mg *Controlled release tablets (OxyContin®):* 10, 15, 20, 30, 40, 60, 80 mg *Oral liquid:* 5 mg/5 mL *Oral concentrate:* 20 mg/mL	Available as combination product with either APAP or ASA Lacks the 6-OH group of morphine, possibly decreasing cross-sensitivity within the phenanthrene group
Oxymorphone	Phenanthrene	*Injectable:* 1, 1.5 mg/mL *Suppository:* 5 mg *Immediate release tablets (Opana®):* 5, 10 mg *Controlled release tablets (Opana ER®):* 5, 10, 20, 40 mg	Lacks the 6-OH group of morphine, possibly decreasing cross-sensitivity within the phenanthrene group
		Partial Agonists	
Buprenorphine	Phenanthrene	*Injectable:* 0.3 mg/mL	Has been used sublingually; oral film available for opioid detoxification Lacks the 6-OH group of morphine, possibly decreasing cross-sensitivity within the phenanthrene group

(continued)

TABLE 18.8 Common Opioid Analgesics *(continued)*

Generic Name	Opioid Chemical Class	Common Available Dosage Forms and Strengths	Comments
Methadone	Diphenylheptane	*Injectable*: 10 mg/mL *Tablets*: 5, 10 mg *Dispersible tablets*: 40 mg *Oral liquid*: 5 mg/5 mL, 10 mg/5 mL, 10 mg/10 mL *Oral concentrate*: 10 mg/mL	Dispersible tablet only available for methadone maintenance clinics
Fentanyl	Phenylpiperidines	*Injectable*: 50 µg/mL *Transdermal patch (Duragesic)*: 25, 50, 75, 100 µg/h *Buccal effervescent (Fentoral)*: 100, 200, 400 µg *Transmucosal (Fentanyl Oralet)*: 100, 200, 300, 400 µg *Transmucosal (Actiq)*: 200, 400, 600, 800, 1,200, 1,600 µg	
Meperidine	Phenylpiperidines	*Injectable*: 50 mg/mL 100 mg/mL *Tablet*: 50 mg 100 mg	Not recommended for use in the elderly or for long-term use

Generic Name	Opioid Chemical Class	Common Available Dosage Forms and Strengths	Comments
		Mixed Agonist–Antagonists	
Butorphanol	Phenanthrene	*Injectable*: 1, 2 mg/mL *Nasal spray*: 10 mg/mL	Lacks the 6-OH group of morphine, possibly decreasing cross-sensitivity within the phenanthrene group
Nalbuphine	Phenanthrene	*Injectable*: 10, 20 mg/mL	—
Pentazocine	Pentazocine	*Injectable*: 30 mg/mL *Tablet*: 50 mg (with 0.5 mg naloxone)	Also in combination with ASA or APAP

APAP, acetaminophen; ASA, acetylsalicylic acid (aspirin).

Then, depending on the pain presentation (e.g., nociceptive, neuropathic, or both), the regimen can be tailored to the patient's needs (see Table 18.6). It is important to remember that this approach is fluid, and as such, it is often necessary to make adjustments throughout the course of an individual patient's care. Additionally, patient care is not a static process. As such, it may be appropriate to titrate patients as indicated. As previously discussed, patient assessment and reassessment is a priority in providing good analgesic care.

In 1986, the World Health Organization (WHO) developed a simple three-step approach to the management of cancer pain (Table 18.9).[15] This approach is often referred to as the WHO analgesic ladder. This simple and well-tested approach to the rational selection, administration, and titration of analgesics is commonly used in pain management. Although designed initially for cancer pain, the general tenets of this approach can be useful when considering drug therapy for patients with other pain presentations.

Opioid Pharmacotherapy

As noted above, opioid analgesics are classified into three classes that arise from our understanding of how these substances occupy and activate primarily the mu and kappa regions of the opioid receptor complex.[16] Full agonists fully occupy and activate the mu and kappa regions of the opioid receptor complex and, as such, have the potential for an unlimited dose/analgesic response. Partial agonists function by

TABLE 18.9 The World Health Organization Analgesic Ladder

Step 1.	Mild pain: pain intensity 1–3 on the NRS Acetaminophen, NSAIDs +/– adjuvant analgesics
Step 2.	Moderate pain: pain intensity of 4–6 on the NRS Simple analgesics (acetaminophen, NSAIDs) *plus* weaker opioids (codeine, hydrocodone, oxycodone) +/– adjuvant analgesics
Step 3.	Severe pain: pain intensity of 7–10 on the NRS Simple analgesics (acetaminophen, NSAIDs) *plus* stronger opioids (morphine, oxycodone, hydromorphone, fentanyl, methadone, levorphanol) +/– adjuvants

occupying only part of the mu region of an opioid receptor and produce a lesser degree of analgesia than a full agonist. Mixed agonist–antagonist opioids activate kappa receptors and either block or antagonize the mu receptor region, yielding a lesser degree of analgesia than full agonists. In the case of partial agonists and mixed agonist–antagonists, a dose ceiling effect occurs. These two classes are known clinically to have a maximal analgesic effect at their FDA-labeled maximum doses. Unfortunately, the adverse effect profile for these two classes continues to worsen when patients use doses in excess of the listed maximum dose. Clinicians should avoid using mixed agonist–antagonists or partial agonists in combination with full agonist opioids, as this combination can lead to an opioid withdrawal and worsening of the patient's pain situation.

Opioid pharmacotherapy is often complicated by various issues related to misunderstanding the actual pharmacologic basis for their use. Understanding the following terms will enable clinicians to better provide analgesic care to their patients:

- Opiophobia—the irrational fear by clinicians and/or patients related to appropriate opioid use for analgesic purposes. This phenomenon appears to be due in part to misunderstanding such terms as addiction, dependence, and tolerance.[17]
- Narcotic—a term many clinicians still inappropriately use when they refer to opioid analgesics. This archaic term was used to describe opium and its derivatives in prior generations. Today, the word *narcotic* is a legal term that includes a wide range of sedating and potentially abused substances and is no longer limited to opioid analgesics.[18]
- Addiction—the use of a substance that causes the user harm, yet the user continues to use the substance. Iatrogenic addiction as a consequence of opioid exposure for analgesic purposes is extremely rare.[19,20]
- Dependence—a pharmacologic situation where removal of a substance from a patient will induce a withdrawal reaction. This phenomenon is common with many medications and is to be expected for all patients with repeated exposure to opioid analgesics.[20]
- Tolerance—a state of adaptation in which exposure to a drug induces changes in the CNS that result in diminution of one or more of the drug's effects over time. Tolerance is a variable experience for patients using opioids and is more pronounced during acute and subacute administration.[20]
- Pseudoaddiction—a behavior defined in terms of patients who have appropriate drug-seeking behavior for the purpose of pain relief, not

for abuse or substance misuse.[21] This type of presentation occurs when a patient requests more opioid for analgesic purposes but has behaviors (e.g., anger, hostility) that are attributed incorrectly to addiction. Appropriate attention to analgesia will unmask this situation.

- Pseudotolerance—a situation where opioid dose escalation occurs and appears consistent with pharmacologic tolerance; however, following careful assessment, this is better attributed to other variables such as progressive disease, the presence of new pathology, or increased or excessive physical activity.[22] Other issues that can manifest as pseudotolerance are nonadherence, drug interactions, or drug diversion.
- Hyperalgesia—Dorland's Medical Dictionary (27th Edition) defines hyperalgesia as excessive sensitiveness or sensibility to pain. Opioid-induced hyperalgesia may be caused by use of long-term or high-dose opioids.

Oral Opioid Pharmacotherapy

Persistent ongoing pain is often best approached by using oral long-acting opioids to provide for a patient's pain requirements throughout the day.[23] This approach is consistent with the WHO guidelines, facilitates compliance, and minimizes the potential for toxicity. Long-acting opioids can be separated into those that are pharmaceutically modified to deliver shorter half-life agents over a longer time period (e.g., MS Contin®, OxyContin®) or those agents with inherently long-acting pharmacokinetic profiles (e.g., methadone). In general, the pharmaceutically modified agents are much easier to dose and titrate. These agents can typically be managed in most primary care settings with little special training. Methadone pharmacokinetics are more complicated, especially in patients with renal clearance concerns. As a consequence, dosing becomes more problematic for those not accustomed to monitoring this therapy. The reader is referred to other sources for a more detailed discussion.[24,25]

Opioid PCA Pharmacotherapy

Opioids are also commonly used in the setting of various pain presentations using an approach called patient-controlled analgesia (PCA).[26] In general terms, this approach uses intravenous or epidural as patient-controlled epidural analgesia (PCEA) opioids in a manner that allows the patient to help titrate the dose they need to manage their pain. PCAs have become commonplace in most hospitals, and pharmacy services are often responsible for many of the components of delivering this type of analgesia. Depending on the patient's presentation, the variables associated with PCA delivery can include a patient-directed dose at clinician preselected time points. Typically, this involves prescribing a set dose, a dosing interval, and maximum or lockout amount per larger time frame. At times, this as-needed component can be augmented by a basal or continuous infusion where warranted. For opioid-naïve patients during the initial phase of acute pain management, it is best to avoid initiating a basal infusion. Table 18.10 lists examples of data found on a typical PCA order sheet.

Opioid Pharmacotherapy Pearls

- Patients already receiving opioid pharmacotherapy for persistent pain: If the patient uses short-acting opioids on a regular basis and it is appropriate to continue with opioid pharmacotherapy, calculate the average 24-hour opioid dose, and then consider using a long-acting opioid alternative to provide around-the-clock analgesia where appropriate. When using long-acting opioid, continue using breakthrough short-acting doses when indicated.
- Opioid-naïve patients with episodic or fluctuating pain: Consider using an opioid analgesic based on the WHO analgesic ladder and

TABLE 18.10 Opioid PCA Setting Information

Drug	Typical Drug Concentration for PCA	Typical Starting Demand Dose (Range)	Typical Lockout Demand Dose Interval (Range)
Fentanyl	50 μg/mL	10 μg (10–50 μg)	6 minutes (5–8 minutes)
Hydromorphone	0.2 mg/mL	0.2 mg (0.05–0.4 mg)	8 minutes (5–10 minutes)
Morphine	1 mg/mL	1 mg (0.5–2.5 mg)	8 minutes (5–10 minutes)

PCA, patient-controlled analgesia.
Source: Ashburn MA, Lipman AG, Carr D, et al. *Principles of Analgesic Use in the Treatment of Acute Pain and Cancer Pain*. Glenview, IL: American Pain Society; 2003.

level of pain. Reassess routinely to determine if pain is appropriately treated, and when indicated, determine if chronic/persistent pain will be better managed with long-acting formulations. If pain remains uncontrolled after 24 hours, increase the routine dose by 25% to 50% for reports of mild to moderate pain, by 50% to 100% for severe to uncontrolled pain, or by an amount at least equal to the total dose of as-needed (PRN) medication used during the previous 24 hours. If pain is severe and uncontrolled after 1 or 2 doses (e.g., crescendo pain), increase the dose by 50% to 100%.

- Breakthrough or PRN analgesia: In most situations, patients using long-acting opioids should also be offered rescue analgesia for breakthrough pain in the event of worsening pain, episodic pain, or pain that is inadequately controlled by the long-acting opioid regimen. A simple approach is to provide doses that are 5% to 15% of the total 24-hour long-acting opioid dose in use.[27] Normally, these doses are offered to the patient on a PRN basis every 3 or 4 hours. *Always* recalculate the breakthrough opioid dose after changing the long-acting regimen so that it is always 5% to 15% of this total daily dose.
- Opioid dose escalation: Patients requiring more than two to four daily breakthrough doses on a routine basis may need to have their long-acting opioid regimen increased.[19,27] A simple approach is to determine the total amount of opioid used in an average 24-hour period (scheduled doses plus breakthrough doses) and administer this new total in divided doses as indicated by the product used.
- Equianalgesic conversion: At times, it is necessary to stop one opioid and initiate an alternative. This can be due to suboptimal relief or the presence of adverse effects. Traditionally, clinicians have used published equianalgesic dose charts (Table 18.11) to determine the effective equianalgesic dose conversion for many commonly prescribed opioids.[28,29] Unfortunately, these tables are based on older data that are primarily associated with single-dose studies and do not compensate for incomplete cross-tolerance and individual variation. In recent years, it has been suggested that for patients with well-controlled pain, it is advisable to use 50% to 75% of the published equianalgesic dose of the new opioid to compensate for incomplete cross-tolerance and individual variation. If the patient has moderate to severe pain, a 25% or less dose reduction is advised. An important exception to this paradigm is methadone, which appears to have higher-than-expected potency during chronic dosing compared

TABLE 18.11 Adult Equianalgesic Dose Comparison

	Equianalgesic Dose (mg)	
Name	**Oral**	**Parenteral**
Full Agonists		
Morphine	30	10
Hydromorphone	7.5	1.5
Oxycodone	20	—
Oxymorphone	10	1
Meperidine	300	75
Mixed Agonist–Antagonists		
Nalbuphine	—	10
Butorphanol	—	2
Pentazocine	50	30
Partial Agonist		
Buprenorphine	—	0.4

Source: Ashburn MA, Lipman AG, Carr D, et al. *Principles of Analgesic Use in the Treatment of Acute Pain and Cancer Pain.* Glenview, IL: American Pain Society; 2003.

with published equianalgesic doses for acute dosing. The reader is referred to other resources for methadone dosing.

- Opioids to avoid: Meperidine is an opioid analgesic that has proven extremely problematic over the years. The principal metabolite is normeperidine, which produces significant adverse effects such as tremulousness, dysphoria, myoclonus, and seizures. Many hospitals and health systems have either severely restricted its use or banned it from their formulary.

Common Opioid Adverse Reactions

- Constipation due to opioids is almost universal, and tolerance very rarely, if ever, develops. Management should be proactive, using stimulant laxatives (e.g., senna, bisacodyl, glycerin, and casanthranol) that are titrated to effect. Stool softeners (e.g., docusate sodium) are not usually effective by themselves but can prove useful in addition to the stimulant laxative for patients with dry hard stools. Bulk-forming agents (e.g., psyllium) should be avoided in the vast majority of patients since they require substantial fluid intake and are poorly tolerated in patients with advanced disease and poor gastrointestinal mobility. For patients unable or unwilling to use a stimulant laxative, the addition of an osmotic agent (e.g., polyethylene glycol, lactulose, or sorbitol) may be useful.

- Nausea and vomiting due to opioids usually disappear as tolerance develops during the first few days of therapy. Effective pharmacotherapies used to treat this problem include ondansetron, prochlorperazine, haloperidol, and metoclopramide. Patients not responding to these agents may require changes in the opioid used, the route the opioid is administered, or both.
- Sedation and/or mental clouding is often an issue during opioid initiation or during dose escalation. Sedation may be the result of prior inadequate sleep due to poor pain control. If the sedation is due to the opioid and continues to be problematic, a different opioid and/or alternate route may improve the problem. However, this may not be in the best interest of the patient if he or she has achieved good analgesia. In this setting, the use of a psychostimulant (e.g., methylphenidate) may be a consideration.
- Agitation, confusion, excessive sedation, hallucinations, myoclonus, nightmares, or seizures may imply that too much opioid is on board or that the patient is unable to effectively eliminate toxic metabolites. Opioid use is often complicated by buildup of metabolites in patients who are dehydrated or have poor renal function. If metabolite buildup is suspected, it is advisable to consider switching the patient to another opioid. If buildup of an opioid metabolite is not suspected (e.g., excessive dosing), reevaluation and titration of the opioid should take precedence.

Pharmacist Role

Pharmacists play a significant role in the management of pain across the entire health care continuum. This is in large part because pharmacotherapy is such a central component to most analgesic regimens. In addition, within the community practice setting, pharmacists are recognized as easily accessible and trusted advisors for pain issues.

In the institutional setting, pharmacists are often members of clinical services that deal with various pain management issues and may be responsible for implementing analgesic pharmacotherapy in accordance with institutional guidelines. In a number of hospitals, pharmacists are primarily responsible for managing PCA programs. Pharmacists play various other roles including development of guidelines, formulary management, and educating patients as well as other health care providers.[30]

References

1. Tsang A, Von Korff M, Lee S, et al. Chronic common pain conditions in developed and developing countries: gender and age differences and comorbidity with depression-anxiety disorders. *J Pain*. 2008;9(10):883–891.
2. Institute of Medicine (IOM). *Relieving Pain in America: A Blueprint for Transforming Prevention, Care, Education and Research*. Washington, DC: The National Academies Press; 2011.
3. Merskey H, Bogduk N. *Classification of Chronic Pain*. 2nd ed. Seattle, WA: IASP Press; 1994.
4. Siddall PJ, Cousins MJ. Persistent pain as a disease entity: implications for clinical management. *Anesth Analg*. 2004;99(2):510–520.
5. Gloth FM III. Principles of perioperative pain management in older adults. *Clin Geriatr Med*. 2001;17(3):553–573.
6. Gilson AM, Joranson DE. U.S. policies relevant to the prescribing of opioid analgesics for the treatment of pain in patients with addictive disease. *Clin J Pain*. 2002;18(4 Suppl):S91–S98.
7. Hadjistavropoulos T, Herr K, Turk DC, et al. An interdisciplinary expert consensus statement on assessment of pain in older persons. *Clin J Pain*. 2007;23(1 Suppl):S1–S43.
8. Acute Pain Management Guideline Panel. *Acute Pain Management: Operative or Medical Procedures and Trauma. Clinical Practice Guideline*. AHCPR Pub. No. 92–0032. Rockville, MD: Agency for Health Care Policy and Research, Public Health Service, U.S. Department of Health and Human Services; 1992.
9. Jacox A, Carr DB, Payne R, et al. *Management of Cancer Pain. Clinical Practice Guideline Number 9*. AHCPR Publication No. 94–0592. Rockville, MD: Agency for Health Care Policy and Research, US Department of Health and Human Services, Public Health Service; 1994.
10. Wong DL, Baker CM. Smiling faces as anchor for pain intensity scales. *Pain*. 2001;89(2–3):295–300.
11. National Institutes of Health Consensus Development Conference. The integrated approach to the management of pain. *J Pain Symptom Manage*. 1987;2:35–44.

12. Portenoy R, Hagen N. Breakthrough pain: definition, prevalence and characteristics. *Pain*. 1990;41:273–281.
13. Cleary J. Pharmacokinetic and pharmacodynamic issues in the treatment of breakthrough pain. *Semin Oncol*. 1997;214:13–19.
14. Eisenberg E, McNicol E, Carr DB. Opioids for neuropathic pain. *Cochrane Database Syst Rev*. 2006;(3):CD006146.
15. World Health Organization (WHO). *Cancer Pain Relief and Palliative Care: Report of a WHO Expert Committee*. Geneva, Switzerland: WHO; 1990.
16. Hare B. The opioid analgesics: rational selection of agents for acute and chronic pain. *Hosp Formul*. 1987;22:64–86.
17. Rhodin A. The rise of opiophobia: is history a barrier to prescribing? *J Pain Palliat Care Pharmacother*. 2006;20(3):31–32.
18. Jackson KC, Lipman AG. Opioid analgesics. In: Tollison CD, Satterwhite JR, Tollison JW, eds. *Practical Pain Management*. 3rd ed. Philadelphia, PA: Lippincott Williams & Wilkins; 2002.
19. The American Society of Addiction Medicine. Public Policy Statement on Definitions Related to the Use of Opioids in Pain Treatment. www.asam.org, 1997.
20. Rinaldi R, Steindler E, Wilford B, et al. Clarification and standardization of substance abuse terminology. *JAMA*. 1988;259:555–557.
21. Weissman DE, Haddox JD. Opioid pseudoaddiction—an iatrogenic syndrome. *Pain*. 1989;36:363–366.
22. Pappagallo M. The concept of pseudotolerance to opioids. *J Pharm Care Pain Symptom Control*. 1998;6:95–98.
23. Pillai Riddell RR, Craig KD. Time-contingent schedules for postoperative analgesia: a review of the literature. *J Pain*. 2003;4(4):169–175.
24. www.cancer.gov/cancertopics/pdg/supportivecare/pain/HealthProfessional/page3
25. Lugo RA, Satterfield KL, Kern SE. Pharmacokinetics of methadone. *J Pain Palliat Care Pharmacother*. 2005;19(4):13–24.
26. Beeton A, Upton P, Shipton E. The case for patient-controlled analgesia. Inter-patient variation in postoperative analgesic requirements. *S Afr J Surg*. 1992;30:1–6.
27. Indelicato RA, Portenoy RK. Opioid rotation in the management of refractory cancer pain. *J Clin Oncol*. 2003;21(9 Suppl):87S–91S.
28. Ashburn MA, Lipman AG, Carr D, et al. *Principles of Analgesic Use in the Treatment of Acute Pain and Cancer Pain*. Glenview, IL: American Pain Society; 2003.
29. Prommer E. Oxymorphone: a review. *Support Care Cancer*. 2006;14:109–115.
30. Strassels SA, McNicol E, Suleman R. Postoperative pain management: a practical review, Part 1. *Am J Health Syst Pharm*. 2005;62(18):1904–1916.

19

Over-the-Counter Drug Therapy and Dietary Supplements/Complementary Care

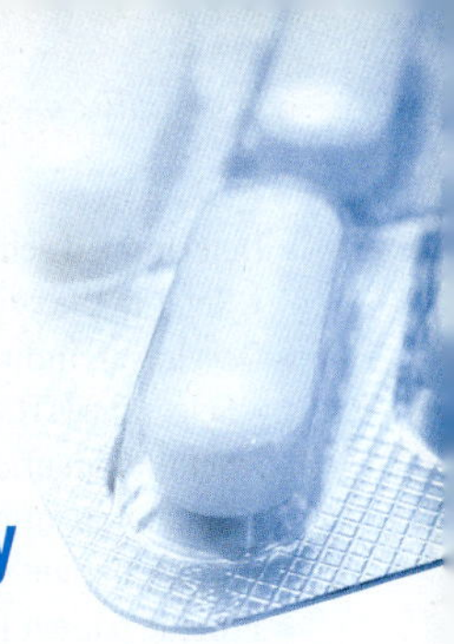

Ty Vo, Melanie Petilla Foeppel,

Marianne Krupicka, and Patricia M. Mossbrucker

Over-the-Counter Drug Therapy

The prevalence of over-the-counter (OTC) drug use has increased significantly over the past 25 years. In 2011, sales of OTC medications in the United States exceeded $17 billion.[1] Sales data mirror the findings of a 2003 National Council on Patient Information and Education survey, which reports that 73% of consumers prefer self-treatment with nonprescription medications.[2] The growing demand for OTC drug therapy may be attributed to patients becoming empowered to take ownership of their own health care and feeling more confident in self-treating their illnesses. However, as a growing number of drugs are switched from prescription to OTC status, the OTC drug market has become complex. It has been estimated that 57% of all health problems can be treated with OTC products.[1] Not surprisingly, 66% of adults find it challenging to choose an appropriate nonprescription medication due to the wide range of OTC products available.[3] This demonstrates a need and an opportunity for pharmacist intervention.[2,4] The pharmacist is viewed by patients as the most accessible health care provider and a reliable source of drug information. This provides the pharmacist with an excellent opportunity to provide patient education and assist with product selection to ensure safe, appropriate, and effective use.

Role of the Pharmacist

- Be familiar with currently available products and product labels
- Gather patient-specific information to make an assessment

- Determine if self-treatment is appropriate
  - Refer to the primary care clinician as appropriate
- Develop an individualized action plan
  - Select the OTC product(s)
  - Set therapeutic goals
  - Set therapeutic end points
- Provide patient education
- Provide patient follow-up
- Document encounter

There are several assessment methods available for collecting patient information and determining the appropriateness of self-care. The Self-Care Institute of the American Pharmacists Association (APhA) recommends the use of a data collection process called QuEST/SCHOLAR.[5] This acronym details the various steps in collecting patient information in a sequential and easily reproducible manner. The steps are as follows: Quickly and accurately assess the patient:

Ask about current complaints (SCHOLAR)
Ask about other medications and other products
Ask about coexisting conditions and allergies

Establish that the patient is an appropriate self-care candidate:

No severe symptoms
No symptoms that persist or return repeatedly without an identifiable cause
No self-treating to avoid medical care

Suggest appropriate self-care strategies:

Medications
General care measures

Talk with the patient:

About medication action
About administration
About adverse effects and how to manage them
About what to expect from treatment
About appropriate follow-up

Symptoms: what are the main and associated symptoms?
Characteristics: what are the symptoms like?
History: has this happened in the past? What has been done so far?

Onset: when did it start?
Location: where is the problem?
Aggravating factors: what makes it worse?
Remitting factors: what makes it better?

In addition to completing QuEST/SCHOLAR, the pharmacist should also selectively elicit the following information[6]:

- Who is the patient? Is the patient the person in the pharmacy or someone else?
- How old is the patient?
- Is the patient male or female? If the patient is female, is she pregnant or breast-feeding?
- Is the patient on a special diet? Does the patient have special nutritional requirements?
- Who is responsible for administering the medication?

Refer the patient to the primary care clinician when[6]

- Symptoms are too severe to be endured by the patient without definitive diagnosis and treatment.
- Symptoms are minor but persistent and do not appear to be the result of some easily identifiable cause.
- Symptoms have repeatedly returned with no readily recognizable cause.
- The pharmacist is in doubt about the patient's medical condition.

Special Populations

Pediatric

- It is important to note that for most OTC products, the Food and Drug Administration recommends against self-medication in infants and children under the age of 2 years.[6,7]
- In 2008, the U.S. Food and Drug Administration (FDA) supported the voluntary actions of OTC cough and cold medication manufacturers to change product labeling to "do not use" in children age 4 and under.[8] Though these updates were made to further prevent the misuse OTC cough and cold products in children, these actions have not changed the official monographs for these medications.[9,10]
- Parents should be educated regarding the lack of antitussive effects, risk for adverse events, and potential for overdose in children from OTC cough and cold medications.
- Consult the *Lexicomp Pediatric & Neonatal Handbook* or *Harriet Lane Handbook* for guidance on specific dosing.

Pregnancy and Lactation

- Be familiar with the risk factors assigned to all drugs based on the level of risk to the fetus[11]:
  - A: Adequate and well-controlled studies in pregnant women have not shown an increased risk to the fetus in any trimester of the pregnancy.
  - B: Animal studies have shown no evidence of harm to the fetus, but there are no adequate and well-controlled studies in pregnant women; or animal studies have shown an adverse effect, but adequate and well-controlled studies in pregnant women have failed to demonstrate a risk to the fetus in any trimester.
  - C: Animal studies have shown an adverse effect, and there are no adequate and well-controlled studies in pregnant women; or no animal studies have been conducted, and there are no adequate and well-controlled studies in pregnant women.
  - D: Evidence of harm to the fetus has been shown in studies, but the benefits of therapy may outweigh the risk, for example, if the drug is needed in a life-threatening situation or for a serious disease for which safer drugs cannot be used or are ineffective.
  - X: Evidence of harm to the fetus has been shown in studies. The use of the drug outweighs any possible benefit. The drug is contraindicated in women who are or may become pregnant.
- Consult *Drugs in Pregnancy and Lactation* by Briggs for guidance.

Geriatric[12]

- Age 65 years or older
- May predispose patients to potential problems with nonprescription drugs due to
  - Altered pharmacokinetic and pharmacodynamic profile
  - Preexisting medical conditions
  - Duplicate therapy or polypharmacy
  - Increased sensitivity to anticholinergic drugs

Common Conditions Treated with Nonprescription Drugs[13]

- Pain
- Cough, cold, flu, sore throat
- Allergies, sinus problems
- Heartburn, indigestion
- Constipation, diarrhea, gas

- Minor infections
- Skin problems

Recommended Pediatric Dosages of Nonprescription Drugs

As a reminder, it is important to note the voluntary changes to the manufacturers' product labeling of OTC cough and cold medications in children age 4 and under.[9]

Pediatric Age Groups[14]

- Neonates: 1 day to 1 month
- Infants: 1 month to 1 year
- Children: 1 year to 11 years
- Adolescents: 12 years to 16 years

Analgesics[15,16]

- Acetaminophen
  - Infants and children
- Use caution with different dosage forms: infant drops versus children's suspension
  - Orally: 10 to 15 mg/kg PO every 4 to 6 hours PRN. Maximum 90 mg/kg/24 h
  - Rectally: 10 to 15 mg/kg PR every 4 to 6 hours PRN. Maximum 90 mg/kg/24 h
- Ibuprofen
  - Infants and children
- Use caution with different dosage forms: infant drops versus children's suspension
  - Orally: 5 to 10 mg/kg PO every 6 to 8 hours PRN. Maximum 40 mg/kg/24 h

Antihistamines[15,16]

- Brompheniramine
  - Not recommended in infants and children younger than 2 years of age. Children under 6 years of age should be consulted by a physician[17]
  - Ages 2 to <6 years: 1 mg PO every 4 hours PRN. Maximum 6 mg/24 h
  - Ages 6 to 12 years: 2 mg PO every 4 hours PRN. Maximum 12 mg/24 h

- Chlorpheniramine maleate
  - Not recommended in infants and children younger than 2 years of age. Children under 6 years of age should be consulted by a physician[17]
  - Ages 2 to <6 years: 1 mg PO every 4 to 6 hours PRN. Maximum 6 mg/24 h
  - Ages 6 to 11 years: 2 mg PO every 4 to 6 hours PRN. Maximum 12 mg/24 h
- Diphenhydramine[15,16]
  - Not recommended in infants and children younger than 2 years of age. Children under 6 years of age should be consulted by a physician[17]
  - Ages 2 to <6 years: 6.25 mg every 4 to 6 hours PRN. Maximum 37.5 mg/24 h
  - Ages 6 to <12 years: 12.5 to 25 mg every 4 to 6 hours PRN. Maximum 150 mg/24 h
- Cetirizine[15,16]
  - Ages 2 to 5 years: 2.5 mg PO once a day. Maximum 5 mg/24 h
  - Ages 6 years or older: 5 to 10 mg PO once a day. Maximum 10 mg/24 h
- Loratadine[17,18]
  - Ages 2 to 5 years: 5 mg PO once a day. Maximum 5 mg/24 h
  - Ages 6 years or older: 10 mg PO once a day. Maximum 10 mg/24 h

Decongestants

- Phenylephrine[15,16]
  - Not recommended in infants and children younger than 2 years of age
  - Ages 4 to 5 years: 2.5 mg PO every 4 to 6 hours PRN up to 7 days. Maximum 15 mg/24 h
  - Ages 6 to 11 years: 5 mg PO every 4 to 6 hours PRN up to 7 days. Maximum 30 mg/24 h
  - ≥12 years: refer to adult dosing
- Pseudoephedrine[15,16]
  - Note individual state legal requirements for the sale and purchase of this product before recommending
  - Not recommended in infants and children younger than 2 years of age
  - Ages 4 to 5 years: 15 mg PO every 4 to 6 hours PRN. Maximum 60 mg/24 h
  - Ages 6 to 12 years: 30 mg PO every 4 to 6 hours PRN. Maximum 120 mg/24 h

Expectorants

- Guaifenesin[15,16]
  - Consult a physician
  - Ages 2 to 5 years: 50 to 100 mg every 4 hours PRN. Maximum 600 mg/24 h
  - Ages 6 to 11 years: 100 to 200 mg every 4 hours PRN. Maximum 1,200 mg/24 h

Cough Suppressants

- Dextromethorphan[15,16]
  - Not recommended in infants or children younger than 2 years of age
  - Ages 2 to 6 years: 2.5 to 7.5 mg every 4 to 8 hours PRN or 15 mg every 12 hours PRN (sustained-release suspension). Maximum 30 mg/24 h
  - Ages 6 to 12 years: 5 to 10 mg every 4 hours PRN or 30 mg every 12 hours PRN (sustained-release suspension). Maximum 60 mg every 24 hours

Note: The American Academy of Pediatrics recommends against its use in children due to lack of proven benefit.[18]

Recommend Adult Dosages of Nonprescription Drugs

Analgesics[19]

- Acetaminophen
  - 325 to 1,000 mg every 4 to 6 hours PRN. Maximum 4,000 mg/d

Note: In 2011, the manufacturer of Tylenol products voluntarily reduced the maximum daily dosage of its OTC products. Labeling for Extra Strength Tylenol now indicates a maximum daily dosage of 3,000 mg, with a lengthened dosing interval of two tablets every 6 hours. The maximum daily dosage of OTC Regular Strength Tylenol is 3,250 mg.

- Ibuprofen
  - 200 to 400 mg every 4 to 6 hours PRN. Maximum 1,200 mg/d
- Naproxen sodium
  - 220 mg every 8 to 12 hours PRN. Maximum 660 mg/d

Antihistamines[9]

- Chlorpheniramine: 4 mg every 4 to 6 hours PRN. Maximum 24 mg/24 h
- Diphenhydramine: 25 to 50 mg every 4 to 6 hours PRN. Maximum 300 mg/24 h

- Loratadine: 10 mg once a day. Maximum 10 mg/24 h
- Cetirizine: 5 to 10 mg once a day. Maximum 10 mg/24 h

Cough Suppressants[9]

- Dextromethorphan: 10 to 20 mg every 4 hours PRN or 30 mg every 6 to 8 hours PRN (sustained-release suspension). Maximum 120 mg/24 h

Decongestants[9]

- Phenylephrine: 10 mg every 4 hours PRN. Maximum 60 mg/24 h
- Pseudoephedrine: 60 mg every 4 to 6 hours PRN. Maximum 240 mg/24 h

Expectorants[9]

- Guaifenesin: 200 to 400 mg every 4 hours. Maximum 2,400 mg/24 h

Useful Resources

1. Krinsky DL, Berardi RR, Ferreri SP, et al., eds. *Handbook of Nonprescription Drugs: An Interactive Approach to Self-Care*. 17th ed. Washington, DC: American Pharmacists Association; 2012.
2. Tschudy MM, Arcara KM, eds. *The Harriet Lane Handbook: A Manual For Pediatric House Officers*. 19th ed. Philadelphia, PA: Mosby Elsevier; 2012.
3. Briggs GG, Freeman RK, Yaffe SJ. *Drugs in Pregnancy and Lactation*. 9th ed. Philadelphia, PA: Lippincott Williams & Wilkins; 2011.
4. Information for Consumers: Understanding Over-the-Counter Medicine. U.S. Food and Drug Administration. Available at www.fda.gov/Drugs/ResourcesForYou/Consumers/BuyingUsingMedicineSafely/UnderstandingOver-the-CounterMedicines/

Dietary Supplements/Complementary Care

It is estimated that 38 million adults in the United States use at least one form of complementary and alternative medicine, but only one-third share this information with their health care clinicians.[20,21] Pharmacists can play a unique role in helping patients make appropriate decisions about supplement use. Reasons for using dietary supplements can vary, including belief that conventional medicine is ineffective, too expensive, or will work better in combination with supplements.[22] Although the focus may be on herbs, dietary supplements also include a wide range of vitamins, minerals, amino acids, enzymes, organ tissues, metabolites, and hormones. This section focuses on the dietary supplements.

Because supplements are derived originally from natural sources, patients may feel that they are safe. It is important for them to understand that dietary supplements are in the category under the general umbrella of foods not drugs regulated by the FDA's Center for Food Safety and Applied Nutrition. As a result, the manufacturers do not need approval from or register their products with the FDA. Under the Dietary Supplement Health and Education Act of 1994 (DSHEA), they are responsible for ensuring that a product is safe before it is marketed.[23] The 2007 enactment of good manufacturing practice (GMP) for dietary supplements requires manufacturers to certify good manufacturing processes and verify that listed label ingredients match package contents. The FDA is responsible for taking actions against any unsafe product after it reaches the market.[23,24]

Role of the Pharmacist

Patients often seek advice in product selection from pharmacists. Key considerations to inform patients in selection and use of dietary supplements include the following[25]:

- Use products with labels containing symbols of United States Pharmacopeia (USP), National Formulary (NF), National Science Foundation (NSF), or good manufacturing practice (GMP) or products that have been evaluated by ComsumerLab.com.
- Use products that identify the following:
  - Source (i.e., the botanical name and part of the plant used)
  - Strength of the preparation or dose
  - Lot number and expiration date
  - Name, address, and phone number of manufacturer
- Use supplements containing only one ingredient.
- Do not take more than the recommended dose.
- Limit how long you take the supplement.
- Tell your health care providers you are using this supplement.
- Report adverse effects related to the supplement to the FDA by calling 1-800-332-1088 or online at www.fda.gov/medwatch.[26]

Medical Condition Considerations

Pharmacists should make note of the individual patient's history before making a recommendation to use dietary supplements. If possible, including the patient's supplement use in his or her medication profile can prevent future adverse outcomes. Before using a dietary supplement, patients should discuss use with their clinicians if they[27]

1. Plan to become pregnant, are pregnant, or are breast-feeding
2. Plan to use the supplement for a child
3. Have a serious medical condition such as diabetes, hypertension, or heart disease
4. Take prescription or OTC medications regularly
5. Have a history of allergic reaction to a specific dietary supplement
6. Have surgery or other procedure scheduled

With an estimated 18% of the US population using supplements on a regular basis,[25] it is important for pharmacists to be familiar with commonly used products. Table 19.1 lists the top 10 supplements used by adults in the United States in 2010.[27] Likewise, Table 19.2 lists 12 supplements that have been associated with serious adverse events and should be avoided.[28]

TABLE 19.1 Top 10 Herbal Supplements Sales in the United States in 2010 (food, drug and mass market channels only, does not include health food store or direct sales channels)

1. Cranberry
2. Saw palmetto
3. Soy
4. Garlic
5. Ginkgo
6. Echinacea
7. Milk thistle
8. Black cohosh
9. St. John's wort
10. Ginseng

Sources: Symphony IRI Group: FDM Market Sales Data for Herbal Supplements, Dec 26, 2010; and American Herbal Products Association. 2011 Annual Report. Available at www.ahpa.org/Portals/0/pdfs/2011/20AHPA/20Annual/20Report_FINAL.pdf. Accessed March 12, 2013.

TABLE 19.2 Dangerous Supplements to Avoid

Aconite
Bitter orange
Chaparral
Colloidal silver
Coltsfoot
Comfrey
Country mallow
Germander
Greater celandine
Kava
Lobelia
Yohimbe

Source: Consumer Reports. Dangerous Supplements—What You Don't Know About These 12 Ingredients Could Hurt You. Available at www.consumerreports.org/cro/2012/05/dangerous-supplements/index.htm. Accessed May 8, 2013.

The following list of frequently used supplements includes some considerations for their use.[29–32] It is important to note that this is not a comprehensive listing of all indications, side effects, or interactions, but is intended as a starting point for pharmacists in answering patients' questions and guiding appropriate use.

Black Cohosh

- Do not confuse with blue cohosh
- Has estrogenic effects

Used for:

- Menopausal symptoms (possibly effective)

Common side effects:

- Gastrointestinal (GI) upset, dizziness, headache, and rash

Possible drug interactions:

- May inhibit CYP2D6
- Cisplatin: may decrease cytotoxic effect
- Hepatotoxic drugs: may increase risk of liver damage

Possible lab changes:

- May cause changes in liver function tests

Avoid or use precaution in patients with:

- Breast and other hormone-sensitive cancers, kidney transplant, liver disease, pregnancy, and lactation

Coenzyme Q-10 (Ubiquinone)

Used for:

- Improving immune function in HIV/AIDS (possibly effective)
- Migraine headache prevention (possibly effective)
- Hypertension (possibly effective)
- Congestive heart failure (possibly effective)
- Statin-induced myopathy (insufficient reliable evidence)

Common side effects:

- Nausea, vomiting, appetite suppression, and heartburn

Possible drug interactions:

- Antihypertensive drugs: may have additive blood pressure–lowering effects
- Chemotherapy: antioxidant effects may protect tumor cells from chemotherapeutic agents.
- Warfarin: may have vitamin K–like procoagulant effects

Possible lab changes:

- May increase cholesterol levels

Avoid or use precaution in patients with:

- Hypotension and hypertension

Cranberry

Used for:

- Reduction or prevention of urinary tract infection (possibly effective)

Common side effects:

- Usually well tolerated
- Nausea, vomiting, and diarrhea (juice)

Possible drug interactions:

- May inhibit CYP2C9
- May increase anticoagulant activity of warfarin

Avoid or use precaution in patients with:

- Nephrolithiasis (kidney stones) due to its high oxalate content

Echinacea

- Most efficacious species are *E. purpurea*, *E. angustifolia*, and *E. pallida*

Used for:

- Reduction of common cold symptoms and duration (possibly effective)

Common side effects:

- Nausea, vomiting, diarrhea, and abdominal pain

Possible drug interactions:

- Caffeine: may increase caffeine plasma concentrations
- Immunosuppressants: may reduce efficacy
- Appears to inhibit CYP1A2
- Appears to inhibit intestinal and induce hepatic CYP3A4

Possible lab changes:

- None known

Avoid or use precaution in patients with:

- Autoimmune diseases including multiple sclerosis, systemic lupus erythematosus, and rheumatoid arthritis
- Allergies to Asteraceae/Compositae family (ragweed, chrysanthemums, marigolds, many others)

Feverfew

Used for:

- Migraine headache

Common side effects:

- Nervousness, insomnia, dizziness, nausea, vomiting, heartburn, and sun sensitivity

Possible drug interactions:

- Anticoagulant/antiplatelet drugs: may increase bleeding risk
- May inhibit CYP1A2, CYP2C9, CYP2C19, and CYP3A4

Possible lab changes:

- None known

Avoid or use precaution in patients with:

- Allergies to Asteraceae/Compositae family (ragweed, chrysanthemums, marigolds, many others)

Fish Oil (Omega-3 Fatty Acids)

- Take with meals or freeze capsules to minimize GI side effects
- Recommend use of brands assayed to avoid contaminants including mercury

Used for:

- Hypertriglyceridemia
- Cardiovascular disease risk reduction (likely effective)

Common side effects:

- Fishy aftertaste, halitosis, heartburn, loose stool, bruising, and bleeding

Possible drug interactions:

- Anticoagulant/antiplatelet drugs: may increase bleeding risk
- Antihypertensives: may have additive effect

Possible lab changes:

- May increase international normalized ratio (INR) and prothrombin time (PT)
- May increase low-density lipoprotein (LDL) cholesterol

Avoid or use precaution in patients with:

- Seafood allergies and implantable defibrillators

Garlic

Used for:

- Slow development of atherosclerosis (possibly effective)
- Hypertension (possibly effective)
- Hyperlipidemia (possibly ineffective)

Common side effects:

- Breath and body odor, mouth and GI irritation, flatulence, nausea, vomiting, diarrhea, and increased bruising and bleeding

Possible drug interactions:

- Anticoagulant/antiplatelet drugs: may increase bleeding risk
- Contraceptive drugs: may decrease effectiveness
- Cyclosporine: may decrease effectiveness
- Isoniazid: may inhibit absorption across intestinal mucosa, decreasing effectiveness
- Nonnucleoside reverse transcriptase inhibitors (NNRTIs) and protease inhibitors (PIs): may decrease plasma concentrations, decreasing effectiveness

Possible lab changes:

- May increase INR and PT

Avoid or use precaution in patients with:

- Bleeding disorders, GI irritation, and upcoming surgery

Ginger

Used for:

- Morning sickness (possibly effective)
- Postoperative nausea/vomiting (possibly effective)
- Vertigo (possibly effective)
- Osteoarthritis (possibly effective)

Common side effects:

- Abdominal discomfort, heartburn, diarrhea, irritation of mouth and throat, and hypoglycemia (high doses)

Possible drug interactions:

- Anticoagulant/antiplatelet drugs: may increase bleeding risk
- Alprazolam: may decrease effectiveness
- Fluoxetine: may cause hypomania

Possible lab changes:

- None known

Avoid or use precaution in patients with:

- Bleeding conditions, diabetes (hypoglycemia), and heart conditions

Ginkgo

- Avoid use of seed, which can increase seizure risk

Used for:

- Age-related memory impairment, cognitive function, dementia, and intermittent claudication (possible effective)
- Altitude sickness and antidepressant-induced sexual dysfunction (possible ineffectiveness)

Common side effects:

- GI upset, restlessness, headache, lack of muscle tone or weakness, and bleeding

Possible drug interactions:

- Anticoagulant/antiplatelet drugs, ibuprofen: may increase bleeding risk
- Trazodone: may lead to coma due to excessive GABAergic activity

Possible lab changes:

- None known

Avoid or use precaution in patients with:

- Bleeding disorders, diabetes, epilepsy, infertility attempting to conceive, and upcoming surgery

Ginseng

- Refers to species of the genus *Panax*; commonly used species Asian and American
- Does not refer to Siberian ginseng, of the genus *Eleutherococcus*

Used for:

- Cognitive function (possibly effective)
- Diabetes (possibly effective)
- Erectile dysfunction (possibly effective)

Common side effects:

- GI upset, nervousness, tachycardia, and insomnia

Possible drug interactions:

- Anticoagulant/antiplatelet drugs: may increase bleeding risk
- Antidiabetes drugs: may increase risk of hypoglycemia
- Caffeine: may have additive stimulant effect

Possible lab changes:

- Activated partial thromboplastin time (aPTT), prothrombin time (PT), and thrombin time (TT) may be prolonged

Avoid or use precaution in patients with:

- Autoimmune disease, bleeding disorders, diabetes, insomnia, organ transplants, schizophrenia, cardiovascular disease, and hormone-sensitive cancers

Glucosamine Sulfate

- Hydrochloride salt form not effective for osteoarthritis
- Sometimes used in combination with chondroitin and/or methylsulfonylmethane (MSM) but with an inconsistent or modest efficacy

Used for:

- Osteoarthritis (likely effective)

Common side effects:

- Nausea, heartburn, diarrhea, constipation, and increases in blood glucose levels

Possible drug interactions:

- Antimitotic chemotherapeutic agents: theoretically might induce resistance
- Warfarin: may change INRs when used in combination with chondroitin at higher than recommended doses

Possible lab changes:

- May increase INRs when taken in combination with warfarin and chondroitin at higher than recommended doses
- Little or no effect noted on blood glucose or lipid levels

Avoid or use precaution in patients with:

- Shellfish allergies, asthma

Green Tea

- Contains caffeine

Used for:

- Mental alertness and performance (likely effective)
- Cholesterol reduction (possibly effective)
- Decreased risk of developing cardiovascular disease (insufficient reliable evidence)
- Diabetes (insufficient reliable evidence)
- Hypertension (insufficient reliable evidence)

Common side effects:

- Nausea, vomiting, abdominal pain, bloating, diuresis, and central nervous system (CNS) stimulation including dizziness, insomnia, agitation, and confusion

Possible drug interactions:

- Anticoagulant/antiplatelet drugs: may increase bleeding risk
- CNS stimulants: may have additive stimulant effect
- Clozapine: may inhibit metabolism, increasing serum concentrations
- Lithium: may change serum levels
- Theophylline: may reduce clearance and increase serum levels
- Alcohol, contraceptives, estrogen, disulfiram, fluconazole, fluvoxamine, mexiletine, nicotine, quinolone antibiotics, terbinafine, and verapamil

Possible lab changes:

- May decrease ferritin, hemoglobin, and iron levels
- May increase liver function tests
- May interfere with dipyridamole thallium imaging

Avoid or use precaution in patients with:

- Iron deficiency anemia, bleeding disorders, cardiac conditions, diabetes, glaucoma, hypertension, liver disease, and osteoporosis

Melatonin

- Avoid products from animal sources

Used for:

- Insomnia (possibly effective)
- Jet lag (possibly effective)

- Attention deficit hyperactivity disorder (ADHD) (insufficient reliable evidence)

Common side effects:

- Daytime drowsiness, headache, dizziness, resumption of spotting or menstrual flow in postmenopausal women, mood changes, and hormonal changes

Possible drug interactions:

- Anticoagulant/antiplatelet drugs: may increase effect, with bleeding and decreased prothrombin activity
- Benzodiazepines, alcohol, and sedatives: may have additive sedating effects
- Immunosuppressants: may stimulate immune function and interfere with therapy
- Nifedipine gastrointestinal therapeutic system (GITS): decreases effectiveness with increase in blood pressure and heart rate

Possible lab changes:

- May increase human growth hormone levels
- May decrease serum luteinizing hormone levels
- May cause dose-dependent increases or decreases in oxytocin levels
- May cause dose-dependent increases or decreases in vasopressin levels

Avoid or use precaution in patients with:

- Depression, diabetes, hypertension, and seizure disorder

Milk Thistle

Used for:

- Treatment of liver damage and disease (insufficient reliable evidence)

Common side effects:

- Laxative effect, nausea, dyspepsia, and anorexia

Possible drug interactions:

- May inhibit CYP2C9
- May reduce clearance of drugs that undergo glucuronidation

Possible lab changes:

- None known

Avoid or use precaution in patients with:

- Allergies to the Asteraceae/Compositae family (ragweed, chrysanthemums, marigolds, many others)
- Hormone-sensitive cancers

Peppermint

Used for:

- Dyspepsia (possibly effective)

Common side effects:

- Heartburn, nausea, vomiting, mouth burning, and ulceration

Possible drug interactions:

- Cyclosporine: may inhibit metabolism, increasing drug levels
- May inhibit CYP1A2, CYP2C19, CYP2C9, and CYP3A4
- Histamine H_2–receptor antagonists and proton pump inhibitors, may cause premature dissolution of enteric coated preparations

Possible lab changes (observed in animal models):

- May increase follicle-stimulating hormone (FSH) levels
- May increase luteinizing hormone (LH) levels
- May reduce testosterone levels

Avoid or use precaution in patients with:

- Achlorhydria, diarrhea, pregnancy, and breast-feeding

Red Clover

- Has estrogenic effects

Used for:

- Menopausal symptoms (insufficient reliable evidence)

Common side effects:

- Myalgia, headache, vaginal spotting, rash, nausea, breast tenderness, and weight gain

Possible drug interactions:

- Anticoagulant/antiplatelet drugs: may increase bleeding risk
- Contraceptive drugs, estrogen, and tamoxifen: may reduce efficacy
- May inhibit CYP1A2, CYP2C19, CYP2C9, and CY3A4

Possible lab changes:

- None known

Avoid or use precaution in patients with:

- Breast and other hormone-sensitive cancers, coagulation disorders, pregnancy, and breast-feeding

Saw Palmetto

- Has antiestrogenic effects

Used for:

- Benign prostatic hyperplasia (BPH) symptoms (likely effective)

Common side effects:

- Dizziness, headache, GI upset, diarrhea, and postural hypotension

Possible drug interactions:

- Anticoagulant/antiplatelet drugs: may increase risk of bleeding

Possible lab changes:

- May change INRs
- Does not appear to significantly affect prostate-specific antigen (PSA) levels

Avoid or use precaution in patients with:

- Planned surgery due to excessive intraoperative bleeding

Soy

- Has estrogenic effects

Used for:

- Menopausal symptoms (possibly effective)
- Reducing risk of developing breast cancer (possibly effective)
- Hyperlipidemia (possibly effective)

Common side effects:

- Constipation, diarrhea, bloating, nausea, and insomnia

Possible drug interactions:

- Monoamine oxidase inhibitors (MAOI): may increase risk of hypertensive crisis when used with fermented soy products
- Tamoxifen: may cause interference due to estrogenic effects
- Warfarin: may decrease INRs and may inhibit platelet aggregation

Possible lab changes:

- Parathyroid levels may be reduced in postmenopausal women
- PSA may be reduced in men with prostate cancer
- Thyroid-stimulating hormone (TSH) may be increased

Avoid or use precaution in patients with:

- Asthma, breast cancer, endometrial cancer, kidney stones, and renal failure

St. John's Wort

Used for:

- Mild to moderate depression (likely effective)

Common side effects:

- Insomnia, vivid dreams, agitation, irritability, GI upset, and dry mouth

Possible drug interactions:

- May increase the risk of serotonin syndrome
  - "Triptans," selective serotonin reuptake inhibitors (SSRIs), monoamine oxidase inhibitors (MAOIs), nefazodone, fenfluramine, meperidine, pentazocine, and tramadol
- May induce cytochrome isoenzyme metabolism (CYP1A2, CYP2C9, CYP2C19, CYP3A4) and P-glycoprotein causing decreased serum concentrations and reduction in therapeutic effect
  - Alprazolam, amitriptyline, nortriptyline, contraceptive, cyclosporine, methylphenidate, simvastatin, imatinib, irinotecan, NNRTIs and PIs, and warfarin
- Phenobarbital and phenytoin: may increase metabolism, decreasing therapeutic levels

- Fexofenadine: may decrease clearance, increasing serum levels
- Clopidogrel: may increase risk of bleeding
- Digoxin and tacrolimus: may decrease serum levels

Possible lab changes:

- May decrease INR and PT levels for warfarin patients
- May increase TSH levels

Avoid or use precaution in patients with:

- Alzheimer disease, ADHD, bipolar disease, schizophrenia, and infertility attempting to conceive

Additional Reliable Sources on Dietary Supplements

- Natural Medicines Comprehensive Database. Available at www.naturaldatabase.com
- The U.S. Food and Drug Administration. Available at www.fda.gov
- National Center for Complementary and Alternative Medicine, National Institutes of Health. Available at www.nccam.nih.gov
- Natural Standard, the Authority on Integrative Medicine. Available at www.naturalstandard.com
- Medline Plus. Available at www.nlm.nih.gov/medlineplus/druginformation.html
- Office of Dietary Supplements, National Institute of Health. Available at www.ods.od.nih.gov
- Dietary Supplement Ingredient Database. Available at www.dietarysupplements.nlm.nih.gov/dietary

References

1. Consumer Healthcare Products Association. *OTC Retail Sales—1964–2011*. Available at http://chpa-info.org/pressroom/Retail_Sales.aspx. Accessed May 11, 2013.
2. Covington TR. Nonprescription drug therapy: issues and opportunities. *Am J Pharm Educ*. 2006;70(6):137.
3. Uses and Attitudes About Taking Over-the-Counter Medicines: Findings of a 2003 National Opinion Survey. Bethesda, MD: National Council of Patient Information and Education; 2003. Available at: http://www.bemedwise.org/survey/summary_survey_findings.pdf. Accessed May 18, 2013.
4. Hong SH, Spadaro D, West D, et al. Patient valuation of pharmacist services for self care with OTC medications. *J Clin Pharm Ther*. 2005;30:193–199.
5. Buring SM, Kirby J, Conrad WF. A structured approach for teaching students to counsel self-care patients. *Am J Pharm Educ*. 2007;71(1):8.

6. Lawrence BM, Isettes B. Patient assessment and consultation. In: Krinsky DL, Berardi RR, Ferreri SP, et al., eds. *Handbook of Nonprescription Drugs: An Interactive Approach to Self-Care*. 17th ed. Washington, DC: American Pharmacists Association; 2012.
7. FDA Center for Drug Evaluation and Research (CDER). Public Health Advisory—Nonprescription Cough and Cold Medicine Use in Children. January 17, 2008. Available at www.fda.gov/cder/drug/advisory/cough_cold_2008.htm. Accessed February 5, 2008.
8. Food and Drug Administration. Consumer Updates. Using Over-the-Counter Cough and Cold Products in Children. Updated April 11, 2013. Available at http://www.fda.gov/ForConsumers/ConsumerUpdates/ucm048515.htm. Accessed May 11, 2013.
9. Scolaro KL. Disorders related to colds and allergy. In: Krinsky DL, Berardi RR, Ferreri SP, et al., eds. *Handbook of Nonprescription Drugs: An Interactive Approach to Self-Care*. 17th ed. Washington, DC: American Pharmacists Association; 2012.
10. Food and Drug Administration. Public Health Advisory: FDA Recommends That Over-the-Counter (OTC) Cough and Cold Products Not Be Used for Infants and Children under 2 Years of Age. Updated April 14, 2013. Available at http://www.fda.gov/ForConsumers/ConsumerUpdates/ucm051137.htm. Accessed May 11, 2013.
11. Briggs GG, Freeman RK, Yaffe SJ. *Drugs in Pregnancy and Lactation*. 9th ed. Philadelphia, PA: Lippincott Williams & Wilkins; 2011.
12. Hajjar ER, Gray SL, Guay DR, et al. Geriatrics. In: Talbert RL, DiPiro JT, Matzke GR, et al., eds. *Pharmacotherapy: A Pathophysiologic Approach*. 8th ed. New York, NY: McGraw-Hill; 2011.
13. Henderson ML. Self-care and nonprescription pharmacotherapy. In: Krinsky DL, Berardi RR, Ferreri SP, et al., eds. *Handbook of Nonprescription Drugs: An Interactive Approach to Self-Care*. 17th ed. Washington, DC: American Pharmacists Association; 2012.
14. Nahata MC, Taketomo C. Pediatrics. In: Talbert RL, DiPiro JT, Matzke GR, et al., eds. *Pharmacotherapy: A Pathophysiologic Approach*. 8th ed. New York, NY: McGraw-Hill; 2011.
15. Lexicomp: Pediatric and Neonatal Lexi-Drugs [Internet]. Hudson, OH: Lexi-Comp, Inc. Available at http://online.lexi.com/lco/action/home. Accessed May 19, 2013.
16. Tschudy MM, Arcara KM, eds. *The Harriet Lane Handbook: A Manual for Pediatric House Officers*. 19th ed. Philadelphia, PA: Mosby Elsevier; 2012.
17. Food and Drug Administration. Code of Federal Regulations. Title 21: Part 341—Cold, Cough, Allergy, Bronchodilator, and Antiasthmatic Products for Over-the-Counter Human Use. Updated April 4, 2012. Available at http://www.accessdata.fda.gov/scripts/cdrh/cfdocs/cfcfr/CFRSearch.cfm?fr=341.72. Accessed May 11, 2013.

18. American Academy of Pediatrics. Use of codeine- and dextromethorphan-containing cough remedies in children. *Pediatrics* 1997;99:918–920.
19. Wilkinson JL. Headache. In: Krinsky DL, Berardi RR, Ferreri SP, et al., eds. *Handbook of Nonprescription Drugs: An Interactive Approach to Self-Care*. 17th ed. Washington, DC: American Pharmacists Association; 2012.
20. National Center for Complementary and Alternative Medicine. The Use of Complementary and Alternative Medicine in the United States. Available at www.nccam.nih.gov/news/camstats/2007/camsurvey_fs1.htm. Accessed May 8, 2013.
21. Eisenberg DM, Kessler RC, Van Rompay MI, et al. Perceptions about complementary therapies relative to conventional therapies among adults who use both: results from a national survey. *Ann Intern Med.* 2001;135:344–351.
22. Kennedy J. Herb and supplement use in the US adult population. *Clin Ther* 2005;27:1847–1858.
23. Food and Drug Administration. Dietary Supplements. Available at www.fda.gov/Food/DietarySupplements/default.htm. Accessed May 8, 2013.
24. FDA issues dietary supplements final rule [press release]. Rockville, MD: US Food and Drug Administration. June 22, 2007. Available at www.fda.gov/bbs/topics/NEWS/2007/NEW01657.html. Accessed May 24, 2013.
25. Tsourounis C, Denneby C. Introduction to dietary supplements. In: Krinsky DL, Berardi RR, Ferreri SP, et al., eds. *Handbook of Nonprescription Drugs: An Interactive Approach to Self-Care*. 17th ed. Washington, DC: American Pharmacists Association; 2012.
26. Food and Drug Administration. Dietary Supplements—Adverse Event Reporting. Available at www.fda.gov/Food/DietarySupplements/ReportAdverseEvent/default.htm. Accessed May 8, 2013.
27. American Herbal Products Association. 2011 Annual Report. Available at www.ahpa.org/Portals/0/pdfs/2011%20AHPA%20Annual%20Report_FINAL.pdf. Accessed March 12, 2013.
28. Consumer Reports. Dangerous Supplements—What You Don't Know About These 12 Ingredients Could Hurt You. Available at www.consumerreports.org/cro/2012/05/dangerous-supplements/index.htm. Accessed May 8, 2013.
29. Natural Medicine Comprehensive Database. Available at www.naturaldatabase.com. Accessed May 8, 2013.
30. Natural Standard, The Authority on Integrative Medicine. Available at www.naturalstandard.com. Accessed January 25, 2008.
31. National Center for Complementary and Alternative Medicine, National Institutes of Health. Available at www.nccam.nih.gov. Accessed May 8, 2013.
32. Medline Plus. Available at www.nlm.nih.gov/medlineplus/druginformation.html. Accessed May 8, 2013.

20

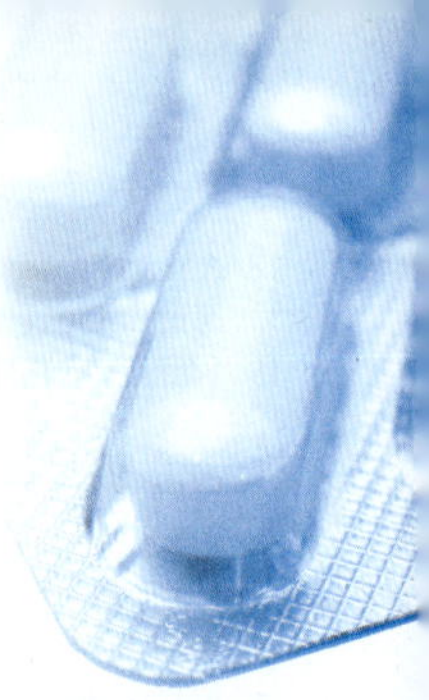

Vaccines and Pharmacists as Immunizers

Jeffery Fortner, Kristine Marcus,
Pauline A. Low, and Brad Fujisaki

The Pharmacist's Involvement in Immunization-Related Activities

All states now allow pharmacists, and a majority allow pharmacy interns under the supervision of their preceptor, to administer vaccines to adults after proper training.[1] Two of the most commonly targeted and reimbursed immunizations given in pharmacies include inactivated influenza and pneumococcal polysaccharide vaccines.[2] However, pharmacists in all settings can have an impact on improving national vaccination rates for at-risk patients through participation in all three levels of vaccine practice: advocacy, facilitation, and vaccine administration (Table 20.1).

Discuss with your colleagues which of these activities are available to participate in at your pharmacy site. Even if it is not a routine part of the site's practice to give immunizations, you can still contribute to the patient's preventative health by including vaccinations in your questioning when taking a medication history and recommending vaccination when appropriate.

Pharmacists as Immunizers

Pharmacists must be aware of whether pharmacy interns are allowed to administer vaccines in the state where they are gaining practice experience, if there are any limitations on which vaccines may be given, if a prescription for vaccination is required, and which patient populations may be served. The requirements and restrictions on providing immunizations are usually outlined in the state's Pharmacy Practice Act that can be found in the Board of Pharmacy's

TABLE 20.1 Examples of Pharmacist Immunization Activities by Practice Setting

Pharmacy Practice Setting	Examples of Immunization Activities
Community pharmacy	• Providing vaccinations • Taking vaccination histories, screening patients, and recommending vaccination • Hosting other licensed health care providers to administer immunizations
Clinic pharmacy	• Providing vaccinations • Taking vaccination histories, screening patients, and recommending vaccination • Establishing standing orders for vaccination of eligible patients • Managing formularies to include all necessary vaccines for the patient population served
Institutional pharmacy	• Taking vaccination histories, screening patients, and recommending vaccination • Establishing standing orders for vaccination of eligible patients • Managing formularies to include all necessary vaccines for the patient population served
All settings	• Educating and motivating patients to obtain timely immunizations • Providing public education on vaccine-preventable diseases and the importance of immunization • Providing vaccine information to patients and other health care providers • Maintaining the cold chain and insuring proper storage conditions of vaccines dispensed or administered

Administrative Rules. These rules will generally include specifics on the training and recordkeeping that is expected when providing immunization in a pharmacy setting. When you are new to a particular pharmacy practice, review and discuss with your supervisor the rules, policies, and standard operating procedures provided by the Board of Pharmacy and your practice site.

Vaccine Administration Steps—Overview

While individual site policies and procedures will be more specific, the usual steps in providing vaccination are shown in Figure 20.1. This figure is the framework for our review on pharmacist-provided vaccinations throughout the rest of this chapter.

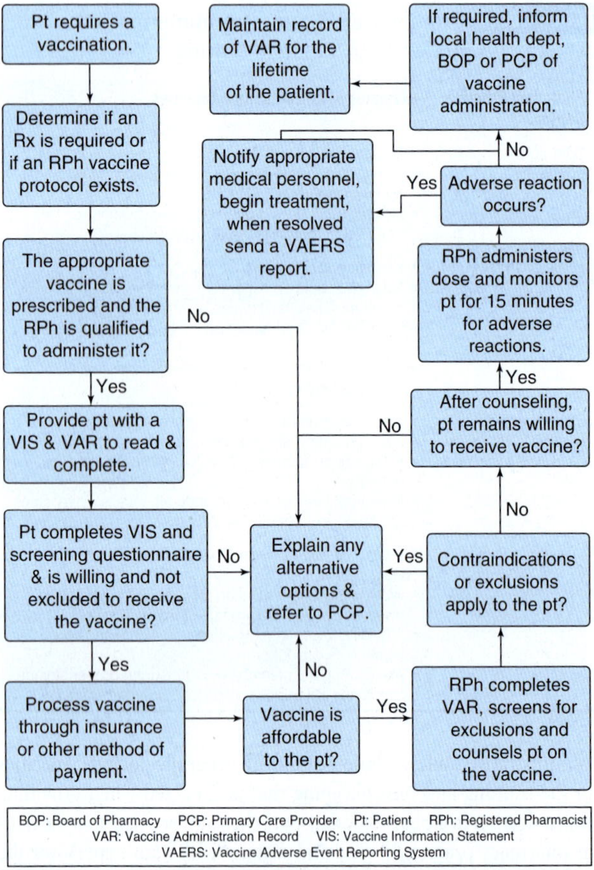

FIGURE 20.1 Steps for administering vaccinations.

Identifying Who Needs Vaccination

Immunization Recommendations

Tables are available from the Centers for Disease Control and Prevention (CDC) to quickly identify patients who are recommended to receive vaccination either by age or by other population target. These tables are referred to as Immunization Schedules and are updated annually. Pharmacists and interns administering or recommending vaccines must insure they are using the most current recommendations by checking the date in the upper right corner of the schedule. Due to the frequency of revision, schedules published in printed or electronic drug information references may be out of date. Changes to the Immunization Schedules are provisionally recommended by the Advisory Committee on Immunization Practices (ACIP) in February, June, and October and then are approved by the CDC and the U.S. Department of Health and Human Services and subsequently published in the CDC's Morbidity and Mortality Weekly Report and to the CDC's National Center for Immunization and Respiratory Diseases (NCIRD, formerly known as the National Immunization Program) Web site. Pharmacists and interns can stay informed of upcoming changes and refer to the most current recommendations in immunization practice through these two key sites:

- Bookmark: CDC's NCIRD Web site: http://www.cdc.gov/vaccines/
- Bookmark and subscribe to Immunization Action Coalition (IAC) Express news service: Immunization Action Coalition: www.immunize.org

Using the CDC Immunization Schedules

The Immunization Schedules indicate when certain vaccines should ideally be given and how many doses are necessary to complete the primary series or to provide a booster dose. Footnotes for each vaccine provide additional detailed information and should be read in conjunction with the schedule. The user can quickly access the relevant schedule by knowing the patient's age and medical conditions. The current schedules (Table 20.2) are available in various formats (office-size poster, brochure size, pocket size, and as a digital download) at: http://www.cdc.gov/vaccines/schedules/index.html

TABLE 20.2 Current CDC Immunization Schedules

- "Childhood" (birth through <7 years old)
- "Adolescent" (7–18 years old)
- "Childhood and Adolescent Catch-Up Schedule" (4 months–18 years old who started late or are more than 1 month behind)
- "Combined Childhood, Adolescent and Catch Up Schedule" (0–18 years old)
- "Adult" (>19 years old)—includes an additional table with vaccines that might be indicated for adults based on medical and other indications

The NCIRD Web site also includes links for targeted population recommendations that are subsets to the Immunization Schedules (e.g., college students; health care workers; pregnant women; patients with immune deficiencies, altered immunocompetence, or hematopoietic stem cell transplant):

- http://www.cdc.gov/vaccines/spec-grps/conditions.htm

Immunization General Rules and Overview

The CDC Pink Book is a frequently updated essential reference that includes chapters on principles of immunization, general recommendations for immunization, and vaccine-preventable diseases and their associated vaccines. Throughout the Pink Book, the CDC highlights general rules of immunization that have been compiled in Table 20.3.

Understanding Available Vaccines

Vaccines can be distinguished from one another by a number of factors such as viability (live or inactive), adult versus pediatric use, inactive ingredients, and methods of administration. When working with vaccines, pharmacists and interns will also need to be aware of vaccine

TABLE 20.3 General Rules for Immunization from the CDC Pink Book

- The more similar a vaccine is to the disease-causing form of the organism, the better the immune response to the vaccine.
- Live attenuated vaccines generally produce long-lasting immunity with a single dose.
- Inactivated vaccines require multiple doses and may require periodic boosting to maintain immunity.
- Live attenuated vaccines may be affected by circulating antibody to the antigen.
- Inactivated vaccines generally are not affected by circulating antibody to the antigen.
- All vaccines can be administered at the same visit as all other vaccines.
- Increasing the interval between doses of a multidose vaccine does not diminish the effectiveness of the vaccine.
- Decreasing the interval between doses of a multidose vaccine may interfere with antibody response and protection.

Adapted from Centers for Disease Control and Prevention. In: Atkinson W, Hamborsky J, Stanton A, et al., eds. *Epidemiology and Prevention of Vaccine-Preventable Diseases [The Pink Book]*. 12th ed. Washington, DC :Public Health Foundation; 2012.[4,16]

nomenclature and abbreviations. Vaccines currently available in the United States are shown in Table 20.4.[3]

Viability—Why It Matters

Certain patient populations (e.g., immunocompromised, pregnant) are excluded from receiving live vaccines because of the theoretical health risk of contracting the disease from the vaccine. In these populations of patients, the risk of vaccine use (even from attenuated vaccines that contain weakened, avirulent, or altered live bacteria or viruses) generally outweighs the perceived benefit of vaccination. Inactivated vaccines that are formulated with killed whole or isolated components of bacteria or virus do not pose this same risk.

The issue of interference of immunogenicity between simultaneous administrations of a live vaccine with other vaccines or circulating antibodies has been a historical concern. Current recommendations state that live vaccines may be coadministered in eligible patients with other live vaccines or inactive vaccines at the same immunization session. However, if two parenteral live vaccines or live intranasal influenza vaccine are not administered at the same visit, then they must be separated by 4 weeks to reduce the chance that the first vaccine may result in a suboptimal response to the second vaccine.[4] Likewise, the presence of circulating antibodies from blood products containing antibody may impair the patient's response to a live vaccine. If the live vaccine was given first, then administration of the antibody should be delayed 2 weeks. If the antibody was given first, then administration of the live vaccine is generally delayed for 3 months or longer with notable exceptions.[4]

Adult Versus Pediatric Vaccines

Confusion among available vaccines can be expected since different formulations of vaccines contain similar active ingredients but may be administered to different age groups or at different doses. The pharmacy student needs to be aware of which vaccines are indicated for which age groups and what the appropriate age-based dose is to avoid errors. One example is diphtheria, tetanus, and acellular pertussis vaccines. DTaP is used exclusively in children aged 2 months to ≤7 years old. Tdap is used in adolescents and adults. Adolescent patients may receive either brand of Tdap depending on age (Boostrix® for 10 through 18 years of age vs. Adacel® if 11 years or older), while adults can only receive the Adacel® brand of Tdap.

TABLE 20.4 Summary of Vaccines Available in the United States

Type of Vaccine	Proprietary Names	Viability	Route	Typical Dose
Meningococcal A, C, Y, W-135				
• Polysaccharide	*Menomune-A/C/Y/W-135*	Inactivated	Subcutaneous	0.5 mL
• Conjugated	*Menactra*	Inactivated	IM	0.5 mL
Mumps	*Mumpsvax*	Live	Subcutaneous	0.5 mL
Papillomavirus, types 6, 11, 16, 18	*Gardasil*	Inactivated	IM	0.5 mL
Pneumococcal, 7-valent	*Prevnar*	Inactivated	IM	0.5 mL
Pneumococcal, 23-valent	*Pneumovax 23*	Inactivated	Subcutaneous IM	0.5 mL
Poliovirus inactivated	*Ipol*	Inactivated	Subcutaneous	0.5 mL
Rabies (various culture media)	*BioRab, Imovax Rabies, RabAvert*	Inactivated	IM	1 mL
Rotavirus vaccine	*RotaTeq*	Live	Oral	0.2 mL
Rubella	*Meruvax II*	Live	Subcutaneous	0.5 mL
	Boostrix, Adacel	Inactivated	IM	0.5 mL
Tetanus toxoid (adsorbed) (TT)	Generic	Inactivated	IM	0.5 mL
Tetanus–diphtheria toxoids (Td)	Generic, *Decavac*	Inactivated	IM	0.5 mL
Typhoid (oral)	*Vivotif Berna*	Live	Oral	Four capsules
Typhoid Vi (parenteral, polysaccharide)	*Typhim Vi*	Inactivated	IM	0.5 mL
Vaccinia	*Dryvax*	Live	Scarification	3 or 15 punctures
Varicella	*Varivax*	Live	Subcutaneous	0.5 mL
Yellow fever	*YF-VAX*	Live	Subcutaneous	0.5 mL
Zoster	*Zostavax*	Live	Subcutaneous	0.65 mL

Reprinted from John D. Grabenstein. *Immunofacts 2013: Vaccines and Immunologic Drugs (Immunofacts Vaccines and Immunologic Drugs)*. Philadelphia, PA: Lippincott Williams & Wilkins; 2012.

Another example is inactivated influenza vaccine where there are multiple brands indicated for different age groups and one brand that covers the full range of indicated age groups. Fluzone® brand has a pediatric unit dose syringe version formulated specifically for patients 6 to 35 months of age that is thimerosal free and delivers the recommended 0.25-mL dose. Fluzone® also has a multidose vial presentation that contains thimerosal and can be used for all indicated ages of patients by withdrawing the appropriate dosage amount (i.e., 0.25 mL for ages 6 to 35 months and 0.5 mL for patients 3 years old or older) from the 5-mL vial.

A final example is pneumococcal vaccine where a polysaccharide and conjugate formulation are available. The conjugate form (Prevnar®) is used in children younger than 2 years old, while the polysaccharide version (Pneumovax® 23) is used in older children and adults.

Vaccine-Inactive Ingredients

Vaccines may contain excipients that may prove problematic for some patients who have allergies or sensitivities to these ingredients used in the formulation or packaging of vaccines. Some common excipients of concern are latex in the vial or syringe components, residual egg protein or antibiotic from the vaccine production process, or added pharmaceutical aids such as thimerosal as a preservative.

Vaccine Acronyms and Nomenclature

Although the use of abbreviations when ordering medications or biologicals is error prone,[5–7] the use of these short codes for different vaccines is still prevalent. Especially with the advent of combination vaccines and vaccines indicated for restricted age groups, recognition of the content differences between brand name products is necessary to avoid errors. Pharmacists and interns will need to be familiar with common acronyms and trade names used when ordering or documenting administration of vaccines.

Electronic flash cards and interactive matching tables to assist practitioners in learning common vaccine names (trade/generic/abbreviation), viability, type, and route of administration are available at

- Childhood and Adolescent Vaccines: http://www.studystack.com/menu-115865
- Adult Vaccines: http://www.studystack.com/menu-115834

Patient Education and Vaccine Information Statements

Federal statute requires all health care providers to provide the most current edition of the CDC vaccine information statements (VIS) to the patient or his or her proxy prior to administration of each dose of certain designated vaccines[8] (Table 20.5). State laws may be more restrictive and must also be followed. Best practice dictates providing VIS even for nondesignated vaccines. The health care provider may provide additional vaccine information materials, but these may not substitute for the CDC-produced VIS. VIS are available in multiple languages and now include a leaflet for combination vaccines and a multivaccine VIS from birth to 6 months. The most current VIS are available at: http://www.cdc.gov/vaccines/pubs/vis/default.htm or http://www.immunize.org/vis/

Vaccine Contraindications and Precautions Screening

As health care practitioners, we routinely ask ourselves, "Will this patient's overall health be worse after I administer this treatment?" This primary concern can be partially addressed by always considering

TABLE 20.5 Vaccines Requiring Provision of Vaccine Information Statement

- Diphtheria–tetanus +/– pertussis (DTaP/DT)
- Haemophilus influenzae type b
- Hepatitis A
- Hepatitis B
- Human papillomavirus (HPV)
- Influenza, inactivated injectable
- Influenza, live, intranasal
- Measles, mumps, rubella (MMR)
- Meningococcal
- Pneumococcal conjugate
- Polio
- Rotavirus
- Tetanus–diphtheria +/– pertussis (Td/Tdap)
- Varicella (chickenpox)
- Or combinations containing any of the above

Adapted from Centers for Disease Control and Prevention. *Mandatory Instructions for the Use of the Vaccine Information Statements.* Atlanta, GA: Centers for Disease Control and Prevention (CDC); May 2013. Available at www.cdc.gov/vaccines/pubs/vis/

a treatment's contraindications and precautions. Consider the following:

- A patient with a history of egg-induced anaphylaxis receives an injection of influenza vaccine.
- A patient with an immune deficiency receives a dose of live zoster vaccine.
- A patient with a febrile respiratory illness receives an injection of pneumococcal vaccine.

Each of these situations could result in the vaccine administrator causing a life-threatening reaction in the patient. And each could be avoided if the administrator used a system to identify patients with contraindications. Systems to identify contraindications include the following:

- Providing the patient with a CDC-published VIS that clearly lists any contraindications using terms a patient understands
- Using a general screening questionnaire or one tailored to a specific vaccine that identifies potential contraindications
- Personally counseling the patient about the vaccine and emphasizing the contraindications

If a practitioner utilizes each of these systems, he or she can reasonably establish whether a patient can safely receive a vaccine.

Part of the pharmacist's role also involves clearing up the patient's and caregiver's misconceptions about contraindications to receiving immunizations (Table 20.6). Luckily, there are few true contraindications or precautions for most vaccinations, and these are often temporary.[4]

Various screening questionnaires are available from the IAC (Table 20.7). Guides and discussions of contraindications and precautions that can form the foundation for patient counseling can also be found at the NCIRD Web site (Table 20.8) and in the CDC Pink Book.[4] By integrating these free resources into a vaccination routine, pharmacists can help to ensure positive patient outcomes with vaccines.

Vaccine Administration

Most vaccines currently on the market are given by parenteral injection. However, there are two vaccines that are given orally and one that is given intranasally. In general, live vaccines are given orally,

TABLE 20.6 Invalid Contraindications to Vaccination

Invalid Contraindication	Suggested Response to Misconception about Contraindication
Mild illness	• Mild acute illnesses, such as low-grade fever, upper respiratory infection, colds, and mild diarrhea do not interfere with vaccine response. • ACIP has not defined a body temperature above which vaccines should not be administered. The decision to vaccinate should be based on the overall evaluation of the person rather than on an arbitrary body temperature.
Antimicrobial therapy	• Antibiotics do not have an effect on the immune response to most vaccines. • No commonly used antimicrobial drug will inactivate a live-virus vaccine. However, antiviral drugs may affect vaccine replication in some circumstances.
Disease exposure or convalescence	• There is no evidence that either disease exposure or convalescence will affect the response to a vaccine or increase the likelihood of an adverse event.
Pregnant or immunosuppressed person in the household	• Vaccination of healthy contacts reduces the chance of exposure of pregnant women and immunosuppressed persons. • With limited exceptions, most vaccines including live vaccines can be administered to infants or children who are household contacts.
Breast-feeding	• Breast-feeding does not decrease the response to routine childhood vaccines and is not a contraindication for any vaccine except smallpox. • Breast-fed infants should be vaccinated according to recommended schedules for protection against vaccine-preventable disease. • The risk of transmission of vaccine virus is unknown but is probably low.
Preterm birth	• Preterm infants have been shown to respond adequately to vaccines used in infancy. Vaccines should be started on schedule on the basis of the child's chronologic age.
Allergy to products not present in vaccine or allergy that is not anaphylactic	• Infants and children with nonspecific allergies, duck, or feather allergy, or allergy to penicillin; children who have relatives with allergies; and children taking allergy shots can and should be immunized. No vaccine available in the United States contains duck antigen or penicillin. • Anaphylactic allergy to a vaccine component (such as egg or neomycin) is a true contraindication to vaccination. If an allergy to a vaccine component is not anaphylactic, it is not a contraindication to that vaccine.

(continued)

TABLE 20.6 Invalid Contraindications to Vaccination *(continued)*

Invalid Contraindication	Suggested Response to Misconception about Contraindication
Family history of adverse events	• The only family history that is relevant in the decision to vaccinate a child is immunosuppression. A family history of adverse reactions unrelated to immunosuppression or family history of seizures or sudden infant death syndrome (SIDS) is not a contraindication to vaccination.
Multiple vaccines	• Administration at the same visit of all vaccines for which a person is eligible is effective and critical to reaching and maintaining high vaccination coverage. • All vaccines (except smallpox) can be administered at the same visit as all other vaccines.

ACIP, Advisory Committee on Immunization Practices.
Adapted from Centers for Disease Control and Prevention. General recommendations on immunization. In: Atkinson W, Hamborsky J, Stanton A, et al., eds. *Epidemiology and Prevention of Vaccine-Preventable Diseases [The Pink Book]*. 12th ed. Washington, DC: Public Health Foundation; 2012.

intranasally, or by subcutaneous (SC or SQ) injection. Inactivated vaccines are generally given by intramuscular (IM) injection. A quick review of injection site location, appropriate needle length selection, and needle insertion techniques are shown in Figure 20.2. Detailed instructions, photographs, and graphics of injection techniques are available in the CDC Pink Book's Appendix D.[9] Refer to Table 20.4 or the product package insert for the recommended route of administration for specific vaccines.

Coadministration of the most common live and inactivated vaccines at the same immunization session results in adequate responses

TABLE 20.7 Links to IAC Adult Screening Questionnaires

General screening for adults	http://www.immunize.org/catg.d/p4065.pdf
Hepatitis A	http://www.immunize.org/catg.d/2190hepa.pdf
Hepatitis B	http://www.immunize.org/catg.d/2191hepb.pdf
Influenza, injectable	http://www.immunize.org/catg.d/p4066.pdf
Influenza, intranasal	http://www.immunize.org/catg.d/p4067.pdf
Additional languages available	http://www.immunize.org/handouts/screening-vaccines.asp

TABLE 20.8 CDC Links to Guides to Vaccine Contraindications

Guide to contraindications to vaccinations • Covers all the US vaccines as of February 2011. Provides contraindications by condition or symptom and has vaccine content listed by vaccine	Download pdf: http://www.cdc.gov/vaccines/recs/vac-admin/contraindications.htm
Contraindications to vaccine chart • Presents true contraindications and precautions by vaccine as of July 2012. Also includes column of invalid contraindications that should not prevent administration	Chart on Web site: http://www.cdc.gov/vaccines/recs/vac-admin/contraindications-vacc.htm

from the individual vaccines and has not been associated with an increased rate of side effects.[4]

Many pharmacists will ask the patient to remain nearby for 15 minutes after administration so that the patient may be observed for the development of a life-threatening or other severe reaction to the vaccine.

Vaccine Adverse Events

Managing and Reporting Vaccine Adverse Reactions

While anaphylaxis from vaccine administration is rare, pharmacists providing immunizations need to be prepared to respond to these situations until other medical help arrives (Table 20.9). All vaccine providers should have an emergency management plan in place and an adequate stock of medications and equipment necessary to respond to a severe vaccine reaction. Maintenance of BLS certification is also required. Appendix D of the CDC Pink Book[9] includes adult and pediatric emergency management protocols and standing order templates from the IAC that can be used by pharmacists providing vaccines.

Pharmacists are more likely to encounter patients with mild local adverse events or psychological reactions to vaccination. Appendix D of the CDC Pink Book also contains sections on the medical management of localized reactions, fright, and syncope.[9]

Customary practice includes documenting all vaccine reactions in the patient's pharmacy record and notifying his or her primary care provider so that the same information can be recorded in the patient's permanent medical record.

Injection Site and Needle Size		
Subcutaneous (SC) Injection Use a 23–25 gauge needle. Choose the injection site that is appropriate to the person's age and body mass.		
Age	**Needle Length**	**Injection Site**
Infants (1–12 mos)	5/6″	Fatty tissue over anterolateral thigh muscle
Children (≥12 mos). adolescents, & adults	5/6″	Fatty tissue over anterolateral thigh muscle or fatty tissue over triceps
Intramuscular (IM) Injection Use a 22–25 gauge needle. Choose the injection site and needle length appropriate to the person's age and body mass.		
Age	**Needle Length**	**Injection Site**
Newborn (1st 28 days)	5/8″	Anterolateral thigh muscle
Infant (1–12 mos)	1″	Anterolateral thigh muscle
Toddler (1–2 yrs)	1″ 1 1/4″ 5/8″–1″	Anterolateral thigh muscle or deltoid muscle of arm
Children 3–18 yrs	5/8″–1″ 1″–1 1/4″	Deltoid muscle of arm or anterolateral thigh muscle
≥19 yrs (Sex/Weight)		
Male/Female less than 130 lbs	5/8″–1″	Deltoid muscle of arm
Female (130–200 lbs) Male (130–260 lbs)	1″–1 1/2″	Deltoid muscle of arm
Female (200+ lbs) Male (260+ lbs)	1 1/2″	Deltoid muscle of arm

***If skin is stretched tight and subcutuneous tissue is not bunched.*

FIGURE 20.2 Vaccine injection basics. (From Immunization Action Coalition, www.immunize.org)

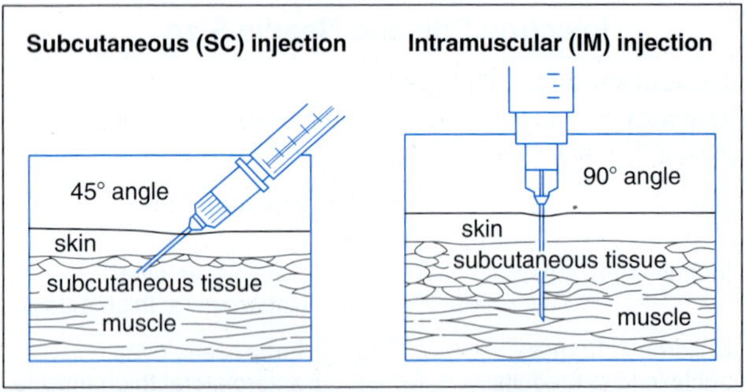

FIGURE 20.2 *(Continued)*

Health care providers and the public are encouraged to report all vaccine adverse events through the national postmarketing safety program, Vaccine Adverse Event Reporting System (VAERS). Health care providers are required by law to report certain problems listed in the Table of Reportable Events that can be found at http://vaers.hhs.gov/resources/VAERS_Table_of_Reportable_Events_Following_Vaccination.pdf.[10] In general, reporting of any problem that resulted in emergency treatment, hospitalization, disability, or death is required. Causation does not need to be established before reporting of adverse events in vaccinated adults and children. Even if the reporter is uncertain if the observed reaction was related to

TABLE 20.9 Example Management of a Generalized Anaphylactic Reaction to Adult Vaccination

1. Have bystander call 911/EMS
2. Administer epinephrine IM
3. Administer diphenhydramine IM or PO
4. Monitor vitals (HR, RR, BP)
5. Administer CPR if necessary
6. Repeat epinephrine IM q10- to 20-minute PRN × three doses until help arrives
7. Document all vitals, medications given, and personnel providing care
8. After event has resolved, contact the protocol physician or patient's PCP to report reaction and patient condition on triage to EMS
9. After event has resolved, document reaction and report to VAERS

EMS, emergency medical services; IM, intramuscularly; PO, by mouth; HR, heart rate; RR, respiratory rate; BP, blood pressure; CPR, cardiopulmonary resuscitation; PRN, as needed; PCP, primary care provider; VAERS, Vaccine Adverse Event Reporting System.

the vaccine, they are encouraged to file a report. Reports can be filed online at www.vaers.hhs.gov or by calling 1-800-822-7967 or faxing 1-877-721-0366.

A federal program called the National Vaccine Injury Compensation Program exists to help pay for the care of anyone who has had a serious reaction to a routinely recommended childhood vaccine. Settlement amounts are predetermined according to the Vaccine Injury Table published in Appendix F of the CDC Pink Book.[10] More information is available at www.hrsa.gov/vaccinecompensation or 1-800-338-2382.

Vaccine Administration Documentation

Vaccine Administration Records (VARs) must be maintained by the immunization provider for all patients receiving vaccination. It is also helpful to update or issue the patient a portable vaccination record such as the yellow Adult Immunization Record pocket card (http://www.immunize.org/shop/). Pharmacists providing immunizations may be subject to additional or special requirements for sharing their documentation with the patient's primary care provider, health division, or licensing board. Individual state rules and standards of practice should be consulted.

Documentation required at the time of vaccination is outlined in federal law (Table 20.10),[8] but state law or insurance adjudication may impose further requirements. Standard practice for documenting dose administration includes date and time of administration, dose/amount given, administration location, method of administration, lot number, and initials of the provider (e.g., MM/DD/YYYY TIME Pneumovax 0.5 mL IM left deltoid, Lot ABC123, INITIALS).

TABLE 20.10 Minimum Federal Requirements for Vaccine Administration Documentation

1. The edition date of the VIS distributed
2. The date the VIS was provided to the patient or his or her proxy
3. The name, address, and title of the individual who administered the vaccine
4. The date of administration
5. The vaccine manufacturer and lot number of the vaccine used

Adapted from Centers for Disease Control and Prevention. *Mandatory Instructions for the Use of the Vaccine Information Statements.* Atlanta, GA: Centers for Disease Control and Prevention (CDC); May 2013. Available at www.cdc.gov/vaccines/pubs/vis/

Vaccination Reimbursement

Unfortunately, insurance coverage for vaccination is not universal and not all insurers recognize pharmacists as vaccination providers that are eligible for payment. Medicare Part B does recognize pharmacists as mass immunization providers that are eligible for reimbursement for both the vaccine product itself and a vaccination administration fee. Enrollment as a Medicare provider is required to bill for covered services.[11,12] Pharmacists and interns should check with their supervisor on the processes used at their site for billing for vaccinations.

Most pharmacists are not currently certified to administer vaccines to children but may be asked by other practitioners about the federally funded Vaccines for Children (VFC) program that provides vaccines at no cost to children who are at risk for not receiving vaccination because of inability to pay. VFC programs are required to be a part of each state's Medicaid plan, and so they are often administered through state/territory health division immunization projects.

- CDC VFC homepage: http://www.cdc.gov/vaccines/programs/vfc/index.html
- State Immunization Program Web site Links are maintained by IAC at: http://www.immunize.org/states/index.htm

Recommended Key Vaccine References

Free Publications or Webpages

General Reference

- Centers for Disease Control and Prevention. Epidemiology and Prevention of Vaccine-Preventable Diseases (The Pink Book) [Book on Internet]. May 2012 [cited May, 2013]; [about 504 p.]. Available from http://www.cdc.gov/vaccines/pubs/pinkbook/index.html
    - Essential reference for health care providers (updated annually or biannually). Chapters are presented on each vaccine-preventable disease and provide a thorough review of epidemiology, disease, transmission, vaccination recommendations, and patient selection. Also contains sections on principles of immunizations, administration technique, immunization strategies, vaccine safety, vaccine storage and handling, practice standards, and resources.

- National Center for Immunization and Respiratory Diseases. Vaccines and immunizations [Homepage on Internet]. Atlanta, GA: Centers for Disease Control and Prevention (CDC); c2012–2013 [2010; cited May, 2013]. Available from: http://www.cdc.gov/vaccines/
  - Portal for the national immunization program for lay and health professional–target audiences. Essential for keeping up to date with the most current recommendations. Full of educational materials and useful links.
- Vaccination information for health care professionals [Homepage on Internet]. St. Paul, MN: Immunization Action Coalition (IAC); [2013; cited May, 2013]. Available from http://www.immunize.org/
  - Portal for health professionals. This nonprofit collaborator with the CDC provides camera-ready immunization information and educational materials, copyright free. Their "Ask the Experts" section is particularly useful for hard to find information. Sign up to get their newsletters or listservs.
- Look for your local state or regional health division's immunization program Webpage
  - These sites usually have a health care provider portal with useful information like pharmacy protocols for immunization and model standing orders (e.g., http://www.oregon.gov/DHS/ph/imm/). These Web sites are also where local VFC vaccine program and ordering information are usually found.

Vaccine Handling and Storage

- Package Inserts [Webpage on Internet]. St. Paul, MN: Immunization Action Coalition (IAC); [2013; cited May, 2013]. Available from: http://www.immunize.org/packageinserts/
  - Provides package inserts for all available vaccines, review each insert to determine vaccine-specific shipping requirements; condition upon arrival; storage requirements; shelf life; instructions for reconstitution and use; shelf life after reconstitution, thawing, and opening; and any special instructions.
- National Center for Immunization and Respiratory Diseases. Vaccine Storage and Handling Toolkit [homepage on internet]. Atlanta, GA: Centers for Disease Control and Prevention (CDC); c2012 [2012; cited May, 2013]. Available from: http://www2a.cdc.gov/nip/isd/shtoolkit/splash.html

Role of Pharmacists

- American Society of Health-Systems Pharmacists. ASHP Guidelines on the Pharmacist's Role in Immunization [guideline on internet]. 2003 [cited May, 2013]; [about 6 p.]. Available from: http://www.ashp.org/s_ashp/docs/files/BP07/Specific_Gdl_Immun.pdf

Establishing a Vaccine Practice

- Association for Professionals in Infection Control and Epidemiology (APIC). Healthcare Personnel Immunization Toolkit [PDF file]. 2012 [2012; cited May, 2013]. Available from: http://www.apic.org/Resource_/TinyMceFileManager/Practice_Guidance/HCW_Immunization_Toolkit_122012.pdf
    - This toolkit provides a compilation of resources for health care personnel who provide or are planning to provide immunization services. Includes sections such as clinic operations, client education, and quality assurance in addition to basics of immunization delivery.
- Hogue MD. Incorporating Adult Immunization Services into Community Pharmacy Practice. Pharmacy Times [continuing education on the internet]. Princeton, NJ: Ascend Media; 2007 [updated 2008; cited May, 2013]. Available from: https://secure.pharmacytimes.com/lessons/200707-02.asp
    - Excellent overview of key aspects for practitioners interested in beginning to offer immunization services in community pharmacy practice.

Publications for Purchase or Subscription

- Grabenstein JD. *Immunofacts 2013: Vaccines and Immunologic Drugs.* 1st ed. St. Louis, MO: Wolters Kluwer Health; 2013.
    - Most detailed, up-to-date reference book available on immunologic drugs.
- American Pharmacists Association. Pharmacy-Based Immunization Delivery: A Certificate Program for Pharmacists [self-study and live seminar certificate training program]. 2013 [updated 2013; cited May, 2013]. Available from: http://www.pharmacist.com/pharmacy-based-immunization-delivery
    - National leader in pharmacist and pharmacy student vaccination certification.
    - American Pharmacists Association (APhA)–Academy of Student Pharmacists (ASP) collaboratively developed the

Operation Immunization Program promoting vaccination and administering vaccines at health fairs, community pharmacies, and student health–sponsored events that many students may be familiar with.

Adult Preventative Health (Nonvaccine Related)

Nationwide Health Promotion

- Various programs and initiatives exist to promote the importance of disease prevention and screening to individuals and health care professionals and eliminate health disparities. Of those most pertinent to pharmacy professionals, two are particularly highlighted:
  - Healthy People 2010—sponsored by The Office of Disease Prevention and Health Promotion. The American College of Clinical Pharmacy (ACCP) produced a White Paper calling for Pharmacist support in 2004.[13]
  - Health-system Pharmacy 2015 is an initiative from the American Society of Health-system Pharmacists designed to enhance pharmacy practice in health systems, including the adoption of evidence-based health screening and pharmacotherapy.[14]

Evidence-Based Recommendations

- The *Agency for Healthcare Research and Quality* (AHRQ) subgroup, *U.S. Preventative Services Task Force* (USPSTF) publishes recommendations for Preventative Services[15] that are updated periodically on almost 60 different health care concerns. Major USPSTF recommendations are summarized in the tables that follow.
- It is important to note that "health screening" recommendations assume a patient is asymptomatic. The presence of symptoms removes a patient from the arena of health screening, into disease-specific therapy, which is outside the scope of this chapter.
- The recommendations included in this section are associated with the requisite USPSTF grading classifications (A, B, C, D, I), as follows:
  - A—The USPSTF recommends the [screening] to eligible patients. The USPSTF found high certainty that the net benefit is substantial. *Offer or provide this [screening].*

- B—The USPSTF recommends the [screening] to eligible patients. There is high certainty that the net benefit is moderate or there is moderate certainty that the net benefit is moderate to substantial. *Offer or provide this [screening].*
- C—The USPSTF recommends selectively offering or providing this service to individual patients based on professional judgment and patient preferences. There is at least moderate certainty that the net benefit is small. *Offer or provide this [screening] for selected patients depending on individual circumstances.*
- D—The USPSTF recommends against the [screening]. There is moderate or high certainty that the service has no net benefit or that the harms outweigh the benefits. *Discourage the use of this [screening].*
- I—The USPSTF concludes that the evidence is insufficient to assess the balance of benefits and harms of the [screening]. Evidence is lack, of poor quality, or conflicting, and the balance of benefits and harms cannot be determined or recommend for or against routinely providing [screening]. Evidence that the [screening] is effective is lacking, of poor quality, or conflicting, and the balance of benefits and harms cannot be determined. *Read the clinical considerations section USPSTF Recommendation Statement. If the [screening] is offered, patients should understand the uncertainty about the balance of benefits and harms.*

U.S. Preventive Services Task Force Grade Definitions. May 2008. http://www.uspreventiveservicestaskforce.org/uspstf/grades.htm

General Adult Heath Screening

Table 20.11 provides a summary of the major health screening recommendations for adult males and females. [a]Guideline update in development.

Female-Specific Health Screening

Table 20.12 summarizes the health screening recommendations for adult females. Health screening recommendations specifically for pregnant women are included in Table 20.13, and those that are adult male specific are covered in Table 20.14.

(Text continued on page 642)

TABLE 20.11 General Adult Health Screening Recommendations Summary

Health Screening Area (Internet Citation[s])	Summary of Key Recommendations	Release Date
Colorectal cancer *Screening for Colorectal Cancer*, Topic Page. October 2008. U.S. Preventive Services Task Force. Agency for Healthcare Research and *Quality, Rockville, MD*. http://www.uspreventiveservicestaskforce.org/uspstf08/colocancer/colors.htm *healthfinder®*: http://www.healthfinder.gov *National Cancer Institute: National Institutes of Health*: http://www.nci.nih.gov	• Class A recommendation ∘ Screen men and women between ages 50 and 75 using any of the following: • High-sensitivity fecal occult blood testing every year • Sigmoidoscopy every 5 years combined with high-sensitivity fecal occult blood testing every 3 years • Colonoscopy every 10 years	2008
Diabetes mellitus *Screening for type 2 Diabetes Mellitus in Adults, Topic Page. June 2008. U.S. Preventive Services Task Force. Agency for Healthcare Research and Quality, Rockville, MD*. http://www.uspreventiveservicestaskforce.org/uspstf/uspsdiab.htm[a] *American Diabetes Association:* http://care.diabetesjournals.org/content/36/Supplement_1	• Class B recommendation ∘ Screen asymptomatic adults with sustained blood pressure (treated or untreated) >135/80 mm Hg • Expert opinion: The American Diabetes Association (ADA) recommends[17]: ∘ Screening patients with a body mass index (BMI) ≥25 kg/m^2 who also have one or more of the following risk factors • Physical inactivity • First-degree relative with diabetes • High-risk race/ethnicity (e.g., African American, Latino, Native American, Asian American, Pacific Islander) • Women who delivered a baby weighing >9 lb or were diagnosed with gestational diabetes mellitus • Hypertension (≥140/90 mm Hg or on therapy for hypertension) • High-density lipoprotein cholesterol (HDL-C) <35 mg/dL and/or triglyceride >250 mg/dL • Women with polycystic ovary syndrome ∘ A1C ≥5.7%, impaired glucose tolerance (IGT), or impaired fasting glucose (IFG) on previous testing • Other clinical conditions associated with insulin resistance (e.g., severe obesity, acanthosis nigricans)	2008[a] 2013

(continued)

TABLE 20.11 General Adult Health Screening Recommendations Summary *(continued)*

Health Screening Area (Internet Citation[s])	Summary of Key Recommendations	Release Date
	▪ History of CVD ◦ In patients without risk factors, begin testing at age 45 years if BMI ≥25 kg/m^2 ◦ Screening every 3 years (or more frequently for high-risk individuals) ◦ Diagnosis of diabetes mellitus if any of: • A1C ≥6.5% • Fasting plasma glucose ≥126 mg/dL • 2-hour plasma glucose ≥200 mg/dL during an oral glucose tolerance test • Random plasma glucose ≥200 mg/dL	
Hypertension *U.S. Preventive Services Task Force. Screening for High Blood Pressure: Clinical Summary of U.S. Preventive Services Task Force Recommendation. December 2007.*[a] *Agency for Healthcare Research and Quality, Rockville, MD.* http://www.uspreventiveservicestaskforce.org/uspstf/uspshype.htm http://www.nhlbi.nih.gov/guidelines/hypertension/jnc7full.htm	• Class A recommendation • Screen adults for hypertension (defined as: systolic blood pressure [SBP] of 140 mm Hg or higher, or diastolic blood pressure [DBP] of 90 mm Hg or higher after two or more elevated readings obtained on at least two visits spanning over at least 1 to several weeks) • The Seventh Report of the Joint National Committee on Prevention, Detection, Evaluation, and Treatment of High Blood Pressure[18] (JNC 7) recommends screening: ◦ Every 2 years with BP <120/80 ◦ Every year with SBP of 120–139 mm Hg or DBP of 80–90 mm Hg	2007[a]
Lipids *Screening for Lipid Disorders in Adults, Topic Page. June 2008. U.S. Preventive Services Task Force. Agency for Healthcare Research and Quality, Rockville, MD.* http://www.uspreventiveservicestaskforce.org/uspstf08/lipid/lipidrs.htm *Third Report of the National Cholesterol Education Program*	• Class A recommendation ◦ Men aged 35 years and older, women aged 45 years and older ◦ Men aged 20–35 years and for women aged 20–45 years in the presence of any of the following: • Diabetes • Previous personal history of CHD or noncoronary atherosclerosis (e.g., abdominal aortic aneurysm, peripheral artery disease, carotid artery stenosis) • A family history of cardiovascular disease before age 50 in male relatives or age 60 in female relatives	2008 2004[a]

TABLE 20.11 General Adult Health Screening Recommendations Summary *(continued)*

Health Screening Area (Internet Citation[s])	Summary of Key Recommendations	Release Date

(NCEP) Expert Panel on Detection, Evaluation, and Treatment of High Blood Cholesterol in Adults (Adult Treatment Panel III). http://www.nhlbi.nih.gov/guidelines/cholesterol/atp3full.pdf[a]	• Tobacco use
	• Hypertension
	• Obesity (BMI ≥30)
	  ◦ Screen for elevated total cholesterol (TC) and decreased HDL-C based on fasting or nonfasting samples
	• Expert opinion
	  ◦ The National Cholesterol Education Program (NCEP)[19] Adult Treatment Panel III recommends screening every 5 years or more frequently for patients with lipid levels approaching treatment threshold	

Obesity *Screening and Interventions to Prevent Obesity in Adults, Topic Page. June 2012. U.S. Preventive Services Task Force. Agency for Healthcare Research and Quality, Rockville, MD.* http://www.uspreventiveservicestaskforce.org/uspstf/uspsobes.htm	• Class B recommendation ◦ Screen for obesity (defined as BMI >30 kg/m^2)	2012
Oral cancer *Screening for Oral Cancer, Topic Page. February 2004. U.S. Preventive Services Task Force. Agency for Healthcare Research and Quality, Rockville, MD.* http://www.ahrq.gov/clinic/uspstf/uspsoral.htm	• Class I recommendation ◦ No evidence to support routine screening	2004
Skin cancer *Screening for Skin Cancer, Topic Page. February 2009. U.S. Preventive Services Task Force. Agency for Healthcare Research and Quality, Rockville, MD.* http://www.ahrq.gov/clinic/uspstf/uspsskca.htm	• Class I recommendation ◦ No evidence to support routine screening	2009

(continued)

TABLE 20.11 General Adult Health Screening Recommendations Summary *(continued)*

Health Screening Area (Internet Citation[s])	Summary of Key Recommendations	Release Date
Thyroid cancer *Screening for Thyroid Cancer, Topic Page. U.S. Preventive Services Task Force. Agency for Healthcare Research and Quality, Rockville, MD.* http://www.ahrq.gov/clinic/uspstf/uspsthca.htm	• New evidence currently under examination. Revised recommendations to be published	1996
Tobacco use *Counseling to Prevent Tobacco Use and Tobacco-Caused Disease, Topic Page. April 2009. U.S. Preventive Services Task Force. Agency for Healthcare Research and Quality, Rockville, MD.* http://www.ahrq.gov/clinic/uspstf/uspstbac.htm	• Class A recommendation ∘ Screen for tobacco use and provide tobacco cessation interventions for those who use tobacco products ∘ All pregnant women should be asked about tobacco use and provide pregnancy-tailored counseling for those who smoke	2009

[a]Update in progress.

TABLE 20.12 Female-Specific Health Screening

Health Screening Area (Internet Citation[s])	Summary of Key Recommendations	Release Date
Breast cancer *Screening for Breast Cancer, Topic Page. December 2009. U.S. Preventive Services Task Force. Agency for Healthcare Research and Quality, Rockville, MD.* http://www.ahrq.gov/clinic/uspstf/uspsbrca.htm	• Class B recommendation ∘ Screening mammography every 2 years for women aged 50–74 years • Class C recommendation ∘ Screening mammography before the age of 50 years should be an individual decision that takes into account the patient context, including the patient's values regarding specific benefits and harms	2009
Cervical cancer *Screening for Cervical Cancer, Topic Page. March 2012. U.S. Preventive Services Task Force. Agency for Healthcare Research and Quality, Rockville, MD.* http://www.ahrq.gov/clinic/uspstf/uspscerv.htm	• Class A recommendation ∘ Screen females with a cervix age 21–65 years with cervical cytology (Pap smears) every 3 years ∘ Women aged 30–65 years who want to lengthen the screening interval, screen with a combination of cytology, and human papillomavirus (HPV) testing every 5 years	2012

TABLE 20.12 Female-Specific Health Screening *(continued)*

Health Screening Area (Internet Citation[s])	Summary of Key Recommendations	Release Date
Chlamydial infection *Screening for Chlamydial Infection, Topic Page. June 2007. U.S. Preventive Services Task Force. Agency for Healthcare Research and Quality, Rockville, MD.* http://www.ahrq.gov/clinic/uspstf/uspschlm.htm[a]	• Class A recommendation ∘ Screen for chlamydial infection: ▪ All sexually active nonpregnant young women aged 24 years and younger ▪ Women aged 25 years or older who are not pregnant but are at increased risk (previous chlamydial infection or other sexually transmitted infections, new or multiple sexual partners, inconsistent condom use, sex work)	2007[a]
Osteoporosis *Screening for Osteoporosis, Topic Page. January 2011. U.S. Preventive Services Task Force. Agency for Healthcare Research and Quality, Rockville, MD.* http://www.ahrq.gov/clinic/uspstf/uspsoste.htm	• Class B recommendation ∘ Screen women aged 65 years and older for osteoporosis and in younger women whose fracture risk is equal to or greater than that of a 65-year-old white woman who has no additional risk factors	2011

[a]Update in progress.

TABLE 20.13 Pregnancy-Specific Health Screening

Health Screening Area (Internet Citation[s])	Summary of Key Recommendations	Release Date
Bacteriuria *Screening for Asymptomatic Bacteriuria, Topic Page. July 2008. U.S. Preventive Services Task Force. Agency for Healthcare Research and Quality, Rockville, MD.* http://www.ahrq.gov/clinic/uspstf/uspsbact.htm	• Class A recommendation ∘ Screen for asymptomatic bacteriuria with urine culture at 12–16 weeks' gestation or at the first prenatal visit, if later	2008
Chlamydial infection *Screening for Chlamydial Infection, Topic Page. June 2007. U.S. Preventive Services Task Force. Agency for Healthcare Research and Quality, Rockville, MD.* http://www.ahrq.gov/clinic/uspstf/uspschlm.htm[a]	• Class B recommendation ∘ Screen all pregnant women aged 24 years and younger ∘ Screen pregnant women aged older than 24 years if at increased risk for a chlamydial infection (previous chlamydial infection or other sexually transmitted infections, new or multiple sexual partners, inconsistent condom use, sex work) ∘ The first screening should occur at the first prenatal visit. Women at continued risk or acquiring new risk factors should receive a second screening during the third trimester	2007[a]

(continued)

TABLE 20.13 Pregnancy-Specific Health Screening *(continued)*

Health Screening Area (Internet Citation[s])	Summary of Key Recommendations	Release Date
Gonorrhea infection *Screening for Gonorrhea, Topic Page. May 2005. U.S. Preventive Services Task Force. Agency for Healthcare Research and Quality, Rockville, MD.* http://www.ahrq.gov/clinic/uspstf/uspsgono.htm[a]	• Class B recommendation ∘ Screen for gonorrhea infection in high-risk pregnant women (history of previous gonorrhea infection, other sexually transmitted infections, new or multiple sexual partners, inconsistent condom use, sex work, and drug use). The first screening should occur at the first prenatal visit. Women at continued risk or acquiring new risk factors should receive a second screening during the third trimester	2005[a]
Hepatitis B virus (HBV) infection *Screening for Hepatitis B Infection, Topic Page. June 2009. Preventive Services Task Force. Agency for Healthcare Research and Quality, Rockville, MD.* http://www.ahrq.gov/clinic/uspstf/uspshepb.htm	• Class A recommendation ∘ Screen all pregnant women for HBV at first prenatal visit	2009
HIV infection *Human Immunodeficiency Virus Infection, Topic Page. April 2013. U.S. Preventive Services Task Force. Agency for Healthcare Research and Quality, Rockville, MD.* http://www.ahrq.gov/clinic/uspstf/uspshivi.htm	• Class A recommendation ∘ Screen all pregnant women for HIV, including those who present in labor who are untested and whose HIV status is unknown	2013
Rh(D) incompatibility *Screening for Rh (D) Incompatibility, Topic Page. February 2004. U.S. Preventive Services Task Force. Agency for Healthcare Research and Quality, Rockville, MD.* http://www.ahrq.gov/clinic/uspstf/uspsdrhi.htm	• Class B recommendation ∘ Complete Rh (D) blood typing and antibody testing for all pregnant women during their first visit for pregnancy-related care	2004

TABLE 20.13 Pregnancy-Specific Health Screening *(continued)*

Health Screening Area (Internet Citation[s])	Summary of Key Recommendations	Release Date
Iron deficiency anemia *Screening for Iron Deficiency Anemia, Topic Page. May 2006 U.S. Preventive Services Task Force. Agency for Healthcare Research and Quality, Rockville, MD.* http://www.ahrq.gov/clinic/uspstf/uspsiron.htm[a]	• Class B recommendation ◦ Screen all pregnant women for iron deficiency anemia	2006[a]
Syphilis infection *Screening for Syphilis Infection, Topic Page. May 2009. U.S. Preventive Services Task Force. Agency for Healthcare Research and Quality, Rockville, MD.* http://www.ahrq.gov/clinic/uspstf/uspssyph.htm	• Class A recommendation ◦ Screen all pregnant women for syphilis infection	2009
Tobacco use *Counseling to Prevent Tobacco Use and Tobacco-Caused Disease, Topic Page. April 2009. U.S. Preventive Services Task Force. Agency for Healthcare Research and Quality, Rockville, MD.* http://www.ahrq.gov/clinic/uspstf/uspstbac.htm	• Class A recommendation ◦ Screen all pregnant women for tobacco use and provide augmented pregnancy-tailored counseling to those who smoke	2009

[a]Update in progress.

TABLE 20.14 Male-Specific Health Screening

Health Screening Area (Internet Citation[s])	Summary of Key Recommendations	Release Date
Prostate cancer *Screening for Prostate Cancer, Topic Page. May 2012. U.S. Preventive Services Task Force. Agency for Healthcare Research and Quality, Rockville, MD.* http://www.ahrq.gov/clinic/uspstf/uspsprca.htm	• Class D recommendation ◦ prostate specific antigen (PSA)-based screening is not recommended	2012

References

1. APhA and AMCP. Pharmacist-provided immunization compensation and recognition: white paper summarizing APhA/AMCP stakeholder meeting. *J Am Pharm Assoc.* 2011;51: 704–712. Available at http://amcp.org/pharmacist_immune_compensation/. Accessed May, 2013.
2. Kamal KM, Madhavan SS, Maine LL. Impact of the American Pharmacists Association's (APhA) immunization training certification program. *Am J Pharm Educ.* 2003;67(4): 1–10.
3. Grabenstein JD. Immunofacts 2013: Vaccines and Immunologic Drugs. 1st ed. St. Louis, MO: Wolters Kluwer Health; 2013.
4. Centers for Disease Control and Prevention. *Chapter 2: General Recommendations on Immunization. Epidemiology and Prevention of Vaccine-Preventable Diseases (The Pink Book).* Atkinson W, Hamborsky J, McIntyre L, et al., eds. 10th ed. Washington, DC: Public Health Foundation; 2007.
5. Results for ISMP Survey on Vaccine Abbreviation Use [webpage on internet]. October 2003 [cited May, 2013]. Available from: http://www.ismp.org/Survey/surveyresults/SurveyHosp.asp
6. ISMP Medication Safety Alert! ISMP Quarterly Action Agenda: July–September 2003 [webpage on internet]. October 2003 [cited May, 2013]. Available from: http://www.ismp.org/Newsletters/acutecare/articles/A4Q03Action.asp?ptr=y
7. The Joint Commission. "Do not use list": Facts About the Official "do not use" List [webpage on internet]. February 2012 [cited May, 2013]. Available from: http://www.jointcommission.org/assets/1/18/Do_Not_Use_List.pdf
8. Centers for Disease Control and Prevention. Instructions for the Use of Vaccine Information Statements [document on internet]. Atlanta, GA: Centers for Disease Control and Prevention (CDC); February 6, 2008 [cited May, 2013]. Available from: http://www.cdc.gov/vaccines/pubs/vis/downloads/vis-Instructions.pdf
9. Centers for Disease Control and Prevention. *Appendix D: Vaccine Administration. Epidemiology and Prevention of Vaccine-Preventable Diseases (The Pink Book).* In: Atkinson W, Hamborsky J, McIntyre L, eds. 10th ed. Washington, DC: Public Health Foundation; 2007.
10. Centers for Disease Control and Prevention. *Appendix F: Vaccine Safety. Epidemiology and Prevention of Vaccine-Preventable Diseases (The Pink Book).* Atkinson W, Hamborsky J, McIntyre L, et al., eds. 10th ed. Washington, DC: Public Health Foundation; 2007.
11. American Society of Health-System Pharmacists. ASHP guidelines on the pharmacist's role in immunization. *Am J Health Syst Pharm.* 2003; 60:1371–1377.
12. Hogue MD. *Incorporating Adult Immunization Services into Community Pharmacy Practice. Pharmacy Times [continuing education on the internet].*

Princeton, NJ: Ascend Media; 2007 [updated 2008; cited 2013 May]. Available from: https://secure.pharmacytimes.com/lessons/200707-02.asp

13. Calis KA, Hutchison LC, Elliott ME, et al. Healthy people 2010: challenges, opportunities, and a call to action for America's pharmacists. *Pharmacotherapy*. 2004;24(9):1241–1294.
14. American Society for Health-System Pharmacists. Health-System Pharmacy 2015 [webpage on internet]. April 2007 [cited May 30, 2013]; Available from http://www.ashp.org/s_ashp/cat1c.asp?CID=218&DID=255
15. The Agency for Healthcare Research and Quality (AHRQ). *U.S. Preventive Services Task Force* [webpage on internet]. Rockville, MD: Agency for Healthcare Research and Quality. April 2007 [cited 2013 May 30]; Available from http://www.ahrq.gov/clinic/uspstf/uspstopics.htm
16. Centers for Disease Control and Prevention. *Chapter 1: Principles of Vaccination. Epidemiology and Prevention of Vaccine-Preventable Diseases (The Pink Book)*. In: Atkinson W, Hamborsky J, McIntyre L, et al., eds. 10th ed. Washington, DC: Public Health Foundation; 2007.
17. American Diabetes Association. Diagnosis and Classification of Diabetes Mellitus. *Diabetes Care*. 2007;30: S42–47S.
18. Chobanian AV, et al. The Seventh Report of the Joint National Committee on Prevention, Detection, Evaluation, and Treatment of High Blood Pressure: The JNC 7 report. *JAMA*. 2003;289:2560–2572.
19. Expert Panel on Detection, Evaluation, and Treatment of High Blood Cholesterol in Adults. Executive summary of the Third Report of the National Cholesterol Education Program (NCEP) Expert Panel on Detection, Evaluation, and Treatment of High Blood Cholesterol in Adults (Adult Treatment Panel III). *JAMA*. 2001;285:2486–2497.

INDEX

Note: Page numbers followed by *b*, *f*, or *t* indicate, respectively, boxes, figures, or tables.